General
Ophthalmology

. . . Now do you not see that the eye embraces the beauty of the whole world? It is the lord of astronomy and the maker of cosmography; it counsels and corrects all the arts of mankind; it leads men to the different parts of the world; it is the prince of mathematics, and the sciences founded on it are absolutely certain. It has measured the distances and sizes of the stars; it has found the elements and their locations; it . . . has given birth to architecture, and to perspective, and to the divine art of painting. Oh excellent thing, superior to all others created by God! . . . What peoples, what tongues will fully describe your true function? The eye is the window of the human body through which it feels its way and enjoys the beauty of the world. Owing to the eye the soul is content to stay in its bodily prison, for without it such bodily prison is torture.

—Leonardo da Vinci (1452–1519)

a LANGE medical book

General
Ophthalmology

fourteenth edition

Daniel Vaughan, MD
Clinical Professor of Ophthalmology
University of California, San Francisco
Governor, Francis I. Proctor Foundation for Research in Ophthalmology

Taylor Asbury, MD
Professor of Ophthalmology, Associate Director
Department of Ophthalmology
College of Medicine
University of Cincinnati

Paul Riordan-Eva, FRCS, FRCOphth
Consultant Neuro-ophthalmologist
Moorfields Eye Hospital and the National Hospital for Neurology and
    Neurosurgery, London, England
Consultant Clinical Scientist, Medical Research Council

Illustrated by
Laurel V. Schaubert

APPLETON & LANGE
Stamford, Connecticut

Copyright © 1995 by Appleton & Lange
A Simon & Schuster Company
Copyright © 1989 by Appleton & Lange

96 97 98 / 10 9 8 7 6 5 4 3

Prentice Hall International (UK) Limited, *London*
Prentice Hall of Australia Pty. Limited, *Sydney*
Prentice Hall Canada, Inc., *Toronto*
Prentice Hall Hispanoamericana, S.A., *Mexico*
Prentice Hall of India Private Limited, *New Delhi*
Prentice Hall of Japan, Inc., *Tokyo*
Simon & Schuster Asia Pte. Ltd., *Singapore*
Editora Prentice Hall do Brasil Ltda., *Rio de Janeiro*
Prentice Hall, *Englewood Cliffs, New Jersey*

ISBN 0-8385-3127-X
ISSN 0891-2084

Acquisitions Editor: Shelley Reinhardt
Production Editor: Chris Langan
Art Coordinator: Becky Hainz-Baxter

PRINTED IN THE UNITED STATES OF AMERICA

ISBN 0-8385-3127-X

This edition of
General Ophthalmology
is dedicated to
the memory of
Dr. Orson Wayne White

Table of Contents

Differential Diagnosis of Common Causes of Inflamed Eye . . . .   Inside Front Cover

Authors   ix

Preface   xi

Acknowledgments   xii

1. Anatomy & Embryology of the Eye   1
   Paul Riordan-Eva, FRCS, FRCOphth

2. Ophthalmologic Examination   29
   David F. Chang, MD

3. Commonly Used Eye Medications   62
   Philip P. Ellis, MD

4. Lids & Lacrimal Apparatus   78
   John H. Sullivan, MD

5. Conjunctiva   95
   Ivan R. Schwab, MD, & Chandler R. Dawson, MD

6. Cornea   123
   Roderick Biswell, MD

7. Uveal Tract & Sclera   147
   William G. Hodge, MD, FRCS(C)

8. Lens   165
   John P. Shock, MD, & Richard A. Harper, MD

9. Vitreous   175
   Conor O'Malley, MD

10. Retina & Intraocular Tumors   186
    Robert A. Hardy, MD

11. Glaucoma   208
    Daniel Vaughan, MD, & Paul Riordan-Eva, FRCS, FRCOphth

12. Strabismus   226
    Taylor Asbury, MD, & Miles J. Burke, MD, MS

13. Orbit   245
    John H. Sullivan, MD

14. Neuro-ophthalmology   255
    Pamela S. Chavis, MD, & William F. Hoyt, MD

15. **Ocular Disorders Associated With Systemic Diseases** 296
M.D. Sanders, FRCP, FRCS, & Elizabeth M. Graham, FRCP, FRCOphth

16. **Immunologic Diseases of the Eye** 330
William G. Hodge, MD, FRCS(C)

17. **Special Subjects of Pediatric Interest** 339
Douglas R. Fredrick, MD

18. **Genetic Aspects** 348
Taylor Asbury, MD, & Paul Riordan-Eva, FRCS, FRCOphth

19. **Trauma** 356
Taylor Asbury, MD, & James J. Sanitato, MD

20. **Optics & Refraction** 364
Paul Riordan-Eva, FRCS, FRCOphth, & Orson W. White, MD

21. **Preventive Ophthalmology** 381
John P. Whitcher, MD, MPH

22. **Low Vision** 388
Eleanor E. Faye, MD

23. **Blindness** 396
John P. Whitcher, MD, MPH

24. **Lasers in Ophthalmology** 401
James B. Wise, MD

Appendix I: Visual Standards 409

Appendix II: Practical Factors in Illumination 413

**Appendix III: Rehabilitation of the Visually Handicapped
   & Special Services Available to the Blind** 415

Glossary of Terms Relating to the Eye 419

Index 423

Abbreviations & Symbols Used in Ophthalmology .... **Inside Back Cover**

The Authors

Taylor Asbury, MD
Professor of Ophthalmology, Associate Director, Department of Ophthalmology, College of Medicine, University of Cincinnati.

Roderick Biswell, MD
Associate Clinical Professor of Ophthalmology, University of California School of Medicine, San Francisco.

Miles J. Burke, MD, MS
Associate Professor of Ophthalmology, College of Medicine, University of Cincinnati; Director, Department of Pediatric Ophthalmology, Cincinnati Children's Hospital Medical Center.

David F. Chang, MD
Associate Clinical Professor of Ophthalmology, University of California School of Medicine, San Francisco.

Pamela S. Chavis, MD
Chief of Neuro-ophthalmology, King Khaled Eye Specialist Hospital, Riyadh, Saudi Arabia.

J. Brooks Crawford, MD
Clinical Professor of Ophthalmology, University of California School of Medicine, San Francisco.

Chandler R. Dawson, MD
Director, Francis I. Proctor Foundation for Research in Ophthalmology, and Professor of Ophthalmology and International Health, University of California, San Francisco.

Philip P. Ellis, MD
Professor of Ophthalmology and Chairman of Department of Ophthalmology, University of Colorado School of Medicine, Denver.

Eleanor E. Faye, MD
Opthalmologic Director, Lighthouse Low Vision Service, New York; Attending Ophthalmologist, Manhattan Eye and Ear Hospital, New York.

Frederick T. Fraunfelder, MD
Professor of Ophthalmology and Chairman of Department of Ophthalmology, Oregon Health Sciences University, Portland; Director, Casey Eye Institute; and Director, National Registry of Drug–Induced Ocular Side Effects.

Douglas R..Fredrick, MD
Assistant Clinical Professor of Ophthalmology, University of California, San Francisco.

Elizabeth M. Graham, FRCP, FRCOphth
Consultant Medical Ophthalmologist, St. Thomas' Hospital and National Hospital for Neurology and Neurosurgery, London.

Robert A. Hardy, MD
Assistant Clinical Professor of Ophthalmology, University of California School of Medicine, San Francisco; Chief of Ophthalmology, Merrithew Memorial Hospital, Martinez, California.

Richard A. Harper, MD
Assistant Professor of Ophthalmology, University of Arkansas College of Medicine, Little Rock.

William G. Hodge, MD, FRCS(C)
Clinical Instructor, Francis I. Proctor Foundation for Research in Ophthalmology, University of California School of Medicine, San Francisco; Clinical Instructor, McGill University Faculty of Medicine, Montreal, Quebec.

William F. Hoyt, MD
Professor of Ophthalmology, Neurology, and Neurosurgery, University of California School of Medicine, San Francisco.

Conor O'Malley, MD
San Jose, California.

Paul Riordan-Eva, FRCS, FRCOphth
Consultant Neuro-ophthalmologist, Moorfields Eye Hospital and the National Hospital for Neurology and Neurosurgery, London; Consultant Clinical Scientist, Medical Research Council.

M. D. Sanders, FRCP, FRCS
Consultant Ophthalmologist, St. Thomas' Hospital and National Hospital for Neurology and Neurosurgery, London; Lecturer, University of London.

James J. Sanitato, MD
Associate Professor of Clinical Ophthalmology, Department of Ophthalmology, University of Cincinnati Medical Center, Cincinnati.

Ivan R. Schwab, MD
Professor of Ophthalmology, University of California, School of Medicine, Davis.

John P. Shock, MD
Professor of Ophthalmology and Chairman of Department of Ophthalmology, University of Arkansas College of Medicine, Little Rock; Director, Harvey & Bernia Jones Eye Institute.

John H. Sullivan, MD
Clinical Professor of Ophthalmology, University of California School of Medicine, San Francisco.

Daniel Vaughan, MD
Clinical Professor of Ophthalmology, University of California School of Medicine, San Francisco, and Governor, Francis I. Proctor Foundation for Research in Ophthalmology, San Francisco.

John P. Whitcher, MD, MPH
Professor of Clinical Ophthalmology, Francis I. Proctor Foundation for Research in Ophthalmology, University of California School of Medicine, San Francisco.

Orson W. White, MD*
Salt Lake City, Utah.

James B. Wise, MD
Clinical Professor of Ophthalmology, University of Oklahoma Health Sciences Center, Oklahoma City.

*Deceased

Preface

For over three decades, *General Ophthalmology* has served as the most concise, current, and authoritative review of the subject for medical students, ophthalmology residents, practicing ophthalmologists, nurses, optometrists, and colleagues in other fields of medicine and surgery as well as allied health personnel. The fourteenth edition has been revised and updated in keeping with that goal. It contains the following changes from the thirteenth edition:

■ Major revisions of the chapter on NEURO-OPHTHALMOLOGY
■ Significant changes in the chapters on the CONJUNCTIVA, TRAUMA, and UVEAL TRACT & SCLERA

As in past revisions, we have relied on the assistance of many authorities in special fields who have given us the benefit of their advice. In particular, we wish to thank our new authors: Douglas R. Fredrick, Richard A. Harper, William Hodge, and John P. Whitcher.

Daniel Vaughan, MD
Taylor Asbury, MD
Paul Riordan-Eva, FRCS, FRCOphth

May 1995

Acknowledgments

Arthur Asbury
Crowell Beard
Karenan Biretta
Laurie Campbell
Patricia Cunnane
Hans Gassman
Margaret Henry
Harry Hind
Geraldine Hruby
Marianne Huslid

Vicente Jocson
Heinrich König
Charles Leiter
Ngoc Nguyen
G. Richard O'Connor
Patricia Pascoe
Kenneth Rogers
Margot Riordan-Eva
Lionel Sorensen
Phillips Thygeson

Anatomy & Embryology of the Eye

1

Paul Riordan-Eva, FRCS, FRCOphth

I. NORMAL ANATOMY

THE ORBIT
(Figures 1–1 and 1–2)

The orbital cavity is schematically represented as a pyramid of four walls that converge posteriorly. The medial walls of the right and left orbit are parallel and are separated by the nose. In each orbit, the lateral and medial walls form an angle of 45 degrees, which results in a right angle between the two lateral walls. The orbit is compared to the shape of a pear, with the optic nerve representing its stem. The anterior circumference is somewhat smaller in diameter than the region just within the rim, which makes a sturdy protective margin.

The volume of the adult orbit is approximately 30 mL, and the eyeball occupies only about one-fifth of the space. Fat and muscle account for the bulk of the remainder.

The anterior limit of the orbital cavity is the **orbital septum,** which acts as a barrier between the eyelids and orbit (see below).

The orbits are related to the frontal sinus above, the maxillary sinus below, and the ethmoid and sphenoid sinuses medially. The thin orbital floor is easily damaged by direct trauma to the globe, resulting in a "blowout" fracture with herniation of orbital contents into the maxillary antrum. Infection within the sphenoid and ethmoid sinuses can erode the paper-thin medial wall (lamina papyracea) and involve the contents of the orbit. Defects in the roof (eg, neurofibromatosis) may result in visible pulsations of the globe transmitted from the brain.

Orbital Walls

The roof of the orbit is composed principally of the orbital plate of the **frontal bone.** The lacrimal gland is

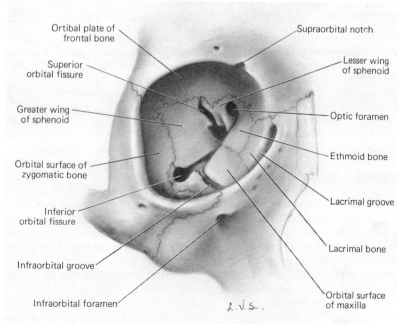

Figure 1–1. Anterior view of bones of right orbit.

Ortibal plate of frontal bone

Superior orbital fissure

Greater wing of sphenoid

Orbital surface of zygomatic bone

Inferior orbital fissure

Infraorbital groove

Infraorbital foramen

Supraorbital notch

Lesser wing of sphenoid

Optic foramen

Ethmoid bone

Lacrimal groove

Lacrimal bone

Orbital surface of maxilla

L.V.S.

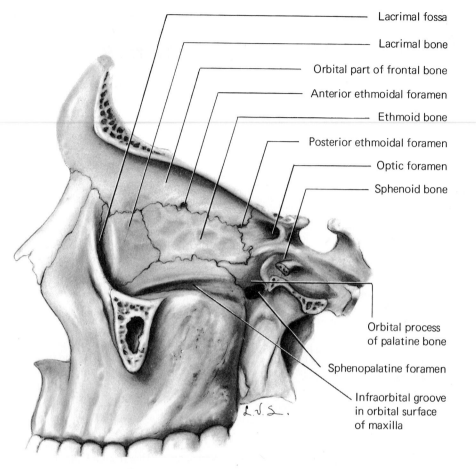

Lacrimal fossa

Lacrimal bone

Orbital part of frontal bone

Anterior ethmoidal foramen

Ethmoid bone

Posterior ethmoidal foramen

Optic foramen

Sphenoid bone

Orbital process
of palatine bone

Sphenopalatine foramen

Infraorbital groove
in orbital surface
of maxilla

Figure 1–2. Medial view of bony wall of left orbit.

located in the lacrimal fossa in the anterior lateral aspect of the roof. Posteriorly, the lesser wing of the **sphenoid bone** containing the optic canal completes the roof.

The lateral wall is separated from the roof by the superior orbital fissure, which divides the lesser from the greater wing of the **sphenoid bone.** The anterior portion of the lateral wall is formed by the orbital surface of the **zygomatic (malar) bone.** This is the strongest part of the bony orbit. Suspensory ligaments, the lateral palpebral tendon, and check ligaments have connective tissue attachments to the lateral orbital tubercle.

The orbital floor is separated from the lateral wall by the inferior orbital fissure. The orbital plate of the **maxilla** forms the large central area of the floor and is the region where blowout fractures most frequently occur. The frontal process of the **maxilla** medially and the **zygomatic bone** laterally complete the inferior orbital rim. The orbital process of the **palatine bone** forms a small triangular area in the posterior floor.

The boundaries of the medial wall are less distinct. The **ethmoid bone** is paper-thin but thickens anteriorly

as it meets the **lacrimal bone.** The body of the **sphenoid** forms the most posterior aspect of the medial wall, and the angular process of the **frontal bone** forms the upper part of the posterior lacrimal crest. The lower portion of the posterior lacrimal crest is made up of the **lacrimal bone.** The anterior lacrimal crest is easily palpated through the lid and is composed of the frontal process of the **maxilla.** The lacrimal groove lies between the two crests and contains the lacrimal sac.

Orbital Apex
(Figure 1–3)

The apex of the orbit is the entry portal for all nerves and vessels to the eye and the site of origin of all extraocular muscles except the inferior oblique. The **superior orbital fissure** lies between the body and the greater and lesser wings of the sphenoid bone. The superior ophthalmic vein and the lacrimal, frontal, and trochlear nerves pass through the lateral portion of the fissure that lies outside the annulus of Zinn. The superior and inferior divisions of the oculomotor nerve and the abducens and nasociliary nerves pass through the

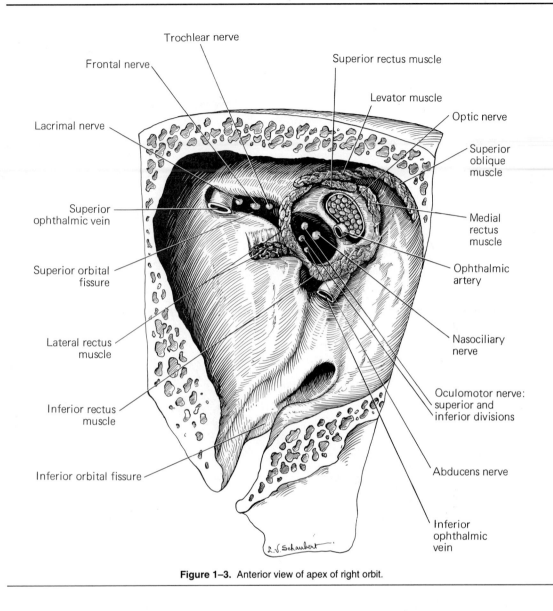

Figure 1–3. Anterior view of apex of right orbit.

medial portion of the fissure within the annulus of Zinn. The optic nerve and ophthalmic artery pass through the optic canal, which also lies within the annulus of Zinn. The inferior ophthalmic vein may pass through any part of the superior orbital fissure, including the portion adjacent to the body of the sphenoid that lies inferomedial to the annulus of Zinn. The inferior ophthalmic vein frequently joins the superior ophthalmic vein before exiting the orbit.

Blood Supply
(Figures 1–4 to 1–6)

The principal arterial supply of the orbit and its structures derives from the ophthalmic artery, the first major branch of the intracranial portion of the internal carotid artery. This branch passes beneath the op-

tic nerve and accompanies it through the optic canal into the orbit. The first intraorbital branch is the central retinal artery, which enters the optic nerve about 8–15 mm behind the globe. Other branches of the ophthalmic artery include the lacrimal artery, supplying the lacrimal gland and upper eyelid; muscular branches to the various muscles of the orbit; long and short posterior ciliary arteries; medial palpebral arteries to both eyelids; and the supraorbital and supratrochlear arteries. The short posterior ciliary arteries supply the choroid and parts of the optic nerve. The two long posterior ciliary arteries supply the ciliary body and anastomose with each other and with the anterior ciliary arteries to form the major arterial circle of the iris. The anterior ciliary arteries are derived from the muscular branches to the rectus muscles.

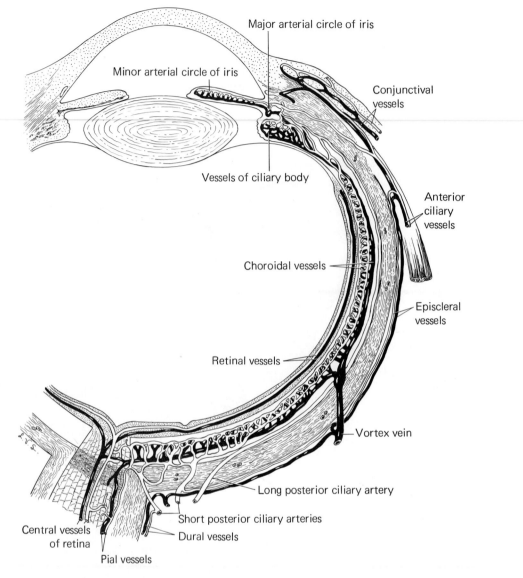

Major arterial circle of iris

Minor arterial circle of iris

Conjunctival vessels

Vessels of ciliary body

Anterior ciliary vessels

Choroidal vessels

Episcleral vessels

Retinal vessels

Vortex vein

Long posterior ciliary artery

Short posterior ciliary arteries

Central vessels of retina

Dural vessels

Pial vessels

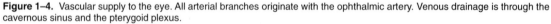

Figure 1–4. Vascular supply to the eye. All arterial branches originate with the ophthalmic artery. Venous drainage is through the cavernous sinus and the pterygoid plexus.

They supply the anterior sclera, episclera, limbus, and conjunctiva as well as contributing to the major arterial circle of the iris. The most anterior branches of the ophthalmic artery contribute to the formation of the arterial arcades of the eyelids, which make an anastomosis with the external carotid circulation via the facial artery.

The venous drainage of the orbit is primarily through the superior and inferior ophthalmic veins, into which drain the vortex veins, the anterior ciliary veins, and the central retinal vein. The ophthalmic veins communicate with the cavernous sinus via the superior orbital fissure and the pterygoid venous plexus via the inferior orbital fissure. The superior

ophthalmic vein is initially formed from the supraorbital and supratrochlear veins and from a branch of the angular vein, all of which drain the skin of the periorbital region. This provides a direct communication between the skin of the face and the cavernous sinus, thus forming the basis of the potentially lethal cavernous sinus thrombosis secondary to superficial infection of the periorbital skin.

THE EYEBALL

The normal adult globe is approximately spherical, with an anteroposterior diameter averaging 24.5 mm.

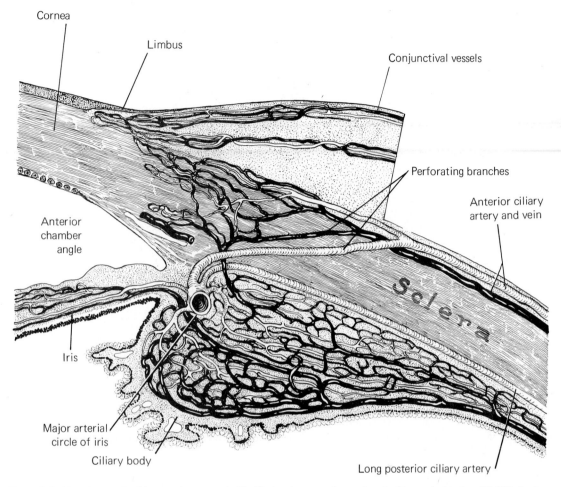

Figure 1–5. Vascular supply of the anterior segment. (Modified, redrawn, and reproduced, with permission, from Wolff E: *Anatomy of the Eye and Orbit,* 4th ed. Blakiston-McGraw, 1954.)

THE CONJUNCTIVA

The conjunctiva is the thin, transparent mucous membrane that covers the posterior surface of the lids (the palpebral conjunctiva) and the anterior surface of the sclera (the bulbar conjunctiva). It is continuous with the skin at the lid margin (a mucocutaneous junction) and with the corneal epithelium at the limbus.

The **palpebral conjunctiva** lines the posterior surface of the lids and is firmly adherent to the tarsus. At the superior and inferior margins of the tarsus, the conjunctiva is reflected posteriorly (at the superior and inferior fornices) and covers the episcleral tissue to become the bulbar conjunctiva.

The **bulbar conjunctiva** is loosely attached to the orbital septum in the fornices and is folded many times. This allows the eye to move and enlarges the secretory conjunctival surface. (The ducts of the lacrimal gland open into the superior temporal fornix.) Except at the limbus (where Tenon's capsule and the conjunctiva are fused for about 3 mm), the bulbar conjunctiva is loosely attached to Tenon's capsule and the underlying sclera.

A soft, movable, thickened fold of bulbar conjunctiva (the **semilunar fold**) is located at the inner canthus and corresponds to the nictitating membrane of some lower animals. A small, fleshy, epidermoid structure (the **caruncle**) is attached superficially to the inner portion of the semilunar fold and is a transition zone containing both cutaneous and mucous membrane elements.

Histology

The **conjunctival epithelium** consists of two to five layers of stratified columnar epithelial cells, superficial and basal. Conjunctival epithelium near the limbus, over the caruncle, and near the mucocutaneous junctions at the lid margins consists of stratified squamous epithelial cells. The **superficial epithelial cells** contain round or oval mucus-secreting goblet cells. The mucus, as it forms, pushes aside the goblet cell nucleus and is necessary for proper dispersion of the precorneal tear film. The **basal epithelial cells** stain more

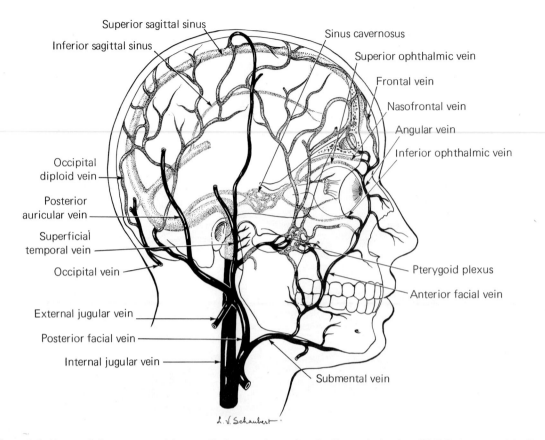

Superior sagittal sinus

Inferior sagittal sinus

Sinus cavernosus

Superior ophthalmic vein

Frontal vein

Nasofrontal vein

Angular vein

Inferior ophthalmic vein

Occipital diploid vein

Posterior auricular vein

Superficial temporal vein

Occipital vein

Pterygoid plexus

Anterior facial vein

External jugular vein

Posterior facial vein

Internal jugular vein

Submental vein

Figure 1–6. Venous drainage system of the eye. (Redrawn and reproduced, with permission, from Wolff E: *Anatomy of the Eye and Orbit,* 4th ed. Blakiston-McGraw, 1954.)

deeply than the superficial cells and near the limbus may contain pigment.

The **conjunctival stroma** is divided into an adenoid (superficial) layer and a fibrous (deep) layer. The **adenoid layer** contains lymphoid tissue and in some areas may contain "follicle-like" structures without germinal centers. The adenoid layer does not develop until after the first 2 or 3 months of life. This explains why inclusion conjunctivitis of the newborn is papillary in nature rather than follicular and why it later becomes follicular. The **fibrous layer** is composed of connective tissue that attaches to the tarsal plate. This explains the appearance of the papillary reaction in inflammations of the conjunctiva. The fibrous layer is loosely arranged over the globe.

The **accessory lacrimal glands** (glands of Krause and Wolfring), which resemble the lacrimal gland in structure and function, are located in the stroma. Most of the glands of Krause are in the upper fornix, the remaining few in the lower fornix. The glands of Wolfring lie at the superior margin of the upper tarsus.

Blood Supply, Lymphatics, & Nerve Supply

The conjunctival arteries are derived from the anterior ciliary and palpebral arteries. The two arteries anastomose freely and—along with the numerous conjunctival veins that generally follow the arterial pattern—form a considerable conjunctival vascular network. The conjunctival lymphatics are arranged in superficial and deep layers and join with the lymphatics of the eyelids to form a rich lymphatic plexus. The conjunctiva receives its nerve supply from the first (ophthalmic) division of the fifth nerve. It possesses a relatively small number of pain fibers.

TENON'S CAPSULE (Fascia Bulbi)

Tenon's capsule is a fibrous membrane that envelops the globe from the limbus to the optic nerve. Adjacent to the limbus, the conjunctiva, Tenon's capsule, and the episclera are fused together. More posteriorly, the inner surface of Tenon's capsule lies against the sclera, and its outer aspect is in contact with orbital fat and other structures within the extraocular muscle cone. At the point where Tenon's capsule is pierced by tendons of the extraocular muscles in their passage to their attachments to the globe, it sends a tubular reflection around each of these muscles. These fascial reflections become continuous with the fascia of the muscles, the fused fasciae sending expansions to the surrounding structures and to the orbital bones. The fascial expansions are quite tough and limit the action of the extraocular muscles and are therefore known as **check ligaments.** The lower segment of Tenon's capsule is thick and fuses with the fascia of the inferior rectus and the inferior oblique muscles to form the suspensory ligament of the eyeball (Lockwood's ligament), upon which the globe rests.

THE SCLERA & EPISCLERA

The **sclera** is the fibrous outer protective coating of the eye (Figure 1–7). It is dense and white and continuous with the cornea anteriorly and the dural sheath of the optic nerve posteriorly. A few strands of scleral tissue pass across the anterior portion of the optic nerve as the **lamina cribrosa.** The outer surface of the anterior sclera is covered by a thin layer of fine elastic tissue, the **episclera,** which contains numerous blood vessels that nourish the sclera. The brown pigment layer on the inner surface of the sclera is the lamina fusca, which forms the outer layer of the suprachoroidal space.

At the insertion of the rectus muscles, the sclera is about 0.3 mm thick; elsewhere it is about 1 mm thick. Around the optic nerve, the sclera is penetrated by the long and short posterior ciliary arteries and the long and short ciliary nerves (Figure 1–8). The long posterior ciliary arteries and long ciliary nerves pass from the optic nerve to the ciliary body in a shallow groove on the inner surface of the sclera at the 3 and 9 o'clock meridians. Slightly posterior to the equator, the four vortex veins draining the choroid exit through the sclera, usually one in each quadrant. About 4 mm posterior to the limbus, slightly anterior to the insertion of the respective rectus muscle, the four anterior ciliary arteries and veins penetrate the sclera. The nerve supply to the sclera is from the ciliary nerves.

Histologically, the sclera consists of many dense bands of parallel and interlacing fibrous tissue bundles, each of which is 10–16 μm thick and 100–140 μm wide. The histologic structure of the sclera is remarkably similar to that of the cornea. The reason for the transparency of the cornea and the opacity of the sclera is the relative deturgescence of the cornea.

THE CORNEA

The cornea is a transparent tissue comparable in size and structure to the crystal of a small wristwatch (Figure 1–9). It is inserted into the sclera at the limbus, the circumferential depression at this junction being known as the scleral sulcus. The average adult cornea is 0.54 mm thick in the center, about 0.65 mm thick at the periphery, and about 11.5 mm in diameter. From anterior to posterior, it has five distinct layers (Figure 1–10): the epithelium (which is continuous with the epithelium of the bulbar conjunctiva), Bowman's layer, the stroma, Descemet's membrane, and the endothelium. The epithelium has five or six layers of cells, the endothelium only one. Bowman's layer is a clear acellular layer, a modified portion of the stroma. Descemet's membrane is a clear elastic membrane that appears amorphous on electron microscopy and represents the basement membrane of the corneal endothelium. The corneal stroma accounts for about 90% of the corneal thickness. It is composed of intertwining lamellae of collagen fibrils about 1 μm wide that run almost the full diameter of the cornea. They run parallel to the surface of the cornea and by virtue of their size and periodicity are optically clear. The lamellae lie within a ground substance of hydrated proteoglycans in association with the keratocytes that produce the collagen and ground substance.

Sources of nutrition for the cornea are the vessels of the limbus, the aqueous, and the tears. The superficial cornea also gets most of its oxygen from the atmosphere. The sensory nerves of the cornea are supplied by the first (ophthalmic) division of the fifth (trigeminal) cranial nerve.

The transparency of the cornea is due to its uniform structure, avascularity, and deturgescence.

THE UVEAL TRACT

The uveal tract is composed of the iris, the ciliary body, and the choroid (Figure 1–7). It is the middle vascular layer of the eye and is protected by the cornea and sclera. It contributes blood supply to the retina.

Iris

The **iris** is the anterior extension of the ciliary body. It presents as a flat surface with a centrally situated round aperture, the pupil. The iris lies in contiguity with the anterior surface of the lens, dividing the anterior chamber from the posterior chamber, each of which contains aqueous humor. Within the stroma of the iris are the sphincter and dilator muscles. The two heavily pigmented layers on the posterior surface of the iris represent anterior extensions of the neuroretina and retinal pigment epithelium.

The blood supply to the iris is from the major circle of the iris (Figure 1–4). Iris capillaries have a nonfenestrated endothelium and hence do not normally leak intravenously injected fluorescein. Sensory nerve supply to the iris is via fibers in the ciliary nerves.

The iris controls the amount of light entering the eye. Pupillary size is principally determined by a balance between constriction due to parasympathetic activity transmitted via the third cranial nerve and dilation due to sympathetic activity. (See Chapter 14.)

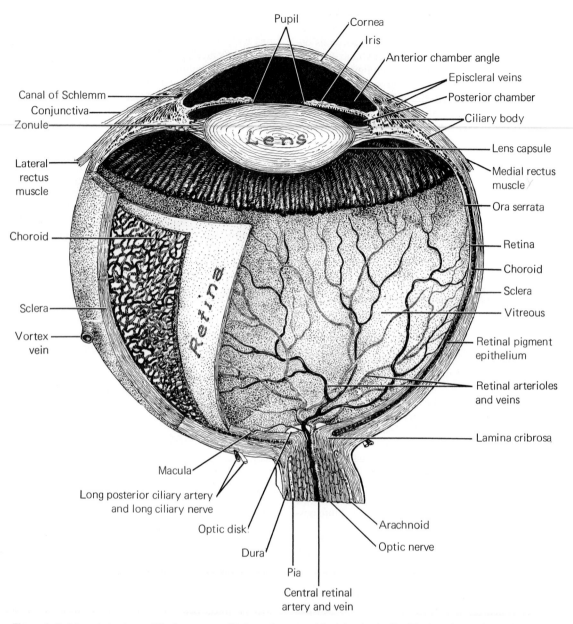

Figure 1–7. Internal structures of the human eye. (Redrawn from an original drawing by Paul Peck and reproduced with permission, from: *The Anatomy of the Eye.* Courtesy of Lederle Laboratories.)

The Ciliary Body

The **ciliary body,** roughly triangular in cross-section, extends forward from the anterior end of the choroid to the root of the iris (about 6 mm). It consists of a corrugated anterior zone, the pars plicata, and a flattened posterior zone, the pars plana. The ciliary processes arise from the pars plicata (Figure 1–11). They are composed mainly of capillaries and veins that drain through the vortex veins. The capillaries are large and fenestrated and hence leak intravenously injected fluorescein. There are two layers of ciliary epithelium:

an internal nonpigmented layer, representing the anterior extension of the neuroretina; and an external pigmented layer, representing an extension of the retinal pigment epithelium. The ciliary processes and their covering ciliary epithelium are responsible for the formation of aqueous.

The **ciliary muscle** is composed of a combination of longitudinal, circular, and radial fibers. The function of the circular fibers is to contract and relax the zonular fibers, which originate in the valleys between the ciliary processes (Figure 1–12). This alters the tension

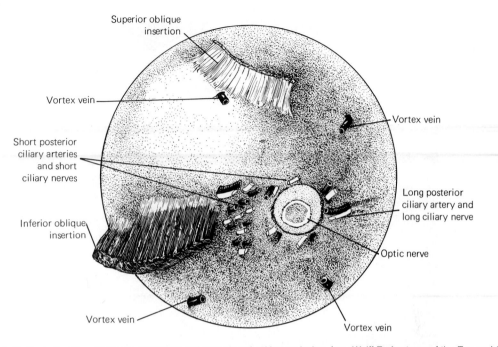

Superior oblique
insertion

Vortex vein

Vortex vein

Short posterior
ciliary arteries
and short
ciliary nerves

Long posterior
ciliary artery and
long ciliary nerve

Inferior oblique
insertion

Optic nerve

Vortex vein

Vortex vein

Figure 1–8. Posterior view of left eye. (Redrawn and reproduced, with permission, from Wolff E: *Anatomy of the Eye and Orbit*, 4th ed. Blakiston-McGraw.)

on the capsule of the lens, giving the lens a variable focus for both near and distant objects in the visual field. The longitudinal fibers of the ciliary muscle insert into the trabecular meshwork to influence its pore size.

The blood vessels supplying the ciliary body are derived from the major circle of the iris. The sensory nerve supply of the iris is via the ciliary nerves.

The Choroid

The choroid is the posterior segment of the uveal tract, between the retina and the sclera. It is composed of three layers of choroidal blood vessels: large, medium, and small. The deeper the vessels are placed in the choroid, the wider their lumens (Figure 1–13). The internal portion of the choroid vessels is known as the choriocapillaris. Blood from the choroidal vessels drains via the four vortex veins, one in each of the four posterior quadrants. The choroid is bounded internally by Bruch's membrane and externally by the sclera. The suprachoroidal space lies between the choroid and the sclera. The choroid is firmly attached posteriorly to the margins of the optic nerve. Anteriorly, the choroid joins with the ciliary body.

The aggregate of choroidal blood vessels serves to nourish the outer portion of the underlying retina (Figure 1–4).

THE LENS

The lens is a biconvex, avascular, colorless and almost completely transparent structure, about 4 mm thick and 9 mm in diameter. It is suspended behind the iris by the zonule, which connects it with the ciliary body. Anterior to the lens is the aqueous; posterior to it, the vitreous. The lens capsule (see below) is a semipermeable membrane (slightly more permeable than a capillary wall) that will admit water and electrolytes.

A subcapsular epithelium is present anteriorly (Figure 1–14). The lens nucleus is harder than the cortex. With age, subepithelial lamellar fibers are continuously produced, so that the lens gradually becomes larger and less elastic throughout life. The nucleus and cortex are made up of long concentric lamellae. The suture lines formed by the end-to-end joining of these lamellar fibers are {Y}-shaped when viewed with the slitlamp (Figure 1–15). The {Y} is upright anteriorly and inverted posteriorly.

Each lamellar fiber contains a flattened nucleus. These nuclei are evident microscopically in the peripheral portion of the lens near the equator and are continuous with the subcapsular epithelium.

The lens is held in place by a suspensory ligament known as the zonule (zonule of Zinn), which is composed of numerous fibrils that arise from the surface of the ciliary body and insert into the lens equator.

The lens consists of about 65% water, about 35% protein (the highest protein content of any tissue of the body), and a trace of minerals common to other body tissues. Potassium is more concentrated in the lens than in most tissues. Ascorbic acid and glutathione are present in both oxidized and reduced forms.

There are no pain fibers, blood vessels, or nerves in the lens.

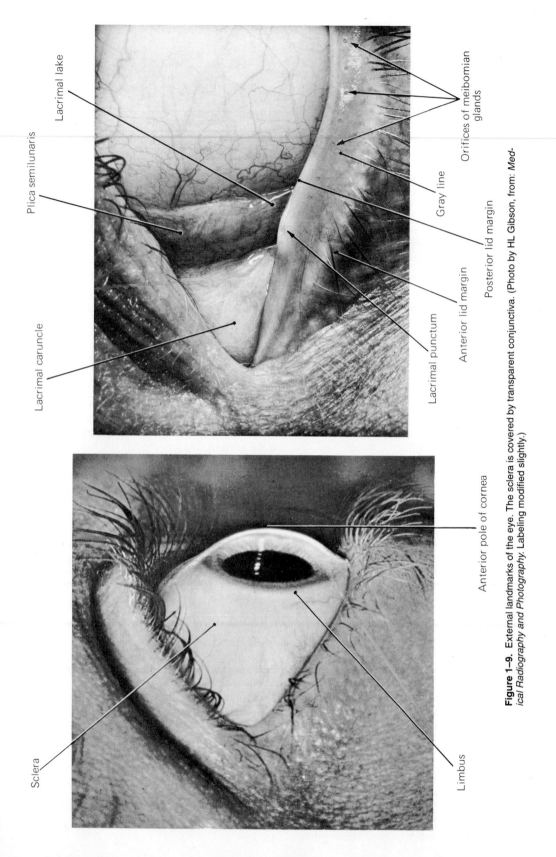

Lacrimal lake

Plica semilunaris

Lacrimal caruncle

Orifices of meibomian glands

Gray line

Posterior lid margin

Anterior lid margin

Lacrimal punctum

Anterior pole of cornea

Sclera

Limbus

Figure 1–9. External landmarks of the eye. The sclera is covered by transparent conjunctiva. (Photo by HL Gibson, from: *Medical Radiography and Photography.* Labeling modified slightly.)

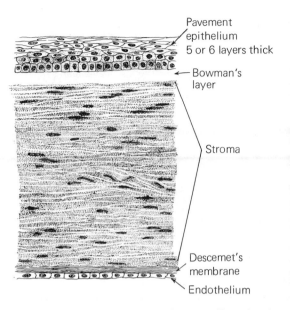

Pavement epithelium
5 or 6 layers thick

Bowman's layer

Stroma

Descemet's membrane

Endothelium

Figure 1–10. Transverse section of cornea. (Reproduced, with permission, from Wolff E: *Anatomy of the Eye and Orbit,* 4th ed. Blakiston-Mcgraw, 1954.)

Ora serrata
Ciliary process
Pars plana
Zonule

Lens

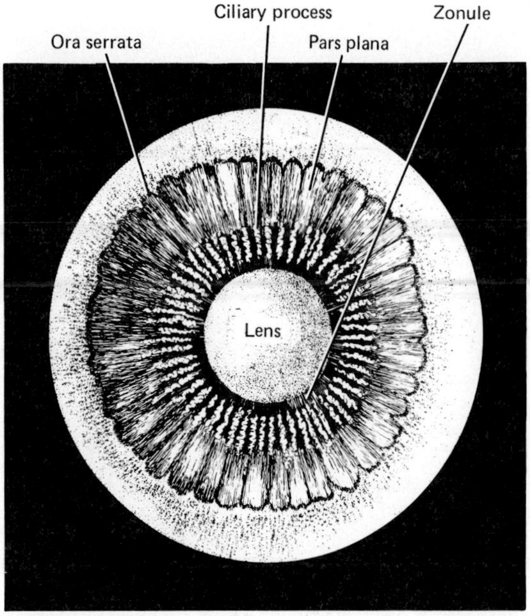

Figure 1–11. Posterior view of ciliary body, zonule, lens, and ora serrata. (Redrawn and reproduced, with permission, from: Wolff E: *Anatomy of the Eye and Orbit,* 4th ed. Blakiston-McGraw, 1954.)

THE AQUEOUS

Aqueous humor is produced by the ciliary body. Entering the posterior chamber, it passes through the pupil into the anterior chamber (Figure 1–7) and then peripherally toward the anterior chamber angle. The physiology of the aqueous is discussed in Chapter 11.

THE ANTERIOR CHAMBER ANGLE

The anterior chamber angle lies at the junction of the peripheral cornea and the root of the iris (Figures 1–12, 1–16, and 11–3). Its main anatomic features are Schwalbe's line, the trabecular meshwork (which overlies Schlemm's canal), and the scleral spur.

Schwalbe's line marks the termination of the corneal endothelium. The trabecular meshwork is triangular in cross-section, with its base directed toward the ciliary body. It is composed of perforated sheets of collagen and elastic tissue, forming a filter with decreasing pore size as the canal of Schlemm is approached. The internal portion of the meshwork, facing the anterior chamber, is known as the uveal meshwork; the external portion, adjacent to the canal of Schlemm, is called the corneoscleral meshwork. The longitudinal fibers of the ciliary muscle insert into the trabecular meshwork. The scleral spur is an inward extension of the sclera between the ciliary body and Schlemm's canal, to which the iris and ciliary body are attached. Efferent channels from Schlemm's canal (about 30 collector channels

and about 12 aqueous veins) communicate with the episcleral venous system.

THE RETINA

The retina is a thin, semitransparent, multilayered sheet of neural tissue that lines the inner aspect of the posterior two-thirds of the wall of the globe. It extends almost as far anteriorly as the ciliary body, ending at that point in a ragged edge, the ora serrata (Figure 1–12). In adults the ora serrata is about 6.5 mm behind Schwalbe's line on the temporal side and 5.7 mm behind it nasally. The outer surface of the sensory retina is apposed to the retinal pigment epithelium and thus related to Bruch's membrane, the choroid, and the sclera. In most areas, the retina and retinal pigment epithelium are easily separated to form the subretinal space, such as occurs in retinal detachment. But at the optic disk and the ora serrata, the retina and retinal pigment epithelium are firmly bound together, thus limiting the spread of subretinal fluid in retinal detachment. This contrasts with the potential suprachoroidal space between the choroid and sclera, which extends to the scleral spur. Choroidal detachments thus extend beyond the ora serrata, under the pars plana and pars plicata. The epithelial layers of the inner surface of the ciliary body and the posterior surface of the iris represent anterior extensions of the retina and retinal pigment epithelium. The inner surface of the retina is apposed to the vitreous.

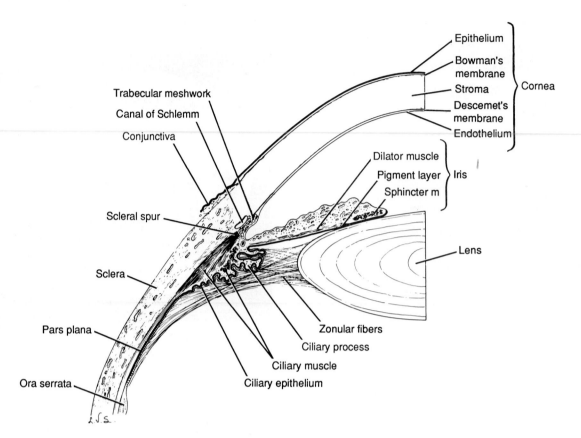

Figure 1–12. Anterior chamber angle and surrounding structures.

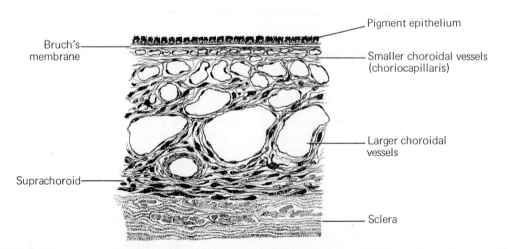

Figure 1–13. Cross section of choroid. (Redrawn and reproduced, with permission, from Wolff E: *Anatomy of the Eye and Orbit,* 4th ed. Blakiston-McGraw, 1954.)

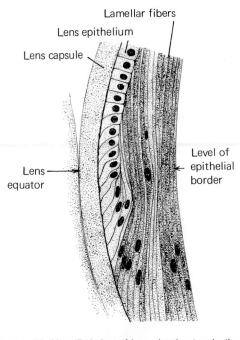

Figure 1–14. Magnified view of lens showing termination of subcapsular epithelium (vertical section).

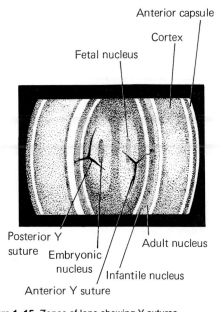

Figure 1–15. Zones of lens showing Y sutures. [Figures 1–14 and 1–15 are redrawn from Duke-Elder WS: *Textbook of Ophthalmology*, vol 1. Mosby, 1942. Drawings first appeared in Salzmann M: *Anatomy and History of the Human Eyeball in the Normal State.* Univ of Chicago Press, 1912.]

The layers of the retina, starting from its inner aspect, are as follows: (1) internal limiting membrane; (2) nerve fiber layer, containing the ganglion cell axons passing to the optic nerve; (3) ganglion cell layer; (4) inner plexiform layer, containing the connections of the ganglion cells with the amacrine and bipolar cells; (5) inner nuclear layer of bipolar, amacrine, and horizontal cell bodies; (6) outer plexiform layer, containing the connections of the bipolar and horizontal cells with the photoreceptors; (7) outer nuclear layer of photoreceptor cell nuclei; (8) external limiting membrane; (9) photoreceptor layer of rod and cone inner and outer segments; and (10) retinal pigment epithelium (Figure 1–17). The inner layer of Bruch's membrane is actually the basement membrane of the retinal pigment epithelium.

The retina is 0.1 mm thick at the ora serrata and 0.23 mm thick at the posterior pole. In the center of the posterior retina is the macula. This can be defined clinically as the area of yellowish pigmentation resulting from the presence of luteal pigment (xanthophyll), which is 1.5 mm in diameter. An alternative histologic definition is that part of the retina in which the ganglion cell layer is more than one cell thick. Clinically, this corresponds to the area bounded by the temporal retinal vascular arcades. In the center of the macula, about 3.5 mm lateral to the optic disk, is the fovea, clinically obvious as a depression that creates a particular reflection when viewed ophthalmoscopically. It corresponds to the retinal avascular zone of fluorescein angiography. Histologically, the fovea is characterized by thinning of the outer nuclear layer and absence of the other parenchymal layers as a result of the oblique course of the photoreceptor cell axons (Henle fiber layer) and the centrifugal displacement of the retinal layers that are closer to the inner retinal surface. The foveola is the most central portion of the fovea, in which the photoreceptors are all cones, and the thinnest part of the retina. All these histologic features provide for fine visual discrimination. The normally empty extracellular space of the retina is potentially greatest at the macula, and diseases that lead to accumulation of extracellular material cause considerable thickening of this area.

The retina receives its blood supply from two sources: the choriocapillaris immediately outside Bruch's membrane, which supplies the outer third of the retina, including the outer plexiform and outer nuclear layers, the photoreceptors, and the retinal pigment epithelium; and branches of the central retinal artery, which supply the inner two-thirds (Figure 1–4). The fovea is supplied entirely by the choriocapillaris and is susceptible to irreparable damage when the retina is detached. The retinal blood vessels have a nonfenestrated endothelium, which forms the inner blood-retinal barrier. The endothelium of choroidal vessels is fenestrated. The outer blood-retinal barrier lies at the level of the retinal pigment epithelium.

THE VITREOUS

The vitreous is a clear, avascular, gelatinous body that comprises two-thirds of the volume and weight of

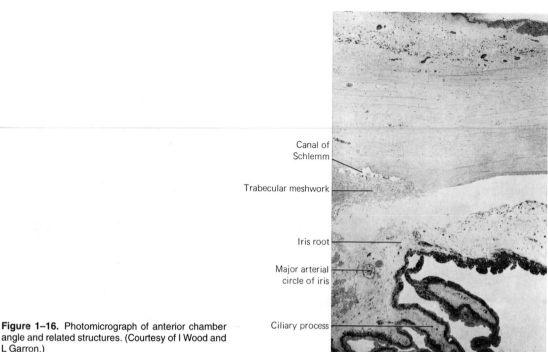

Canal of Schlemm

Trabecular meshwork

Iris root

Major arterial circle of iris

Ciliary process

Figure 1–16. Photomicrograph of anterior chamber angle and related structures. (Courtesy of I Wood and L Garron.)

the eye. It fills the space bounded by the lens, retina, and optic disk (Figure 1–7). The outer surface of the vitreous—the hyaloid membrane—is normally in contact with the following structures: the posterior lens capsule, the zonular fibers, the pars plana epithelium, the retina, and the optic nerve head. The base of the vitreous maintains a firm attachment throughout life to the pars plana epithelium and the retina immediately behind the ora serrata. The attachment to the lens capsule and the optic nerve head is firm in early life but soon disappears.

The vitreous is about 99% water. The remaining 1% includes two components, collagen and hyaluronic acid, which give the vitreous a gel-like form and consistency because of their ability to bind large volumes of water.

THE EXTERNAL ANATOMIC LANDMARKS

Accurate localization of the position of internal structures with reference to the external surface of the globe is important in many surgical procedures. The external distance of structures from the limbus is greater than their extent as measured on the internal surface of the globe. Externally, the ora serrata is situated approximately 6 mm from the limbus on the medial side and 7 mm on the temporal side of the globe. This corresponds to the level of insertion of the rectus muscles. Extending for 4 mm anterior to the ora serrata is the pars plana, and injections into the vitreous cavity should be given through this region, 4–5 mm from the limbus in the phakic eye. In the aphakic eye,

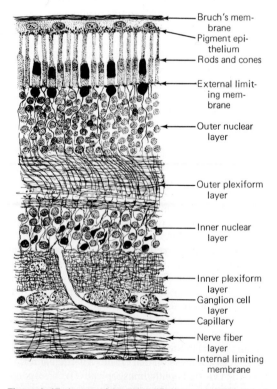

Bruch's membrane
Pigment epithelium
Rods and cones

External limiting membrane

Outer nuclear layer

Outer plexiform layer

Inner nuclear layer

Inner plexiform layer
Ganglion cell layer
Capillary
Nerve fiber layer
Internal limiting membrane

Figure 1–17. Layers of the retina. (Redrawn and reproduced, with permission, from Wolff E: *Anatomy of the Eye and Orbit,* 4th ed. Blakiston-McGraw, 1954.)

it is possible to inject 0.5–1 mm more anteriorly. The pars plicata, which is the target for cyclodestructive procedures in the treatment of intractable glaucoma, occupies the 2–3 mm directly posterior to the limbus.

THE EXTRAOCULAR MUSCLES

Six extraocular muscles control the movement of each eye: four rectus and two oblique muscles.

Rectus Muscles

The four rectus muscles originate at a common ring tendon (annulus of Zinn) surrounding the optic nerve at the posterior apex of the orbit (Figure 1–3). They are named according to their insertion into the sclera on the medial, lateral, inferior, and superior surfaces of the eye. The principal action of the respective muscles is thus to adduct, abduct, depress, and elevate the globe (see Chapter 12). The muscles are about 40 mm long, becoming tendinous 4–9 mm from the point of insertion, where they are about 10 mm wide. The approximate distances of the points of insertion from the corneal limbus are as follows: medial rectus, 5 mm: inferior rectus, 6 mm; lateral rectus, 7 mm; and superior rectus, 8 mm (Figure 1–18). With the eye in the primary position, the vertical rectus muscles make an angle of about 23 degrees with the optic axis.

Oblique Muscles

The two oblique muscles control primarily torsional movement and, to a lesser extent, upward and downward movement of the globe (see Chapter 12).

The **superior oblique** is the longest and thinnest of the ocular muscles. It originates above and medial to the optic foramen and partially overlaps the origin of the levator palpebrae superioris muscle. The superior oblique has a thin, fusiform belly (40 mm long) and passes anteriorly in the form of a tendon to its trochlea, or pulley. It is then reflected backward and downward to attach in a fan shape to the sclera beneath the superior rectus. The trochlea is a cartilaginous structure attached to the frontal bone 3 mm behind the orbital rim. The superior oblique tendon is enclosed in a synovial sheath as it passes through the trochlea.

The **inferior oblique** muscle originates from the nasal side of the orbital wall just behind the inferior orbital rim and lateral to the nasolacrimal duct. It passes beneath the inferior rectus and then under the lateral rectus muscle to insert onto the sclera with a short tendon. The insertion is into the posterotemporal segment of the globe and just over the macular area. The muscle is 37 mm long.

In the primary position, the muscle plane of the superior and inferior oblique muscles forms an angle of 51–54 degrees with the optic axis.

Fascia

All the extraocular muscles are ensheathed by fascia. Near the points of insertion of these muscles the fascia is continuous with Tenon's capsule, and fascial condensations to adjacent orbital structures serve as check ligaments (Figures 1–19 and 1–20).

Nerve Supply

The oculomotor nerve (III) innervates the medial, inferior, and superior rectus muscles and the inferior

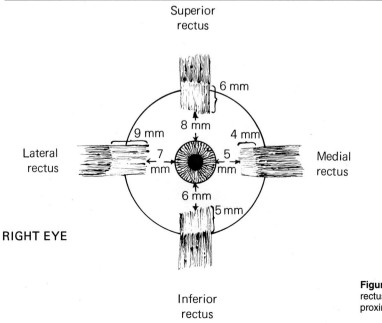

Figure 1–18. Approximate distances of the rectus muscles from the limbus, and the approximate lengths of tendons.

oblique muscle. The abducens nerve (VI) innervates the lateral rectus muscle; the trochlear nerve (IV) innervates the superior oblique muscle.

Blood Supply

The blood supply to the extraocular muscles is derived from the muscular branches of the ophthalmic artery. The lateral rectus and inferior oblique muscles are also supplied by branches from the lacrimal artery and the infraorbital artery, respectively.

THE OCULAR ADNEXA

1. EYEBROWS

The eyebrows are folds of thickened skin covered with hair. The skin fold is supported by underlying muscle fibers. The glabella is the hairless prominence between the eyebrows.

2. EYELIDS

The upper and lower eyelids (palpebrae) are modified folds of skin that can close to protect the anterior eyeball (Figure 1—21). Blinking helps spread the tear film, which protects the cornea and conjunctiva from dehydration. The upper lid ends at the eyebrows; the lower lid merges into the cheek.

The eyelids consist of five principal planes of tissues. From superficial to deep, they are the skin layer, a layer of striated muscle (orbicularis oculi), areolar tissue, fibrous tissue (tarsal plates), and a layer of mucous membrane (palpebral conjunctiva) (Figure 1–22).

Structures of the Eyelids

A. Skin Layer: The skin of the eyelids differs from skin on most other areas of the body in that it is thin, loose, and elastic and possesses few hair follicles and no subcutaneous fat.

B. Orbicularis Oculi Muscle: The function of the orbicularis oculi muscle is to close the lids. Its muscle fibers surround the palpebral fissure in concentric fashion and spread for a short distance around the orbital margin. Some fibers run onto the cheek and the forehead. The portion of the muscle that is in the lids is known as its pretarsal portion; the portion over the orbital septum is the preseptal portion. The segment outside the lid is called the orbital portion. The orbicularis oculi is supplied by the facial nerve.

C. Areolar Tissue: The submuscular areolar tissue that lies deep to the orbicularis oculi muscle communicates with the subaponeurotic layer of the scalp.

D. Tarsal Plates: The main supporting structure of the eyelids is a dense fibrous tissue layer that—along with a small amount of elastic tissue—is called the tarsal plate. The lateral and medial angles and extensions of the tarsal plates are attached to the orbital margin by the lateral and medial palpebral ligaments. The upper and lower tarsal plates are also attached by a condensed, thin fascia to the upper and lower orbital margins. This thin fascia forms the orbital septum.

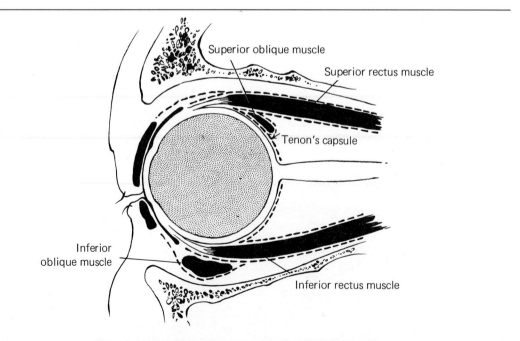

Figure 1–19. Fascia about muscles and eyeball (Tenon's capsule).

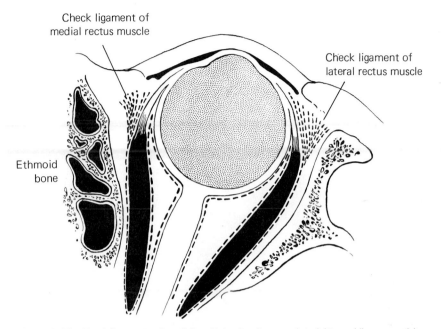

Figure 1–20. Check ligaments of medial and lateral rectus muscles, right eye (diagrammatic).

E. Palpebral Conjunctiva: The lids are lined posteriorly by a layer of mucous membrane, the **palpebral conjunctiva,** which adheres firmly to the tarsal plates. A surgical incision through the gray line of the lid margin (see below) splits the lid into an anterior lamella of skin and orbicularis muscle and a posterior lamella of tarsal plate and palpebral conjunctiva.

Lid Margins

The free lid margin is 25–30 mm long and about 2 mm wide. It is divided by the gray line (mucocutaneous junction) into anterior and posterior margins.

A. Anterior Margin:

1. Eyelashes–The eyelashes project from the margins of the eyelids and are arranged irregularly. The upper lashes are longer and more numerous than the lower lashes and turn upward; the lower lashes turn downward.

2. Glands of Zeis–These are small modified sebaceous glands that open into the hair follicles at the base of the eyelashes.

3. Glands of Moll–These are modified sweat glands that open in a row near the base of the eyelashes.

B. Posterior Margin: The posterior lid margin is in close contact with the globe, and along this margin are the small orifices of modified sebaceous glands (meibomian, or tarsal, glands).

C. Lacrimal Punctum: At the medial end of the posterior margin of the lid, a small elevation with a central small opening can be seen on the upper and lower lids. The puncta serve to carry the tears down through the corresponding canaliculus to the lacrimal sac.

Palpebral Fissure

The palpebral fissure is the elliptic space between the two open lids. The fissure terminates at the medial and lateral canthi. The lateral canthus is about 0.5 cm from the lateral orbital rim and forms an acute angle. The medial canthus is more elliptic than the lateral canthus and surrounds the lacrimal lake (Figure 1–21).

Two structures are identified in the lacrimal lake: the **lacrimal caruncle,** a yellowish elevation of modified skin containing large modified sweat glands and sebaceous glands that open into follicles which contain fine hair (Figure 1–9); and the **plica semilunaris,** a vestigial remnant of the third eyelid of lower animal species.

In Orientals, a skin fold known as **epicanthus** passes from the medial termination of the upper lid to the medial termination of the lower lid, hiding the caruncle. Epicanthus may be present normally in young infants of all races and disappears with development of the nasal bridge but persists throughout life in Orientals.

Orbital Septum

The orbital septum is the fascia behind that portion of the orbicularis muscle that lies between the orbital rim and the tarsus and serves as a barrier between the lid and the orbit.

The orbital septum is pierced by the lacrimal vessels and nerves, the supratrochlear artery and nerve, the supraorbital vessels and nerves, the infratrochlear nerve (Figure 1–23), the anastomosis between the angular and ophthalmic veins, and the levator palpebrae superioris muscle.

The **superior orbital septum** blends with the ten-

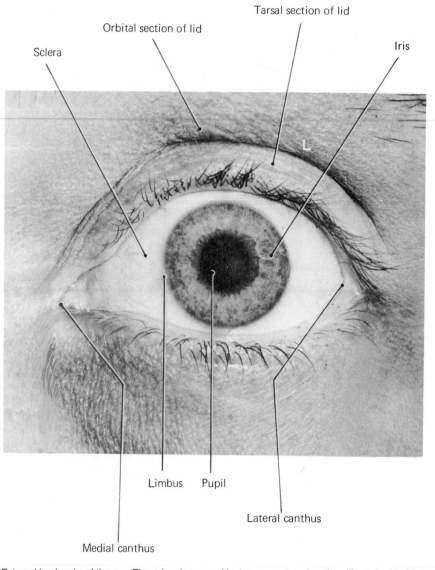

Tarsal section of lid

Orbital section of lid

Iris

Sclera

Limbus   Pupil

Lateral canthus

Medial canthus

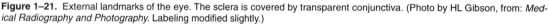

Figure 1–21. External landmarks of the eye. The sclera is covered by transparent conjunctiva. (Photo by HL Gibson, from: *Medical Radiography and Photography.* Labeling modified slightly.)

don of the levator palpebrae superioris and the superior tarsus; the **inferior orbital septum** blends with the inferior tarsus.

Lid Retractors

The lid retractors are responsible for opening the eyelids. They are formed by a musculofascial complex, with both striated and smooth muscle components, known as the levator complex in the upper lid and the capsulopalpebral fascia in the lower lid.

In the upper lid, the striated muscle portion is the **levator palpebrae superioris,** which arises from the apex of the orbit and passes forward to divide into an aponeurosis and a deeper portion that contains the smooth muscle fibers of **Müller's (superior tarsal)**

muscle (Figure 1–22). The aponeurosis elevates the anterior lamella of the lid, inserting into the posterior surface of the orbicularis oculi and through this into the overlying skin to form the upper lid skin crease. Müller's muscle inserts into the upper border of the tarsal plate and the superior fornix of the conjunctiva, thus elevating the posterior lamella.

In the lower lid, the main retractor is the inferior rectus muscle, from which fibrous tissue extends to enclose the inferior oblique muscle and insert into the lower border of the tarsal plate and the orbicularis oculi. Associated with this aponeurosis are the smooth muscle fibers of the inferior tarsal muscle.

The smooth muscle components of the lid retractors are innervated by sympathetic nerves. The levator and

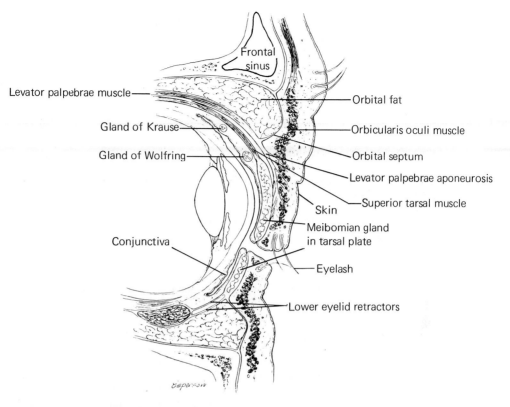

Figure 1–22. Cross section of the eyelids. (Courtesy of C Beard.)

inferior rectus muscles are supplied by the third cranial (oculomotor) nerve. Ptosis is thus a feature of both Horner's syndrome and third nerve palsy.

Levator Palpebrae Superioris Muscle

The levator palpebrae muscle arises with a short tendon from the undersurface of the lesser wing of the sphe-noid above and ahead of the optic foramen. The tendon blends with the underlying origin of the superior rectus muscle. The levator belly passes forward, forms an aponeurosis, and spreads like a fan. The muscle, including its smooth muscle component (Müller's muscle), and its aponeurosis form an important part of the upper lid retractor (see above). The palpebral segment of the orbicularis oculi muscle acts as its antagonist.

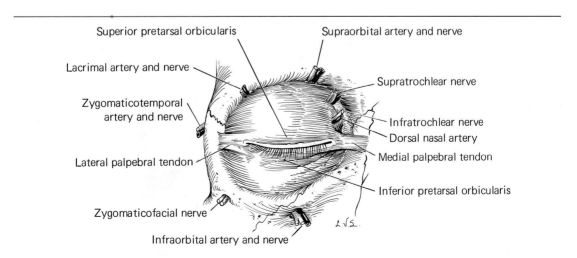

Figure 1–23. Vessels and nerves to extraocular structures.

The two extremities of the levator aponeurosis are called its medial and lateral horns. The medial horn is thin and is attached below the frontolacrimal suture and into the medial palpebral ligament. The lateral horn passes between the orbital and palpebral portions of the lacrimal gland and inserts into the orbital tubercle and the lateral palpebral ligament.

The sheath of the levator palpebrae superioris is attached to the superior rectus muscle inferiorly. The superior surface, at the junction of the muscle belly and the aponeurosis, forms a thickened band that is attached medially to the trochlea and laterally to the lateral orbital wall, the band forming the check ligaments of the muscle. The band is also known as Whitnall's ligament.

The levator is supplied by the superior branch of the oculomotor nerve (III). Blood supply to the levator palpebrae superioris is derived from the lateral muscular branch of the ophthalmic artery.

Sensory Nerve Supply

The sensory nerve supply to the eyelids is derived from the first and second divisions of the trigeminal nerve (V). The small lacrimal, supraorbital, supratrochlear, infratrochlear, and external nasal nerves are branches of the ophthalmic division of the fifth nerve. The infraorbital, zygomaticofacial, and zygomaticotemporal nerves are branches of the maxillary (second) division of the trigeminal nerve.

Blood Supply & Lymphatics

The blood supply to the lids is derived from the lacrimal and ophthalmic arteries by their lateral and medial palpebral branches. Anastomoses between the lateral and medial palpebral arteries form the tarsal arcades that lie in the submuscular areolar tissue.

Venous drainage from the lids empties into the ophthalmic vein and the veins that drain the forehead and temple. The veins are arranged in pre- and posttarsal plexuses (Figure 1–6).

Lymphatics from the lateral segment of the lids run into the preauricular and parotid nodes. Lymphatics draining the medial side of the lids empty into the submandibular lymph nodes.

3. THE LACRIMAL APPARATUS

The lacrimal complex consists of the lacrimal gland, the accessory lacrimal glands, the canaliculi, the lacrimal sac, and the nasolacrimal duct (Figure 1–24).

The lacrimal gland consists of the following structures:

(1) The almond-shaped **orbital portion,** located in the lacrimal fossa in the anterior upper temporal segment of the orbit, is separated from the palpebral portion by the lateral horn of the levator palpebrae muscle. To reach this portion of the gland surgically, one must incise the skin, the orbicularis oculi muscle, and the orbital septum.

(2) The smaller **palpebral portion** is located just above the temporal segment of the superior conjunctival fornix. Lacrimal secretory ducts, which open by approximately ten fine orifices, connect the orbital and palpebral portions of the lacrimal gland to the superior conjunctival fornix. Removal of the palpebral portion of the gland cuts off all of the con-

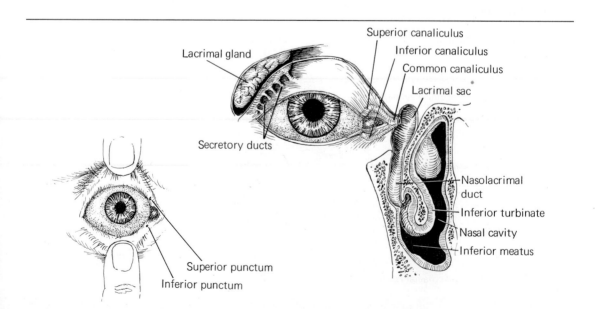

Figure 1–24. The lacrimal drainage system. (Redrawn with modifications and reproduced, with permission, from Thompson J, Elstrom ER: Radiography of the nasolacrimal passageways. Med Radiogr Photogr 1949;25[3]:66.)

necting ducts and thus prevents secretion by the entire gland.

The accessory lacrimal glands (glands of Krause and Wolfring) are located in the substantia propria of the palpebral conjunctiva.

Tears drain from the lacrimal lake via the upper and lower puncta and canaliculi to the **lacrimal sac,** which lies in the lacrimal fossa. The nasolacrimal duct continues downward from the sac and opens into the inferior meatus of the nasal cavity, lateral to the inferior turbinate. Tears are directed into the puncta by capillary attraction and gravity and by the blinking action of the eyelids. The combined forces of capillary attraction in the canaliculi, gravity, and the pumping action of Horner's muscle, which is an extension of the orbicularis oculi muscle to a point behind the lacrimal sac, all tend to continue the flow of tears down the nasolacrimal duct into the nose.

Blood Supply & Lymphatics

The blood supply of the lacrimal gland is derived from the lacrimal artery. The vein that drains the gland joins the ophthalmic vein. The lymphatic drainage joins with the conjunctival lymphatics to drain into the preauricular lymph nodes.

Nerve Supply

The nerve supply to the lacrimal gland is by (1) the lacrimal nerve (sensory), a branch of the trigeminal first division; (2) the great superficial petrosal nerve (secretory), which comes from the superior salivary nucleus; and (3) sympathetic nerves accompanying the lacrimal artery and the lacrimal nerve.

Related Structures

The **medial palpebral ligament** connects the upper and lower tarsal plates to the frontal process at the inner canthus anterior to the lacrimal sac. The portion of the lacrimal sac below the ligament is covered by a few fibers of the orbicularis oculi muscle. These fibers offer little resistance to swelling and distention of the lacrimal sac. The area below the medial palpebral ligament becomes swollen in acute dacryocystitis, and fistulas commonly open in the area.

The angular vein and artery lie just deep to the skin, 8 mm to the nasal side of the inner canthus. Skin incisions made in surgical procedures on the lacrimal sac should always be placed 2–3 mm to the nasal side of the inner canthus to avoid these vessels.

THE OPTIC NERVE

The trunk of the optic nerve consists of about 1 million axons that arise from the ganglion cells of the retina (nerve fiber layer). The optic nerve emerges from the posterior surface of the globe through a short, circular opening in the sclera about 1 mm below and 3 mm nasal to the posterior pole of the eye (Figure 1–8). The nerve fibers become myelinated on leaving the eye, increasing the diameter from 1.5 mm (within the sclera) to 3 mm (within the orbit). The orbital segment of the nerve is 25–30 mm long; it travels within the optic muscle cone, via the bony optic canal, and thus gains access to the cranial cavity. The intracanalicular portion measures 4–9 mm. After a 10 mm intracranial course, the nerve joins the opposite optic nerve to form the optic chiasm.

Eighty percent of the optic nerve consists of visual fibers that synapse in the lateral geniculate body on neurons whose axons terminate in the primary visual cortex of the occipital lobes. Twenty percent of the fibers are pupillary and bypass the geniculate body en route to the pretectal area. Since the ganglion cells of the retina and their axons are part of the central nervous system, they will not regenerate if severed.

Sheaths of the Optic Nerve (Figure 1–25)

The fibrous wrappings that ensheathe the optic nerve are continuous with the meninges. The pia mater is loosely attached about the nerve near the chiasm and only for a short distance within the cranium, but it is closely attached around most of the intracanalicular and all of the intraorbital portions. The pia consists of some fibrous tissue with numerous small blood vessels (Figure 1–26). It divides the nerve fibers into bundles by sending numerous septa into the nerve substance. The pia continues to the sclera, with a few fibers running into the choroid and lamina cribrosa.

The arachnoid comes in contact with the optic nerve at the intracranial end of the optic canal and accompanies the nerve to the globe, where it ends in the sclera and overlying dura. This sheath is a diaphanous connective tissue membrane with many septate connections with the pia mater, which it closely resembles. It is more intimately associated with pia than with dura.

The dura mater lining the inner surface of the cranial vault comes in contact with the optic nerve as it leaves the optic canal. As the nerve enters the orbit from the optic canal, the dura splits, one layer (the periorbita) lining the orbital cavity and the other forming the outer dural covering of the optic nerve. The dura becomes continuous with the outer two-thirds of the sclera. The dura consists of tough, fibrous, relatively avascular tissue lined by endothelium on the inner surface.

The subdural space is between the dura and the arachnoid; the subarachnoid space is between the pia and the arachnoid. Both are more potential than actual spaces under normal conditions but are direct continuations of their corresponding intracranial spaces. Subarachnoid or subdural fluid under sufficient pressure will fill these potential spaces about the optic

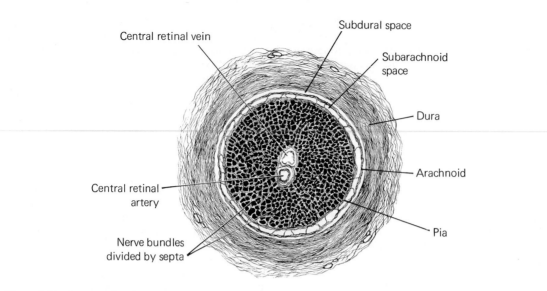

Figure 1–25. Cross section of the optic nerve (Redrawn and reproduced, with permission, from Wolff E: *Anatomy of the Eye and Orbit,* 6th ed. Blakiston-McGraw, 1968.)

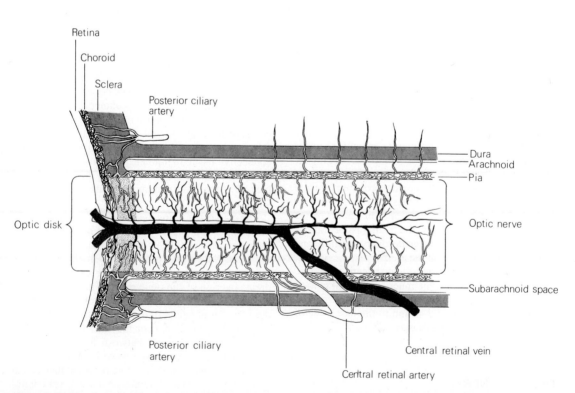

Figure 1–26. Blood supply of the optic nerve. (Redrawn and reproduced, with permission, from: Hayreh SS: Trans Am Acad Ophthalmol Otolaryngol 1974;78:240.)

nerve. The meningeal layers are adherent to each other and to the optic nerve and the surrounding bone within the optic foramen, making the optic nerve resistant to traction from either end.

Blood Supply
(Figure 1–26)

The surface layer of the optic disk receives blood from branches of the retinal arterioles. The rest of the nerve in front of the lamina cribrosa is supplied by branches from the peripapillary choroidal vessels. In the region of the lamina cribrosa, the arterial supply is from the short posterior ciliary arteries. The retrolaminar optic nerve receives some blood from branches of the central retinal artery. The remainder of the intraorbital nerve, as well as the intracanalicular and intracranial portions, are supplied by a pial network of vessels derived from the various branches of the ophthalmic artery and other branches of the internal carotids.

THE OPTIC CHIASM

The optic chiasm is variably situated near the top of the diaphragm of the sella turcica, most often posteriorly, projecting 1 cm above it and at a 45-degree angle upward from the optic nerves as they emerge from the optic canals (Figure 1–27). The lamina terminalis forms the anterior wall of the third ventricle. The internal carotid arteries lie just laterally, adjacent to the cavernous sinuses. The chiasm is made up of the junction of the two optic nerves and provides for crossing of the nasal fibers to the opposite optic tract and passage of temporal fibers to the ipsilateral optic tract. The macular fibers are arranged similarly to the rest of the fibers except that their decussation is farther posteriorly and superiorly. The chiasm receives many small blood vessels from the neighboring circle of Willis.

THE RETROCHIASMATIC
VISUAL PATHWAYS

Each optic tract begins at the posterolateral angle of the chiasm and sweeps around the upper part of the cerebral peduncle to end in the lateral geniculate nucleus. Afferent pupillary fibers leave the tract just anterior to the nucleus and pass via the brachium of the superior colliculus to the midbrain. (The pupillary pathway is diagrammed in Figure 14–2.) Afferent visual fibers terminate on cells in the lateral geniculate nucleus that give rise to the geniculocalcarine tract. This tract traverses the posterior limb of the internal capsule and then fans out into a broad bundle called the optic radiation. The fibers in this bundle curve backward around the anterior aspect of the temporal horn

of the lateral ventricle and then medially to reach the calcarine cortex of the occipital lobe, where they terminate. The most inferior fibers, which carry projections from the superior aspect of the contralateral half of the visual field, course anteriorly into the temporal lobe in a configuration known as Meyer's loop. Lesions of the temporal lobe that extend 5 cm back from the anterior tip involve these fibers and can produce superior quadrantanopic field defects.

The primary visual cortex (area V1) occupies the upper and lower lips and the depths of the calcarine fissure on the medial aspect of the occipital lobe. Each lobe receives input from the two ipsilateral half-retinas, representing the contralateral half of the binocular visual field. Projection of the visual field onto the visual cortex occurs in a precise and orderly retinotopic pattern. The macula is represented at the medial posterior pole, and the peripheral parts of the retina project to the most anterior part of the calcarine cortex. On either side of area V1 lies area V2, and then area V3. V2 appears to function in a manner very similar to V1. Area V4, situated on the medial surface of the cerebral hemisphere but more anterior and inferior than V1 in the region of the fusiform gyrus, seems to be primarily concerned with color processing. Motion detection localizes to an area at the junction of the occipital and temporal lobes, lateral to area V1 and known as area V5 or MT.

THE OCULOMOTOR NERVE (III)

The oculomotor nerve originates from between the cerebral peduncles and passes near the posterior communicating artery of the circle of Willis. Lateral to the pituitary gland, it is closely approximated to the optic tract, and here it pierces the dura to course in the lateral wall of the cavernous sinus. As the nerve leaves the cavernous sinus, it divides into superior and inferior divisions. The superior division enters the orbit within the annulus of Zinn at its highest point and adjacent to the trochlear nerve (Figure 1–3). The inferior division enters the annulus of Zinn low and passes below the optic nerve to supply the medial and inferior rectus muscles. A large branch from the inferior division extends forward to supply the inferior oblique. A small twig from the proximal end of the nerve to the inferior oblique carries parasympathetic fibers to the ciliary ganglion.

THE TROCHLEAR NERVE (IV)

Although the thinnest of the cranial nerves, the trochlear nerve (Figure 1–3) has the longest intracranial course, and it is also the only nerve to originate on the dorsal surface of the brain stem. The fibers de-

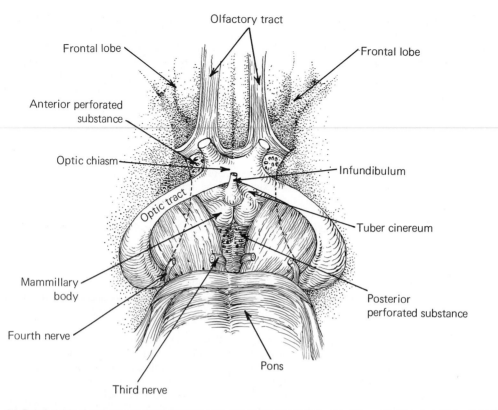

Figure 1–27. Relationship of optic chiasm from inferior aspect. (Redrawn and reproduced, with permission, from Duke-Elder WS: *System of Ophthalmology.* Vol 2. Mosby, 1961.)

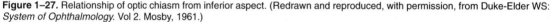

cussate before they emerge from the brainstem just before the inferior colliculi, where they are subject to injury from the tentorium. The nerve pierces the dura behind the sella turcica and travels within the lateral walls of the cavernous sinus to enter the superior orbital fissure medial to the frontal nerve. From this point it travels within the periorbita of the roof over the levator muscle to the upper surface of the superior oblique muscle.

THE TRIGEMINAL NERVE (V)
(Figure 1–3)

The trigeminal nerve originates from the pons, and its sensory roots form the trigeminal ganglion. The first (ophthalmic) of the three divisions passes through the lateral wall of the cavernous sinus and divides into the lacrimal, frontal, and nasociliary nerve. The **lacrimal nerve** passes through the upper lateral aspect of the superior orbital fissure, outside the annulus of Zinn, and continuing its lateral course in the orbit to terminate in the lacrimal gland, providing its sensory innervation. Slightly medial to the lacrimal nerve within the superior orbital fissure is the frontal nerve, which is the

largest of the first division of branches of the trigeminal nerve. It also crosses over the annulus of Zinn and follows a course over the levator to the medial aspect of the orbit, where it divides into the supraorbital and supratrochlear nerves. These provide sensation to the brow and forehead. The nasociliary nerve is the sensory nerve of the eye. After entering through the medial portion of the annulus of Zinn, it lies between the superior rectus and the optic nerve. Branches to the ciliary ganglion and those forming the ciliary nerves provide sensory supply to the cornea, iris, and ciliary body. The terminal branches are the infratrochlear nerve, which supplies the medial portion of the conjunctiva and eyelids, and the anterior ethmoidal nerve, which provides sensation to the tip of the nose. Thus, the skin on the tip of the nose may be affected with vesicular lesions prior to the onset of herpes zoster ophthalmicus.

The second (maxillary) division of the trigeminal nerve passes through the foramen rotundum and enters the orbit through the inferior orbital fissure. It passes through the infraorbital canal, becoming the **infraorbital nerve,** and exits via the infraorbital foramen, supplying sensation to the lower lid and adjacent cheek. It is frequently damaged in fractures of the orbital floor.

THE ABDUCENS NERVE (VI)

The abducens nerve (Figure 1–3) originates between the pons and medulla and pursues an extended course up the clivus to the posterior clinoid, penetrates the dura, and passes within the cavernous sinus. (All other nerves course through the lateral wall of the cavernous sinus.) After passing through the superior orbital fissure within the annulus of Zinn, the nerve continues laterally to innervate the lateral rectus muscle.

II. EMBRYOLOGY OF THE EYE

The eye is derived from three of the primitive embryonic layers: surface ectoderm, including its derivative the neural crest; neural ectoderm; and mesoderm. Endoderm does not enter into the formation of the eye. Mesenchyme is the term for embryonic connective tissue. Ocular and adnexal connective tissues previously were thought to be derived from mesoderm, but it has now been shown that most of the mesenchyme of all of the head and neck region is derived from the cranial neural crest.

The **surface ectoderm** gives rise to the lens, the lacrimal gland, the epithelium of the cornea, conjunctiva, and adnexal glands, and the epidermis of the eyelids.

The **neural crest,** which arises from the surface ectoderm in the region immediately adjacent to the neural folds of neural ectoderm, is responsible for formation of the corneal keratocytes, the endothelium of the cornea and the trabecular meshwork, the stroma of the iris and choroid, the ciliary muscle, the fibroblasts of the sclera, the vitreous, and the optic nerve meninges. It is also involved in formation of the orbital cartilage and bone, the orbital connective tissues and nerves, the extraocular muscles, and the subepidermal layers of the eyelids.

The **neural ectoderm** gives rise to the optic vesicle and optic cup and is thus responsible for the formation of the retina and retinal pigment epithelium, the pigmented and nonpigmented layers of ciliary epithelium, the posterior epithelium, the dilator and sphincter muscles of the iris, and the optic nerve fibers and glia.

The **mesoderm** is now thought to contribute only to the extraocular muscles and the orbital and ocular vascular endothelium.

Optic Vesicle Stage

The embryonic plate is the earliest stage in fetal development during which ocular structures can be differentiated. At the 2.5 mm (2 week) stage, the edges of the neural groove thicken to form the neural folds (Figure 1–28). The folds then fuse to form the neural tube, which sinks into the underlying mesoderm and detaches itself from the surface epithelium. The site of the optic groove or optic sulcus is in the cephalic neural folds on either side of and parallel to the neural groove. This occurs when neural folds begin to close at 3 weeks.

At the 9 mm (4 week) stage, just before the anterior portion of the neural tube closes completely, neural ectoderm grows outward and toward the surface ectoderm on either side to form the spherical optic vesicles. The optic vesicles are connected to the forebrain by the optic stalks. At this stage also, a thickening of the surface ectoderm (lens plate) begins to form opposite the ends of the optic vesicles.

Optic Cup Stage

As the optic vesicle invaginates to produce the optic cup, the original outer wall of the vesicle approaches its inner wall. The invagination of the ventral surface of the optic stalk and of the optic vesicle occurs simultaneously and creates a groove, the optic (embryonic) fissure. The margins of the optic cup then grow around the optic fissure. At the same time, the lens plate invaginates to form first a cup and then a hollow sphere known as the lens vesicle. By the 9 mm (4 week) stage, the lens vesicle separates from the surface ectoderm and lies free in the rim of the optic cup.

The optic fissure allows the vascular mesoderm to enter the optic stalk and eventually to form the hyaloid system of the vitreous cavity. As invagination is completed, the optic fissure narrows and closes during the 13 mm (6 week) stage, leaving one small permanent opening at the anterior end of the optic stalk through which the hyaloid artery passes. At the 100 mm (4 month) stage, the retinal artery and vein pass through this opening. At this stage also, the ultimate general structure of the eye has been determined.

Further development of the eye consists in differentiation of the individual optic structures. In general, differentiation of the optic structures occurs more rapidly in the posterior than in the anterior segment of the eye during the early stages and more rapidly in the anterior segment during the later stages of gestation.

EMBRYOLOGY OF SPECIFIC STRUCTURES

Lids & Lacrimal Apparatus

The lids develop from mesenchyme except for the epidermis of the skin and the epithelium of the conjunctiva, which are derivatives of surface ectoderm. The lid buds are first seen at 16 mm (6 weeks) growing in front of the eye, where they meet and fuse at the 37 mm (8 week) stage. They separate during the fifth month. The lashes and meibomian and other lid glands develop as downgrowths from the epidermis.

The lacrimal and accessory lacrimal glands develop from the conjunctival epithelium. The lacrimal drainage system (canaliculi, lacrimal sac, and naso-

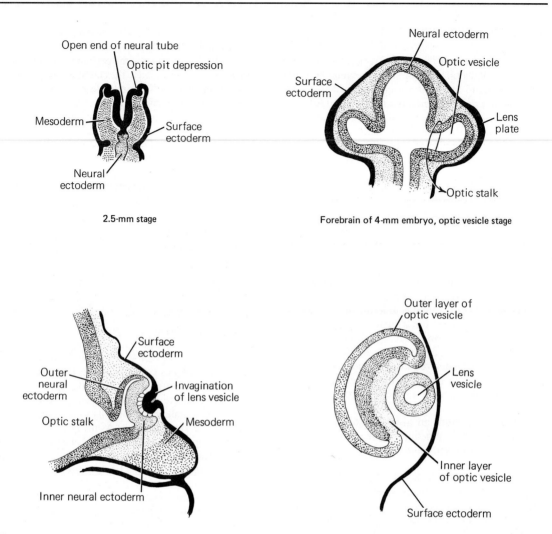

2.5-mm stage

Forebrain of 4-mm embryo, optic vesicle stage

5-mm stage. Beginning formation of optic cup by invagination.

9-mm stage. Lens vesicle has separated from surface ectoderm and lies free in rim of optic cup.

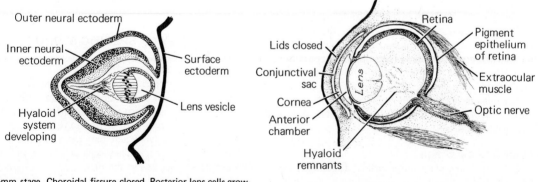

13-mm stage. Choroidal fissure closed. Posterior lens cells growing forward.

65-mm stage (3 months)

Figure 1–28. Embryologic development of ocular structures. (Redrawn and reproduced, with permission, from Mann IC: *The Development of the Human Eye,* 2nd ed. British Medical Association, 1950.)

lacrimal duct) are also surface ectodermal derivatives, which develop from a solid epithelial cord that becomes buried between the maxillary and nasal processes of the developing facial structures. This cord canalizes just before birth.

Sclera & Extraocular Muscles

The sclera and extraocular muscles are formed from condensations of mesenchyme encircling the optic cup and are first identifiable at the 20 mm (7 week) stage. Development of these structures is well advanced by the fourth month. Tenon's capsule appears about the insertions of the rectus muscles at the 80 mm (12 week) stage and is complete at 5 months.

Anterior Segment

The anterior segment of the globe is formed by invasion of neural crest cells into the space between the surface ectoderm, which develops into the corneal epithelium, and the lens vesicle, which has become separated from it. The invasion of neural crest cells occurs in three stages: The first is responsible for formation of the corneal endothelium, the second for formation of the corneal stroma, and the third for formation of the iris stroma. The anterior chamber angle is formed from a residual condensation of mesenchyme at the anterior rim of the optic cup. The mechanism of formation of the anterior chamber itself—and hence the angle structures—is still debated but certainly seems to involve patterns of migration of neural crest cells and subsequent changes in their structure rather than cleavage of mesodermal tissue as previously thought.

The corneal epithelium and endothelium are first apparent at the 12 mm (5 week) stage. Descemet's membrane is secreted by the flattened endothelial cells by the 75 mm (13 week) stage. The stroma slowly thickens and forms an anterior condensation just under the epithelium that is recognizable at 100 mm (4 months) as Bowman's layer. A definite corneoscleral junction is present at 4 months.

The double row of posterior iris epithelium is a forward extension of the anterior rim of the optic cup. This grows forward during the third month (50 mm stage) to lie posterior to the neural crest cells that form the iris stroma. These two epithelial layers become pigmented in the iris, whereas only the outer layer is pigmented in the ciliary body. By the fifth month (150 mm) stage, the sphincter muscle of the pupil is developing from a bud of nonpigmented epithelium derived from the anterior epithelial layer of the iris near the pupillary margin. Soon after the sixth month, the dilator muscle appears in the anterior epithelial layer near the ciliary body.

The anterior chamber of the eye first appears at 20 mm (7 weeks) and remains very shallow until birth. At 65 mm (9–10 weeks), Schlemm's canal appears as a vascular channel at the level of the recess of the angle and gradually assumes a relatively more anterior location as the angle recess develops. The iris, which in the early stages of development is quite anterior, gradually lies relatively more posteriorly as the chamber angle recess develops, most likely because of the difference in rate of growth of the anterior segment structures. The trabecular meshwork develops from the loose vascular mesenchymal tissue lying originally at the margin of the optic cup. The aqueous drainage system is ready to function before birth.

Lens

Soon after the lens vesicle lies free in the rim of the optic cup (13 mm or 6 week stage), the cells of its posterior wall elongate, encroach on the empty cavity, and finally fill it in (26 mm or 7 week stage). At about this stage (13 mm or 6 week), a hyaline capsule is secreted by the lens cells. Secondary lens fibers elongate from the equatorial region and grow forward under the subcapsular epithelium, which remains as a single layer of cuboidal epithelial cells, and backward under the lens capsule. These fibers meet to form the lens sutures (upright {Y} anteriorly and inverted {Y} posteriorly), which are complete by the seventh month. (This growth and proliferation of secondary lens fibers continues at a decreasing rate throughout life; the lens therefore continues to enlarge slowly, causing compression of the lens fibers.)

Ciliary Body & Choroid

The ciliary epithelium is formed from the same anterior extension of the optic cup that is responsible for the posterior iris epithelium. Only the outer layer becomes pigmented. The ciliary muscle and blood vessels are derived from mesenchyme.

At the 6 mm (3{½} week) stage, a network of capillaries encircles the optic cup and develops into the choroid. By the third month, the intermediate and large venous channels of the choroid are developed and drain into the vortex veins to exit from the eye.

Retina

The outer layer of the optic cup remains as a single layer and becomes the pigment epithelium of the retina. Pigmentation begins at the 10 mm (5 week) stage. Secretion of the inner layer of Bruch's membrane occurs by the 13 mm (6 week) stage. The inner layer of the optic cup undergoes a complicated differentiation into the other nine layers of the retina. This occurs slowly throughout gestation. By the seventh month, the outermost cell layer (consisting of the nuclei of the rods and cones) is present as well as the bipolar, amacrine, and ganglion cells and nerve fibers. The macular region is thicker than the rest of the retina until the eighth month, when macular depression begins to develop. Macular development is not complete in anatomic terms until 6 months after birth.

Vitreous

A. First Stage: (Primary vitreous, 4.5 to 13 mm or 3 to 6 week stage.) At about the 4.5 mm stage, mesenchymal cells and fibroblasts derived from mesenchyme at the rim of the optic cup or associated with the hyaloid vascular system, together with minor contributions from the embryonic lens and the inner layer of the optic vesicle, form the vitreous fibrils of the primary vitreous. Ultimately, the primary vitreous comes to lie just behind the posterior pole of the lens in association with remnants of the hyaloid vessels (Cloquet's canal).

B. Second Stage: (Secondary vitreous, 13 to 65 mm or 6 to 10 week stage.) The fibrils and cells (hyalocytes) of the secondary vitreous are thought to originate from the vascular primary vitreous. Anteriorly, the firm attachment of the secondary vitreous to the internal limiting membrane of the retina constitutes the early stages of formation of the vitreous base. The hyaloid system develops a set of vitreous vessels as well as vessels on the lens capsule surface (tunica vasculosa lentis). The hyaloid system is at its height at 40 mm and then atrophies from posterior to anterior.

C. Third Stage: (Tertiary vitreous, 65 mm or 10 weeks on.) During the third month, the marginal bundle of Drualt is forming. This consists of vitreous fibrillar condensations extending from the future ciliary epithelium of the optic cup to the equator of the lens. Condensations then form the suspensory ligament of the lens, which is well developed by the 100 mm or 4 month stage. The hyaloid system atrophies completely during this stage.

Optic Nerve

The axons of the ganglion cells of the retina form the nerve fiber layer. The fibers slowly form the optic stalk and then the optic nerve (26 mm stage). Mesenchymal elements enter the surrounding tissue to form the vascular septa of the nerve. Medullation extends from the brain peripherally down the optic nerve, and at birth has reached the lamina cribrosa. Medullation is completed by age 3 months.

Blood Vessels

Long ciliary arteries bud off from the hyaloid at the 16 mm (6 week) stage and anastomose around the optic cup margin with the major circle of the iris by the 30 mm (7 week) stage.

The hyaloid system (see Vitreous, above) atrophies completely by the eighth month. The hyaloid artery gives rise to the central retinal artery and its branches (100 mm or 4 month stage). Buds begin to grow into the retina and develop the retinal circulation, which reaches the ora serrata at 8 months. The branches of the central retinal vein develop simultaneously

III. GROWTH & DEVELOPMENT OF THE EYE

Eyeball

At birth, the eye is larger in relation to the rest of the body than is the case in children and adults. In relation to its ultimate size (reached at 7–8 years), it is comparatively short, averaging 16.5 mm in anteroposterior diameter (the only optically significant dimension). This would make the eye quite hyperopic if it were not for the refractive power of the nearly spherical lens.

Cornea

The newborn infant has a relatively large cornea that reaches adult size by the age of 2 years. It is flatter than the adult cornea, and its curvature is greater at the periphery than in the center. (The reverse is true in adults.)

Lens

At birth, the lens is more nearly spherical in shape than later in life, producing a greater refractive power that helps to compensate for the short anteroposterior diameter of the eye. The lens grows throughout life as new fibers are added to the periphery, making it flatter.

The consistency of the lens material changes throughout life. At birth, it may be compared with soft plastic; in old age, the lens is of a glass-like consistency. This accounts for the greater resistance to change of shape in accommodation as one grows older.

Iris

At birth, there is little or no pigment on the anterior surface of the iris; the posterior pigment layer showing through the translucent tissue gives the eyes of most infants a bluish color. As the pigment begins to appear on the anterior surface, the iris assumes its definitive color. If considerable pigment is deposited, the eyes become brown. Less iris stroma pigmentation results in blue, hazel, or green coloration.

Ophthalmologic Examination

2

David F. Chang, MD

Of all the organs of the body, the eye is most accessible to direct examination. Visual function can be quantified by simple subjective testing. The external anatomy of the eye is visible to inspection with the unaided eye and with fairly simple instruments. Even the interior of the eye is visible through the clear cornea. The eye is the only part of the body where blood vessels and central nervous system tissue (retina and optic nerve) can be viewed directly. Important systemic effects of infectious, autoimmune, neoplastic, and vascular diseases may be visible from the internal eye examination.

The purpose of sections I and II of this chapter is to provide an overview of the ocular history and basic complete eye examination as performed by an ophthalmologist. In section III, more specialized examination techniques will be presented.

I. OCULAR HISTORY

The **chief complaint** is characterized according to its duration, frequency, intermittency, and rapidity of onset. The location, the severity, and the circumstances surrounding onset are important as well as any associated symptoms. Current eye medications being used and all other current and past ocular disorders are recorded, and a review of other pertinent ocular symptoms is performed.

The **past medical history** centers on the patient's general state of health and principal systemic illnesses if any. Vascular disorders commonly associated with ocular manifestations—such as diabetes and hypertension—should be asked about specifically. Just as a medical history should include ocular medications being used, the eye history should list the patient's systemic medications. This provides a general indication of health status and may include medications that affect ocular health, such as corticosteroids. Finally, any drug allergies should be recorded.

The **family history** is pertinent for ocular disorders

such as strabismus, amblyopia, glaucoma, cataracts, and retinal problems, such as retinal detachment or macular degeneration. Medical diseases such as diabetes may be relevant as well.

COMMON OCULAR SYMPTOMS

A basic understanding of ocular symptomatology is necessary for performing a proper ophthalmic examination. Ocular symptoms can be divided into three basic categories: abnormalities of vision, abnormalities of ocular appearance, and abnormalities of ocular sensation—pain and discomfort.

Symptoms and complaints should always be fully characterized. Was the **onset** gradual, rapid, or asymptomatic? (For example, was blurred vision in one eye not discovered until the opposite eye was inadvertently covered?) Was the **duration** brief, or has the symptom continued until the present visit? If the symptom was intermittent, what was the frequency? Is the **location** focal or diffuse, and is involvement unilateral or bilateral? Finally, is the **degree** characterized by the patient as mild, moderate, or severe?

One should also determine what therapeutic measures have been tried and to what extent they have helped. Has the patient identified circumstances that trigger or worsen the symptom? Have similar instances occurred before, and are there any other associated symptoms?

The following is a brief overview of common ocular complaints. Representative examples of some causes are given here and discussed more fully elsewhere in this book.

ABNORMALITIES OF VISION

Visual Loss

Loss of visual acuity may be due to abnormalities anywhere along the optical and neurologic visual pathway. One must therefore consider refractive (focusing) error, lid ptosis, clouding or interference from the ocular media (eg, corneal edema, cataract, or hemorrhage in the vitreous or aqueous space), and malfunction of the retina (macula), optic nerve, or intracranial visual pathway.

A distinction should be made between decreased central acuity and peripheral vision. The latter may be focal, such as a scotoma, or more expansive as with hemianopia. With the exception of cortical blindness and amblyopia, abnormalities of the intracranial visual pathway usually disturb the visual field rather than central visual acuity.

Transient loss of central or peripheral vision is frequently due to circulatory changes anywhere along the neurologic visual pathway from the retina to the occipital cortex. Examples would be amaurosis fugax or migrainous scotoma.

The degree of visual impairment may vary under different circumstances. For example, uncorrected nearsighted refractive error may seem worse in dark environments. This is because pupillary dilation allows more misfocused rays to reach the retina, increasing the blur. A central focal cataract may seem worse in sunlight. In this case, pupillary constriction prevents more rays from entering and passing around the lens opacity. Blurred vision from corneal edema may improve as the day progresses owing to corneal dehydration from surface evaporation.

Visual Aberrations

Glare or **haloes** may result from uncorrected refractive error, scratches on spectacle lenses, excessive pupillary dilation, and hazy ocular media, such as corneal edema or cataract. **Visual distortion** (apart from blurring) may be manifested as an irregular pattern of dimness, wavy or jagged lines, and image magnification or minification. Causes may include the aura of migraine, optical distortion from strong corrective lenses, or lesions involving the macula and optic nerve. **Flashing** or **flickering** lights may indicate retinal traction (if instantaneous) or migrainous scintillations that last for several seconds or minutes. **Floating spots** may represent normal vitreous strands due to vitreous "syneresis" or separation (see Chapter 9), or the pathologic presence of pigment, blood, or inflammatory cells. **Oscillopsia** is a shaking field of vision that may be due to harmless lid twitching ("myokymia") or to certain forms of nystagmus.

It must be determined whether **double vision** is monocular or binocular (ie, disappears if one eye is covered). **Monocular diplopia** is often a split shadow or ghost image. Causes include uncorrected refractive error, such as astigmatism, or focal media abnormalities such as cataracts or corneal irregularities (eg, scars, keratoconus). **Binocular diplopia** (see Chapters 12 and 14) can be vertical, horizontal, diagonal, or torsional. If the deviation occurs or increases in one gaze direction as opposed to others, it is called "incomitant." Neuromuscular dysfunction or mechanical restriction of globe rotation is suspected. "Comitant" deviation is one that remains constant regardless of the direction of gaze. It is usually due to childhood strabismus.

ABNORMALITIES OF APPEARANCE

Complaints of "red eye" call for differentiation between redness of the lids and periocular area versus redness of the globe. The latter can be caused by subconjunctival hemorrhage or by vascular congestion of the conjunctiva, sclera, or episclera (connective tissue between the sclera and conjunctiva). Causes of such congestion may be either external surface inflammation, such as conjunctivitis and keratitis, or intraocular inflammation such as iritis and acute glaucoma. Color abnormalities other than redness may include jaundice and hyperpigmented spots on the iris or outer ocular surface.

Other changes in appearance of the **globe** that may be noticeable to the patient include focal lesions of the ocular surface, such as a pterygium, and asymmetry of pupil size, called "anisocoria." The **lids** and **periocular tissues** may be the source of visible signs such as edema, redness, focal growths and lesions, and abnormal position or contour, such as ptosis. Finally, the patient may notice bulging or displacement of the globe, as with exophthalmos.

PAIN & DISCOMFORT

"Eye pain" may be periocular, ocular, retrobulbar (behind the globe), or poorly localized. Examples of **periocular** pain may be tenderness of the lid, tear sac, sinuses, or temporal artery. **Retrobulbar** pain can be due to orbital inflammation of any kind. Certain locations of inflammation, such as optic neuritis or orbital myositis, may produce pain on eye movement. Many **nonspecific** complaints such as "eyestrain," "pulling," "pressure," "fullness," and certain kinds of "headaches" are poorly localized. Causes may include fatigue from ocular accommodation or binocular fusion, or referred discomfort from nonocular muscle tension or fatigue.

Ocular pain itself may seem to emanate from the surface or from deeper within the globe. Corneal epithelial damage typically produces a superficial sharp pain or foreign body sensation exacerbated by blinking. Topical anesthesia will immediately relieve this pain. Deeper internal aching pain occurs with acute glaucoma, iritis, endophthalmitis, and scleritis. The globe is often tender to palpation in these situations. Reflex spasm of the ciliary muscle and iris sphincter can occur with iritis or keratitis, producing brow ache and painful "photophobia" (light sensitivity). This discomfort is markedly improved by instillation of cycloplegic dilating drops (see Chapter 3).

Eye Irritation

Superficial ocular discomfort usually results from surface abnormalities. **Itching,** as a primary symptom, is often a sign of allergic sensitivity. Symptoms of **dryness,** burning, grittiness, and mild foreign body sensation can occur with dry eyes or other types of mild corneal irritation. **Tearing** may be of two general types. Sudden reflex tearing is usually due to irritation of the ocular surface. In contrast, chronic watering and "epiphora" (tears rolling down the cheek) may indicate abnormal lacrimal drainage (see Chapter 4).

Ocular **secretions** are often diagnostically nonspecific. Severe amounts of discharge that cause the lids to be glued shut upon awakening usually indicate viral or bacterial conjunctivitis. More scant amounts of mucoid discharge can also be seen with allergic and noninfectious irritations. Dried matter and crusts on the lashes may occur acutely with conjunctivitis or chronically with blepharitis (lid margin inflammation).

II. BASIC OPHTHALMOLOGIC EXAMINATION

The purpose of the ophthalmologic physical examination is to evaluate both the function and the anatomy of the two eyes. Function includes vision and nonvisual functions, such as eye movements and alignment. Anatomically, ocular problems can be subdivided into three areas: those of the adnexa (lids and periocular tissue), the globe, and the orbit. A complete basic examination would include all of these areas except for the orbit. Detailed examination of the orbit requires the aid of specialized techniques discussed later in this chapter.

VISION

Just as assessment of vital signs is a part of every physical examination, any ocular examination must include assessment of vision, regardless of whether vision is mentioned as part of the chief complaint. Good vision results from a combination of an intact neurologic visual pathway, a structurally healthy eye, and proper focus of the eye. An analogy might be made to a video camera, requiring a functioning cable connection to the monitor, a mechanically intact camera body, and a proper focus setting. Measurement of visual acuity is subjective rather than objective, since it requires responses on the part of the patient.

Refraction

The unaided distant focal point of the eye varies among normal individuals depending on the shape of the globe and the cornea (Figure 2–1). An **emmetropic** eye is naturally in optimal focus for distance vision. An **ametropic** eye (ie, one with myopia, hyperopia, or astigmatism) needs corrective lenses to be in proper focus for distance. This optical requirement is called **refractive error. Refraction** is the procedure by which this natural optical error is characterized and quantified (Figure 2–2) (see Chapter 20).

Refraction is often necessary to distinguish between blurred vision caused by refractive (ie, optical) error or by medical abnormalities of the visual system. Thus, in addition to being the basis for prescription of corrective glasses or contact lenses, refraction serves a diagnostic function.

Testing Central Vision

Vision can be divided into central vision and peripheral vision. Central visual acuity is measured with a display of different-sized targets shown at a standard distance from the eye. For example, the familiar "Snellen chart" is composed of a series of progres-

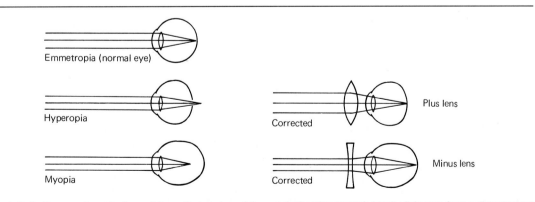

Figure 2–1. Common imperfections of the optical system of the eye **(refractive errors).** Ideally, light rays from a distant target should automatically arrive in focus on the retina if the retina is situated precisely at the eye's natural focal point. Such an eye is called **emmetropic.** In **hyperopia** ("farsightedness"), the light rays from a distant target instead come to a focus behind the retina, causing the retinal image to be blurred. A biconvex (+) lens corrects this by increasing the refractive power of the eye, and shifting the focal point forward. In **myopia** ("nearsightedness"), the light rays come to a focus in front of the retina, as though the eyeball is too long. Placing a biconcave (–) lens in front of the eye diverges the incoming light rays; this effectively weakens the optical power of the eye enough so that the focus is shifted backward and onto the retina. (Modified and reproduced, with permission, from Ganong WF: *Review of Medical Physiology,* 15th ed. Lange, 1991.)

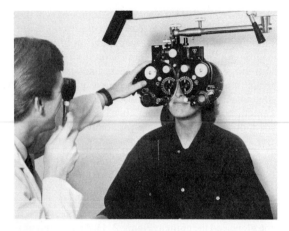

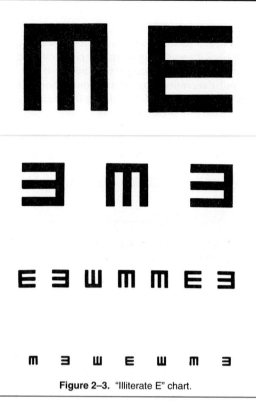

Figure 2–2. Refraction being performed using a "phoropter." This device contains the complete range of corrective lens powers which can quickly be changed back and forth, allowing the patient to subjectively compare various combinations while viewing the eye chart at a distance. (Photo by M Narahara.)

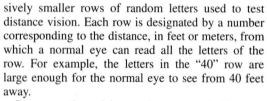

Figure 2–3. "Illiterate E" chart.

sively smaller rows of random letters used to test distance vision. Each row is designated by a number corresponding to the distance, in feet or meters, from which a normal eye can read all the letters of the row. For example, the letters in the "40" row are large enough for the normal eye to see from 40 feet away.

By convention, vision can be measured either at a distance at 20 feet (6 meters) or at near, 14 inches away. For diagnostic purposes, distance acuity is the standard for comparison and is always tested separately for each eye. Acuity is scored as a set of two numbers (eg, "20/40"). The first number represents the testing distance in feet between the chart and the patient, and the second number represents the smallest row of letters that the patient's eye can read from the testing distance. 20/20 vision is normal; 20/60 vision indicates that the patient's eye can only read from 20 feet letters large enough for a normal eye to read from 60 feet.

Charts containing numerals can be used for patients not familiar with the English alphabet. The "illiterate E" chart is used to test small children or if there is a language barrier. "E" figures are randomly rotated in each of four different orientations throughout the chart. For each target, the patient is asked to point in the same direction as the three "bars" of the E (Figure 2–3). Most children can be tested in this manner beginning at about age 3½.

Uncorrected visual acuity is measured without glasses or contact lenses. **Corrected** acuity means that these aids were worn. Since poor uncorrected distance acuity may simply be due to refractive (ie, focusing) error, corrected visual acuity is a more relevant assessment of ocular health.

Pinhole Test

If the patient needs glasses or if they are unavailable, the corrected acuity can be estimated by testing vision through a "pinhole." Refractive blur (eg, myopia, hyperopia, astigmatism) is caused by multiple misfocused rays entering through the pupil and reaching the retina. This prevents formation of a sharply focused image.

Viewing the Snellen chart through a placard of multiple tiny pinhole-sized openings prevents most of the misfocused rays from entering the eye. Only a few centrally aligned focused rays will reach the retina, resulting in a sharper image. In this manner, the patient may be able to read within one or two lines of what would be possible if proper corrective glasses were being used.

Testing Poor Vision

The patient unable to read the largest letter on the chart (eg, the "20/200" letter) should be moved closer to the chart until that letter can be read. The distance from the chart is then recorded as the first number. Visual acuity of "5/200" means that the patient can just make out the largest letter from a distance of 5 feet. An eye unable to read any letters is tested by the ability to count fingers. A notation on the chart that reads "CF at 2 ft" indicates that the eye was able to count fingers held 2 feet away but not farther away.

If counting fingers is not possible, the eye may be

able to detect a hand moving vertically or horizontally ("HM," or "hand motions" vision). The next lower level of vision would be the ability to perceive light ("LP," or "light perception"). An eye that cannot perceive light is considered totally blind ("NLP," or "no light perception").

Testing Peripheral Vision

Because it is much grosser than central acuity, side vision is harder to test quantitatively. Specialized tests described in the next section are used when peripheral vision measurements are needed, such as for the diagnosis of early glaucoma.

Gross screening of the peripheral field of vision can be quickly performed using **confrontation testing.** Since the visual fields of the two eyes overlap, each eye must be tested separately. The patient is seated facing the examiner several feet away and begins by covering the left eye while the right eye fixes on the examiner's left eye.

The examiner then briefly shows several fingers of one hand (usually one, two, or four fingers) peripherally in one of the four quadrants. The patient must identify the number of fingers flashed while maintaining straight-ahead fixation. Since patient and examiner are staring eye to eye, any loss of fixation by the patient will be noticed. The upper and lower temporal and the upper and lower nasal quadrants are all tested in this fashion for each eye.

If the examiner closes the right eye while the patient covers the left eye—and if the targets (fingers) are presented at a distance halfway between the patient and the examiner—their respective peripheral fields should be the same. This allows comparison of the patient's field with the examiner's own. Consistent errors indicate gross deficiencies in the quadrant tested, as seen with retinal detachments, optic nerve abnormalities, and ischemic or mass injuries to the intracranial visual pathway. Since dense visual field abnormalities are often asymptomatic, confrontation testing should be included in complete ophthalmologic examinations.

A subtle form of right or left homonymous hemianopia may exist that can only be elicited by simultaneously presenting targets on both sides of the midline—not when targets are presented on one side at a time. To perform **simultaneous confrontation testing,** the examiner holds both hands out peripherally, one on each side. The patient must signify on which side (right, left, or both) the examiner is intermittently wiggling the fingers. Surprisingly, a patient with a mild left hemianopia may still be able to detect one hand wiggling fingers to the left side and may fail to see them (to the left) only when the examiner is simultaneously wiggling the fingers on both hands. This interesting finding indicates partial or relative inattention to the left side as both sides are being equally—and simultaneously—stimulated.

More sophisticated means of visual field testing are discussed later in this chapter.

PUPILS

Basic Examination

The pupils should appear symmetric, and each one should be examined for size, shape (circular or irregular), and reactivity to both light and accommodation. Pupillary abnormalities may be due to (1) neurologic disease, (2) acute intraocular inflammation causing either spasm or atony of the pupillary sphincter, (3) previous inflammation causing adhesions of the iris, (4) prior surgical alteration, (5) the effect of systemic or eye medications, and (6) benign variations of normal.

To avoid accommodation, the patient is asked to stare in the distance as a penlight is directed toward each eye. Dim lighting conditions help to accentuate the pupillary response and may best demonstrate an abnormally small pupil. Likewise, an abnormally large pupil may be more apparent in brighter background illumination. The **direct response** to light refers to constriction of the illuminated pupil. The reaction may be graded as either brisk or sluggish. Normally, a **consensual** constriction will simultaneously occur in the opposite nonilluminated pupil. This is usually a slightly weaker response. The neuroanatomy of the pupillary pathway is discussed in Chapter 14.

Swinging Penlight Test for Marcus Gunn Pupil

As a light is swung back and forth in front of the two pupils, one can compare the direct and consensual reactions of each pupil. Since the direct reaction is usually stronger than the consensual, each pupil as the light falls directly on it should immediately constrict slightly more. Start by shining the light into the right eye, causing consensual constriction of the left pupil. As the light is then swung toward the left eye, the left pupil should constrict slightly more due to the direct light response. The right pupil should behave similarly as the light is swung back toward the right eye.

If the afferent conduction of light in the left optic nerve is impaired as a consequence of disease, the left pupil will have a weak direct response but its consensual efferent response will remain unchanged. As the light is swung from the right to the left eye, the left pupil will then paradoxically *widen* (since its abnormal direct response is weaker than the consensual response initiated by the healthy right optic nerve). This phenomenon is called a Marcus Gunn pupil, or relative afferent pupillary defect, since the paradoxic dilation in response to direct illumination occurs in the eye with the abnormal afferent pathway (ie, optic nerve or retina). Because the Marcus Gunn pupil still reacts and is often of normal size, the swinging flashlight test may be the only means of demonstrating it.

Marcus Gunn pupil is further discussed and illustrated in Chapter 14.

OCULAR MOTILITY

The objective of ocular motility testing is to evaluate the alignment of the eyes and their movements, both individually ("ductions") and in tandem ("versions"). A more complete discussion of motility testing and abnormalities is presented in Chapter 12.

Testing Alignment

Normal patients have binocular vision. Since each eye generates a visual image separate from and independent of that of the other eye, the brain must be able to fuse the two images in order to avoid "double vision." This is achieved by having each eye positioned so that both foveas are simultaneously fixating on the object of regard.

A simple test of binocular alignment is performed by having the patient look toward a penlight held several feet away. A pinpoint light reflection, or "reflex," should appear on each cornea and should be centered over each pupil if the two eyes are straight in their alignment. If the eye positions are convergent, such that one eye points inward ("esotropia"), the light reflex will appear temporal to the pupil in that eye. If the eyes are divergent, such that one eye points outward ("exotropia"), the light reflex will be located more nasally in that eye. This test can be used with infants.

The **cover test** (see Figure 12–3) is a more accurate method of verifying normal ocular alignment. The test requires good vision in both eyes. The patient is asked to gaze at a distant target with both eyes open. If both eyes are fixating together on the target, covering one eye should not affect the position or continued fixation of the other eye.

To perform the test, the examiner suddenly covers one eye and carefully watches to see that the second eye does not move (indicating that it was fixating on the same target already). If the second eye was not identically aligned but was instead turned abnormally inward or outward, it could not have been simultaneously fixating on the target. Thus, it will have to quickly move to find the target once the previously fixating eye is covered. Fixation of each eye is tested in turn.

An abnormal cover test is expected in patients with diplopia. However, diplopia is not always present in many patients with long-standing ocular malalignment. When the test is abnormal, prism lenses of different power can be used to neutralize the refixation movement of the misaligned eye. In this way, the amount of eye deviation can be quantified based on the amount of prism power needed. A more complete dis-

cussion of this test and its variations is presented in Chapter 12.

Testing Extraocular Movements

The patient is asked to follow a target with both eyes as it is moved in each of the four cardinal directions of gaze. The examiner notes the speed, smoothness, range, and symmetry of movements and observes for unsteadiness of fixation (eg, nystagmus).

Impairment of eye movements can be due to neurologic problems (eg, cranial nerve palsy), primary extraocular muscular weakness (eg, myasthenia gravis), or mechanical constraints within the orbit limiting rotation of the globe (eg, orbital floor fracture with entrapment of the inferior rectus muscle). If the amount of deviation of ocular alignment is the same in all directions of gaze, is called "comitant." It is "incomitant" if the amount of deviation varies with the direction of gaze.

EXTERNAL EXAMINATION

Before studying the eye under magnification, a general external examination of the ocular adnexa (eyelids and periocular area) is performed. Skin lesions, growths, and inflammatory signs such as swelling, erythema, warmth, and tenderness are evaluated by gross inspection and palpation.

The positions of the eyelids are checked for abnormalities such as ptosis or lid retraction. Asymmetry can be quantified by measuring the central width (in millimeters) of the "palpebral fissure"—the space between the upper and lower lid margins. Abnormal motor function of the lids, such as impairment of upper lid elevation or forceful lid closure, may be due to either neurologic or primary muscular abnormalities.

Gross malposition of the globe, such as proptosis, may be seen with certain orbital diseases. Palpation of the bony orbital rim and periocular soft tissue should always be done in instances of suspected orbital trauma, infection, or neoplasm. The general facial examination may contribute other pertinent information as well. Depending on the circumstances, checking for enlarged preauricular lymph nodes, sinus tenderness, temporal artery prominence, or skin or mucous membrane abnormalities may be diagnostically relevant.

SLITLAMP EXAMINATION

Basic Slitlamp Biomicroscopy

The slitlamp (Figure 2–4) is a table-mounted binocular microscope with a special adjustable illumination source attached. A linear slit beam of incandescent light is projected onto the globe, illuminating an optical cross section of the eye (Figure 2–5). The angle of illumination can be varied along with the width, length, and intensity of the light beam. The magnification can

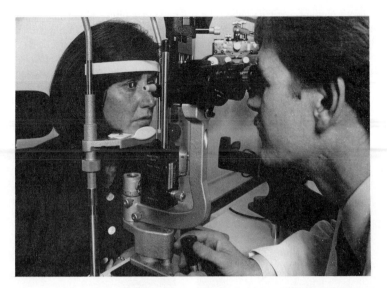

Figure 2–4. Slitlamp examination. (Photo by M Narahara.) (Courtesy of the American Academy of Ophthalmology.)

be adjusted as well (normally $10\times$ to $16\times$ power). Since the slitlamp is a binocular microscope, the view is "stereoscopic," or three-dimensional.

The patient is seated while being examined, and the head is stabilized by an adjustable chin rest and forehead strap. Using the slitlamp alone, the anterior half of the globe—the "anterior segment"—can be visualized. Details of the lid margins and lashes, the palpebral and bulbar conjunctival surfaces, the tear film and cornea, the iris, and the aqueous can be studied. Through a dilated pupil, the crystalline lens and the anterior vitreous can be examined as well.

Because the slit beam of light provides an optical cross section of the eye, the precise anteroposterior location of abnormalities can be determined within each of the clear ocular structures (eg, cornea, lens, vitreous

body). The highest magnification setting is sufficient to show the abnormal presence of cells within the aqueous, such as red or white blood cells or pigment granules. Aqueous turbidity, called "flare," resulting from increased protein concentration can be detected in the presence of intraocular inflammation. Normal aqueous is optically clear, without cells or flare.

Adjunctive Slitlamp Techniques

The eye examination with the slitlamp is supplemented by the use of various techniques. Tonometry is discussed separately in a subsequent section.

A. Lid Eversion: Lid eversion to examine the undersurface of the upper lid can be performed either at the slitlamp or without the aid of that instrument. It should always be done if the presence of a foreign body

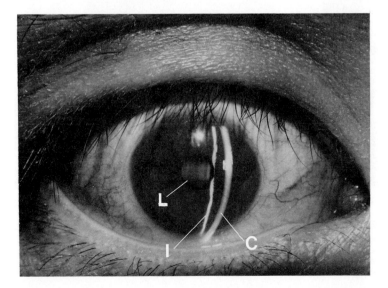

Figure 2–5. Slitlamp photograph of a normal right eye. The curved slit of light to the right is reflected off of the cornea (C), while the slit to the left is reflected off of the iris (I). As the latter slit passes through the pupil, the anterior lens (L) is faintly illuminated in cross section. (Photo by M Narahara.)

is suspected. A semirigid plate of cartilage called the tarsus gives each lid its contour and shape. In the upper lid, the superior edge of the tarsus lies centrally about 8–9 mm above the lashes. On the undersurface of the lid, it is covered by the tarsal palpebral conjunctiva.

Following topical anesthesia, the patient is positioned at the slitlamp and instructed to look down. The examiner gently grasps the upper lashes with the thumb and index finger of one hand while using the other hand to position an applicator handle just above the superior edge of the tarsus (Figure 2–6). The lid is everted by applying slight downward pressure with the applicator as the lash margin is simultaneously lifted. The patient continues to look down, and the lashes are held pinned to the skin overlying the superior orbital rim, as the applicator is withdrawn. The tarsal conjunctiva is then

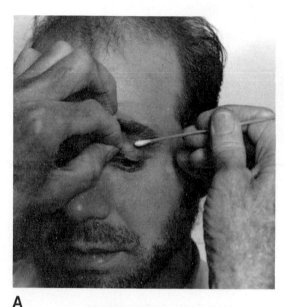

A

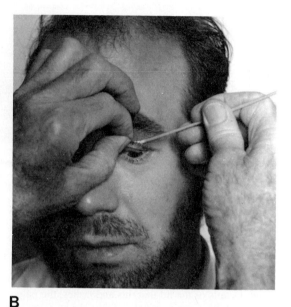

B

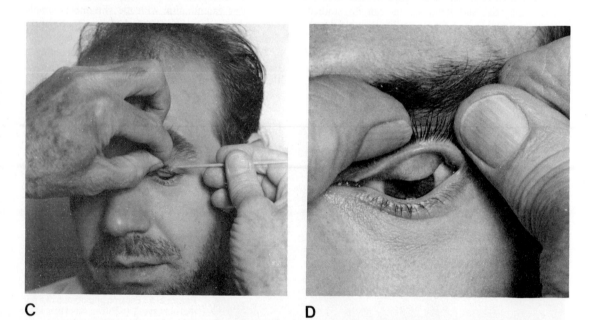

C

D

Figure 2–6. Technique of lid eversion. **A:** With the patient looking down, the upper lashes are grasped with one hand as an applicator stick is positioned at the superior edge of the upper tarsus (at the upper lid crease). **B and C:** As the lashes are lifted, slight downward pressure is simultaneously applied with the applicator stick. **D:** The thumb pins the lashes against the superior orbital rim, allowing examination of the undersurface of the tarsus. (Photos by M Narahara.)

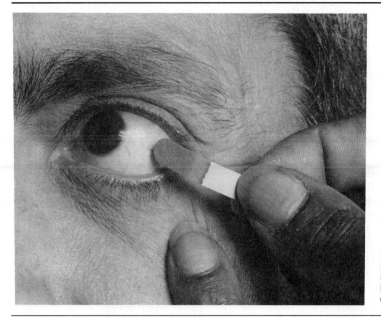

Figure 2–7. Instillation of fluorescein dye. (Photo by M Narahara.) Fluorescein staining of a dendritic epithelial defect due to herpes simplex keratitis is shown in Figure 6–5.

examined under magnification. To undo eversion the lid margin is gently stroked downward as the patient looks up.

B. Fluorescein Staining: Fluorescein is a specialized dye that stains the cornea and highlights any irregularities of its epithelial surface. Sterile paper strips containing fluorescein are wetted and touched against the inner surface of the lower lid, instilling the yellowish dye into the tear film (Figure 2–7). The illuminating light of the slitlamp is made blue with a filter, causing the dye to fluoresce.

A uniform film of dye should cover the normal cornea. If the corneal surface is abnormal, excessive amounts of dye will absorb into or collect within the affected area. Abnormalities can range from tiny punctate dots, such as those resulting from excessive dryness or ultraviolet light damage, to large geographic defects in the epithelium such as those seen in corneal abrasions or infectious ulcers (see Figure 6–6).

C. Special Lenses: Special examining lenses can expand and further magnify the slitlamp examination of the eye's interior. A goniolens (Figure 2–8) pro-

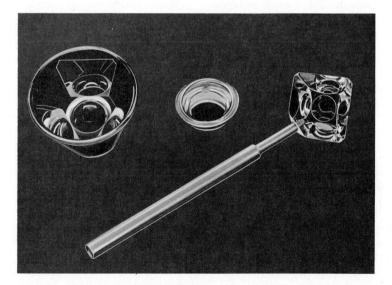

Figure 2–8. Three types of goniolenses. ***Left:*** Goldmann three-mirror lens. Besides the goniomirror, there are also two peripheral retinal mirrors and a central fourth mirror for examining the central retina. ***Center:*** Koeppe lens. ***Right:*** Posner/Zeiss-type lens. (Photo by M Narahara.)

vides visualization of the anterior chamber "angle" formed by the iridocorneal junction. Other lenses placed on or in front of the dilated eye allow slitlamp evaluation of the posterior half of the globe's interior—the "posterior segment." Since the slitlamp is a binocular microscope, these lenses provide a magnified three-dimensional view of the posterior vitreous, the fundus, and the disk. Examples are the Goldmann-style three-mirror lens (Figure 2–8), the Hruby lens, and the Volk-style 90-diopter biconvex lens.

D. Special Attachments: Special attachments to the slitlamp allow it to be used with a number of techniques requiring microscopic visualization. Special camera bodies can be attached for photographic documentation and for special applications such as corneal endothelial cell studies. Special instruments for study of visual potential require attachment to the slitlamp. Finally, laser sources are attached to a slitlamp to allow microscopic visualization and control of eye treatment.

TONOMETRY

The globe can be thought of as an enclosed compartment through which there is a constant circulation of aqueous humor. This fluid maintains the shape and a relatively uniform pressure within the globe. Tonometry is the method of measuring the intraocular fluid pressure using calibrated instruments that indent or flatten the corneal apex. As the eye becomes firmer, a greater force is required to cause the same amount of indentation. Pressures between 10 and 24 mm Hg are considered within the normal range.

Two common types of tonometry are the **Schiotz** and **applanation** methods. The Schiotz tonometer measures the amount of corneal indentation produced by a preset weight or force. The softer the eye, the more a given force will be able to indent the cornea. As the eye becomes firmer, less corneal indentation will result from the same amount of force.

In contrast to the Schiotz tonometer, the applanation tonometer can vary and measure the amount of force applied. The ocular pressure is determined by the force required to flatten the cornea by a predetermined standard amount. At lower intraocular pressures, less tonometer force is needed to achieve the standard degree of corneal flattening than at higher intraocular pressures. Since both methods employ devices that touch the patient's cornea, they require topical anesthetic and disinfection of the instrument tip prior to use. (Tonometer disinfection techniques are discussed in Chapter 21.) While retracting the lids with any method of tonometry, care must be taken to avoid pressing on the globe and artificially increasing its pressure.

Schiotz Tonometry

The advantage of this method is that it is simple, requiring only a portable hand-held instrument—the

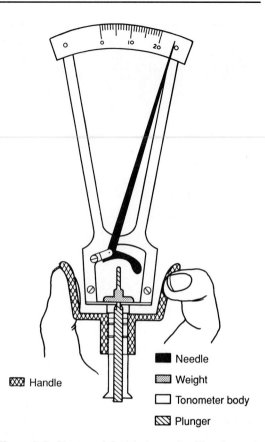

Figure 2–9. Diagram of Schiotz tonometer. The plunger is shown with the 5.5-g weight attached at one end.

Schiotz tonometer (Figure 2–9). It can be used in any clinic or emergency room setting, at the hospital bedside, or in the operating room. It is a practical device for the nonophthalmologist, who might use it to screen patients for glaucoma or to diagnose acute angle closure glaucoma in an emergency situation.

The three separate components of the tonometer should be cleaned, assembled, and then disassembled with each use. The tonometer **body** consists of a cylindric hollow plunger barrel fixed to a measuring scale with an indicator needle. The attached handle, which can slide along the outside of the cylindric barrel, supports the weight of the tonometer when it is not resting on the eye. The **plunger** is a slender blunt-tipped rod that is inserted into the barrel shaft, where it can slide back and forth. One end will touch the cornea, while the other end will deflect the needle of the measuring scale. The 5.5-g **weight** screwed onto the upper end of the plunger (farthest from the patient) keeps it from falling out of the shaft.

The patient is placed supine, and topical anesthetic is instilled into each eye. As the patient looks straight ahead, the lids are kept gently opened by lightly retracting the skin against the bony orbital rims. The tonometer is lowered with the other hand until the concave "end" of the barrel balances on the cornea (Figure 2–10). With a force determined by the attached weight, the blunt protruding plunger will press into and slightly indent the central cornea. The corneal resistance, which is proportionate to the intraocular pressure, will displace the plunger upward. As the plunger slides upward within the barrel, it will deflect the needle on the scale. The higher the intraocular pressure, the greater the corneal resistance to indentation, the more the plunger will be displaced upward, and the farther the needle will be deflected along the calibrated scale.

A conversion chart is used to translate the reading from the scale into millimeters of mercury. If the eye is firm, additional weights (7.5 g and 10 g) can be added to the plunger to increase the force brought to bear on the cornea. Calibration is checked by placing the tonometer on a "cornea-shaped" metal block that should deflect the needle maximally so that it aligns with the "0" end of the scale.

Applanation Tonometry

The Goldmann applanation tonometer (Figure 2–11) is attached to the slitlamp and measures the amount of force required to flatten the corneal apex by a standard amount. The higher the intraocular pressure, the greater the force required. Since Goldmann applanation tonometer is a more accurate method than Schiotz tonometry, it is preferred by ophthalmologists.

Following topical anesthesia and instillation of fluorescein, the patient is positioned at the slitlamp and the tonometer is swung into place. To visualize the fluorescein, the cobalt blue filter is used with the brightest illumination setting. After grossly aligning the tonometer in front of the cornea, the examiner looks through the slitlamp ocular just as the tip contacts the cornea. A manually controlled counterbalanced spring varies the force applied by the tonometer tip.

Upon contact, the tonometer tip flattens the central cornea and produces a thin circular outline of fluorescein. A prism in the tip visually splits this circle into two semicircles that appear green while viewed through the slitlamp oculars. The tonometer force is adjusted manually until the two semicircles just overlap, as shown in Figure 2–12. This visual end point indicates that the cornea has been flattened by the set standard amount. The amount of force required to do this is translated by the scale into a pressure reading in millimeters of mercury.

A portable electronic applanation tonometer, the

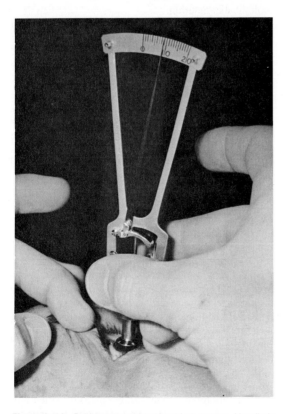

Figure 2–10. Schiotz tonometer placed on cornea. Handle is being held by thumb and third finger of right hand in this photo. (Photo by Diane Beeston.)

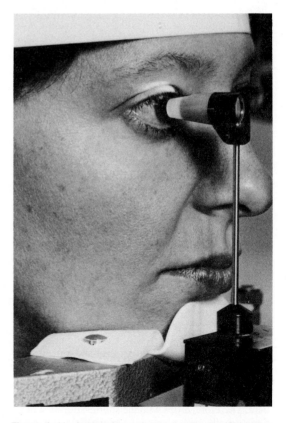

Figure 2–11. Applanation tonometry, using the Goldmann tonometer attached to the slit lamp. (Photo by M Narahara. Courtesy of the American Academy of Ophthalmology.)

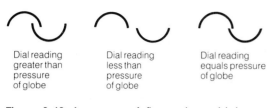

Dial reading
greater than
pressure
of globe

Dial reading
less than
pressure
of globe

Dial reading
equals pressure
of globe

Figure 2–12. Appearance of fluorescein semicircles, or "mires," through the slit lamp ocular, showing the end point for applanation tonometry.

Tono-Pen, has been developed. Although accurate, it requires daily recalibration. It is more expensive than the Schiotz tonometer and therefore is less often found in clinics and emergency departments. The **Perkins tonometer** is a portable mechanical applanation tonometer with a mechanism similar to the Goldmann tonometer. The **pneumatotonometer** is another applanation tonometer, particularly useful when the cornea has an irregular surface.

Noncontact Tonometry

The **noncontact ("air-puff") tonometer** is not as accurate as applanation tonometers. A small puff of air is blown against the cornea. The air rebounding from the corneal surface hits a pressure-sensing membrane in the instrument. This method does not require anesthetic drops, since no instrument touches the eye. Thus, it can be more easily used by technicians and is useful in screening programs.

DIAGNOSTIC MEDICATIONS

Topical Anesthetics

Eye drops such as proparacaine, tetracaine, and benoxinate provide rapid onset, short-acting topical anesthesia of the cornea, and conjunctiva. They are used prior to ocular contact with diagnostic lenses and instruments such as the tonometer. Other diagnostic manipulations utilizing topical anesthetics will be discussed later. These include corneal and conjunctival scrapings, lacrimal canalicular and punctal probing, and scleral depression.

Mydriatic (Dilating) Drops

The pupil can be pharmacologically dilated by either stimulating the iris dilator muscle with a sympathomimetic agent (eg, 2.5% phenylephrine) or by inhibiting the sphincter muscle with an anticholinergic eye drop (eg, 0.5% or 1% tropicamide). Anticholinergic medications also inhibit accommodation, an effect called "cycloplegia." This may aid the process of refraction but causes further inconvenience for the patient. Therefore, drops with the shortest duration of action (usually several hours) are used for diagnostic applications. Combining drops from both pharmaco-

logic classes produces the fastest onset (15–20 minutes) and widest dilation.

Because dilation can cause a small rise in intraocular pressure, tonometry should always be performed before these drops are instilled. There is also a risk of precipitating an attack of acute angle-closure glaucoma if the patient has preexisting narrow anterior chamber angles (between the iris and cornea). Such an eye can be identified using the technique illustrated in Figure 12–8. Finally, excessive instillation of these drops should be avoided because of the systemic absorption that can occur through the nasopharyngeal mucous membranes following lacrimal drainage.

A more complete discussion of diagnostic drops is found in Chapter 3.

DIRECT OPHTHALMOSCOPY

Instrumentation

The hand-held direct ophthalmoscope provides a magnified (15×) monocular image of the ocular media and fundus. Because of its portability and the detailed view of the disk and retinal vasculature it provides, direct ophthalmoscopy is a standard part of the general medical examination as well as the ophthalmologic examination.

Darkening the room usually causes enough natural pupillary dilation to allow evaluation of the central fundus, including the disk, the macula, and the proximal retinal vasculature. Pharmacologically dilating the pupil greatly enhances the view and permits a more extensive examination of the peripheral retina. The fundus examination is also optimized by holding the ophthalmoscope as close to the patient's pupil as possible (approximately 1–2 inches), just as one can see more through a keyhole by getting as close to it as possible. This requires using the examiner's right eye and hand to examine the patient's right eye and the left eye and hand to examine the patient's left eye (Figure 2–13). If the examiner wears spectacles, they can either be left on or off.

The intensity, color, and spot size of the illuminating light can be adjusted as well as the ophthalmoscope's point of focus. The latter is changed using a wheel of progressively higher power lenses that the examiner dials into place. These lenses are sequentially arranged and numbered according to their power in units called "diopters." The descending scale of black numbers designates the (+) converging lenses, whereas the ascending scale of red numbers designates the (–) divergent lenses.

As one dials this focusing wheel counterclockwise from high plus (+) lenses down to zero and on through increasingly minus (–) lenses, the focus is shifted progressively farther away from the ophthalmoscope toward the patient. By starting with a higher (+) lens and

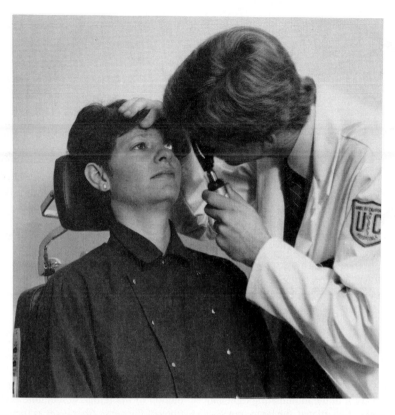

Figure 2–13. Direct ophthalmoscopy. The examiner uses the left eye to evaluate the patient's left eye. (Photo by M Narahara. Courtesy of the American Academy of Ophthalmology.)

dialing in this direction, the examiner will eventually bring the cornea and iris into focus, followed several steps later by the retina. The refractive error (ie, "prescriptions") of the patient's and the examiner's eyes will determine the lens power needed to bring the fundus into optimal focus.

Fundus Examination

The primary value of the direct ophthalmoscope is in examination of the fundus (Figure 2–14). The view may be impaired by cloudy ocular media, such as a cataract, or by insufficient pupillary dilation. As the patient fixates on a distant target with the opposite eye, the examiner first brings retinal details into sharp focus. Since the retinal vessels all arise from the disk, the latter is located by following any major vascular branch back to this common origin. At this point, the ophthalmoscope beam will be aimed slightly nasal to the patient's line of vision, or "visual axis." One should study the shape, size, and color of the disk, the distinctness of its margins (Figure 14–6), and the size of the pale central "physiologic cup." The ratio of cup size to disk size is of diagnostic importance in glaucoma (Figures 2–15 and 2–16).

The macular area (Figure 2–14) is located approxi-

mately two "disk diameters" temporal to the edge of the disk. A small pinpoint white reflection or "reflex" marks the central fovea. This is surrounded by a more darkly pigmented and poorly circumscribed area called the macula. The retinal vascular branches approach from all sides but stop short of the fovea. Thus, its location can be confirmed by the focal absence of retinal vessels or by asking the patient to stare directly into the light.

The major retinal vessels are then examined and followed as far distally as possible in each of the four quadrants (superior, inferior, temporal, and nasal). The veins are darker and wider than their paired arteries. The vessels are examined for color, tortuosity, and caliber as well as for associated abnormalities such as aneurysms, hemorrhages, or exudates. Sizes and distances within the fundus are often measured in "disk diameters (DD)." (The typical optic disk is approximately 1.5 mm in diameter.) Thus, one might describe a "1 DD area of hemorrhage located 2.5 DD inferotemporal to the fovea."

Dilating the pupil pharmacologically enables more of the periphery to be visualized. The patient is asked to look in the direction of the quadrant one wishes to examine. Thus, the temporal retina of the right eye is seen when the patient looks temporally to the right, while the superior retina is seen when the patient looks

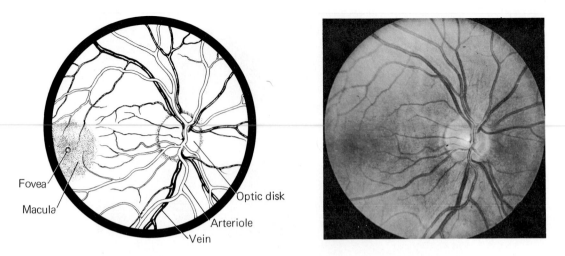

Figure 2–14. Photo and corresponding diagram of a normal fundus. Note that the retinal vessels all stop short of and do not cross the fovea. (Photo by Diane Beeston.)

up. This principle works because as the globe rotates about a point in the center of the eye, the retina and the cornea move in opposite directions. As the patient looks up, the superior retina rotates downward into the examiner's line of vision.

The spot size and color of the illuminating light can be varied. If the pupil is well dilated, the large spot size of light affords the widest area of illumination. With a smaller pupil, however, much of this light would be reflected back toward the examiner's eye by the patient's iris, interfering with the view. For this reason, the smaller spot size of light is selected for undilated pupils. The green "red-free" filter assists in the examination of the retinal vasculature and the subtle striations of the nerve fiber layer as they course toward the disk (see Figure 14–5).

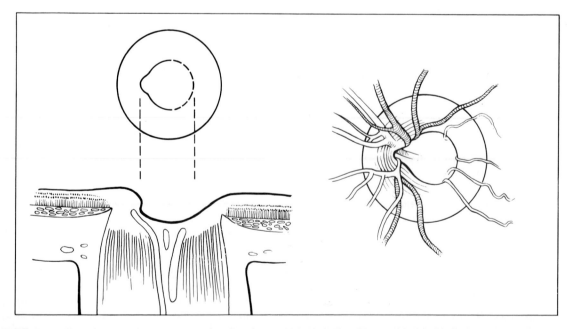

Figure 2–15. Diagram of a moderately cupped disk viewed on end and in profile, with an accompanying sketch for the patient's record. The width of the central cup divided by the width of the disk is the "cup-to-disk ratio." The cup-to-disk ratio of this disk is approximately 0.5.

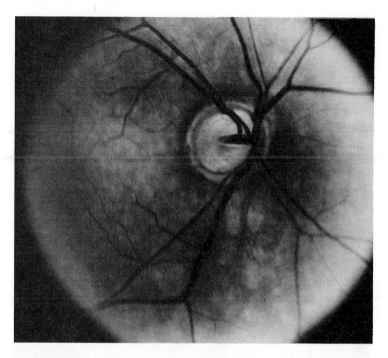

Figure 2–16. Cup-to-disk ratio of 0.9 in a patient with end-stage glaucoma. The normal disk tissue is compressed into a peripheral thin rim surrounding a huge pale cup.

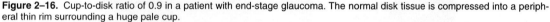

Anterior Segment Examination

As discussed earlier, the direct ophthalmoscope can be focused more anteriorly so as to provide a magnified view of the conjunctiva, cornea, and iris. The slit-lamp allows a far superior and more magnified examination of these areas, but it is not portable and may be unavailable.

Red Reflex Examination

If the illuminating light is aligned directly along the visual axis of a dilated pupil, the pupillary space will appear as a homogeneous bright reddish-orange color. This so-called red reflex is a reflection of the fundus color (actually the combined color of the choroidal vasculature and pigmentation) back through clear ocular media—the vitreous, lens, aqueous, and cornea. The red reflex is best observed by holding the ophthalmoscope at arm's length from the patient as he looks toward the illuminating light. By dialing the lens wheel, the bright red reflex will appear when the ophthalmoscope is focused on the plane of the pupil.

Any opacity located along this central optical pathway will block all or part of this bright reflex and appear as a dark spot or shadow. If a small opacity is seen, have the patient look momentarily away and then back toward the light. If the opacity is still moving or floating, it is located within the vitreous (eg, small hemorrhage). If it is stationary, it is probably in the lens (eg,

focal cataract) or on the cornea (eg, scar). Less red reflex is visible with a small pupil, limiting the usefulness of this test.

INDIRECT OPHTHALMOSCOPY

Instrumentation

The binocular indirect ophthalmoscope (Figure 2–17) complements and supplements the direct ophthalmoscopic examination. Since it requires wide pupillary dilation and is difficult to learn, this technique is used primarily by ophthalmologists. The patient can be examined while seated, but the supine position is preferable.

The indirect ophthalmoscope is worn on the examiner's head and allows binocular viewing through a set of lenses of fixed power. A bright adjustable light source attached to the headband is directed toward the patient's eye. As with direct ophthalmoscopy, the patient is told to look in the direction of the quadrant being examined. A convex lens is hand-held several inches from the patient's eye in precise orientation so as to simultaneously focus light onto the retina and an image of the retina in midair between the patient and the examiner. Using the preset head-mounted ophthalmoscope lenses, the examiner can then "focus on" and visualize this midair image of the retina.

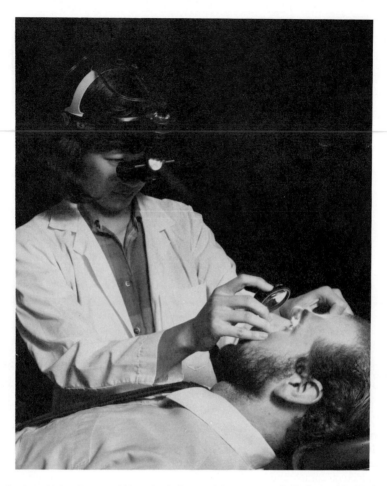

Figure 2–17. Examination with head-mounted binocular indirect ophthalmoscope. A 20-diopter hand-held condensing lens is used. (Photo by M Narahara.)

Comparison of Indirect & Direct Ophthalmoscopy

Indirect ophthalmoscopy is so called because one is viewing an "image" of the retina formed by a hand-held "condensing lens." In contrast, direct ophthalmoscopy allows one to focus on the retina itself. Compared with the direct ophthalmoscope (15× magnification), indirect ophthalmoscopy provides a much wider field of view (Figure 2–18) with less overall magnification (approximately 3.5× using a standard 20-diopter hand-held condensing lens). Thus, it presents a wide panoramic fundus view from which specific areas can be selectively studied under higher magnification using either the direct ophthalmoscope or the slitlamp with special auxiliary lenses.

Indirect ophthalmoscopy has three distinct advantages over direct ophthalmoscopy. One is the brighter light source that permits much better visualization through cloudy media. A second advantage is that by using both eyes, the examiner enjoys a stereoscopic view, allowing visualization of elevated masses or retinal detachment in three dimensions. Finally, indirect

ophthalmoscopy can be used to examine the entire retina even out to its extreme periphery, the ora serrata. This is possible for two reasons. Optical distortions caused by looking through the peripheral lens and cornea interfere very little with the indirect ophthalmoscopic examination, compared with the direct ophthalmoscope. In addition, the adjunct technique of scleral depression can be used.

Scleral depression (Figure 2–19) is performed as the peripheral retina is being examined with the indirect ophthalmoscope. A smooth, thin metal probe is used to gently indent the globe externally through the lids at a point just behind the corneoscleral junction (limbus). As this is done, the ora serrata and peripheral retina are pushed internally into the examiner's line of view. By depressing around the entire circumference, the peripheral retina can be viewed in its entirety.

Because of all of these advantages, indirect ophthalmoscopy is used preoperatively and intraoperatively in the evaluation and surgical repair of retinal detachments. A minor disadvantage of indirect ophthalmoscopy is that it provides an inverted image of the

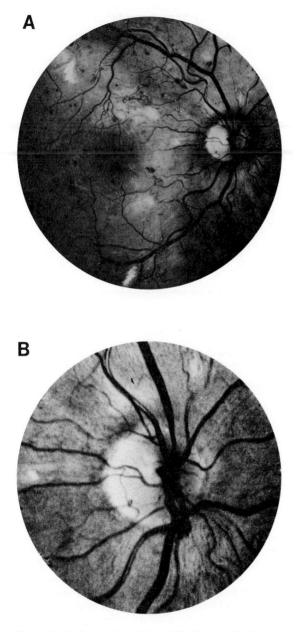

A

B

Figure 2–18. Comparison of view within the same fundus using the indirect ophthalmoscope **(A)** and the direct ophthalmoscope **(B).** The field of view with the latter is approximately 10 degrees, compared with approximately 37 degrees using the indirect ophthalmoscope. In this patient with diabetic retinopathy, an important overview is first seen with the indirect ophthalmoscope. The direct ophthalmoscope can then provide magnified details of a specific area. (Photos by M Narahara.)

fundus, which requires a mental adjustment on the examiner's part. Its brighter light source can also be more uncomfortable for the patient.

EYE EXAMINATION BY THE NONOPHTHALMOLOGIST

The preceding sequence of tests would comprise a complete routine or diagnostic ophthalmologic evaluation. A general medical examination would often include many of these same testing techniques.

Assessment of pupils, extraocular movements, and confrontation visual fields is part of any complete neurologic assessment. Direct ophthalmoscopy should always be performed to assess the appearance of the disk and retinal vessels. Separately testing the visual acuity of each eye (particularly with children) may uncover either a refractive or a medical cause of decreased vision. Finally, screening tonometry measurements using the Schiotz tonometer may detect the asymptomatic elevated intraocular pressure of glaucoma, a prevalent condition among the elderly.

The three most common preventable causes of permanent visual loss in developed nations are amblyopia, diabetic retinopathy, and glaucoma. All can remain asymptomatic while the opportunity for preventive measures is gradually lost. During this time, the pediatrician or general medical practitioner may be the only physician the patient visits.

By testing children for visual acuity in each eye, examining and referring diabetics for regular dilated fundus ophthalmoscopy, and referring patients with suspicious discs or tonometry readings to the ophthalmologist, the nonophthalmologist may indeed be the one who truly "saves" that patient's eyesight. This represents both an important opportunity and responsibility for every primary care physician.

III. SPECIALIZED OPHTHALMOLOGIC EXAMINATIONS

This section will discuss ophthalmologic examination techniques with more specific indications that would not be performed on a routine basis. They will be grouped according to the function or anatomic area of primary interest.

DIAGNOSIS OF VISUAL ABNORMALITIES

1. PERIMETRY

Perimetry is used to examine the central and peripheral visual fields. This technique, which is per-

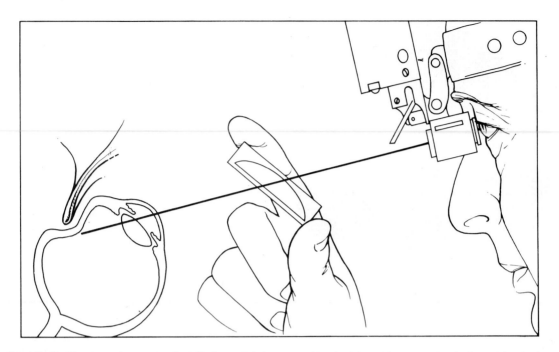

Figure 2–19. Diagrammatic representation of indirect ophthalmoscopy with scleral depression to examine the far peripheral retina. Indentation of the sclera through the lids brings the peripheral edge of the retina into visual alignment with the dilated pupil, the hand-held condensing lens, and the head-mounted ophthalmoscope.

formed separately for each eye, measures the combined function of the retina, the optic nerve, and the intracranial visual pathway. It is used clinically to detect or monitor field loss due to disease at any of these locations. Damage to specific parts of the neurologic visual pathway may produce characteristic patterns of change on serial field examinations.

The visual field of the eye is measured and plotted in degrees of arc. Measurement of degrees of arc remains constant regardless of the distance from the eye the field is checked. The sensitivity of vision is greatest in the center of the field (corresponding to the fovea) and least in the periphery. Perimetry relies on subjective patient responses, and the results will depend on the patient's psychomotor as well as visual status. Perimetry must always be performed and interpreted with this in mind.

The Principles of Testing

Although perimetry is subjective, the methods discussed below have been standardized to maximize reproducibility and permit subsequent comparison. Perimetry requires (1) steady fixation and attention by the patient; (2) a set distance from the eye to the screen or testing device; (3) a uniform, standard amount of background illumination and contrast; (4) test targets of standard size and brightness; and (5) a universal protocol for administration of the test by examiners.

As the patient's eye fixates on a central target, test objects are randomly presented at different locations throughout the field. If they are seen, the patient responds either verbally or with a hand-held signaling device. Varying the target's size or brightness permits quantification of visual sensitivity of different areas in the field. The smaller or dimmer the target seen, the better the sensitivity of that location.

There are two basic methods of target presentation—static and kinetic—that can be used alone or in combination during an examination. In **static perimetry,** different locations throughout the field are tested one at a time. A difficult test object, such as a dim light, is first presented at a particular location. If it is not seen, the size or intensity of the light is incrementally increased until it is just large enough or bright enough to be detected. This is called the "threshold" sensitivity level of that location. This sequence is repeated at a series of other locations, so that the light sensitivity of multiple points in the field can be evaluated and combined to form a profile of the visual field.

In **kinetic perimetry,** the sensitivity of the entire field to one single test object (of fixed size and brightness) is first tested. The object is slowly moved toward the center from a peripheral area until it is first spotted. By moving the same object inward from multiple different directions, a boundary called an **"isopter"** can be mapped out which is specific for that target. The isopter outlines the area within which the target can be seen and beyond which it cannot be seen. Thus, the larger the isopter, the better the visual field of that eye.

The boundaries of the isopter are measured and plotted in degrees of arc. By repeating the test using objects of different size or brightness, multiple isopters can then be plotted for a given eye. The smaller or dimmer test objects will produce smaller isopters.

Methods of Perimetry

The **tangent screen** is the simplest apparatus for standardized perimetry. It utilizes different-sized white pins on a black wand presented against a black screen and is used primarily to test the central 30 degrees of visual field. The advantages of this method are its simplicity and rapidity, the possibility of changing the subject's distance from the screen, and the option of using any assortment of fixation and test objects, including different colors.

The more sophisticated **Goldmann perimeter** (Figure 2–20) is a hollow white spherical bowl positioned a set distance in front of the patient. A light of variable size and intensity can be presented by the examiner (seated behind the perimeter) in either static or kinetic fashion. This method can test the full limit of peripheral vision and was for years the primary method for plotting fields in glaucoma patients.

Computerized automated perimeters (Figure 2–21) now constitute the most sophisticated and sensitive equipment available for visual field testing. Using a bowl similar to the Goldmann perimeter, these instruments display test lights of varying brightness and size but use a quantitative static threshold testing format that is more precise and comprehensive than other methods. Numerical scores (Figure 2–22) corresponding to the threshold sensitivity of each test location can be stored in the computer memory and compared statistically with results from previous examinations or from other normal patients. The higher the numerical score, the better the visual sensitivity of that location in the field. Another important

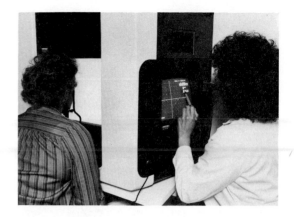

Figure 2–21. Computerized automated perimeter. (Photo by M Narahara.)

advantage is that the test presentation is programmed and automated, eliminating any variability on the part of the examiner.

2. AMSLER GRID

The Amsler grid is used to test the central 20 degrees of the visual field. The grid (Figure 2–23) is viewed by each eye separately at normal reading distance and with reading glasses on if the patient uses them. It is most commonly used to test macular function.

While fixating on the central dot, the patient checks to see that the lines are all straight, without distortion, and that no spots or portions of the grid are missing. One eye is compared with the other. A scotoma or blank area—either central or paracentral—can indicate disease of the macula or optic nerve. Wavy distortion of the lines (metamorphopsia) can indicate macular edema or submacular fluid.

The grid can be used by patients at home to test their own central vision. For example, patients with age-related macular degeneration (see Chapter 10) can use the grid to monitor for sudden metamorphopsia. This often is the earliest symptom of acute fluid accumulation beneath the macula arising from leaking subretinal neovascularization. Since these abnormal vessels maybe treatable with the laser, early detection is important.

3. BRIGHTNESS ACUITY TESTING

The visual abilities of patients with media opacities may vary depending on conditions of lighting. For example, when dim illumination makes the pupil larger, one may be able to "see around" a central focal cataract, whereas bright illumination causing pupillary constriction would have the contrary effect. Bright

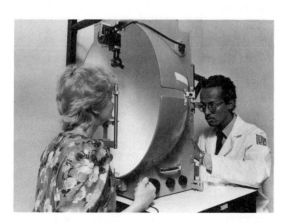

Figure 2–20. Goldmann perimeter. (Photo by M Narahara.)

A

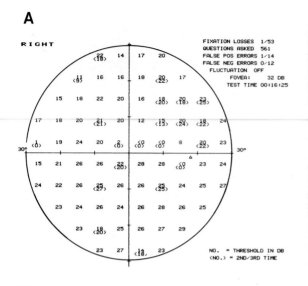

B

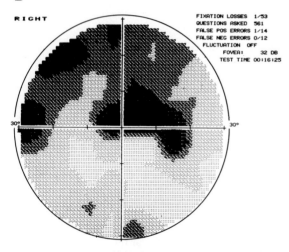

Figure 2–22. A: Numerical printout of threshold sensitivity scores derived by using the static method of computerized perimetry. This is the 30-degree field of a patient's right eye with glaucoma. The higher the numbers, the better the visual sensitivity. The computer retests many of the points (bracketed numbers) to assess consistency of the patient's responses. **B:** Diagrammatic "gray scale" display of these same numerical scores. The darker the area, the poorer the visual sensitivity at that location.

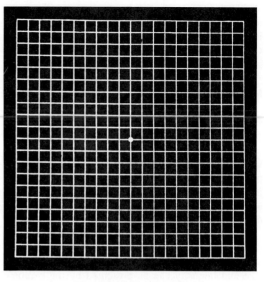

Figure 2–23. Amsler grid.

lights may also cause disabling glare in patients with corneal edema or diffuse clouding of the crystalline lens due to light scattering.

Because the darkened examining room may not accurately elicit the patient's functional difficulties in real life, instruments have been developed to test the effect of varying levels of brightness or glare on visual acuity. Distance acuity with the Snellen chart is usually tested under standard levels of incrementally increasing illumination, and the information may be helpful in making therapeutic or surgical decisions. Asking cataract patients specific questions about how their vision is affected by various lighting conditions is even more important.

4. COLOR VISION TESTING

Normal color vision requires healthy function of the macula and optic nerve. The most common abnormality is X-linked red-green "color blindness," which is present in approximately 8% of the male population. This is due to an X-linked congenital deficiency of one specific type of retinal photoreceptor. Depressed color vision may also be a sensitive indicator of certain kinds of acquired macular or optic nerve disease. For example, in optic neuritis or optic nerve compression (eg, by a mass), abnormal color vision is often an earlier indication of disease than visual acuity, which may still be 20/20.

The most common testing technique utilizes a series of polychromatic plates, such as those of Ishihara or Hardy-Rand-Rittler (Figure 2–24). The plates are made up of dots of the primary colors printed on a background mosaic of similar dots in a confusing variety of secondary colors. The primary dots are arranged in simple patterns (numbers or geometric shapes) that cannot be recognized by patients with deficient color perception.

5. CONTRAST SENSITIVITY TESTING

Contrast sensitivity is the ability of the eye to discern subtle degrees of contrast. Retinal and optic nerve

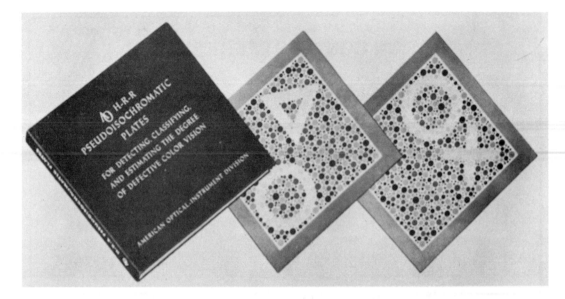

Figure 2–24. Hardy-Rand-Rittler (H-R-R) pseudoisochromatic plates for testing color vision.

disease and clouding of the ocular media (eg, cataracts) can impair this ability. Like color vision, contrast sensitivity may become depressed before Snellen visual acuity is affected in many situations.

Contrast sensitivity is best tested by using standard preprinted charts with a series of test targets (Figure 2–25). Since illumination greatly affects contrast, it must be standardized and checked with a light meter. Each separate target consists of a series of dark parallel lines in one of three different orientations. They are displayed against a lighter, contrasting gray background. As the contrast between the lines and their background is progressively reduced from one target to the next, it becomes more difficult for the patient to judge the orientation of the lines. The patient can be scored according to the lowest level of contrast at which the pattern of lines can still be discerned.

6. ASSESSING POTENTIAL VISION

When opacities of the cornea or lens coexist with disease of the macula or optic nerve, the visual potential of the eye is often in doubt. The benefit of corneal transplantation or cataract extraction will depend on the severity of coexisting retinal or optic nerve impairment. Several methods are available for assessing central visual potential under these circumstances.

Even with a totally opaque cataract that completely prevents a view of the fundus, the patient should still be able to identify the direction of a light directed into the eye from different quadrants. When a red lens is held in front of the light, the patient should be able to differentiate between white and red light. The presence

of a Marcus Gunn afferent pupillary defect indicates significant disease of the retina or optic nerve and thus a poor visual prognosis.

A gross test of macular function involves the patient's ability to perceive so-called **entoptic phenomena.** For example, as the eyeball is massaged with a rapidly moving penlight through the closed lids, the patient should be able to visualize an image of the paramacular vascular branches if the macula is healthy. These may be described as looking like "the veins of a leaf." Because this test is highly subjective and subject to interpretation, it is only helpful if the patient is able to recognize the vascular pattern in at least one eye. Absence of the pattern in the opposite eye then suggests macular impairment.

In addition to these gross methods, sophisticated quantitative instruments have been developed for more direct determination of visual potential in eyes with media opacities. These instruments project a narrow beam of light containing a pattern of images through any relatively clear portion of the media (eg, through a less dense region of a cataract) and onto the retina. The patient's vision is then graded according to the size of the smallest patterns that can be seen.

Two different types of patterns are used. **Laser interferometry** employs laser light to generate interference fringes or gratings, which the patient sees as a series of parallel lines. Progressively narrowing the width and spacing of the lines causes an end point to be reached where the patient can no longer discern the orientation of the lines. The narrowest image width the patient can resolve is then correlated with a Snellen acuity measurement to determine the visual potential of that eye. The **potential acuity meter** projects a stan-

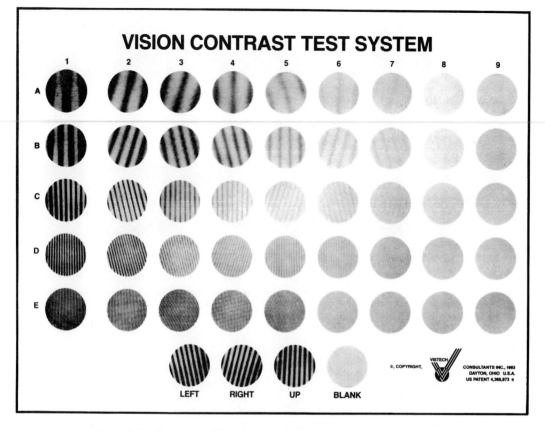

Figure 2–25. Contrast sensitivity test chart. (Courtesy of Vistech Consultants, Inc.)

dard Snellen acuity chart onto the retina. The patient is then graded in the usual fashion, according to the smallest line of letters read.

Although both instruments appear useful in measuring potential visual acuity, false-positive and false-negative results do occur, with a frequency dependent on the type of disease present. Thus, these methods are helpful but not completely reliable in determining the visual prognosis of eyes with cloudy media.

7. TESTS FOR FUNCTIONAL VISUAL LOSS

The measurement of vision is subjective, requiring responses on the part of the patient. The validity of the test may therefore be limited by the alertness or cooperation of the patient. "Functional" visual loss is a subjective complaint of impaired vision without any demonstrated organic or objective basis. Examples include hysterical blindness and malingering.

Recognition of functional visual loss or malingering depends on the use of testing variations in order to elicit inconsistent or contradictory responses. An example would be eliciting "tunnel" visual fields using the tangent screen.

A patient claiming "poor vision" and tested at the standard distance of 1 meter may map out a narrow central zone of intact vision beyond which even large objects—such as a hand—allegedly cannot be seen. The borders ("isopter") of this apparently small area are then marked.

The patient is then moved back to a position 2 meters from the tangent screen. From this position, the field should be twice as large as the area plotted from 1 meter away. If the patient outlines an area of the same size from both testing distances, he will have produced a response that is not physically possible. This would raise a strong suspicion of malingering.

A variety of other different tests can be chosen to assess the validity of different degrees of visual loss that may be in question.

DIAGNOSIS OF OCULAR ABNORMALITIES

1. MICROBIOLOGY & CYTOLOGY

Like any mucous membrane, the conjunctiva can be cultured with swabs for the identification of bacterial infection. Specimens for cytologic examination are obtained by lightly scraping the palpebral conjunctiva (ie, lining the inner aspect of the lid) with a small platinum spatula following topical anesthesia. For the cytologic evaluation of conjunctivitis, Giemsa's stain is used to identify the types of inflammatory cells present, while Gram's stain may demonstrate the presence (and type) of bacteria. These applications are discussed at length in Chapter 5.

The cornea is normally sterile. The base of any suspected infectious corneal ulcer should be scraped with the platinum spatula for Gram staining and culture. This procedure is performed at the slitlamp following topical anesthesia. Because in many cases only trace quantities of bacteria are recoverable, the spatula should be used to plate the specimen directly onto the culture plate without the intervening use of transport media. Any amount of culture growth, no matter how scant, is considered significant, but many cases of infection may still be "culture-negative."

Culture of intraocular fluids is the only reliable method of diagnosing or ruling out infectious endophthalmitis. Aqueous can be tapped by inserting a short 25-gauge needle on a tuberculin syringe through the limbus parallel to the iris. Care must be taken not to traumatize the lens. The diagnostic yield is better if vitreous is cultured. Vitreous specimens can be obtained by a needle tap through the pars plana or by doing a surgical vitrectomy. In the evaluation of noninfectious intraocular inflammation, cytology specimens are occasionally obtained using similar techniques.

2. TECHNIQUES FOR CORNEAL EXAMINATION

Several additional techniques are available for more specialized evaluation of the cornea. The **keratometer** is a calibrated instrument that measures the radius of curvature of the cornea in two meridians 90 degrees apart. If the cornea is not perfectly spherical, the two radii will be different. This is called **astigmatism** and is quantified by measuring the difference between the two radii of curvature. Keratometer measurements are used in contact lens fitting and for intraocular lens power calculations prior to cataract surgery.

Many corneal diseases result in distortion of the otherwise smooth surface of the cornea, which impairs its optical quality. The **photokeratoscope** is an instrument that assesses the uniformity and evenness of the surface by reflecting a pattern of concentric circles onto it. This pattern, which can be visualized and photographed through the instrument, should normally appear perfectly regular and uniform. Focal corneal irregularities will instead distort the circular patterns reflected from that particular area.

Computerized corneal topography is the most advanced technique of mapping the anterior corneal surface. Whereas keratometry provides only a single corneal curvature measurement and photokeratoscopy provide only qualitative information, these computer systems combine and improve on the features of both. A real time video camera records the concentric keratoscopic rings reflected from the cornea. A personal computer digitizes these data from thousands of locations across the corneal surface and displays these measurements in a color-coded map (Figure 2–26). This enables one to quantify and analyze minute changes in shape and refractive power across the entire cornea induced by disease or surgery.

The endothelium is an irreplaceable monolayer of cells lining the posterior corneal surface. These cells function as fluid pumps and are responsible for keeping the cornea thin and dehydrated, thereby maintaining its optical clarity. If these cells become impaired or depleted, corneal edema and thickening result, ultimately decreasing vision. Central corneal thickness can be accurately measured with a **pachymeter,** a device for quantifying and monitoring these changes. The endothelial cells themselves can be photographed with a special slitlamp camera, enabling one to study cell morphology and perform cell counts.

3. GONIOSCOPY

The anterior chamber—the space between the iris and the cornea—is filled with liquid aqueous humor. The aqueous, which is produced behind the iris by the ciliary body, exits the eye through a tiny sieve-like drainage network called the trabecular meshwork. The meshwork is arranged as a thin circumferential band of tissue just anterior to the base of the iris and within the angle formed by the iridocorneal junction (Figure 11–3). This angle recess can vary in its anatomy, pigmentation, and width of opening—all of which may affect aqueous drainage and be of diagnostic relevance for glaucoma.

Gonioscopy is the method of examination of the anterior chamber angle anatomy using binocular magnification and a special **goniolens.** The Goldmann and Posner/Zeiss types of goniolenses (Figure 2–8) have special mirrors angled so as to provide a line of view parallel with the iris surface and directed peripherally toward the angle recess.

After topical anesthesia, the patient is seated at the slitlamp and the goniolens is placed on the eye (Figure 2–27). Magnified details of the anterior chamber angle are viewed stereoscopically. By rotating the mirror, the entire 360-degree circumference of the angle can be examined. The same lens can be used to direct laser treatment toward the angle as therapy for glaucoma.

A third type of goniolens, the Koeppe lens, requires a special illuminator and a separate handheld binocular microscope. It is used with the patient lying supine and can thus be used either in the office or in the operating room (either diagnostically or for surgery).

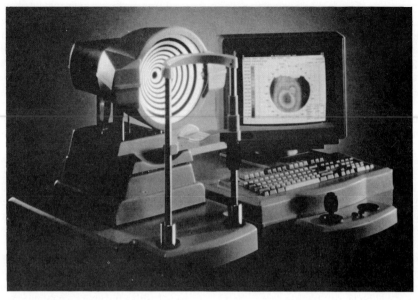

A

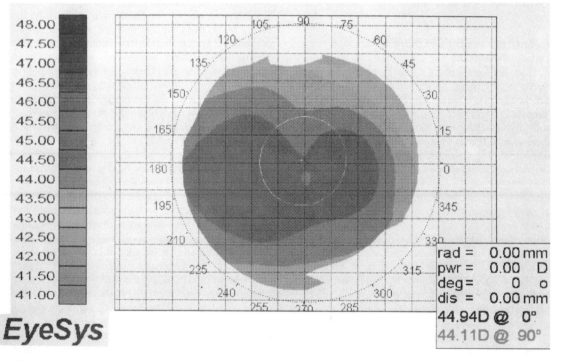

EyeSys

rad =	0.00 mm
pwr =	0.00 D
deg =	0 o
dis =	0.00 mm

44.94D @ 0°
44.11D @ 90°

B

Figure 2–26. *A:* Computerized corneal topography system utilizing video keratoscope and personal computer. *B:* Color-coded topographic display of curvature and refractive power (in diopters) across the entire corneal surface. (Photos courtesy of EyeSys Technologies, Inc.)

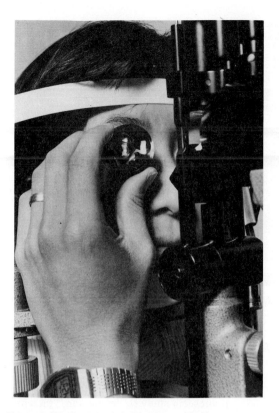

Figure 2–27. Gonioscopy with slitlamp and Goldmann type lens. (Photo by M Narahara.)

4. GOLDMANN THREE-MIRROR LENS

The Goldmann lens is a versatile adjunct to the slit-lamp examination (Figure 2–8). Three separate mirrors, all with different angles of orientation, allow the examiner's line of sight to be directed peripherally at three different angles while using the standard slit-lamp. The most anterior and acute angle of view is achieved with the goniolens, discussed above.

Through a dilated pupil, the other two mirrored lenses angle the examiner's view toward the retinal mid periphery and far periphery, respectively. As with gonioscopy, each lens can be rotated 360 degrees circumferentially and can be used to aim laser treatment. A fourth central lens (no mirror) is used to examine the posterior vitreous and the centralmost area of the retina. The stereoscopic magnification of this method provides the greatest three-dimensional detail of the macula and disk.

The patient's side of the lens has a concavity designed to fit directly over the topically anesthetized cornea. A clear, viscous solution of methylcellulose is placed in the concavity of the lens prior to insertion onto the patient's eye. This eliminates interference from optical interfaces, such as bubbles, and provides mild adhesion of the lens to the eye for stabilization.

5. FUNDUS PHOTOGRAPHY

Special retinal cameras are used to document details of the fundus for study and future comparison. Standard film is used for 35 mm color slides which can be easily stored. As with any form of ophthalmoscopy, a dilated pupil and clear ocular media provide the most optimal view. All of the fundus photographs in this textbook were taken with such a camera.

One of the most common applications is disk photography, used in the evaluation for glaucoma. Since the slow progression of glaucomatous optic nerve damage may be evident only by subtle alteration of the disk's appearance over time (see Chapter 11), precise documentation of its morphology is needed. By slightly shifting the camera angle on two consecutive shots, a "stereo" pair of slides can be produced which will provide a three-dimensional image when studied through a stereoscopic slide viewer. Stereo disk photography thus provides the most sensitive means of detecting increases in glaucomatous cupping.

6. FLUORESCEIN ANGIOGRAPHY

The capabilities of fundus photographic imaging can be tremendously enhanced by fluorescein, a dye whose molecules emit green light when stimulated by blue light. When photographed, the dye highlights vascular and anatomic details of the fundus. Fluorescein angiography has become indispensable in the diagnosis and evaluation of many retinal conditions. Because it can so precisely delineate areas of abnormality, it is an essential guide for planning laser treatment of retinal vascular disease.

Technique

The patient is seated in front of the retinal camera following pupillary dilation (Figure 2–28). After a small amount of fluorescein is injected into a vein in the arm, it circulates throughout the body before eventually being excreted by the kidneys. As the dye passes through the retinal and choroidal circulation, it can be visualized and photographed because of its properties of fluorescence. Two special filters within the camera produce this effect. A blue **"excitatory"** filter bombards the fluorescein molecules with blue light from the camera flash, causing them to emit a green light. The **"barrier"** filter allows only this emitted green light to reach the photographic film, blocking out all other wavelengths of light. A black and white photograph results in which only the fluorescein image is seen.

Because the fluorescein molecules do not diffuse out of normal retinal vessels, the latter are highlighted photographically by the dye, as seen in Figure 2–29. The diffuse, background "ground glass" appearance results from fluorescein filling of the separate underlying

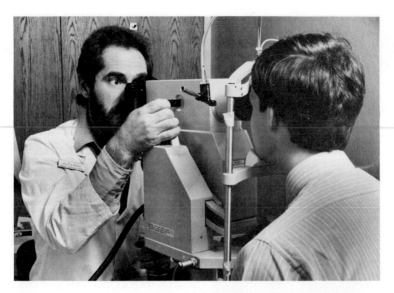

Figure 2–28. Fluorescein angiography with fundus camera. (Photo by M Narahara.)

choroidal circulation. The choroidal and retinal circulations are anatomically separated by a thin, homogeneous monolayer of pigmented cells—the "retinal pigment epithelium." Denser pigmentation located in the macula obscures more of this background choroidal fluorescence (Figure 2–29) causing the darker central zone on the photograph. In contrast, focal atrophy of the pigment epithelium causes an abnormal increase in visibility of the background fluorescence (Figure 2–30).

Applications

A high-speed motorized film advance allows for rapid sequence photography of the dye's transit through the retinal and choroidal circulations over time. A fluorescein study or "angiogram" therefore consists of multiple black and white photos of the fundi taken at different times following dye injection (Figure 2–31). Early phase photos document the dye's initial rapid, sequential perfusion of the choroid, the retinal arteries, and the retinal veins. Later phase photos may, for example, demonstrate

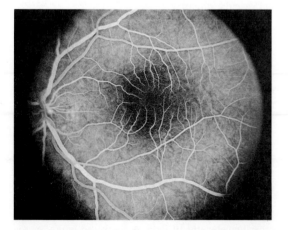

Figure 2–29. Normal angiogram of the central retina. The photo has been taken after the dye (appearing white) has already sequentially filled the choroidal circulation (seen as a diffuse, mottled whitish background), the arterioles and the veins. The macula appears dark due to heavier pigmentation which obscures the underlying choroidal fluorescence that is visible everywhere else. (Photo courtesy of R Griffith and T King.)

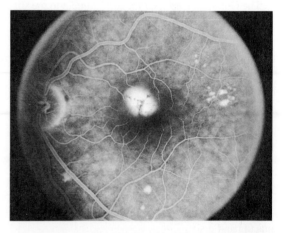

Figure 2–30. Abnormal angiogram in which dye-stained fluid originating from the choroid has pooled beneath the macula. This is one type of abnormality associated with age-related macular degeneration (see Chapter 10). Secondary atrophy of the overlying retinal pigment epithelium in this area causes heightened, unobscured visibility of this increased fluorescence. (Photo courtesy of R Griffith and T King.)

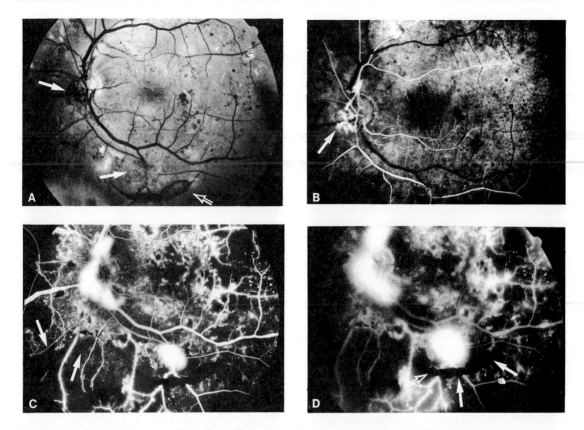

Figure 2–31. Fluorescein angiographic study of an eye with proliferative diabetic retinopathy demonstrating variations in the dye pattern over several minutes' time. **A:** Fundus photograph of left eye (before fluorescein) showing neovascularization (abnormal new vessels) on the disk and inferior to the macula (arrows). This latter area has bled, producing the arcuate preretinal hemorrhage at the bottom of the photo (open arrow). **B:** Early phase angiogram of the same eye, in which fluorescein has initially filled the arterioles and highlighted the area of the disk neovascularization. **C:** Midphase angiogram of the same eye in which dye has begun to leak out of the hyperpermeable areas of neovascularization. In addition to the irregular venous caliber and the microaneurysms (white dots), extensive areas of ischemia are apparent by virtue of the gross absence of vessels (and therefore dye) in many areas (see arrows). **D:** Late-phase photo demonstrating increasing amounts of dye leakage over time. Although the preretinal hemorrhage does not stain with dye, it is detectable as a solid black area since it obscures all underlying fluorescence (arrows). (Photos courtesy of University of California, San Francisco.)

the gradual, delayed leakage of dye from abnormal vessels. This extravascular dye-stained edema fluid will persist long after the intravascular fluorescein has exited the eye.

Figure 2–31 illustrates several of the retinal vascular abnormalities that are well demonstrated by fluorescein angiography. The dye delineates structural vascular alterations, such as aneurysms or neovascularization. Changes in blood flow such as ischemia and vascular occlusion are seen as an interruption of the normal perfusion pattern. Abnormal vascular permeability is seen as a leaking cloud of dye-stained edema fluid increasing over time. Hemorrhage does not stain with dye but rather appears as a dark, sharply demarcated void. This is due to blockage and obscuration of the underlying background fluorescence.

7. ELECTROPHYSIOLOGIC TESTING

Physiologically, "vision" results from a series of electrical signals initiated in the retina and ending in the occipital cortex. Electroretinography, electro-oculography, and visual evoked response testing are methods of evaluating the integrity to the neural circuitry.

Electroretinography (ERG) & Electro-oculography (EOG)

Electroretinography measures the electrical response of the retina to flashes of light, the **flash electroretinogram (ERG),** or to a reversing checkerboard stimulus, the **pattern ERG (PERG).** The recording electrode is placed on the surface of the eye and a reference electrode on the skin of the face. The amplitude of the electrical signal is less than 1 mV, and amplification of the signal and computer averaging of the response to repeated trials are thus necessary to achieve reliable results.

The flash ERG has two major components: the "a wave" and the "b wave". An early receptor potential (ERP) preceding the "a wave" and oscillatory potentials superimposd on the "b wave" may be recorded under certain circumstances. The early part of the flash ERG reflects photoreceptor function, whereas the later response particularly reflects the function of the Müller cells, which are glial cells within the retina. Varying the intensity, wavelength, and frequency of the light stimulus and recording under conditions of light or dark adaptation modulates the waveform of the flash ERG and allows examination of rod and cone photoreceptor function. The flash ERG is a diffuse response from the whole retina and is thus sensitive only to widespread, generalized diseases of the retina—eg, inherited retinal degenerations (retinitis pigmentosa), in which flash ERG abnormalities precede visual loss; congenital retinal dystrophies, in which flash ERG abnormalities may precede ophthalmoscopic abnormalities; and toxic retinopathies from drugs or chemicals (eg, iron intraocular foreign bodies). It is not sensitive to focal retinal disease even when the macula is affected, and is not sensitive to abnormalities of the retinal ganglion cell layer such as in optic nerve disease.

The PERG also has two major components: a positive wave at about 50 msec (P50) and a negative wave at about 95 msec (N95) from the time of the pattern reversal. The P50 seems to reflect macular retinal function, whereas the N95 appears to reflect ganglion cell function. Thus, the PERG is useful in distinguishing retinal and optic nerve dysfunction and in diagnosing macular disease.

Electro-oculography (EOG) measures the standing corneoretinal potential. Electrodes are placed at the medial and lateral canthi to record the changes in electrical potential while the patient performs horizontal eye movements. The amplitude of the corneoretinal potential is least in the dark and maximal in the light. The ratio of the maximum potential in the light to the minimum in the dark is known as the **Arden index.** Abnormalities of the EOG principally occur in diseases diffusely affecting the retinal pigment epithelium and the photoreceptors and often parallel abnormalities of the flash ERG. Certain diseases such as Best's vitelliform dystrophy produce a normal ERG but a characteristically abnormal EOG. EOG is also used to record eye movements.

Visual Evoked Response (VER)

Like electroretinography, the visual evoked response measures the electrical potential resulting from a visual stimulus. However, because it is measured by scalp electrodes placed over the occipital cortex, the entire visual pathway from retina to cortex must be in-

tact in order to produce a normal electrical waveform reading. Like the ERG wave, the VER pattern is plotted on a scale displaying both amplitude and latency (Figure 2–32).

Interruption of neuronal conduction by a lesion will result in reduced amplitude of the VER. Reduced speed of conduction, such as with demyelination, abnormally prolongs the latency of the VER. Unilateral prechiasmatic (retinal or optic nerve) disease can be diagnosed by stimulating each eye separately and comparing the responses. Postchiasmatic disease (eg, homonymous hemianopia) can be identified by comparing the electrode responses measured separately over each hemisphere.

Proportionately, the majority of the occipital lobe area is devoted to the macula. This large cortical area representing the macula is also in close proximity to the scalp electrode, so that the clinically measured VER is primarily a response generated by the macula and optic nerve. An abnormal VER would thus indi-

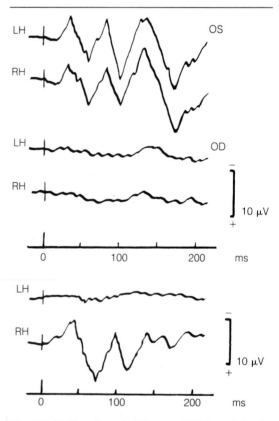

Figure 2–32. ***Top:*** Normal VER generated by stimulating the left eye ("OS") is contrasted with the absent response form the right eye ("OD"), which has a severe optic nerve lesion. "LH" and "RH" signify recordings from electrodes over the left and right hemispheres of the occipital lobe. ***Bottom:*** VER with right homonymous hemianopia. No response is recorded from over the left hemisphere. (Courtesy of M Feinsod.)

cate poor central visual acuity, making it a valuable objective test in situations where subjective testing is unreliable. Such patients might include infants, unresponsive individuals, and suspected malingerers.

8. DARK ADAPTATION

In going from conditions of bright light to darkness, a certain period of time must pass before the retina regains its maximal sensitivity to low amounts of light. This phenomenon is called dark adaptation. It can be quantified by measuring the recovery of retinal sensitivity to low light levels over time following a standard period of bright light exposure. Dark adaptation is often abnormal in retinal diseases characterized by rod photoreceptor dysfunction and impaired night vision.

DIAGNOSIS OF EXTRAOCULAR ABNORMALITIES

1. LACRIMAL SYSTEM EVALUATION

Evaluation of Tear Production

Tears and their components are produced by the lacrimal gland and accessory glands in the lid and conjunctiva (see Chapter 4). The **Schirmer test** is a simple method for assessing gross tear production. Schirmer strips are disposable dry strips of filter paper in standard 5 × 35 mm sizes. The tip of one end is folded at the preexisting notch so that it can drape over the lower lid margin just lateral to the cornea.

Tears in the conjunctival sac will cause progressive wetting of the paper strip. The distance between the leading edge of wetness and the initial fold can be measured after 5 minutes, using a millimeter ruler. The ranges of normal measurements vary depending on whether or not topical anesthetic is used. Without anesthesia, irritation from the Schirmer strip itself will cause reflex tearing, thereby increasing the measurement. With anesthesia, less than 5 mm of wetting after 5 minutes is considered abnormal.

Significant degrees of chronic dryness cause surface changes in the exposed areas of the cornea and conjunctiva. **Fluorescein** will stain punctate areas of epithelial loss on the cornea. Another dye, **rose bengal,** is able to stain devitalized cells of the conjunctiva and cornea before they actually degenerate and drop off.

Evaluation of Lacrimal Drainage

The anatomy of the lacrimal drainage system is discussed in Chapters 1 and 4. The pumping action of the lids draws tears nasally into the upper and lower canalicular channels through the medially located "punctal" openings in each lid margin. After collecting in the lacrimal sac, the tears then drain into the nasopharynx via the nasolacrimal duct. Symptoms of watering are frequently due to increased tear production as a reflex response to some type of ocular irritation. However, the patency and function of the lacrimal drainage system must be checked in the evaluation of otherwise unexplained tearing.

The **Jones I** test evaluates whether the entire drainage system as a whole is functioning. Concentrated fluorescein dye is instilled into the conjunctival sac on the side of the suspected obstruction. After 5 minutes, a cotton Calgiswab is used to attempt to recover dye from beneath the inferior nasal turbinate. Alternatively, the patient blows his nose into a tissue which is checked for the presence of dye. Recovery of any dye indicates that the drainage system is functioning.

The **Jones II** test is performed if no dye is recovered, indicating some abnormality of the system. Following topical anesthesia, a smooth-tipped metal probe is used to gently dilate one of the puncta (usually lower). A 3-mL syringe with sterile water or saline is prepared and attached to a special lacrimal irrigating cannula. This blunt-tipped cannula is used to gently intubate the lower canaliculus, and fluid is injected as the patient leans forward. With a patent drainage system, fluid should easily flow into the patient's nasopharynx without resistance.

If fluorescein can now be recovered from the nose following irrigation, a partial obstruction might have been present. Recovery of clear fluid without fluorescein, however, may indicate inability of the lids to initially pump dye into the lacrimal sac with an otherwise patent drainage apparatus. If no fluid can be irrigated through to the nasopharynx using the syringe, total occlusion is present. Finally, some drainage problems may be due to stenosis of the punctal lid opening, in which case the preparatory dilation may be therapeutic.

2. METHODS OF ORBITAL EVALUATION

Exophthalmometry

A method is needed to measure the anteroposterior location of the globe with respect to the bony orbital rim. The lateral orbital rim is a discrete, easily palpable landmark and is used as the reference point.

The exophthalmometer (Figure 2–33) is a hand-held instrument with two identical measuring devices (one for each eye), connected by a horizontal bar. The distance between the two devices can be varied by sliding one toward or away from the other, and each has a notch that fits over the edge of the corresponding lateral orbital rim. When properly aligned, an attached set of mirrors reflects a side image of each eye profiled alongside a measuring scale, calibrated in millimeters. The tip of the corneal image aligns with a scale reading representing its distance from the orbital rim.

The patient is seated facing the examiner. The distance between the two measuring devices is adjusted

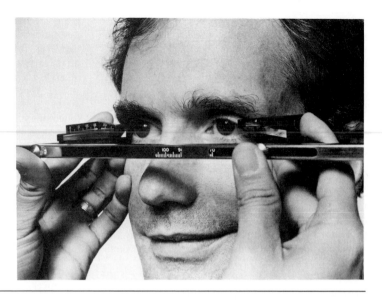

Figure 2–33. Hertel exophthalmometer. (Photo by M Narahara.)

so that each aligns with and abuts against its corresponding orbital rim. To allow reproducibility for repeat measurements in the future, the distance between the two devices is recorded from an additional scale on the horizontal bar. Using the first mirror scale, the patient's right eye position is measured as it fixates on the examiner's left eye. The patient's left eye is measured while fixating on the examiner's right eye.

The distance from the cornea to the orbital rim typically ranges from 12 to 20 mm, and the two eye measurements are normally within 2 mm of each other. A greater distance is seen in exophthalmos, which can be unilateral or bilateral. This abnormal forward protrusion of the eye can be produced by any significant increase in orbital mass, because of the fixed size of the bony orbital cavity. Causes might include orbital hemorrhage, neoplasm, inflammation, or edema.

Ultrasonography

Ultrasonography utilizes the principle of sonar to study structures that may not be directly visible. It can be used to evaluate either the globe or the orbit. High-frequency sound waves are emitted from a special transmitter toward the target tissue. As the sound waves bounce back off the various tissue components, they are collected by a receiver that amplifies and displays them on an oscilloscope screen.

A single probe that contains both the transmitter and receiver is placed against the eye and used to aim the beam of sound (Figure 2–34). Various structures in its path will reflect separate echoes (which arrive at different times) back toward the probe. Those derived from the most distal structures arrive last, having traveled the farthest.

There are two methods of clinical ultrasonography:

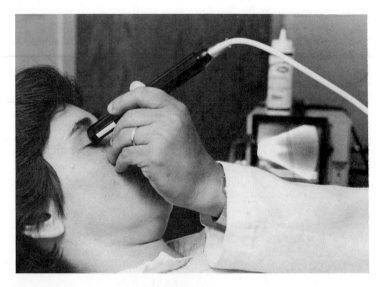

Figure 2–34. Ultrasonography using B-scan probe. The image will appear on the oscilloscope screen, visible in the background. (Photo by M Narahara.)

A scan and B scan. In **A scan ultrasonography,** the sound beam is aimed in a straight line. Each returning echo is displayed as a spike whose amplitude is dependent on the density of the reflecting tissue. The spikes are arranged in temporal sequence, with the latency of each signal's arrival correlating with that structure's distance from the probe (Figure 2–35). If the same probe is now swept across the eye, a continuous series of individual A scans is obtained. From spatial summation of these multiple linear scans, a two-dimensional image, or **B scan,** can be constructed.

Both A and B scans can be used to image and differentiate orbital disease or intraocular anatomy concealed by opaque media. In addition to defining the size and location of intraocular and orbital masses, A and B scans can provide clues to the tissue characteristics of a lesion (eg, solid, cystic, vascular, calcified).

For purposes of measurement, the A scan is the most accurate method. Sound echoes reflected from two separate locations will reach the probe at different times. This temporal separation can be used to calculate the distance between the points, based on the speed of sound in the tissue medium. The most commonly used ocular measurement is the axial length (cornea to retina). This is important in cataract surgery in order to calculate the power for an intraocular lens implant. A scans can also be used to quantify tumor size and monitor growth over time.

The application of pulsed ultrasound and spectral Doppler techniques to orbital ultrasonography provides information on the orbital vasculature. It is certainly possible to determine the direction of flow in the ophthalmic artery and the ophthalmic veins, reversal of flow in these vessels occurring in internal carotid artery occlusion and carotid-cavernous fistula, respectively. As yet, the value of measuring flow velocities in various vessels, including the posterior ciliary arteries, without being able to measure blood vessel diameter is not fully established.

3. OPHTHALMIC RADIOLOGY (X-Ray, CT Scan)

Plain x-rays and CT scans (Figures 13–1 and 13–2) are useful in the evaluation of **orbital** and **intracranial** conditions. CT scan in particular has become the most widely used method for localizing and characterizing structural disease in the extraocular visual pathway. Common orbital abnormalities demonstrated by CT scan include neoplasms, inflammatory masses, fractures, and extraocular muscle enlargement associated with Graves' disease.

The **intraocular** applications of radiology are primarily in the detection of foreign bodies following trauma and the demonstration of intraocular calcium in tumors such as retinoblastoma. CT scan is useful for foreign body localization because of its multidimensional reformatting capabilities and its ability to image the ocular walls.

4. MAGNETIC RESONANCE IMAGING

The technique of magnetic resonance imaging (MRI) has many applications in orbital and intracranial diagnosis. Improvements such as surface receiver coils and thin section techniques have improved the anatomic resolution in the eye and orbit.

Unlike CT, the MRI technique does not expose the patient to ionizing radiation. Multidimensional views

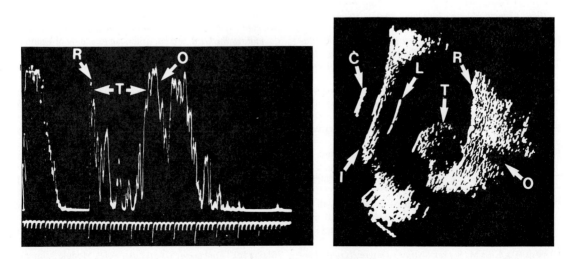

Figure 2–35. A scan *(left)* and B scan *(right)* of an intraocular tumor (melanoma). C = cornea; I = iris; L = posterior lens surface; O = optic nerve; R = retina; T = tumor. (Courtesy of RD Stone.)

(axial, coronal, and sagittal) are possible without having to reposition the patient. Since MRI might cause movement of metal, it should not be used if a metallic foreign body is suspected.

Because it can better differentiate between tissues of different water content, MRI is superior to CT in its ability to image edema, areas of demyelination, and vascular lesions. Bone generates a weak MRI signal, allowing improved resolution of intraosseous disease and a clearer view of the intracranial posterior fossa. Examples of MRI scans are presented in Chapters 13 and 14.

5. OPHTHALMODYNAMOMETRY

Ophthalmodynamometry gives an approximate measurement of the relative pressures in the central retinal arteries and is an indirect means of assessing carotid artery flow on either side. The test consists of exerting pressure on the sclera with a spring plunger while observing with an ophthalmoscope the vessels emerging from the optic disk. Ophthalmodynamometry is useful in the neurologic evaluation of patients who complain of "blacking out" (amaurosis fugax) in one eye, spells of weakness on one side of the body, or other symptoms of transient cerebral ischemia. A difference of more than 20% in the diastolic pressures between the two eyes suggests insufficiency of the carotid arterial system on the side with the lower reading.

The test is often performed in conjunction with angiography and ultrasonography of the carotid arteries.

REFERENCES

Anderson DR: *Automated Static Perimetry.* Mosby, 1992.

Berkow JW et al: *Fluorescein Angiography: Technique and Interpretation.* American Academy of Ophthalmology, 1991.

Boothe WA et al: The Tono-Pen: A manometric and clinical study. Arch Ophthalmol 1988;106:1214.

Carr RE, Siegel IM: *Visual Electrodiagnostic Testing: A Practical Guide for the Clinician,* 2nd ed. Williams & Wilkins, 1990.

Drake M: *A Primer on Automated Perimetry.* Vol 11, No. 8, in: *Focal Points 1993: Clinical Modules for Ophthalmologists.* American Academy of Ophthalmology, 1993.

Ehrlich MI et al: Preschool vision screening for amblyopia and strabismus: Programs, methods, guidelines, 1983. Surv Ophthalmol 1983;28:145.

Faulkner W: *Macular Function Testing Through Opacities.* Vol 4, Module 2, in: *Focal Points 1986: Clinical Modules for Ophthalmologists.* American Academy of Ophthalmology, 1986.

Fellman RL et al: *Gonioscopy: Key to Successful Management of Glaucoma.* Vol 2, Module 7, in: *Focal Points 1984: Clinical Modules for Ophthalmologists.* American Academy of Ophthalmology, 1984.

Fishman GA, Marmor MF: *Clinical Retinal Function Testing.* Vol 9, Module 2, in: *Focal Points 1984: Clinical Modules for Ophthalmologists.* American Academy of Ophthalmology, 1991.

Flaharty PM et al: Color Doppler imaging: A new noninvasive technique to diagnose and monitor carotid cavernous sinus fistulas. Arch Ophthalmol 1991;109:522.

Harrington DO, Drake MV: *The Visual Fields: A Textbook and Atlas of Clinical Perimetry,* 6th ed. Mosby, 1989.

Hirst LW: Clinical evaluation of the corneal endothelium. Vol 4, Module 8, in: *Focal Points 1986: Clinical Modules for Ophthalmologists.* American Academy of Ophthalmology, 1986.

Holder GE: Pattern electroretinography in patients with delayed pattern visual evoked potentials due to distal anterior visual pathway dysfunction. J Neurol Neurosurg Psychiatry 1989;52:1364.

Hoskins HD, Kass M: *Becker-Shaffer's Diagnosis and Therapy of the Glaucomas,* 6th ed. Mosby, 1989.

Hoyt CS, Paks MM: *How to Examine the Eye of the Neonate.* Vol 7, Module 1, in: *Focal Points 1989: Clinical Modules for Ophthalmologists.* American Academy of Ophthalmology, 1989.

Hoyt CS et al: Ophthalmological examination of the infant. Surv Ophthalmol 1982;26:177.

Kline LB: *Computed Tomography in Ophthalmology.* Vol 3, Module 9, in: *Focal Points 1985: Clinical Modules for Ophthalmologists.* American Academy of Ophthalmology, 1985.

Koch DD: *The Role of Glare Testing in Managing the Cataract Patient.* Vol 6, Module 4, in: *Focal Points 1988: Clinical Modules for Ophthalmologists.* American Academy of Ophthalmology, 1988.

Lieberman MF, Drake M: *Computerized Perimetry: A Simplified Guide,* 2nd ed. Slack, 1992.

Mannis MJ: Making sense of contrast sensitivity testing. Arch Ophthalmol 1987;105:627.

Masters BR: *Noninvasive Diagnostic Techniques in Ophthalmology.* Springer, 1990.

Miller BW: A review of practical tests for ocular malingering and hysteria. Surv Ophthalmol 1973;17:241.

Richard JM (editor): *A Manual for the Beginning Ophthalmology Resident,* 3rd ed. American Academy of Ophthalmology, 1980.

Riordan-Eva P et al: Orbital ultrasound in the ocular ischaemic syndrome. Eye 1994;8:93.

Rosenthal ML, Fradin S: The technique of binocular indirect ophthalmoscopy. Highlights Ophthalmol 1966;9:179. (Reprinted as Appendix in: Hilton GF et al: *Retinal Detachment,* 5th ed. American Academy of Ophthalmology, 1989.)

Sanders DR, Koch DD: *An Atlas of Corneal Topography.* Slack, 1993.

Schwartz B: *Optic Disc Evaluation in Glaucoma.* Vol 8, Module 12, in: *Focal Points 1990: Clinical Modules for Ophthalmologists.* American Academy of Ophthalmology, 1990.

Shaffer RN et al: The use of diagrams to record changes in glaucomatous discs. Am J Ophthalmol 1975;80:460.

Slavin ML: *Functional Visual Loss.* Vol 9, Module 2, in: *Focal Points 1991: Clinical Modules for Ophthalmologists.* American Academy of Ophthalmology, 1991.

Stein HA et al: *The Ophthalmic Assistant: Fundamentals and Clinical Practice,* 5th ed. Mosby, 1988.

Thompson HS, Kardon RH: *Clinical Importance of Pupillary Inequality.* Vol 10, No. 10, in: *Focal Points 1992: Clinical Modules for Ophthalmologists.* American Academy of Ophthalmology, 1992.

Thompson HS et al: How to measure the relative afferent pupillary defect. Surv Ophthalmol 1981;26:39.

Tomsak RL: *Magnetic Resonance Imaging in Neuro-ophthalmology.* Vol 4, Module 10, in: *Focal Points 1986: Clinical Modules for Ophthalmologists.* American Academy of Ophthalmology, 1986.

von Noorden GK: *Burian-von Noorden's Binocular Vision and Ocular Motility,* 4th ed. Mosby, 1990.

Wirtschafter JD, Taylor S: *Computed Tomography: An Atlas for Ophthalmologists.* American Academy of Ophthalmology, 1982.

Wirtschafter JD et al: *Magnetic Resonance Imaging and Computed Tomography: Clinical Neuro-orbital Anatomy.* American Academy of Ophthalmology, 1992.

3

Commonly Used Eye Medications

Philip P. Ellis, MD

The following is intended to serve as a concise formulary of commonly used ophthalmic drugs. Standard pharmacology and physiology texts should be consulted for more detailed information.

TOPICAL ANESTHETICS

Topical anesthetics are useful for several diagnostic and therapeutic procedures, including tonometry, removal of foreign bodies or sutures, gonioscopy, conjunctival scraping, and minor surgical operations on the cornea and conjunctiva. One or two instillations are usually sufficient, but the dosage may be repeated during the procedure.

Proparacaine, tetracaine, and benoxinate are the most commonly used topical anesthetics. For practical purposes, they can be said to have equivalent anesthetic potency.

Cocaine 1–4% solution is also used for topical anesthesia.

Note: *Topical anesthetics should never be prescribed for home use,* since prolonged application may cause corneal complications and mask serious ocular disease.

Proparacaine Hydrochloride (Ophthaine, others)

Preparation: Solution, 0.5%. A combined preparation of proparacaine and fluorescein is available as Fluoracaine.
Dosage: 1 drop and repeat as necessary.
Onset and duration of action: Anesthesia begins within 20 seconds and lasts 10–15 minutes.
Comment: Least irritating of the topical anesthetics.

Tetracaine Hydrochloride (Pontocaine)

Preparations: Solution, 0.5%, and ointment, 0.5%.
Dosage: 1 drop and repeat as necessary.
Onset and duration of action: Anesthesia occurs within 1 minute and lasts for 15–20 minutes.
Comment: Stings considerably on instillation.

Benoxinate Hydrochloride

Preparation (as Fluress): Solution, 0.4%.

Dosage: 1 drop and repeat as necessary.
Onset and duration of action: Anesthesia begins within 1 or 2 minutes and lasts for 10–15 minutes.
Comment: Benoxinate 0.4% and fluorescein 0.25% (Fluress) may be used prior to applanation tonometry.

LOCAL ANESTHETICS FOR INJECTION

Lidocaine, procaine, and mepivacaine are commonly used local anesthetics for eye surgery. Longer-acting agents such as bupivacaine and etidocaine are often mixed with other local anesthetics to prolong the duration of effect. Local anesthetics are extremely safe when used with discretion, but the physician must be aware of the potential systemic toxic action when rapid absorption occurs from the site of the injection, with excessive dosage, or following inadvertent intravascular injection.

The addition of hyaluronidase encourages spreading of the anesthetic and shortens the onset to as little as 1 minute. For these reasons, hyaluronidase is commonly used in retrobulbar injections prior to cataract extraction. Up to 4–5 mL may be injected behind the globe with relative safety. Injectable anesthetics are used by ophthalmologists most commonly in older patients, who may be susceptible to cardiac arrhythmias; therefore, epinephrine should not be used in concentrations greater than 1:200,000.

Lidocaine Hydrochloride (Xylocaine)

Owing to its rapid onset and longer action (1–2 hours), lidocaine has become the most commonly used local anesthetic. It is approximately twice as potent as procaine. Up to 30 mL of 1% solution, without epinephrine, may be used safely. In cataract surgery, 15–20 mL is usually more than adequate. The maximum safe dose is 4.5 mg/kg without epinephrine and 7 mg/kg with epinephrine.

Procaine Hydrochloride
(Novocaine)

Preparations: Solution, 1%, 2%, and 10%.

Dosage: Approximately 50 mL of a 1% solution can be injected without causing systemic effects. The maximum safe dose is 10 mg/kg.

Duration of action: 45–60 minutes.

Mepivacaine Hydrochloride
(Carbocaine, others)

Preparations: Solution, 1%, 1.5%, and 2%.

Dosage: Infiltration and nerve block, up to 20 mL of 1% or 2% solution.

Duration of action: Approximately 2 hours.

Comment: Carbocaine is similar to lidocaine in potency. It is usually used in patients who are allergic to lidocaine. The maximum safe dose is 7 mg/kg.

Bupivacaine Hydrochloride
(Marcaine, Sensorcaine)

Preparations: Solution, 0.25%, 0.5%, and 0.75%.

Dosage: The 0.75% solution has been used most frequently in ophthalmology. The maximum safe dose in an adult is 250 mg with epinephrine and 200 mg without epinephrine. Bupivacaine is frequently mixed with an equal amount of lidocaine.

Onset and duration of action: The onset of action is slower than that of lidocaine, but it persists much longer (up to 6–10 hours).

Etidocaine Hydrochloride
(Duranest)

Preparations: Solution, 1% and 1.5%.

Dosage: The maximum safe dose of etidocaine is 4 mg/kg without epinephrine and 5.5 mg/kg with epinephrine. This agent is frequently mixed with lidocaine for local anesthesia in ophthalmic surgery.

Onset and duration of action: The onset of action is slower than that of lidocaine but more rapid than that of bupivacaine. The duration of action is approximately twice as long as that of lidocaine (4–8 hours).

MYDRIATICS & CYCLOPLEGICS

Mydriatics and cycloplegics both dilate the pupil. In addition, cycloplegics cause paralysis of accommodation (patient unable to see near objects, eg, printed words). They are commonly used drugs in ophthalmology, singly and in combination. Their prime uses are (1) for dilating the pupils to facilitate ophthalmoscopy; (2) for paralyzing the muscles of accommodation, particularly in young patients, as an aid in refraction; and (3) for dilating the pupil and paralyzing the muscles of accommodation in uveitis to prevent synechia formation and relieve pain and photophobia. Since mydriatics and cycloplegics both dilate the pupil, they should be used with extreme caution in eyes with narrow anterior chamber angles since either a mydriatic or a cycloplegic can cause angle-closure glaucoma in such eyes.

1. MYDRIATICS
(Sympathomimetics)

Phenylephrine is a mydriatic with no cycloplegic effect.

Phenylephrine Hydrochloride
(Neo-Synephrine, others)

Preparations: Solution, 2.5% and 10%.

Dosage: 1 drop and repeat in 5–10 minutes.

Onset and duration of action: The effect usually occurs within 30 minutes after instillation and lasts 2–3 hours.

Comment: Phenylephrine is used both singly and with cycloplegics to facilitate ophthalmoscopy, in treatment of uveitis, and to dilate the pupil prior to cataract surgery. It is used almost to the exclusion of all other mydriatics. If a patient is allergic to phenylephrine, hydroxyamphetamine hydrobromide (Paredrine) may be substituted. The 10% solution should not be used in newborn infants, in cardiac patients, or in patients receiving reserpine, guanethidine, or tricyclic antidepressants, because of increased susceptibility to the vasopressor effects.

2. CYCLOPLEGICS
(Parasympatholytics)

Atropine Sulfate

Preparations: Solution, 0.5–3%; ointment, 0.5% and 1%.

Dosage: For refraction in children, instill 1 drop of 0.25–0.5% solution in each eye twice a day for 1 or 2 days before the examination and then 1 hour before the examination; ointment, ¼-inch ribbon twice a day for 2 days prior to examination.

Onset and duration of action: The onset of action is within 30–40 minutes. A maximum effect is reached in about 2 hours. The effect lasts for up to 2 weeks in a normal eye, but in the presence of acute inflammation the drug must be instilled two or three times daily to maintain its effect.

Toxicity: Atropine drops must be used with caution to avoid toxic reactions resulting from systemic absorption. Restlessness and excited behavior with dryness and flushing of the skin of the face, dry mouth, fever, inhibition of sweating, and tachycardia are prominent toxic symptoms, particularly in young children.

Comment: Atropine is an effective and long-acting cycloplegic. In addition to its use for cycloplegia in children, atropine is applied topically two or three times daily in the treatment of iritis. It is also used to maintain a dilated pupil after intraocular surgical procedures.

Scopolamine Hydrobromide

Preparation: Solution, 0.25%.

Dosage: 1 drop two or three times daily.

Onset and duration of action: Cycloplegia occurs in about 40 minutes and lasts for 3–5 days when scopolamine is used as an aid to refraction in normal eyes. The duration of action is much shorter in inflamed eyes.

Toxicity: Scopolamine occasionally causes dizziness and disorientation, mainly in older people.

Comment: Scopolamine is an effective cycloplegic. It is used in the treatment of uveitis, in refraction of children, and postoperatively.

Homatropine Hydrobromide

Preparations: Solution, 2% and 5%.

Dosage: For refraction, 1 drop in each eye and repeat two or three times at intervals of 10–15 minutes.

Onset and duration of action: Maximal cycloplegic effect lasts for about 3 hours, but complete recovery time is about 36–48 hours. In certain cases, the shorter action is an advantage over scopolamine and atropine.

Toxicity: Sensitivity and side effects associated with the topical instillation of homatropine are rare.

Cyclopentolate Hydrochloride
(Cyclogyl, others)

Preparations: Solution, 0.5%, 1%, and 2%.

Dosage: For refraction, 1 drop in each eye and repeat after 10 minutes.

Onset and duration of action: The onset of dilatation and cycloplegia is within 30–60 minutes. The duration of action is less than 24 hours.

Comment: Cyclopentolate is more popular than homatropine and scopolamine in refraction because of its shorter duration of action. Occasionally, neurotoxicity may occur, manifested by incoherence, visual hallucinations, slurred speech, and ataxia. These reactions are more common in children.

Tropicamide
(Mydriacyl, others)

Preparations: Solution, 0.5% and 1%.

Dosage: 1 drop of 1% solution two or three times at 5-minute intervals.

Onset and duration of action: The time required to reach the maximum cycloplegic effect is usually

20–25 minutes, and the duration of this effect is only 15–20 minutes; therefore, the timing of the examination after instilling tropicamide is important. Complete recovery requires 5–6 hours.

Comment: Tropicamide is an effective mydriatic with weak cycloplegic action and is therefore most useful for ophthalmoscopy.

Cyclopentolate Hydrochloride-
Phenylephrine Hydrochloride
(Cyclomydril)

Preparation: Solution, 0.2% cyclopentolate hydrochloride and 1% phenylephrine hydrochloride.

Dosage: 1 drop every 5–10 minutes for two or three doses. Pressure should be applied over the nasolacrimal sac after drop instillation to minimize systemic absorption.

Onset and duration of action: Mydriasis and some cycloplegia occur within the first 3–6 minutes. The duration of action is usually less than 24 hours. This drug combination is of particular value for pupillary dilation in examination of premature and small infants.

DRUGS USED IN THE TREATMENT OF GLAUCOMA

The concentration used and the frequency of instillation should be individualized on the basis of tonometric measurements. Use the smallest dosage that effectively controls the intraocular pressure and prevents optic nerve damage.

1. DIRECT-ACTING CHOLINERGIC (PARASYMPATHOMIMETIC) DRUGS

Pilocarpine Hydrochloride
& Nitrate

Preparations: Solution, 0.25%, 0.5–10%, 8%, and 10%; gel, 4%. Also available in a sustained-release system (Ocusert).

Dosage: 1 drop up to six times a day; a ½-inch strip of gel in lower conjunctival cul-de-sac at bedtime.

Comment: Pilocarpine was introduced in 1876 and is still a commonly used antiglaucoma drug.

Carbachol, Topical

Preparations: Solution, 0.75%, 1.5%, 2.25%, and 3%.

Dosage: 1 drop in each eye three or four times a day.

Comment: Carbachol is poorly absorbed through the cornea and usually is used if pilocarpine is ineffective. Its duration of action is 4–6 hours. If benzalkonium chloride is used as the vehicle, the penetration of carbachol is significantly increased.

2. INDIRECT-ACTING REVERSIBLE ANTICHOLINESTERASE DRUGS

Physostigmine Salicylate & Sulfate (Eserine)

Preparations: Solution, 0.25% and 0.5%, and ointment, 0.25%.

Dosage: 1 drop three or four times a day or ¼-inch strip of ointment once or twice a day.

Comment: A high incidence of allergic reactions has limited the use of this old but effective antiglaucoma drug. It can be combined in the same solution with pilocarpine.

3. INDIRECT-ACTING IRREVERSIBLE ANTICHOLINESTERASE DRUGS

These drugs are strong and long-lasting and are used when other antiglaucoma medications fail to control the intraocular pressure. They are employed less frequently than in the past. The miosis produced is extreme; ciliary spasm and myopia are common. Local irritation is common, and phospholine iodide is believed to be cataractogenic in some patients. Pupillary block may occur.

Echothiophate Iodide (Phospholine Iodide)

Preparations: Solution, 0.03%, 0.06%, 0.125%, and 0.25%

Dosage: 1 drop once or twice daily or less often, depending upon the response.

Comment: Echothiophate iodide is a long-acting drug similar to isoflurophate that has the advantages of being water-soluble and causing less local irritation. Systemic toxicity may occur in the form of cholinergic stimulation, including salivation, nausea, vomiting, and diarrhea. Ocular side effects include cataract formation, spasm of accommodation, and iris cyst formation.

Demecarium Bromide (Humorsol)

Preparations: Solution, 0.125% and 0.25%.

Dosage: 1 drop once or twice a day.

Comment: Systemic toxicity similar to that associated with echothiophate iodide may occur.

Isoflurophate (Floropryl)

Preparation: Ointment, 0.025%.

Dosage: A ¼-inch strip of ointment inside lower eyelid once or twice daily.

4. ADRENERGIC (SYMPATHOMIMETIC) DRUGS

In the treatment of glaucoma, epinephrine has the advantages of long duration of action (12–72 hours) and no miosis, which is especially important in patients with incipient cataracts (effect on vision not accentuated). At least 25% of patients develop local allergies; others complain of headache and heart palpitation (less common with dipivefrin).

Epinephrine acts by increasing outflow of aqueous humor.

Some of the preparations available for use in open-angle glaucoma are listed below. The dosage is the same for all, ie, 1 drop once or twice daily:

Epinephrine borate (Eppy/N), 0.5%, 1%, and 2%.

Epinephrine hydrochloride (Epifrin, Glaucon), 0.25%, 0.5%, 1%, and 2%.

Dipivefrin hydrochloride (Propine), 0.1%.

5. BETA-ADRENERGIC BLOCKING DRUGS

Timolol Maleate (Timoptic; Timoptic XE)

Preparations: Solution, 0.25% and 0.5%; gel, 0.025% and 0.5%.

Dosage: 1 drop of 0.25% solution once or twice daily. Increase to 1 drop of 0.5% solution in each eye once or twice daily if needed. One drop of gel once daily.

Comment: Timolol maleate is a nonselective beta-adrenergic blocking agent applied topically for treatment of open-angle glaucoma, aphakic glaucoma, and some types of secondary glaucoma. A single application can lower the intraocular pressure for 12–24 hours. Timolol has been found to be effective in some patients with severe glaucoma inadequately controlled by maximum tolerated antiglaucoma therapy with other drugs. The drug does not affect pupillary size or visual acuity. Although timolol is usually well tolerated, it should be prescribed cautiously for patients with known contraindications to systemic use of beta-adrenergic blocking drugs (eg, asthma, heart failure). (See discussion of side effects, below.)

Betaxolol Hydrochloride (Betoptic; Betoptic S)

Preparations: Solution, 0.25% (Betoptic S) and 0.5%.

Dosage: 1 drop once or twice daily.

Comment: Betaxolol has comparable efficacy to timolol in the treatment of glaucoma. Its relative β_1 receptor selectivity reduces the risk of pulmonary side effects, particularly in patients with reactive airway disease.

Levobunolol Hydrochloride (Betagan)

Preparations: Solution, 0.25% and 0.5%.

Dosage: 1 drop once or twice daily.

Comment: Levobunolol is a nonselective β_1 and β_2 blocker. It has effects comparable to those of timolol in the treatment of glaucoma.

Metipranolol Hydrochloride (OptiPranolol)

Preparation: Solution, 0.3%.

Dosage: 1 drop once or twice daily.

Comment: Metipranolol is a nonselective β_1 and β_2 blocker with ocular effects similar to those of timolol.

Carteolol Hydrochloride (Ocupress)

Preparation: Solution, 0.5% and 1%.

Dosage: One drop once or twice daily.

Comment: Carteolol is a nonselective beta-blocker with pharmacologic effects similar to those of other topical beta-blockers used for the treatment of glaucoma.

6. ALPHA-ADRENERGIC AGONISTS

Apraclonidine Hydrochloride (Iopidine)

Preparation: Solution, 0.5% and 1%.

Dosage: 1 drop of 1% solution before anterior segment laser treatment and a second drop upon completion of the procedure. One drop of 0.5% solution three times a day as short-term adjunctive treatment in glaucoma patients receiving other medications.

Comment: Apraclonidine hydrochloride is a selective α-adrenergic agonist that has been applied topically for prevention and management of intraocular pressure elevations after anterior segment laser procedures. It is also used as short-term adjunctive therapy in patients on maximally tolerated medical therapy who need further reduction of intraocular pressure. Apraclonidine lowers intraocular pressure by decreasing aqueous humor formation, the exact mechanism of which is not clearly understood. Unlike clonidine, apraclonidine does not appear to penetrate blood-tissue barriers easily and produces few side effects. The reported systemic side effects include occasional decreases in diastolic blood pressure, bradycardia, and central nervous system symptoms of insomnia, irritability, and decreased libido. Ocular side effects include conjunctival blanching, upper lid elevation, mydriasis, and burning.

7. CARBONIC ANHYDRASE INHIBITORS

Inhibition of carbonic anhydrase in the ciliary body reduces the secretion of aqueous. The oral administration of carbonic anhydrase inhibitors is especially useful in reducing the intraocular pressure in selected cases of open-angle glaucoma and can be used with some effect in angle-closure glaucoma.

The carbonic anhydrase inhibitors in use are sulfonamide derivatives. Oral administration produces the maximum effect in approximately 2 hours; intravenous administration, in 20 minutes. The duration of maximal effect is 4–6 hours following oral administration.

The carbonic anhydrase inhibitors are used in patients whose intraocular pressure cannot be controlled with eye drops. They are valuable for this purpose but have many undesirable side effects, including potassium depletion, gastric distress, diarrhea, exfoliative dermatitis, renal stone formation, shortness of breath, fatigue, acidosis, and tingling of the extremities. Since the advent of timolol and laser therapy, carbonic anhydrase inhibitors are being used less frequently.

Acetazolamide (Diamox)

Preparations and dosages:

Oral: Tablets, 125 mg and 250 mg; give 125–250 mg two to four times a day (dosage not to exceed 1 g in 24 hours). Sustained-release capsules, 500 mg; give 1 capsule once or twice a day.

Parenteral: May give 500-mg ampules intramuscularly or intravenously for short periods in patients who cannot tolerate the drug orally.

Methazolamide (Neptazane)

Preparation: Tablets, 25 and 50 mg.

Dosage: 50–100 mg two or three times daily (total not to exceed 600 mg/d).

Dichlorphenamide (Daranide)

Preparation: Tablets, 50 mg.

Dosage: Give a priming dose of 100–200 mg followed by 100 mg every 12 hours until the desired response is obtained. The usual maintenance dosage for glaucoma is 25–50 mg three or four times daily. The total daily dosage should not exceed 300 mg daily.

Investigational Topical Agents (MK-927, Sezolamide Hydrochloride, Dorzolamide Hydrochloride)

Topical carbonic anhydrase inhibitors have been studied on an investigational basis for their effectiveness in lowering intraocular pressure. In contrast to the older agents, these drugs are able to penetrate into the eye after topical application, reach the secretory epithelium of the ciliary body, and reduce intraocular pressure by decreasing aqueous secretion. They do not appear to cause substantial ocular or systemic side effects, though they are somewhat irritating.

8. OSMOTIC AGENTS

Hyperosmotic agents such as urea, mannitol, and glycerin are used to reduce intraocular pressure by making the plasma hypertonic to aqueous humor. These agents are generally used in the management of acute (angle-closure) glaucoma and occasionally in pre- or postoperative surgery when reduction of intraocular pressure is indicated. The dosage for all is approximately 1.5 g/kg.

Glycerin
(Glyrol, Osmoglyn)
Preparations and dosage: Glycerin is usually given orally as 50% and 75% solution with water, orange juice, or flavored normal saline solution over ice (1 mL of glycerin weighs 1.25 g). Dose is 1–1.5 g/kg.

Onset and duration of action: Maximum hypotensive effect occurs in 1 hour and lasts 4–5 hours.

Toxicity: Nausea, vomiting, and headache occasionally occur.

Comment: Oral administration and the absence of diuretic effect are significant advantages of glycerin over the other hyperosmotic agents.

Isosorbide
(Ismotic)
Preparation: 45% solution.

Dosage: 1.5 g/kg orally.

Onset and duration of action: Similar to glycerin.

Comment: Unlike glycerin, isosorbide does not produce calories or elevated blood sugar. Other side reactions similar to glycerin. Each 220 mL of isosorbide contains 4.6 meq of sodium.

Mannitol
(Osmitrol)
Preparation: 20% solution in water.

Dosage: 1.5–2 g/kg intravenously.

Onset and duration of action: Maximum hypotensive effect occurs in about 1 hour and lasts 5–6 hours.

Comment: Problems with cardiovascular overload and pulmonary edema are more common with this agent because of the large fluid volumes required.

Urea
(Ureaphil)
Preparation: 30% solution of lyophilized urea in invert sugar.

Dosage: 1–1.5 g/kg intravenously.

Onset and duration of action: Maximum hypotensive effect occurs in about 1 hour and lasts 5–6 hours.

Toxicity: Accidental extravasation at the injection site may cause local reactions ranging from mild irritation to tissue necrosis.

TOPICAL CORTICOSTEROIDS

Indications
Topical corticosteroid therapy is indicated for inflammatory conditions of the anterior segment of the globe. Some examples are allergic conjunctivitis, uveitis, episcleritis, scleritis, phlyctenulosis, superficial punctate keratitis, interstitial keratitis, and vernal conjunctivitis.

Administration & Dosage
The corticosteroids and certain derivatives vary in their anti-inflammatory activity. The relative potency of prednisolone to hydrocortisone is 4 times; of dexamethasone and betamethasone, 25 times. The side effects are not decreased with the higher-potency drugs even though the therapeutic dosage is lower.

The duration of treatment will vary with the type of lesion and may extend from a few days to several months.

Initial therapy for a severely inflamed eye consists of instilling drops every 1 or 2 hours while awake. When a favorable response is observed, gradually reduce the dosage and discontinue as soon as possible.

Caution: The steroids enhance the activity of the herpes simplex virus, as shown by the fact that perforation of the cornea occasionally occurs when they are used in the eye for treatment of herpes simplex keratitis. Corneal perforation was an extremely rare complication of herpes simplex keratitis before the steroids came into general use. Other side effects of local steroid therapy are fungal overgrowth, cataract formation (unusual), and open-angle glaucoma (common). These effects are produced to a lesser degree with systemic steroid therapy. Any patient receiving local ocular corticosteroid therapy or long-term systemic corticosteroid therapy should be under the care of an ophthalmologist.

The following is a partial list of the available topical corticosteroids for ophthalmologic use:

Hydrocortisone ointment, 0.5%.

Prednisolone acetate suspension, 0.125% and 1%.

Prednisolone sodium phosphate solution, 0.125% and 1%.

Dexamethasone sodium phosphate suspension, 0.1%; ointment, 0.05%.

Medrysone suspension, 1%.

Fluorometholone suspension, 0.1% and 0.25%.

MIXTURES OF CORTICOSTEROIDS & ANTI-INFECTIVE AGENTS

There are numerous commercial products containing fixed-dose combinations of corticosteroids and one or more anti-infective agents. They are used by ophthalmologists chiefly to treat conditions in which both agents may be required, eg, marginal keratitis due to a combined staphylococcal infection and allergic reaction, blepharoconjunctivitis, and phlyctenular keratoconjunctivitis. They are also used postoperatively.

These mixtures should not be used to treat conjunctivitis or blepharitis due to unknown causes. They should not be used as substitutes solely for anti-infective agents but only when a clear indication for corticosteroids exists as well. Mixtures of steroids and anti-infective agents may cause all of the same complications that occur with the topical steroid preparations alone.

NONSTEROIDAL ANTI-INFLAMMATORY AGENTS (NSAIDs)

In the past, orally administered NSAIDs, including aspirin and indomethacin, sometimes were given to control ocular inflammation. While a few patients were helped with this therapy, systemic toxicity often occurred. Topical ophthalmic preparations of several NSAIDs have been developed and have become popular in the past few years. They provide ocular bioavailability with little toxicity. These agents act primarily by blocking prostaglandin synthesis through inhibition of cyclooxygenase, the enzyme catalyzing the conversion of arachidonic acid to prostaglandins. Certain NSAIDs also may limit the arachidonic acid available for leukotriene production.

Some ophthalmologists use combinations of topical corticosteroids and NSAIDs to manage ocular inflammation, but the value of adding NSAIDs to adequate steroid therapy is not established. A number of ophthalmologists believe that by using an NSAID, the steroid treatment can be reduced.

Currently, flurbiprofen (Ocufen), 0.03%, and suprofen (Profenal), 1%, have been approved by the Food and Drug Administration for the inhibition of miosis during cataract surgery. Ketorolac (Acular), 0.5%, is approved for use in seasonal allergic conjunctivitis. Diclofenac (Voltaren), 0.1%, is approved for treatment of postoperative inflammation following cataract surgery. Another preparation, indomethacin suspension (Indocid), 1%, is not available in USA but is used in some parts of the world to treat cystoid macular edema, to reduce miosis during cataract surgery, and to treat inflammation following trauma, including cataract surgery.

OTHER DRUGS USED IN THE TREATMENT OF ALLERGIC CONJUNCTIVITIS

Cromolyn Sodium (Opticrom)

Preparation: Solution, 4%.

Dosage: 1 drop four to six times a day.

Comment: Cromolyn is useful in the treatment of many types of allergic conjunctivitis. Response to therapy usually occurs within a few days but sometimes not until treatment is continued for several weeks. Cromolyn acts by inhibiting the release of histamine and SRS-A (slow-reacting substance of anaphylaxis) from mast cells. It is not useful in the treatment of acute symptoms. Soft contact lenses should not be worn during treatment with cromolyn. This product is not currently available in the USA.

Lodoxamide Tromethamine (Alomide)

Preparation: Solution, 0.1%.

Dosage: 1 drop four times a day.

Comment: Lodoxamide is a mast cell stabilizer that inhibits type 1 immediate hypersensitivity reactions. It is indicated in the treatment of allergic reactions of the external ocular tissues, including vernal conjunctivitis and vernal keratitis. As with cromolyn, a therapeutic response does not usually occur until after a few days of treatment.

Levocabastine Hydrochloride (Livostin)

Preparation: Suspension, 0.05%.

Dosage: One drop four times a day.

Comment: Levocabastine is a selective, potent histamine H_1-receptor antagonist. It is useful in reducing acute symptoms of allergic conjunctivitis. Relief of symptoms occurs within minutes after application and lasts up to 2 hours.

Vasoconstrictors & Decongestant

These categories of drugs (see below) are also of interest in the treatment of allergic conjunctivitis.

ANTI-INFECTIVE OPHTHALMIC DRUGS

1. TOPICAL ANTIBIOTIC SOLUTIONS & OINTMENTS

Antibiotics are commonly used in the treatment of external ocular infection, including bacterial conjunctivitis, hordeola, marginal blepharitis, and bacterial corneal ulcers. The frequency of use is related to the severity of the condition. Antibiotic treatment of intraocular infection is set forth in Table 3–1.

Bacitracin, neomycin, polymyxin, erythromycin, tetracycline, gentamicin, and tobramycin are the most commonly used topical antibiotics. They are used separately and in combination as solutions and as ointments.

Bacitracin

Preparation: Ointment, 500 units/g. Commercially available in combinations with polymyxin B.

Comment: Most gram-positive organisms are sensitive to bacitracin. It is not used systemically because of its nephrotoxicity.

Erythromycin

Erythromycin ointment, 0.5% is an effective agent, particularly in staphylococcal conjunctivitis. It may be used instead of silver nitrate in prophylaxis of ophthalmia neonatorum.

Neomycin

Preparations: Solution, 2.5 and 5 mg/mL; ointment, 3.5–5 mg/g. Commercially available in combinations with bacitracin and polymyxin B.

Dosage: Apply ointment or drops three or four times daily. Solutions containing 50–100 mg/mL have been used for corneal ulcers.

Comment: Effective against gram-negative and gram-positive organisms. Neomycin is usually combined with some other drug to widen its spectrum of activity. It is best known in ophthalmologic practice as Neosporin, both in ointment and solution form, in which it is combined with polymyxin and bacitracin. Contact skin sensitivity develops in 5% of patients if the drug is continued for longer than a week.

Table 3–1. Usual adult doses of selected antimicrobials in endophthalmitis.[1,2]

	Subconjunctival Dose (0.5 mL)	Intravenous Dose	Intravitreal Dose (0.1 mL)
Amikacin (Amikin)	25 mg	6 mg/kg every 12 hours	0.4 mg
Amphotericin B (Fungizone)	1–2 mg	Varies (determined on case-by-case basis)	0.005–0.01 mg
Cefamandole (Mandol)	75 mg	1 g every 6–8 hours[3]	1–2 mg
Cefazolin (Ancef, Kefzol)	100 mg	1 g every 6–8 hours	2 mg
Ceftazidime (Fortaz, others)	100 mg	1 g every 8–12 hours	2.25 mg
Clindamycin (Cleocin)	30 mg	0.5–1 g every 8 hours	0.25–1 mg
Gentamicin (Garamycin, Jenamycin)	20 mg	70–100 mg every 8 hours[3]	0.1–0.2 mg
Methicillin (Staphcillin)	100 mg	1–2 g every 6 hours	2 mg
Miconazole (Monistat)	5 mg	200–600 mg every 8 hours	0.025 mg
Tobramycin (Nebcin)	20 mg	70–100 mg every 8 hours[3]	0.5 mg
Vancomycin (Vancocin, others)	25 mg	1 g every 12 hours	1 mg

[1]Modified and reproduced, with permission, from Parke DW, Brinton GS: Endophthalmitis. In: *Infections of the Eye.* Tabbara KF, Hyndiuk RA (editors). Little, Brown, 1986.
[2]Higher doses have been recommended in some cases. The doses listed here are considered appropriate by the present author based on drug toxicity studies.
[3]Nephrotoxic. Dose adjusted based on creatinine clearance and body weight.

Polymyxin B

Preparations: Ointment, 10,000 units/g; suspension, 10,000 units/mL. Commercially available in combination with bacitracin and neomycin.

Comment: Effective against many gram-negative organisms.

2. TOPICAL PREPARATIONS OF SYSTEMIC ANTIBIOTICS

Topical use of the antibiotics commonly used systemically should be avoided if possible, because sensitization of the patient may interfere with future systemic use. However, in certain instances clinical judgment overrides this principle if the drug is particularly effective locally and the disorder is serious. A prime example of this is tetracycline in the treatment of trachoma, the commonest eye infection in the world.

Fluoroquinolones (ciprofloxacin, norfloxacin) have recently become available for ophthalmic use. These agents are effective against a wide variety of gram-positive and gram-negative ocular pathogens, including *Pseudomonas aeruginosa.* They have been used principally for the treatment of corneal ulcers but have also been administered for the treatment of resistant bacterial conjunctivitis.

Tetracyclines

Preparations: Suspension, 10 mg/mL; ointment, 10 mg/g.

Comment: Tetracycline, oxytetracycline, and chlortetracycline have limited uses in ophthalmology because their effectiveness is so often impaired by the development of resistant strains. Solutions of these compounds are unstable with the exception of Achromycin in sesame oil, which is widely used in the treatment of trachoma. Ointment may be used for prophylaxis of ophthalmia neonatorum.

Gentamicin (Garamycin, Genoptic, Gentacidin)

Preparations: Solution, 3 mg/mL; ointment, 3 mg/g.

Comment: Gentamicin is widely accepted for use in serious ocular infections, especially corneal ulcers caused by gram-negative organisms. It is also effective against many gram-positive staphylococci but is not effective against streptococci.

Tobramycin (Tobrex)

Preparations: Solution, 3 mg/mL; ointment, 3 mg/g.

Comment: Similar antimicrobial activity to gentamicin but more effective against streptococci. Best reserved for treatment of *Pseudomonas* keratitis, for which it is more effective.

Chloramphenicol

Preparations: Solution, 5 and 10 mg/mL; ointment, 10 mg/g.

Comment: Chloramphenicol is effective against a wide variety of gram-positive and gram-negative organisms. It rarely causes local sensitization, but cases of aplastic anemia have occurred with long-term therapy.

Ciprofloxacin (Ciloxan)

Preparation: Solution, 3 mg/mL.

Dosage: For treatment of conjunctivitis, 1 drop every 2–4 hours. For treatment of corneal ulcers, 1 drop every 15–30 minutes for the first day, 1 drop every hour the second day, and 1 drop every 4 hours thereafter.

Norfloxacin (Chibroxin)

Preparation: Solution, 3 mg/mL.

Dosage: For conjunctivitis, same as that of ciprofloxacin.

Ofloxacin (Ocuflox)

Preparation: Solution, 3 mg/mL.

Dosage: For treatment of bacterial conjunctivitis, 1 drop every 2–4 hours for 2 days, then 1 drop four times a day. Not currently approved for treatment of corneal ulcers.

3. COMBINATION ANTIBIOTIC AGENTS

Several ophthalmic preparations are available that contain a mixture of antibiotics and bacteriostatic agents (Table 3–2).

4. SULFONAMIDES

The sulfonamides are the most commonly used drugs in the treatment of bacterial conjunctivitis. Their advantages include (1) activity against both gram-

Table 3–2. Some combination antibiotic preparations.

Generic Name	Trade Name
Bacitracin and polymyxin B	Ak-Poly-Bac, Polysporin
Bacitracin (or gramicidin), neomycin, and polymyxin B	Various
Oxytetracycline and polymyxin B	Terramycin w/Polymyxin B
Polymyxin B and trimethoprim	Polytrim

positive and gram-negative organisms, (2) relatively low cost, (3) low allergenicity, and (4) the fact that their use is not complicated by secondary fungal infections, as sometimes occurs following prolonged use of antibiotics.

The commonest sulfonamides employed are sulfisoxazole and sulfacetamide sodium.

Sulfacetamide Sodium
(Sulamyd, others)

Preparations: Ophthalmic solution, 10%, 15%, and 30%; ointment, 10%.

Dosage: Instill 1 drop frequently, depending upon the severity of the conjunctivitis.

Sulfisoxazole
(Gantrisin)

Preparations: Ophthalmic solution, 4%; ointment, 4%.

Dosage: As for sulfacetamide sodium (above).

5. TOPICAL ANTIFUNGAL AGENTS

Natamycin
(Natacyn)

Preparation: Suspension, 5%.

Dosage: Instill 1 drop every 1–2 hours.

Comment: Effective against filamentary and yeast forms. Initial drug of choice for most mycotic corneal ulcers.

Nystatin
(Mycostatin)

Nystatin is not available in ophthalmic ointment form, but the dermatologic preparation (100,000 units/g) is not irritating to ocular tissues and can be used in the treatment of fungal infection of the eye.

Amphotericin B
(Fungizone)

Amphotericin B is more effective than nystatin but not available in ophthalmic ointment form. The dermatologic preparation is highly irritating. A solution (1.5–8 mg/mL of distilled water in 5% dextrose) must be made up in the pharmacy from the powdered drug. Many patients have extreme ocular discomfort following application of this drug.

Miconazole
(Monistat)

A 1% solution is available in the form of an intravenous preparation that may be applied directly into the eye. The drug is not available in an ophthalmologic form.

6. ANTIVIRAL AGENTS

Idoxuridine
(Herplex, Stoxil)

Preparations: Ophthalmic solution, 0.1%; ointment, 0.5%.

Dosage: 1 drop every hour during the day and every 2 hours at night. With improvement (as determined by fluorescein staining), the frequency of instillation is gradually reduced. The ointment may be used four to six times daily, or the solution may be used during the day and the ointment at bedtime.

Comment: Used in the treatment of herpes simplex keratitis. Epithelial infection usually improves within a few days. Therapy should be continued for 3 or 4 days after apparent healing. Many ophthalmologists still prefer to denude the affected corneal epithelium and not use idoxuridine.

Vidarabine
(Vira-A)

Preparation: Ophthalmic ointment, 3%.

Dosage: In herpetic epithelial keratitis, apply four times daily for 7–10 days.

Comment: Vidarabine is effective against herpes simplex virus but not other RNA or DNA viruses. It is effective in some patients unresponsive to idoxuridine. Vidarabine interferes with viral DNA synthesis. The principal metabolite is arabinosylhypoxanthine (Ara-Hx). The drug is effective against herpetic corneal epithelial disease and has limited efficacy in stromal keratitis or uveitis. It may cause cellular toxicity and delay corneal regeneration. The cellular toxicity is less than that of idoxuridine.

Trifluridine
(Viroptic)

Preparation: Solution, 1%.

Dosage: 1 drop every 2 hours (maximum total, 9 drops daily).

Comment: Acts by interfering with viral DNA synthesis. More soluble than either idoxuridine or vidarabine and probably more effective in stromal disease.

Acyclovir
(Zovirax)

Preparation: Capsules, 200 mg.

Comment: Acyclovir is an antiviral agent with inhibitory activity against herpes simplex types 1 and 2, varicella-zoster virus, Epstein-Barr virus, and cytomegalovirus. It is phosphorylated initially by virus-specific thymidine kinase to acyclovir monophosphate and then by cellular kinases to acyclovir triphosphate, which inhibits viral DNA polymerase. Thus, there is a marked selectivity for virus-infected cells. Acyclovir has low toxicity. No commercial ophthalmic preparation is currently available in the USA; a topical product available for treatment of genital herpes should not be used in the eye. An oral preparation is available that may be used for treatment of selected herpes zoster ocular infections.

DIAGNOSTIC DYE SOLUTIONS

Fluorescein Sodium
Preparations: Solution, 2%, in single-use disposable units; as sterile paper strips; as 10% sterile solution for intravenous use in fluorescein angiography.
Dosage: 1 drop.
Comment: Used as a diagnostic agent for detection of corneal epithelial defects, in applanation tonometry, and in fitting contact lenses.

Rose Bengal
Preparation: Solution, 1%, and strips, 1.3 mg.
Dosage: 1 drop.
Comment: Used in diagnosis of keratoconjunctivitis sicca; the mucous shreds and devitalized corneal epithelium stain with rose bengal.

TEAR REPLACEMENT & LUBRICATING AGENTS

Methylcellulose and related chemicals, polyvinyl alcohol and related chemicals, and gelatin are used in the formulation of artificial tears, ophthalmic lubricants, contact lens solutions, and gonioscopic lens solutions. These agents are particularly useful in the treatment of keratoconjunctivitis sicca. (See Chapter 4.)

To increase viscosity and prolong corneal contact time, methylcellulose is sometimes added to eye solutions (eg, pilocarpine). Preservative-free preparations are available for use in patients with sensitivities to these substances.

VASOCONSTRICTORS & DECONGESTANTS

There are many commercially available OTC (over-the-counter) ophthalmic vasoconstrictive agents. The active ingredients in these agents usually are either ephedrine 0.123%, naphazoline 0.012–0.1%, phenylephrine 0.12%, or tetrahydrozoline 0.05–0.15%.

These agents constrict the superficial vessels of the conjunctiva and relieve redness. They also relieve minor surface irritation and itching of the conjunctiva, which can represent a response to noxious or irritating agents such as smog, swimming pool chlorine, etc. Products also are available that contain an antihistamine, antazoline phosphate 0.25–0.5%, or pheniramine maleate 0.3%.

CORNEAL DEHYDRATING AGENTS

Dehydrating solutions and ointments applied topically to the eye reduce corneal edema by creating an osmotic gradient in which the tear film is made hypertonic to the corneal tissues. Temporary clearing of corneal edema results.
Preparations: Anhydrous glycerin solution (Ophthalgan), hypertonic sodium chloride 2% and 5% ointment and solution (Absorbonac, Ak-NaCl, Hypersal, Muro-128).
Dosage: 1 drop of solution or ¼-inch strip of ointment to clear cornea. May be repeated every 3–4 hours.

OCULAR & SYSTEMIC SIDE EFFECTS OF DRUGS

F.T. Fraunfelder, MD

Both systemically and topically administered drugs can produce adverse ocular effects, and topical ophthalmic preparations occasionally lead to systemic effects if too much active ingredient is absorbed. Preservatives in topical ocular medications may also be associated with side effects.

Tables 3–3 to 3–5 list possible ocular and systemic side effects of some ocular and systemic medications. This is not in any way a complete listing of all drugs and their side effects. The information has been compiled from various sources. Physicians are advised to consult product labels, the references at the end of this chapter, and other appropriate sources for further information.

SYSTEMIC SIDE EFFECTS OF TIMOLOL

One example of an ocular drug with which serious side effects may occur is timolol. Timolol by topical administration is the most commonly used antiglaucoma medication in the world and has been associated with severe—even fatal—reactions. Plasma drug concentrations sufficient to cause systemic β-

Table 3–3. Possible adverse effects of systemic drugs.

Drug	Adverse Effects
Allopurinol	Cataract
Amiodarone	Corneal opacity
Amphetamines	Elevation of intraocular pressure
Antibiotics	Conjunctivitis, keratitis
Anticholinergics	Retinal hemorrhage
Barbiturates	Conjunctivitis, Stevens-Johnson syndrome, ptosis, optic atrophy
Busulfan	Cataract
Cardiac glycosides	Retinal degeneration
Chloral hydrate	Conjunctivitis
Chlorambucil	Papilledema
Chloramphenicol	Optic atrophy, optic neuritis
Chloroquine	Corneal opacity, retinal degeneration
Chlorpropamide	Stevens-Johnson syndrome, corneal opacity, extraocular muscle paralysis
Clofazimine	Conjuncitval deposits, corneal opacity
Corticosteroids	Elevation of intraocular pressure, cataract
Diazepam	Nystagmus
Disulfiram	Optic neuritis
Ethambutol	Optic neuritis
Gold salts	Conjunctival deposits, corneal opacity, nystagmus, pigmentation of lens
Guanethidine	Ptosis
Haloperidol	Cataract
Hexamethonium	Retinal vasodilation
Indomethacin	Corneal opacity
Iodoquinol	Optic atrophy
Isoniazid	Optic neuritis
Isotretinoin	Conjunctivitis, corneal opacity, papilledema
Ketamine	Nystagmus
Methyldopa	Conjunctivitis
Monoamine oxidase inhibitors	Optic atrophy
Morphine	Optic neuritis
Nalidixic acid	Papilledema
Naproxen	Corneal opacity
Oral contraceptives	Retinal hemorrhage, retinal edema, retinal vasospasm, corneal edema, nystagmus, papilledema
Penicillamine	Extraocular muscle paralysis, ptosis, optic neuritis
Phenothiazines	Conjunctival deposits, corneal opacity, oculogyric crisis, pigmentation of lens, retinal degeneration
Phenylbutazone	Conjunctivitis, keratitis, retinal hemorrhage
Phenytoin	Nystagmus, extraocular muscle paralysis
Quinacrine	Conjunctival deposits
Quinine	Retinal edema, retinal vasodilation followed by vasoconstriction
Rifampin	Optic neuritis
Salicylates	Nystagmus, retinal hemorrhage
Streptomycin	Conjunctivitis, Stevens-Johnson syndrome, retinal hemorrhage
Tetracycline	Papilledema
Tricyclic antidepressants	Elevation of intraocular pressure
Vitamin A	Conjunctival deposits, papilledema
Vitamin D	Conjunctival deposits, corneal opacity

Table 3–4. Possible adverse systemic effects of topical ocular medications.

Medication	Adverse Effects
Anesthetics, topical local Benoxinate Proparacaine Tetracaine	Allergic reactions, anaphylactic reactions, convulsions, faintness, hypotension, syncope
Antibiotics Chloramphenicol	Allergic reactions; bone marrow depression, including aplastic anemia; gastrointestinal symptoms

Sulfacetamide,
  sulfamethizole,
  sulfisoxazole
	Photosensitivity, Stevens-Johnson syndrome

Tetracycline, chlortetracycline	Photosensitivity, skin discoloration
Anticholinergics Atropine, homatropine, scopolamine	Confusion, dermatitis, dry mouth, excitement, fever, flushed skin, hallucinations, psychosis, tachycardia, thirst
Cyclopentolate, tropicamide	Amnesia, ataxia, convulsions, disorientation, dysarthria, fever
Anticholinesterases, long-acting Demecarium, echothiophate, isoflurophate	Abdominal cramps, diarrhea, fatigue, nausea, rhinorrhea, weight loss
Anticholinesterases, short-acting Neostigmine, physostigmine	Abdominal cramps, depigmentation, diarrhea, vomiting
Beta-adrenoceptor blocker Timolol	Asthma, bradycardia, cardiac arrhythmia, confusion, depression, dizziness, dyspnea, hallucinations, impotence, myasthenia, psychosis
Parasympathomimetics Carbachol, pilocarpine	Abdominal cramps, diarrhea, hypotension, increased salivation, muscle tremors, nausea, respiratory distress, rhinorrhea, slurred speech, sweating, vomiting, weakness

Sympathomimetics
Ephedrine, epinephrine,
  hydroxyamphetamine,
  phenylephrine
	Cardiac arrhythmias, hypertension, palpitations, subarachnoid hemorrhage, tachycardia

adrenoceptor blocking effects can occasionally result from ocular administration. When topical ocular timolol is administered in infants, blood levels are often more than six times what minimum therapeutic levels would be if the drug were given orally for some other condition; these high blood levels may be present for many hours after administration. If the lacrimal system is not closed during administration, an estimated 80% of a timolol eye drop is absorbed from the nasal mucosa and passes almost directly into the vascular system. Because the drug can reach target organs before it is detoxified in the liver, the blood level following topical ophthalmic administration is proportionately higher than when the drug is given orally, as in hypertension. A genetic fault in the oxidative metabolism of beta-blockers has been detected in some patients, and significantly higher levels of plasma concentrations develop in poor metabolizers.

Cardiopulmonary histories should be taken for candidates for beta-blocker glaucoma therapy. Pulmonary function studies should be considered in patients with bronchoconstrictive disease, and electrocardiograms should be ordered on selected patients with cardiac disease. Specifically, the precautions set forth in the package insert should be heeded carefully. Patients with known bronchial asthma, chronic respiratory or cardiovascular disease, or sinus bradycardia should avoid using timolol. The drug should be used with caution in patients receiving other systemic beta-blocking agents.

WAYS TO DIMINISH SYSTEMIC SIDE EFFECTS

One important principle in avoiding systemic side effects from topical ophthalmic medications is to prevent overdosing. The physician should prescribe the lowest concentration of medication that will be therapeutically effective. Only 1 drop of medication is needed at each dosage, since the volume the external eye can hold is less than 1 drop.

Table 3–5. Possible adverse ocular effects of topical ocular medications.

Medication	Adverse Effects
Anesthetics, local Butacaine, proparacaine, tetracaine	Allergic reactions, corneal opacity, decreased corneal wound healing, iritis
Antibiotics Chlortetracycline Neomycin	Allergic reactions, corneal discoloration Allergic reactions, follicular conjunctivitis, keratitis
Anticholinergics Cyclopentolate, tropicamide	Angle-closure glaucoma, blurred vision, photophobia
Anticholinesterases Demecarium, echothiophate, isoflurophate	Accommodative spasm, cataract, depigmentation of lids, iris cysts, lacrimal outflow obstruction
Anti-inflammatory agents Corticosteroids	Cataracts, corneal thinning, decreased corneal wound healing, glaucoma, infection
Antivirals Idoxuridine, trifluridine, vidarabine	Cicatricial pseudopemphigoid, keratitis, lacrimal outflow obstruction
Beta-adrenoceptor blocker Timolol	Blepharoconjunctivitis, corneal anesthesia, diplopia, dry eyes, keratitis, ptosis
Parasympathomimetic Pilocarpine	Accommodative spasm, cicatricial pseudopemphigoid, corneal haze (gel), myopia, retinal detachment
Preservatives Benzalkonium chloride, phenylmercuric nitrate, thimerosal	Allergic reactions, corneal opacity, keratitis
Sympathomimetics Dipivefrin Epinephrine	Allergic reactions, angle-closure glaucoma, follicular conjunctivitis Cicatricial pseudopemphigoid; cystoid macular edema; discoloration of cornea, conjunctiva, and soft contact lens; lacrimal outflow obstruction

The proper method of topical administration of ophthalmic medications is as follows:

(1) Position the patient with head tilted back toward the ceiling.

(2) Grasp the lower eyelid below the lashes, and gently pull the lid away from the eye (Figure 3–1).

(3) Instill 1 drop of medication into the inferior cul-de-sac nearest the involved area, being careful that the tip of the medication bottle does not touch the lashes or eyelids, thus avoiding contamination (Figure 3–2).

(4) To deepen the inferior cul-de-sac, the lower eyelid should then be gently lifted upward to make contact with the upper lid as the eye looks down (Figure 3–3).

(5) Patients should position their heads so that gravity will keep the drug where medically indicated. The eyelids should be kept closed for 3 minutes to prevent blinking, which pumps the drug into the nose and increases systemic absorption. The patient may be shown how to obstruct the lacrimal drainage system with firm pressure over the inner corner of the closed eyelids; however, this is not as important as lid closure (Figure 3–4).

(6) Excess medication in the medial canthus should be blotted away before pressure is released or the eyelids opened. The patient receiving multiple topical medications should wait 10 minutes between doses, so that the first drug will not be washed out of the eye by the second.

NATIONAL REGISTRY OF DRUG-INDUCED OCULAR SIDE EFFECTS

The National Registry of Drug-Induced Ocular Side Effects is a clearinghouse of drug information on ocular toxicology. The principle underlying its establishment is the assumption that the suspicions of practicing clinicians regarding possible ocular toxicity of drugs can be pooled to increase the data base and decrease the lag time in recognizing adverse responses. Physicians who wish to report suspected adverse drug reactions or would like to receive references pertaining to the data in Tables 3–3 to 3–5 should call or write the Casey Eye Institute, Oregon Health Sciences University, 3375 S.W. Terwilliger Blvd., Portland, OR 97201, (503) 494–5686.

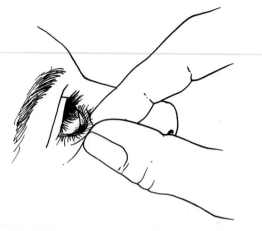

Figure 3–1. With the patient's head tilted back toward the ceiling, grasp the lower eyelid below the lashes and gently pull the lid away from the eye.

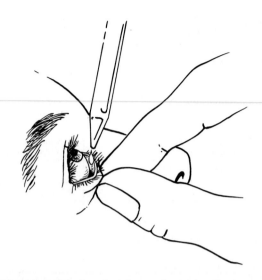

Figure 3–2. One drop of solution or a "match head" amount of ointment should be placed in the inferior cul-de-sac, without touching the bottle to the lashes or eyelids (to prevent contamination).

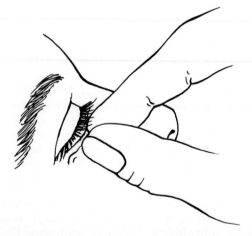

Figure 3–3. While the patient is looking downward, gently lift the lower eyelid to make contact with the upper lid.

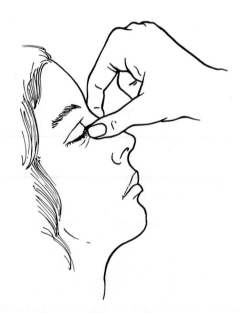

Figure 3–4. For 2 minutes or more, firm pressure is maintained with the forefinger or thumb over the inner corner of the closed eyelids. Lid closure is more important than pressure over the lacrimal sac in decreasing systemic absorption. Any excess medication should be blotted away before pressure is released or the eye is opened.

REFERENCES

American Medical Association: *Drug Evaluations Subscription,* Ophthalmology Drugs, Vol 3, AMA Publishers, 1992.

Bartlett JD, Jaanus SD: *Clinical Ocular Pharmacology,* 2nd ed. Butterworths, 1989.

Caldwell DR et al: Efficacy and safety of lodoxamide 0.1% vs cromolyn sodium 4% in patients with vernal keratoconjunctivitis. Am J Ophthalmol 1992;113:632.

Davidson SI et al: Ocular toxicity from systemic drug therapy: An overview of clinically important adverse reactions. Med Toxicol 1986;1:217.

Doft BH et al: Ceftazidime or amikacin: Choice of intravitreal antimicrobials in the treatment of postoperative endophthalmitis. Arch Ophthalmol 1994;112:17.

Dukes MN, Meyler L (editors): *Side Effects of Drugs,* 16th ed. Elsevier, 1993.

Ellis PP: *Ocular Therapeutics and Pharmacology,* 7th ed. Mosby, 1985.

Flach AJ: Cyclo-oxygenase inhibitors in ophthalmology. Surv Ophthalmol 1992;36:259.

Fraunfelder FT: *Drug-Induced Ocular Side Effects and Drug Interactions,* 4th ed. Lea & Febiger, 1995.

Fraunfelder FT, Roy FH (editors): *Current Ocular Therapy,* 4th ed. Saunders, 1995.

Grant WM, Schuman JS: *Toxicology of the Eye,* 4th ed. Thomas, 1993.

Gwon A et al: Ofloxacin vs tobramycin for the treatment of external ocular infection. Arch Ophthalmol 1992; 110:1234.

Koneru PB et al: Oculotoxicities of systemically administered drugs. J Ocul Pharmacol 1986;2:385.

Lamberts DW, Potter DE (editors): *Clinical Ocular Pharmacology.* Little, Brown, 1987.

Lee VH: Review: New directions in the optimization of ocular drug delivery. J Ocul Pharmacol 1990;6:157.

Leibowitz HM: Clinical evaluation of ciprofloxacin 0.3% ophthalmic solution for treatment of bacterial keratitis. Am J Ophthalmol 1991;112:34S.

McCloskey RV: Topical antimicrobial agents and antibiotics for the eye. Med Clin North Am 1988;72:717.

Nagasubramanian S et al: Comparisons of apraclonidine and timolol in chronic open-angle glaucoma: A three-month study. Ophthalmology 1993;100:1318.

Neu HC: Microbiologic aspects of fluoroquinolones. Am J Ophthalmol 1991;112:15S.

Ophthalmic Drug Facts. Lippincott, 1994.

Palmer EA: How safe are ocular drugs in pediatrics? Ophthalmology 1986;93:1038.

Pavan-Langston D, Dunkel EC: *Handbook of Ocular Drug Therapy and Ocular Side Effects of Systemic Drugs.* Little, Brown, 1991.

Pipkorn U et al: A double-blind evaluation of topical levocabastine, a new specific H_1 antagonist in patients with allergic conjunctivitis. Allergy 1985;40:491.

Salminen L: Review: Systemic absorption of topically applied ocular drugs in humans. J Ocul Pharmacol 1990;6:243.

Wilkerson M et al: Four-week safety and efficacy study of dorzolamide, a novel, active topical carbonic anhydrase inhibitor. Arch Ophthalmol 1993;111:1343.

Zun LS et al: Formulary of commonly used ophthalmologic medications. Emerg Med Clin North Am 1988;6:121.

4

Lids & Lacrimal Apparatus

John H. Sullivan, MD

I. LIDS

SURGICAL ANATOMY OF THE LIDS

The eyelids are thin folds of skin, muscle, and fibrous tissue that serve to protect the delicate structures of the eye. The great mobility of the lids is possible because the skin is among the thinnest anywhere on the body. Fine hairs, visible only under magnification, are present on the eyelids. Beneath the skin lies loose areolar tissue which is capable of massive edematous distention. The orbicularis oculi muscle is adherent to the skin. It is innervated on its deep surface by the facial (VII) cranial nerve, and its function is to close the lids. It is divided into orbital, preseptal, and pretarsal divisions. The orbital portion, which functions primarily in forcible closure, is a circular muscle with no temporal insertion. The preseptal and pretarsal muscles have superficial and deep medial heads that participate in the lacrimal pump (see below).

The lid margins are supported by the tarsi, rigid fibrous plates connected to the orbital rim by the medial and lateral canthal tendons. The orbital septum, which originates from the orbital rim, attaches to the levator aponeurosis, which then joins the tarsus. On the lower lid, it joins the inferior border of the tarsus. The septum is an important barrier between the eyelids and the orbit. Behind it lies the preaponeurotic fat pad, a helpful surgical landmark. An additional fat pad lies medially in the upper lid. The lower lid has two anatomically distinct fat pads beneath the orbital septum.

Deep to the fat lies the levator muscle complex—the principal retractor of the upper eyelid—and its equivalent, the capsulopalpebral fascia in the lower lid. The levator muscle originates in the apex of the orbit. As it enters the eyelid, it forms an aponeurosis that attaches to the lower third of the superior tarsus. In the lower lid, the capsulopalpebral fascia originates from the in-

ferior rectus muscle and inserts on the inferior border of the tarsus. It serves to retract the lower lid in downgaze. The superior and inferior tarsal muscles form the next layer, which is adherent to the conjunctiva. These sympathetic muscles are also lid retractors. Conjunctiva lines the inner surface of the lids. It is continuous with that of the eyeball and contains glands essential for lubrication of the cornea.

The upper lid is larger and more mobile than the lower. A deep crease usually present in the mid position of the upper lid in Caucasians represents the attachment of levator muscle fibers. The crease is much lower or is absent in the Asian eyelid. With age, the thin skin of the upper lid tends to hang over the lid crease and may touch the eyelashes. Aging also thins the orbital septum and reveals the underlying fat pads.

The lateral canthus is 1–2 mm higher than the medial. Because of a loose tendinous insertion to the orbital rim, the lateral canthus is elevated slightly with upgaze.

INFECTIONS & INFLAMMATIONS OF THE LIDS

HORDEOLUM

Hordeolum is infection of the glands of the eyelid. When the meibomian glands are involved, a large swelling occurs called internal hordeolum (Figure 4–1). The smaller and more superficial external hordeolum (sty) is an infection of Zeis's or Moll's glands.

Pain, redness, and swelling are the principal symptoms. The intensity of the pain is a function of the amount of lid swelling. An internal hordeolum may point to the skin or to the conjunctival surface. An external hordeolum always points to the skin.

Most hordeola are caused by staphylococcal infections, usually *Staphylococcus aureus*. Culture is seldom required. Treatment consists of warm compresses three or four times a day for 10–15 minutes. If the process does not begin to resolve within 48 hours, incision and drainage of the purulent material is indi-

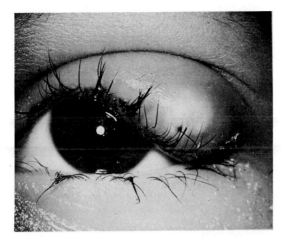

Figure 4–1. Internal hordeolum, left upper eyelid, pointing on skin side. This should be opened by a horizontal skin incision. (Courtesy of A Rosenberg.)

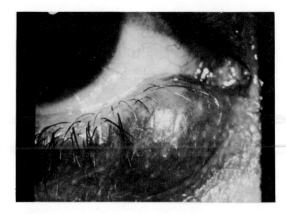

Figure 4–2. Chalazion, right lower eyelid. (Courtesy of K Tabbara.)

cated. A vertical incision should be made on the conjunctival surface to avoid cutting across the meibomian glands. The incision should not be squeezed to express residual pus. If the hordeolum is pointing externally, a horizontal incision should be made on the skin to minimize scar formation.

Antibiotic ointment applied to the conjunctival sac every 3 hours is beneficial. Systemic antibiotics are indicated if cellulitis develops.

CHALAZION

A chalazion (Figure 4–2) is an idiopathic sterile chronic granulomatous inflammation of a meibomian gland, usually characterized by painless localized swelling that develops over a period of weeks. It may begin with mild inflammation and tenderness resembling hordeolum—differentiated from hordeolum by the absence of acute inflammatory signs. Most chalazia point toward the conjunctival surface, which may be slightly reddened or elevated. If sufficiently large, a chalazion may press on the eyeball and cause astigmatism. If large enough to distort vision or to be a cosmetic blemish, excision is indicated.

Laboratory study is seldom indicated, but on pathologic examination there is proliferation of the endothelium of the acinus and a granulomatous inflammatory response that includes Langerhans-type gland cells. Biopsy is indicated for recurrent chalazion, since meibomian gland carcinoma may mimic the appearance of chalazion.

Surgical excision is performed via a vertical incision into the tarsal gland from the conjunctival surface followed by careful curettement of the gelatinous material and glandular epithelium. Intralesional steroid in-

jections alone may be useful for small lesions, and in combination with surgery in difficult cases.

ANTERIOR BLEPHARITIS

Anterior blepharitis is a common chronic bilateral inflammation of the lid margins. There are two main types: staphylococcal and seborrheic. Staphylococcal blepharitis may be due to infection with *Staphylococcus aureus,* in which case it is often ulcerative, or *Staphylococcus epidermidis* or coagulase-negative staphylococci. Seborrheic blepharitis (nonulcerative) is usually associated with the presence of *Pityrosporum ovale,* although this organism has not been shown to be causative. Often, both types are present (mixed infection). Seborrhea of the scalp, brows, and ears is frequently associated with seborrheic blepharitis.

The chief symptoms are irritation, burning, and itching of the lid margins. The eyes are "red-rimmed." Many scales or "granulations" can be seen clinging to the lashes of both the upper and lower lids. In the staphylococcal type, the scales are dry, the lids are red, tiny ulcerated areas are found along the lid margins, and the lashes tend to fall out. In the seborrheic type, the scales are greasy, ulceration does not occur, and the lid margins are less red. In the more common mixed type, both dry and greasy scales are present and the lid margins are red and may be ulcerated. *S aureus* and *P ovale* can be seen together or singly in stained material scraped from the lid margins.

Staphylococcal blepharitis may be complicated by hordeola, chalazia, epithelial keratitis of the lower third of the cornea, and marginal corneal infiltrates (see Chapter 7). Both forms of anterior blepharitis predispose to recurrent conjunctivitis.

The scalp, eyebrows, and lid margins must be kept clean, particularly in the seborrheic type of blepharitis, by means of soap and water shampoo. Scales must be removed from the lid margins daily with a damp cotton applicator and baby shampoo.

Staphylococcal blepharitis is treated with antistaphylococcal antibiotic or sulfonamide eye ointment applied on a cotton applicator once daily to the lid margins.

The seborrheic and staphylococcal types usually become mixed and may run a chronic course over a period of months or years if not treated adequately; associated staphylococcal conjunctivitis or keratitis usually disappears promptly following local antistaphylococcal medication.

POSTERIOR BLEPHARITIS

Posterior blepharitis is inflammation of the eyelids secondary to dysfunction of the meibomian glands. Like anterior blepharitis, it is a bilateral, chronic condition. Anterior and posterior blepharitis may coexist. Seborrheic dermatitis is commonly associated with meibomian gland dysfunction. Colonization or frank infection with strains of staphylococci is frequently associated with meibomian gland disease and may represent one reason for the disturbance of meibomian gland function. Bacterial lipases may cause inflammation of the meibomian glands and conjunctiva and disruption of the tear film.

Posterior blepharitis is manifested by a broad spectrum of symptoms involving the lids, tears, conjunctiva, and cornea. Meibomian gland changes include inflammation of the meibomian orifices (meibomianitis), plugging of the orifices with inspissated secretions, dilatation of the meibomian glands in the tarsal plates, and production of abnormal soft, cheesy secretion upon pressure over the glands. Hordeola and chalazia may also occur. The lid margin shows hyperemia and telangiectasia. It also becomes rounded and rolled inward as a result of scarring of the tarsal conjunctiva, causing an abnormal relationship between the precorneal tear film and the meibomian gland orifices. The tears may be frothy or abnormally greasy. Hypersensitivity to staphylococci may produce epithelial keratitis. The cornea may also develop peripheral vascularization and thinning, particularly inferiorly, sometimes with frank marginal infiltrates. The gross changes of posterior blepharitis are identical to the ocular findings in acne rosacea (see Chapter 15).

Treatment of posterior blepharitis is determined by the associated conjunctival and corneal changes. Frank inflammation of these structures calls for active treatment, including long-term low-dose systemic antibiotic therapy—usually with tetracycline (250 mg twice daily) or erythromycin (250 mg three times daily), but guided by results of bacterial cultures from the lid margins—and (preferably) short-term treatment with weak topical steroids, eg, prednisolone, 0.125% twice daily. Topical therapy with antibiotics or tear substitutes is usually unnecessary and may lead to further disruption of the tear film or toxic reactions to their preservatives.

Periodic meibomian gland expression may be helpful, particularly in patients with mild disease that does not warrant long-term therapy with oral antibiotics or topical steroids. Hordeola and chalazia should be treated appropriately.

ANATOMIC DEFORMITIES OF THE LIDS

ENTROPION

Entropion—turning inward of the lid (Figure 4–3)—may be involutional (spastic, senile), cicatricial, or congenital. Involutional entropion is most common and by definition occurs as a result of aging. It always affects the lower lid and is the result of a combination of laxity of the lower lid retractors, upward migration of the preseptal orbicularis muscle, and buckling of the upper tarsal border.

Cicatricial entropion may involve the upper or lower lid and is the result of conjunctival and tarsal scar formation. It is most often found with chronic inflammatory diseases such as trachoma.

Congenital entropion is rare and should not be confused with congenital **epiblepharon,** which usually afflicts Asians. In congenital entropion, the lid margin is rotated toward the cornea, whereas in epiblepharon the pretarsal skin and muscle cause the lashes to rotate around the tarsal border.

Trichiasis is impingement of eyelashes on the cornea and may be due to entropion, epiblepharon, or simply misdirected growth. It causes corneal irritation and encourages ulceration. Chronic inflammatory lid diseases such as blepharitis may cause scarring of the lash follicles and subsequent misdirected growth.

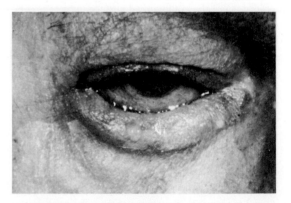

Figure 4–3. Entropion. (Courtesy of M Quickert.)

Distichiasis is a condition manifested by accessory eyelashes, often growing from the orifices of the meibomian glands. It may be congenital or the result of metaplastic changes in the glands of the eyelid margin.

Surgery to evert the lid is effective in all kinds of entropion. A useful temporary measure in involutional entropion is to tape the lower lid to the cheek, with tension exerted temporally and inferiorly. Trichiasis without entropion can be temporarily relieved by plucking the offending eyelashes. Permanent relief may be achieved with electrolysis, laser or knife surgery, or cryosurgery.

ECTROPION

Ectropion (sagging and eversion of the lower lid) (Figure 4–4) is usually bilateral and is a frequent finding in older persons. Ectropion may be caused by relaxation of the orbicularis oculi muscle, either as part of the aging process or following seventh nerve palsy. The symptoms are tearing and irritation. Exposure keratitis may occur.

Involutional ectropion is treated surgically by horizontal shortening of the lid. Cicatricial ectropion is caused by contracture of the anterior lamella of the lid. Treatment requires surgical revision of the scar and often skin grafting for relief. Minor degrees of ectropion can be treated by several fairly deep electrocautery penetrations through the conjunctiva 4–5 mm from the lid margins at the inferior aspect of the tarsal plate. The fibrotic reaction that follows will often draw the lid up to its normal position.

COLOBOMA

Congenital coloboma is the result of incomplete fusion of fetal maxillary processes. The consequence is a lid margin cleft of variable size. The medial aspect of the upper lid is most often involved, and there is often an associated dermoid tumor. Surgical reconstruction can usually be delayed for years but should be done immediately if the cornea is at risk. A full-thickness eyelid defect from any cause is sometimes referred to as a coloboma.

EPICANTHUS

Epicanthus (Figure 4–5) is characterized by vertical folds of skin over the medial canthi. It is typical of Asians and is present to some degree in most children of all races. The skinfold is often large enough to cover part of the nasal sclera and cause "pseudoesotropia." The eye appears to be crossed when the medial aspect of the sclera is not visible. The most frequent type is **epicanthus tarsalis,** in which the superior lid fold is continuous medially with the epicanthal fold. In **epicanthus inversus,** the skinfold blends into the lower lid. Other types are less common. The cause of epicanthus is lack of vertical skin between the canthus and the nose. Surgical correction is directed at vertical lengthening and horizontal shortening. Epicanthal folds in normal children, however, diminish gradually and are seldom apparent by puberty. Epicanthal skinfolds may also be acquired after surgery or trauma of the medial eyelid and nose.

TELECANTHUS

The distance between the medial canthus of each eye—the intercanthal distance—is the same as the length of each palpebral fissure (approximately 30 mm in adults). A wide intercanthal distance may be the result of traumatic disinsertion or congenital craniofacial dysgenesis. Minor degrees of telecanthus (eg, blepharophimosis syndrome) can be corrected with skin and soft tissue surgery. Major craniofacial reconstruction, however, is required when the orbits are widely separated, as in Crouzon's disease (see Chapter 18).

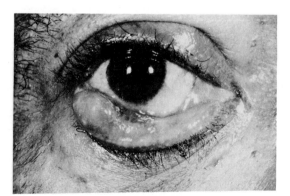

Figure 4–4. Ectropion. (Courtesy of M Quickert.)

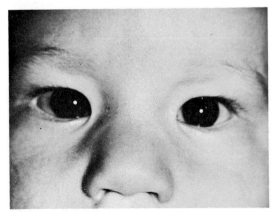

Figure 4–5. Epicanthus tarsalis.

BLEPHAROCHALASIS

Blepharochalasis (Figure 4–6) is a rare condition of unknown cause, sometimes familial, which resembles angioneurotic edema. Repeated attacks begin near puberty, diminish during adulthood, and cause atrophy of periorbital structures. Eyelid skin appears thin, wrinkled, and redundant and is described as resembling cigarette paper. A sunken appearance is the result of fat atrophy. Involvement of the levator aponeurosis produces moderate to severe ptosis. Medical management is limited to symptomatic treatment of edema. Surgical repair of levator dehiscence and excision of redundant skin is most likely to be successful after attacks have abated.

DERMATOCHALASIS

Dermatochalasis (Figure 4–7) is eyelid skin redundancy and loss of elasticity, usually as a result of aging. In the upper lid, the preseptal skin and orbicularis muscle, which normally forms a crease near the upper tarsal border in Caucasians, hangs over the pretarsal portion of the lid. When dermatochalasis is severe, the superior visual field is obstructed. Weakness of the orbital septum causes the medial and preaponeurotic fat pads to bulge. "Bags" in the preseptal region of the lower lid represent herniated orbital fat. Redundant skin may also be present.

Surgery may be indicated for visual or cosmetic reasons. In the upper lid, superfluous eyelid skin is removed as well as muscle and fat for optimum aesthetics. Lower lid surgery is performed for cosmetic reasons unless extreme redundancy contributes to ectropion of the lid margin.

BLEPHAROSPASM

Benign essential blepharospasm is an uncommon type of involuntary muscle contraction characterized by persistent or repetitive spasm of the orbicularis oculi muscle. It is almost always bilateral and is most common in the elderly. The spasms tend to progress in force and frequency, resulting in a grimacing expression and closure of the eyes. Patients may be incapacitated—able to experience only brief intervals of vision between spasms. When the entire face and neck are involved, the condition is known as Meigs' syndrome.

The cause is not known. Emotional stress and fatigue sometimes make the condition worse, leading to speculation that this is a psychogenic affliction. Psychotherapy and psychoactive drugs, however, have had very limited success. A small percentage of patients have psychogenically induced spasms, but in most cases the dysfunction is thought to originate in the basal ganglia.

It is important to differentiate benign essential blepharospasm from hemifacial spasm. The latter condition tends to be unilateral and to involve the upper and lower face. Hemifacial spasm is thought to be related to compression of the facial nerve by an artery or posterior fossa tumor. Jenetta's neurosurgical decompression is the definitive mode of treatment; however, temporary neuromuscular blockade (see below) is less invasive and now more frequently employed.

Other types of involuntary facial movements include **tardive dyskinesia,** which results from prolonged phenothiazine therapy and seldom affects the orbicularis muscle selectively; and **facial tics,** common in children, which are thought to be psychogenic.

Treatment of blepharospasm begins with an attempt to identify the unusual instances of psychoneurotic behavior. Psychotherapy, neuroleptic drug treatment, biofeedback training, and hypnosis have occasionally been used with success. Most patients, however, require either repeated injections for neuromuscular blockade or surgery to ablate the action of the facial nerve.

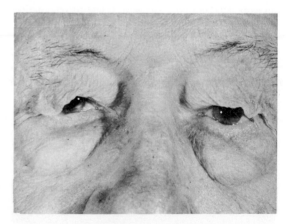

Figure 4–7. Dermatochalasis of upper lids and herniation of orbital fat of lower lids. (Courtesy of M Quickert.)

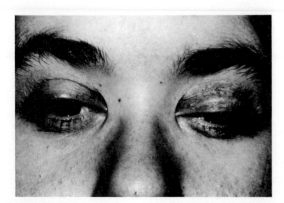

Figure 4–6. Blepharochalasis.

Botulinum toxin type A (Botox) has replaced alcohol as the preferred substance for intramuscular injection to produce temporary neuromuscular paralysis. When intolerance or unresponsiveness to the toxin occurs, the only recourse is selective surgical ablation of the facial nerve or extirpation of the orbicularis musculature.

BLEPHAROPTOSIS

Blepharoptosis is abnormally low position of one or both upper lids. The normal position of the upper lid is midway between the superior limbus and the upper pupillary margin. This may vary by 2 mm provided the lids are symmetric. Blepharoptosis may be congenital or acquired and can be hereditary in either case.

Classification

Classification is important for proper treatment. Beard's revised scheme (Table 4–1) attempts to classify ptosis by etiology.

A. Levator Maldevelopment: Ptosis from levator maldevelopment—formerly classified as true congenital ptosis—is the result of an isolated dystro-

Table 4–1. Beard's revised classification of ptosis.

Levator maldevelopment
  Simple
  With superior rectus weakness
Other myogenic ptosis
  Blepharophimosis syndrome
  Chronic progressive external ophthalmoplegia
  Oculopharyngeal syndrome
  Progressive muscular dystrophy
  Myasthenia gravis
  Congenital fibrosis of the extraocular muscles
Aponeurotic ptosis
  Senile ptosis
  Late-developing hereditary ptosis
  Stress or trauma to levator aponeurosis
    Following cataract surgery
    Following other local trauma
    Blepharochalasis
    Associated with pregnancy
    Associated with Graves' disease
Neurogenic ptosis
  Ptosis caused by lesions of the oculomotor nerve
  Posttraumatic ophthalmoplegia
  Misdirected third nerve ptosis
  Marcus Gunn jaw-winking syndrome
  Horner's syndrome
  Ophthalmoplegic migraine
  Multiple sclerosis
Mechanical ptosis
Apparent ptosis
  Due to lack of posterior eyelid support
  Due to hypotropia
  Due to dermatochalasis

phy of the levator muscle affecting both contraction and relaxation of the fibers. Ptosis is present in the primary position of gaze, and there is reduced movement of the lid in upgaze and impaired closure on downgaze. Lid lag on downgaze is an important clue to diagnosis of levator maldevelopment. Other ocular abnormalities such as strabismus are sometimes associated with this form of congenital ptosis. In 25% of cases, the superior rectus muscle shares the same dystrophic changes as the levator, resulting in weakness of upgaze. It is important to identify this finding. Successful surgical outcome in the presence of superior rectus weakness requires the resection of an additional length of levator.

The distinction between levator maldevelopment and other forms of ptosis is an important one that cannot always be made by the history. Neurologic and other myogenic ptosis may be present at birth. Application of the surgical principles intended for levator maldevelopment to these types of ptosis patients would result in a gross overcorrection.

B. Other Types of Myogenic Ptosis: Blepharophimosis accounts for 5% of cases of congenital ptosis. Poor levator function and severe ptosis are accompanied by telecanthus, epicanthal folds, and cicatricial ectropion of the lower lids. The condition is familial.

Chronic progressive external ophthalmoplegia is a slowly progressive hereditary neuromuscular disease that begins in mid life. All extraocular muscles including the levator and the muscles of facial expression gradually become affected. Other neurodegenerative disorders may be present. In the form known as oculopharyngeal dystrophy, myopathy of the laryngeal muscles produces dysphagia. In Kearns-Sayre syndrome, ophthalmoplegia is associated with retinitis pigmentosa and heart block.

Ptosis and facial weakness may also be found in **myotonic dystrophy.** Other findings include cataract, pupillary abnormalities, frontal baldness, testicular atrophy, and diabetes.

Ptosis associated with the rare and sometimes familial **congenital fibrosis of the extraocular muscles** may be unilateral.

Ptosis and diplopia are often the initial manifestations of **myasthenia gravis.** The orbicularis oculi muscles are also frequently involved. Cogan's lid twitch is sometimes present—on rapid movements of the eyes from downgaze to the primary position, the upper lid twitches upward. Demonstration of lid fatigue, however, is more consistent. The diagnosis can be confirmed by intravenous administration of edrophonium, which temporarily reverses the weakness. Another useful test is the detection of circulating anti-acetylcholine receptor autoantibodies.

Medical management is usually effective initially, but ptosis surgery often becomes necessary. Thymectomy may be helpful in refractory cases. When lid closure and Bell's phenomenon have been impaired, difficult problems with exposure keratitis may complicate ptosis surgery.

C. Aponeurotic Ptosis: A common form of ptosis occurs late in life and results from partial disinsertion or dehiscence of the levator aponeurosis from the tarsal plate. Typically, there are sufficient residual attachments to the tarsus to maintain full excursion of the lid with upgaze. Retention of the attachment of the retracted levator aponeurosis to the skin and orbicularis muscle creates an unusually high lid fold. Thinning of the lid may also occur, and on occasion the image of the iris may be seen through the skin of the upper lid. Trauma is often a precipitating cause of disinsertion of the levator. Ptosis following cataract surgery is thought to be due to this mechanism. A hereditary variant is known as "late-developing hereditary ptosis." The mechanism of ptosis associated with ocular surgery, blepharochalasis, pregnancy, and Graves' disease is usually damage to the aponeurosis.

D. Neurogenic Ptosis: In *(***Marcus Gunn syndrome;** "jaw-winking phenomenon.") the eye opens when the mandible is opened or is deviated to the opposite side. The ptotic levator muscle is innervated by motor branches of the trigeminal nerve as well as the oculomotor nerve.

Partial or complete **oculomotor palsy** is most often a result of trauma. **Aberrant regeneration** is not uncommon and results in bizarre movements of the globe, eyelid, and pupil. Congenital oculomotor nerve paralysis, however, is not associated with aberrant regeneration. If the lid is completely closed, deprivational amblyopia will develop unless the ptosis is corrected. Visually immature children with oculomotor nerve paralysis, even after successful ptosis repair, are almost certain to develop strabismic amblyopia without vigorous and early treatment.

Paralysis of Müller's muscle is almost always associated with **Horner's syndrome** and is usually acquired. Rarely is there more than 2 mm of ptosis, and amblyopia is never a threat.

E. Mechanical Ptosis: The upper lid may be prevented from opening completely because of the mass effect of a neoplasm or the tethering effect of scar formation. Excessive horizontal shortening of the upper lid is a common cause of mechanical ptosis. Another form is that seen following enucleation, when absence of support to the levator by the globe permits the lid to drop.

F. Apparent Ptosis: Hypotropia may give the appearance of ptosis. When the eye looks down, the upper lid drops more than the lower lid. The narrowed palpebral fissure and the ptotic upper lid are much more apparent than the hypotropic globe. Occlusion of the opposite eye, however, reveals the true condition. In severe dermatochalasis, a fold of pretarsal orbicularis and skin may conceal the lid margin and give the appearance of blepharoptosis.

Treatment
(Figure 4–8)

With the exception of myasthenia gravis, all types of ptosis are treated surgically. In children, surgery can be performed when accurate evaluation can be obtained and the child is able to cooperate postoperatively. Astigmatism and myopia may be associated with childhood ptosis. Early surgery might be helpful in preventing anisometropic amblyopia, but this has not been proved. Deprivational amblyopia probably occurs only with complete ptosis, as in oculomotor nerve palsy.

Symmetry is the goal of surgery, and symmetry in all positions of gaze is possible only if levator function is unimpaired. In most cases, the best result that can be achieved is to balance the lids in the primary position. With unilateral ptosis, achievement of symmetry in other positions of gaze is proportionate to levator function.

Most ptosis operations involve resection of the levator aponeurosis or superior tarsal muscle (or both). The superior portion of the tarsus is often resected for additional elevation. Many approaches, from both skin and conjunctiva, are currently in use. In recent years, emphasis has been placed on the advantages of con-

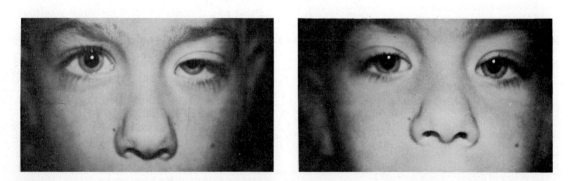

Figure 4–8. Surgical correction of ptosis. *Left:* Before operation, ptosis of the upper lid was present. *Right:* After the operation (levator resection), the ptosis was well corrected and a natural-appearing upper lid fold produced. (Courtesy of C Beard.)

fining the operation to advancement and resection of the levator aponeurosis, especially in acquired ptosis.

Patients with little or no levator function require an alternative elevating source. Suspension of the lids to the brow allows the patient to elevate the lids with the natural movement of the frontalis muscle. Autogenous fascia lata is usually considered the best means of suspension.

COSMETIC MICROPIGMENTATION OF THE LIDS

Tattooing the lids of women is a controversial procedure whose purpose is to eliminate the need for applying eyeliner. The procedure is also occasionally used to simulate cilia following reconstruction of the lid margin. It is performed under local anesthesia using a power-driven handpiece to implant various pigments adjacent to the eyelashes or eyebrow. Because subcutaneous impregnation of certain mercury-based dyes can cause a local inflammatory reaction, these dyes have been abandoned. Carbon particle tattooing appears to be harmless, but the long-term consequences of dye impregnation at the lid margin are unknown.

As is true also of tattoos elsewhere on the body, the intensity and crispness of the image tends to fade with time. Complete removal of the pigmentation because of misplacement or change in fashion is difficult.

TUMORS OF THE EYELIDS

J. Brooks Crawford, MD

BENIGN LID TUMORS

Benign tumors of the lids are very common and increase in frequency with age. Most are readily distinguished clinically, and excision is done for cosmetic reasons. However, it is often impossible to recognize malignant lesions clinically, and biopsy should always be performed if there is any doubt about the diagnosis.

Nevus

Melanocytic nevi of the eyelids are common benign tumors with the same pathologic structure as nevi found elsewhere. They are usually congenital but may be relatively unpigmented at birth, enlarging and darkening during adolescence. Many never acquire visible pigment, and many resemble benign papillomas. Nevi rarely become malignant.

Nevi may be removed by shave excision if desired for cosmetic reasons.

Papillomas

Papillomas are the most common benign eyelid tumors. Two types occur: squamous papillomas and seborrheic keratoses (basal cell papillomas, senile verrucae). In both, fibrovascular cores permeate thickened (acanthotic and hyperkeratotic) surface epithelium, giving it a papillomatous appearance. Seborrheic keratoses occur in middle-aged and older individuals. They have a friable, verrucous surface and are often pigmented because melanin accumulates in the keratocytes.

Molluscum Contagiosum (Figure 4–9)

The typical lesion of this unusual disorder is a small, flat, symmetric, centrally umbilicated growth along the lid margin. It is caused by a large virus and may produce conjunctivitis and even keratitis if the lesion sheds into the conjunctival space.

Cure can usually be achieved by curettement, cautery, or excision.

Xanthelasma (Figure 4–10)

Xanthelasma is a common disorder that occurs on the anterior surface of the eyelid, usually bilaterally near the inner angle of the eye. The lesions appear as yellow, wrinkled patches on the skin and occur most commonly in elderly people. Xanthelasma represents lipid deposits in histiocytes in the dermis of the lid. Clinical evaluation of serum lipid levels is indicated, but only rarely is an abnormality found.

Treatment is indicated for cosmetic reasons. Some lesions can be excised; small lesions can sometimes be cauterized. Recurrence following removal is not unusual.

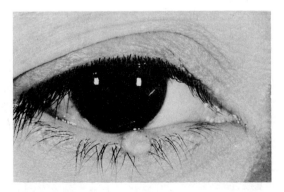

Figure 4–9. Molluscum contagiosum. Note central umbilication.

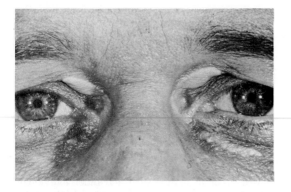

Figure 4–10. Xanthelasma. (Courtesy of M Quickert.)

Hemangioma
(Figure 4–11)

The most common congenital vascular tumor of the eyelids is the **capillary hemangioma,** composed of proliferating capillaries and endothelial cells. They arise at or shortly after birth, often grow rapidly, and usually involute spontaneously by age 7 years. If superficial, they may be bright red (strawberry nevus); deeper lesions may be bluish or violet. Secondary anisometropia, refractive amblyopia, and strabismus are common and must be appropriately treated. Treatment of the tumor is rarely indicated unless it blocks the pupil. If it does, intralesional injection of steroids may produce rapid resolution; if this fails, partial surgical excision is indicated.

Capillary hemangiomas should be differentiated from the much rarer **nevus flammeus (port wine stain),** which is often associated with Sturge-Weber syndrome. These lesions are composed of dilated, cavernous vascular channels; they do not grow or regress like the capillary hemangiomas.

A third type of angioma is the **cavernous hemangioma,** composed of large, endothelium-lined vascular channels with smooth muscle in their walls. They are developmental rather than congenital and tend to arise after the first decade. Unlike capillary hemangiomas, they do not usually regress.

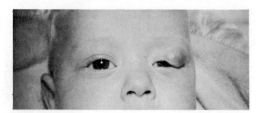

Figure 4–11. Cavernous hemangioma of left upper lid.

PRIMARY MALIGNANT TUMORS OF THE LIDS

Carcinoma
(Figures 4–12 and 4–13)

Basal cell and squamous cell carcinomas of the lids are the most common malignant ocular tumors. These tumors occur most frequently in fair-complexioned individuals who have had chronic exposure to the sun. Ninety-five percent of lid carcinomas are of the basal cell type. The remaining 5% consist of squamous cell carcinomas and meibomian gland carcinomas.

Treatment of all these carcinomas is by complete excision, which is best achieved by controlling the surgical margins with frozen sections. Many of these malignant tumors and many benign ones as well can have the same appearance; biopsy is usually required to establish the correct diagnosis.

A. Basal Cell Carcinoma: Basal cell carcinoma usually grows slowly and painlessly as a nodule that may or may not become ulcerated. It slowly invades adjacent tissues but does not metastasize. A rare type— sclerosing or morphea basal cell carcinoma—tends to extend insidiously and surreptitiously beneath the surface, sometimes producing ectropion, entropion, lid notching or retraction, dimpling of the overlying skin, or loss of eyelashes.

Frozen section study of the surgical margins is particularly important for sclerosing basal cell carcinomas, since the tumor margins are seldom clinically apparent. Microscopically controlled excision (a modified Mohs technique) is used by some dermatologists to achieve complete excision. Selected cases may be treated by other methods such as radiotherapy or cryotherapy with liquid nitrogen.

B. Squamous Cell Carcinoma: Squamous cell carcinomas also grow slowly and painlessly, often starting as a hyperkeratotic nodule that may become

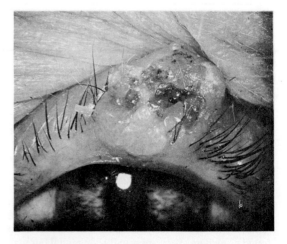

Figure 4–12. Squamous cell carcinoma of upper lid. (Courtesy of A Rosenberg.)

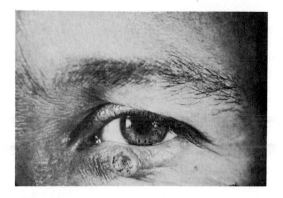

Figure 4–13. Basal cell carcinoma of left lower lid. (Courtesy of S Mettier, Jr.)

ulcerated. Benign inflammatory tumors such as keratoacanthomas may closely resemble carcinomas. The correct diagnosis may depend on biopsy. Like basal cell carcinomas, these tumors can invade and erode through adjacent tissue; they can also spread to regional lymph nodes via the lymphatic system.

C. Sebaceous Gland Carcinoma: Sebaceous gland carcinomas most often arise from the meibomian glands and the glands of Zeis but can also occur in the sebaceous glands of the eyebrow or caruncle. About half resemble benign inflammatory lesions and disorders such as chalazia and chronic blepharitis. They are more aggressive than squamous cell carcinomas, often extending into the orbit, invading lymphatics, and metastasizing.

Carcinoma Associated With Xeroderma Pigmentosum

This rare disease is characterized by the appearance of a large number of freckles in sun-exposed areas of the skin. These are followed by telangiectases, atrophic patches, and eventually a warty growth that may undergo carcinomatous degeneration. The eyelids are frequently affected and may be the first area to show degenerative changes, causing atrophy and ectropion with secondary inflammatory changes of the conjunctiva, symblepharon, corneal ulceration, and carcinoma of the lids. Malignant tumors include basal cell carcinomas, squamous cell carcinomas, and malignant melanomas. This condition is inherited as an autosomal recessive trait. Carriers can often be identified by excessive freckling.

The disease appears early in life and in most cases is fatal by adolescence as a result of metastasis. Life may be prolonged by carefully protecting the skin from actinic rays and treating carcinomatous tumors as rapidly as they appear.

Sarcoma

Soft tissue sarcomas of the orbit are rare and usually are anterior extensions of orbital tumors. Rhabdomyosarcomas involving the lids and orbit are the most common primary malignant tumors found in these tissues in the first decade of life. The lid tumor may be the first sign. A combination of radiotherapy and chemotherapy is usually effective in preserving ocular function and preventing death.

Malignant Melanoma

Malignant melanomas of the eyelids are similar to those elsewhere in the skin and include three distinct varieties: superficial spreading melanoma, lentigo maligna melanoma, and nodular melanoma. Not all malignant melanomas are pigmented. Most pigmented lesions on the eyelid skin are not melanomas. Therefore, biopsy should be used to establish the diagnosis. The prognosis for melanomas of the skin depends upon the depth of invasion or the thickness of the lesion. Tumors less than 0.76 mm in thickness rarely metastasize.

II. LACRIMAL APPARATUS

The lacrimal system incorporates structures involved in the production and drainage of tears. The secretory component consists of the glands that produce the various ingredients of tear fluid. The nasolacrimal ductules form the excretory element of the system, depositing these secretions into the nose. The tear fluid is distributed over the surface of the eye by the action of blinking.

LACRIMAL SECRETORY SYSTEM

The largest volume of tear fluid is produced by the major lacrimal gland located in the lacrimal fossa in the superior temporal quadrant of the orbit. This almond-shaped gland is divided by the lateral horn of the levator aponeurosis into a larger orbital lobe and a smaller palpebral lobe, each with its own ductule system emptying into the superior temporal fornix (Chapter 1). The palpebral lobe can sometimes be visualized by everting the upper lid. The secretions from the main lacrimal gland are triggered by emotion or physical irritation and cause tears to flow copiously over the lid margin (epiphora). Innervation of the main gland is from the pontine lacrimal nucleus through the nervus intermedius and along an elaborate pathway of the maxillary division of the trigeminal nerve. Denervation is a common consequence of acoustic neuroma and other tumors of the cerebellopontine angle.

The accessory lacrimal glands, although only one-tenth the mass of the major gland, have an essential role. The glands of Krause and Wolfring are identical to the major gland but lack a ductile system. These glands are located in the conjunctiva, mainly in the superior fornix. Unicellular goblet cells, also scattered throughout the conjunctiva, secrete glycoprotein in the form of mucin. Modified sebaceous meibomian and zeisian glands of the lid margin contribute lipid to the tears. The glands of Moll are modified sweat glands that also add to the tear film.

The accessory glands are known as the "basic secretors." Their emissions are sufficient to maintain the cornea without those of the main lacrimal gland. Loss of goblet cells, however, leads to drying of the cornea despite profuse tearing from the lacrimal gland.

DISORDERS OF THE SECRETORY SYSTEM

Alacrima

Congenital absence of tearing occurs in Riley-Day syndrome (familial dysautonomia) and anhidrotic ectodermal dysplasia. Although initially asymptomatic, patients may develop signs typical of keratoconjunctivitis sicca. Absence of tears may also occur after disruption of the lacrimal secretory nerve by acoustic neuroma or following surgery of the cerebellopontine angle. Tumors or inflammation of the lacrimal gland may reduce tear production.

Lacrimal Hypersecretion

Primary hypersecretion is rare and must be distinguished from tearing due to obstruction of the excretory ductules. Secondary hypersecretion may be psychogenic or reflex from irritation of surface epithelium or retina. It is possible to stop hypersecretion by blocking the lacrimal secretory nerve in the sphenopalatine ganglion.

Paradoxic Lacrimation ("Crocodile Tears")

This condition is characterized by tearing while eating. Although it may be congenital, it is usually acquired after Bell's palsy and is the result of aberrant regeneration of the facial nerve.

Bloody Tears

This is a rare clinical entity attributed to a variety of causes. It has been associated with menstruation ("vicarious menses"). Blood-tinged tears may be secondary to conjunctival hemorrhage due to any cause (trauma, blood dyscrasia, etc) or to tumors of the lacrimal sac. They have also been reported in a hypertensive patient suffering from epistaxis with extension through the nasolacrimal duct.

Dacryoadenitis

Acute inflammation of the lacrimal gland is a rare condition most often seen in children as a complica-

tion of mumps, measles, or influenza and in adults in association with gonorrhea. Chronic dacryoadenitis may be the result of benign lymphocytic infiltration, lymphoma, leukemia, or tuberculosis (Chapter 16). It is occasionally seen bilaterally as a manifestation of sarcoidosis. When combined with parotid gland swelling, it is called Mikulicz's syndrome.

Considerable pain, swelling, and injection occur over the temporal aspect of the upper eyelid, which often imparts to it an {S}-shaped curve. If bacterial infection is present, systemic antibiotics are given. It is rarely necessary to surgically drain the infection.

LACRIMAL EXCRETORY SYSTEM

The excretory system is composed of the puncta, canaliculi, lacrimal sac, and nasolacrimal duct (see Chapter 1). With each blink, the eyelids close like a zipper—beginning laterally, distributing tears evenly across the cornea, and delivering them to the excretory system on the medial aspect of the lids. Under normal circumstances, tears are produced at about their rate of evaporation, and for that reason few pass through the excretory system. When tears flood the conjunctival sac, they enter the puncta partially by capillary attraction. With lid closure, the specialized portion of pretarsal orbicularis surrounding the ampulla tightens to prevent their escape. Simultaneously, the lid is drawn toward the posterior lacrimal crest, and traction is placed on the fascia surrounding the lacrimal sac, causing the canaliculus to shorten and creating negative pressure within the sac. This dynamic pumping action draws tears into the sac which then pass by gravity and tissue elasticity through the nasolacrimal duct into the inferior meatus of the nose. Valve-like folds of the epithelial lining of the sac tend to resist the retrograde flow of tears and air. The most developed of these flaps is the "valve" of Hasner at the distal end of the nasolacrimal duct. This structure is important because when imperforate in infants it is the cause of congenital obstruction and chronic dacryocystitis.

DISORDERS OF THE EXCRETORY SYSTEM

1. DACRYOCYSTITIS (Figure 4–14)

Infection of the lacrimal sac is a common disease that usually occurs in infants or postmenopausal women. It is most often unilateral and always secondary to obstruction of the nasolacrimal duct. In many adult cases, the cause of obstruction remains unknown.

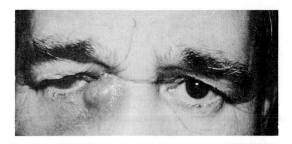

Figure 4–14. Acute dacryocystitis.

Dacryocystitis is uncommon in the intermediate age groups unless it follows trauma or is caused by a dacryolith. Spontaneous improvement follows passage of a dacryolith, but recurrence is the rule.

In infants, chronic infection accompanies nasolacrimal duct obstruction, but acute dacryocystitis is uncommon. Acute dacryocystitis in children is often a result of *Haemophilus influenzae* infection. Prompt and aggressive treatment should be instituted because of the risk of orbital cellulitis.

Acute dacryocystitis in adults is usually caused by *Staphylococcus aureus* or occasionally β-hemolytic streptococci. In chronic dacryocystitis, *Streptococcus pneumoniae* or, rarely, *Candida albicans* is the predominant organism—mixed infections do not occur. The infectious agent can be identified microscopically by staining a conjunctival smear taken after expression of the tear sac.

Clinical Findings

The chief symptoms of dacryocystitis are tearing and discharge. In the acute form, inflammation, pain, swelling, and tenderness are present in the tear sac area. Purulent material can be expressed from the sac. In the chronic form, tearing is usually the only sign. Mucoid material can usually be expressed from the sac. It is curious that dacryocystitis is seldom complicated by conjunctivitis even though the conjunctival sac is constantly being bathed with pus exuding through the lacrimal puncta. Corneal ulcer occasionally occurs following minor corneal trauma in the presence of pneumococcal dacryocystitis.

Treatment

Acute dacryocystitis usually responds to appropriate systemic antibiotics, and the chronic form can often be kept latent with antibiotic drops. However, relief of obstruction is the only cure.

In adults, the presence of a mucocele is evidence that the site of obstruction is in the nasolacrimal duct and that **dacryocystorhinostomy** is indicated. The patency of the canalicular system is ensured if mucus or pus is regurgitated through the puncta on compression of the sac. Examination of the nose is important to ensure adequate drainage space between the septum and the lateral nasal wall. Dacryocystorhinostomy consists of forming a permanent anastomosis between the lacrimal sac and the nose. Exposure is gained by an incision over the anterior lacrimal crest. A bony opening is made in the lateral wall of the nose, and the nasal mucosa is sutured to the mucosa of the lacrimal sac. An endoscopic approach through the nose using laser to help form the opening between the lacrimal sac and the nasal cavity is an alternative.

Excessive tearing (epiphora) is occasionally due to canalicular stenosis (see below) or obstruction at the junction of the common canaliculus and lacrimal sac. In either case, compression of the sac does not cause regurgitation of fluid, mucus, or pus through the puncta, and no mucocele is present. Intubation and irrigation of the canalicular system with a lacrimal cannula and x-ray studies with contrast media (dacryocystography) may identify the site of obstruction. Common canalicular obstruction may be treated by intubation of the passages with silicone stents for 3–6 months. A thick obstructing scar, however, will necessitate dacryocystorhinostomy and canaliculoplasty with silicone intubation of the canalicular system.

In **infantile dacryocystitis,** the site of stenosis is usually at the valve of Hasner. Failure of canalization is a common occurrence (4–7% of newborns), but normally the duct opens spontaneously within the first month. Forceful compression of the lacrimal sac will sometimes rupture the membrane and establish patency. If stenosis persists more than 6 months or if dacryocystitis develops, probing of the duct is indicated. One probing is effective in 75% of cases. In the remainder, cure can almost always be achieved by repeated probing, by inward fracture of the inferior turbinate, or by a temporary silicone lacrimal splint. Probing should not be attempted in the presence of acute infection. Probing is notably unsuccessful in adults.

2. CANALICULAR DISORDERS

Congenital anomalies of the canalicular system include imperforate puncta, accessory puncta, canalicular fistulas, and, rarely, agenesis of the canalicular system. Most cases of canalicular stenosis are acquired, usually the result of viral infections—notably varicella, herpes simplex, and adenovirus infection. Obstruction—even obliteration—may occur with Stevens-Johnson syndrome, pemphigoid, and other conjunctival shrinkage diseases. Systemic chemotherapy with fluorouracil and topical idoxuridine may also cause obstruction. Canaliculitis is an uncommon chronic unilateral infection caused by *Actinomyces israelii* (Figure 4–15), *Candida albicans,* or *Aspergillus* species. It affects the lower canaliculus more often than the upper, occurs exclusively in adults, and causes a secondary purulent conjunctivitis that frequently escapes etiologic diagnosis. Untreated, it will result in canalicular stenosis. The patient complains of a mildly

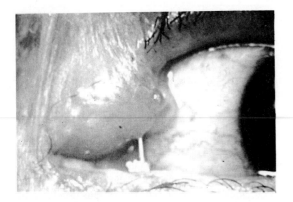

Figure 4–15. *Actinomyces israelii* canaliculitis, left eye. (Courtesy of P Thygeson.)

red and irritated eye with a slight discharge. The punctum usually pouts, and material can be expressed from the canaliculus. The organism can be seen microscopically on a direct smear taken from the canaliculus. Curettage of the necrotic material in the involved canaliculus, followed by irrigation, is usually effective in establishing patency. Canaliculotomy is sometimes necessary. Tincture of iodine may be applied to the lining of the canaliculus after canaliculotomy. Recurrence is common.

Total canalicular obstruction necessitates use of an artificial tear duct for relief of epiphora (conjunctivodacryocystorhinostomy). A Pyrex glass tube is placed between the conjunctival sac and the nasal cavity.

Closure of the punctum is sometimes performed in patients with keratitis sicca to allow tears to remain in the conjunctival sac. Temporary closure may be done with silicone or collagen plugs in the canaliculi or by sealing the punctum with a hot cautery. The temporary obstruction will provide an opportunity to evaluate the effect. Permanent closure may be accomplished by deep cautery within the ampulla with thermal, electrocautery, or laser energy or by dividing the canaliculus surgically.

III. TEARS

John P. Whitcher, MD

Tears form a thin layer approximately 7–10 μm thick that covers the corneal and conjunctival epithelium. The functions of this ultrathin layer are (1) to make the cornea a smooth optical surface by abolishing minute surface epithelial irregularities; (2) to wet and protect the delicate surface of the corneal and conjunctival epithelium; (3) to inhibit the growth of microorganisms by mechanical flushing and antimicrobial action; and (4) to provide the cornea with necessary nutrient substances.

LAYERS OF THE TEAR FILM

The tear film is composed of three layers (Figure 4–16): (1) The superficial layer is a monomolecular film of lipid derived from meibomian glands. It is thought to retard evaporation and form a watertight seal when the lids are closed. (2) The middle aqueous layer is elaborated by the major and minor lacrimal glands and contains water-soluble substances (salts and proteins). (3) The deep mucinous layer is composed of glycoprotein and overlies the corneal and conjunctival epithelial cells. The epithelial cell membranes are composed of lipoproteins and are therefore relatively hydrophobic. Such a surface cannot be wetted with an aqueous solution alone. Mucin is partly adsorbed onto the corneal epithelial cell membranes and is anchored by the microvilli of the surface epithelial cells. This provides a new hydrophilic surface for the aqueous tears to spread over which is wetted by a lowering of surface tension.

COMPOSITION OF TEARS

The normal tear volume is estimated to be 7 ± 2 μL in each eye. Albumin accounts for 60% of the total protein in tear fluid. Globulin and lysozymes are divided equally in the remainder. Immunoglobulins IgA, IgG, and IgE are present. IgA predominates, and differs from serum IgA in that it is not transudated from serum only but is produced by plasma cells located in the

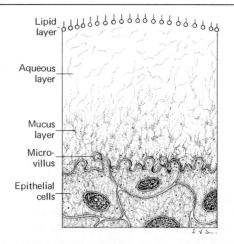

Figure 4–16. The three layers of the tear film covering the superficial epithelial layer of the cornea.

lacrimal gland. In certain allergic conditions such as vernal conjunctivitis, the IgE concentration of tear fluid increases. Tear lysozymes form 21–25% of the total protein and—acting synergistically with gamma globulins and other nonlysozyme antibacterial factors—represent an important defense mechanism against infection. Other tear enzymes may also play a role in diagnosis of certain clinical entities, eg, hexoseaminidase assay for diagnosis of Tay-Sachs disease.

K$^+$, Na$^+$, and Cl$^-$ occur in higher concentrations in tears than in plasma. Tears also contain a small amount of glucose (5 mg/dL) and urea (0.04 mg/dL), and changes in blood concentration parallel changes in tear glucose and urea levels. The average pH of tears is 7.35, though a wide normal variation exists (5.20–8.35). Under normal conditions, tear fluid is isotonic. Tear film osmolality ranges from 295 to 309 mosm/L.

DRY EYE SYNDROME
(Keratoconjunctivitis Sicca)

Dryness of the eye may result from any disease associated with deficiency of the tear film components (aqueous, mucin, or lipid), lid surface abnormalities, or epithelial abnormalities. Although there are many forms of keratoconjunctivitis sicca, those connected with rheumatoid arthritis and other autoimmune diseases are commonly referred to as Sjögren's syndrome.

Etiology

Many of the causes of dry eye syndrome affect more than one component of the tear film or lead to ocular surface alterations that secondarily cause tear film instability. Histopathologic features include the appearance of dry spots on the corneal and conjunctival epithelium, formation of filaments, loss of conjunctival goblet cells, abnormal enlargement of nongoblet epithelial cells, increased cellular stratification, and increased keratinization. The etiology and diagnosis of keratoconjunctivitis sicca are summarized in Table 4–2.

Clinical Findings

Patients with dry eyes complain most frequently of a scratchy or sandy (foreign body) sensation. Other common symptoms are itching, excessive mucus secretion, inability to produce tears, a burning sensation, photosensitivity, redness, pain, and difficulty in moving the lids. In most patients, the most remarkable feature of the eye examination is the grossly normal appearance of the eye. The most characteristic feature on slitlamp examination is the interrupted or absent tear meniscus at the lower lid margin. Tenacious yellowish mucus strands are sometimes seen in the lower conjunctival fornix. The bulbar conjunctiva loses its normal luster and may be thickened, edematous, and hyperemic.

The corneal epithelium shows varying degrees of fine punctate stippling in the interpalpebral fissure. The damaged corneal and conjunctival epithelial cells stain with 1% rose bengal (Figure 4–17), and defects in the corneal epithelium stain with fluorescein. In the late stages of keratoconjunctivitis sicca, filaments may be seen—one end of each filament attached to the corneal epithelium and the other end moving freely (Figure 4–18).

In patients with Sjögren's syndrome, conjunctival scrapings may show increased numbers of goblet cells. Lacrimal gland enlargement occurs uncommonly in patients with Sjögren's syndrome. Diagnosis and grading of the dry eye condition can be achieved with good accuracy using the following diagnostic methods:

A. Schirmer Test: This test is done by drying the tear film and inserting Schirmer strips (Whatman filter paper No. 41) into the lower conjunctival cul-de-sac at the junction of the mid and temporal thirds of the lower lid. The moistened exposed portion is measured 5 minutes after insertion. Less than 10 mm of wetting without anesthesia is considered abnormal.

When performed without anesthesia, the test measures the function of the main lacrimal gland, whose secretory activity is stimulated by the irritating nature of the filter paper. Schirmer tests performed after topical anesthesia (0.5% tetracaine) measure the function of the accessory lacrimal glands (the basic secretors). Less than 5 mm in 5 minutes is abnormal.

The Schirmer test is a screening test for assessment of tear production. False-positive and false-negative results occur. Low readings are sporadically found in normals, and normal tests may occur in dry eyes—especially those secondary to mucin deficiency.

B. Tear Film Break-Up Time: Measurement of the tear film break-up time may sometimes be useful to estimate the mucin content of tear fluid. Deficiency in mucin may not affect the Schirmer test but may lead to instability of the tear film. This causes the film's rapid break-up. "Dry spots" (Figure 4–19) are formed in the tear film, and exposure of the corneal or conjunctival epithelium follows. This process ultimately damages the epithelial cells, which can then be stained with rose bengal. Damaged epithelial cells may be shed from the cornea, leaving areas susceptible to punctate staining when the corneal surface is flooded with fluorescein.

The tear film break-up time can be measured by applying a slightly moistened fluorescein strip to the bulbar conjunctiva and asking the patient to blink. The tear film is then scanned with the aid of the cobalt filter on the slitlamp while the patient refrains from blinking. The time that elapses before the first dry spot appears in the corneal fluorescein layer is the tear film break-up time. Normally, the break-up time is over 15 seconds, but it will be reduced appreciably by the use of local anesthetics, by manipulating the eye, or by hold-

Table 4–2. Etiology and diagnosis of dry eye syndrome.

I. Etiology

A. Conditions Characterized by Hypofunction of the Lacrimal Gland:
  1. Congenital–
    a. Familial dysautonomia (Riley-Day syndrome)
    b. Aplasia of the lacrimal gland (congenital alacrima)
    c. Trigeminal nerve aplasia
    d. Ectodermal dysplasia
  2. Acquired–
    a. Systemic diseases–
      (1) Sjögren's syndrome
      (2) Progressive systemic sclerosis
      (3) Sarcoidosis
      (4) Leukemia, lymphoma
      (5) Amyloidosis
      (6) Hemochromatosis
    b. Infection–
      (1) Trachoma
      (2) Mumps
    c. Injury–
      (1) Surgical removal of lacrimal gland
      (2) Irradiation
      (3) Chemical burn
    d. Medications–
      (1) Antihistamines
      (2) Antimuscarinics: atropine, scopolamine
      (3) General anesthetics: halothane, nitrous oxide
      (4) Beta-adrenergic blockers: timolol, practolol
    e. Neurogenic–Neuroparalytic (facial nerve palsy)

B. Conditions Characterized by Mucin Deficiency:
  1. Avitaminosis A
  2. Stevens-Johnson syndrome
  3. Ocular pemphigoid
  4. Chronic conjunctivitis, eg, trachoma
  5. Chemical burns

6. Medications–Antihistamines, antimuscarinic agents, beta-adrenergic blocking agents (eg, practolol)
  7. Folk remedies, eg, kermes

C. Conditions Characterized by Lipid Deficiency:
  1. Lid margin scarring
  2. Blepharitis

D. Defective Spreading of Tear Film Caused by the Following:
  1. Eyelid abnormalities–
    a. Defects, coloboma
    b. Ectropion or entropion
    c. Keratinization of lid margin
    d. Decreased or absent blinking
      (1) Neurologic disorders
      (2) Hyperthyroidism
      (3) Contact lens
      (4) Drugs
      (5) Herpes simplex keratitis
      (6) Leprosy
    e. Lagophthalmos–
      (1) Nocturnal lagophthalmos
      (2) Hyperthyroidism
      (3) Leprosy
  2. Conjunctival abnormalities–
    a. Pterygium
    b. Symblepharon
  3. Proptosis

II. Diagnostic Tests:

A. Biomicroscopy
B. Rose bengal staining
C. Fluorescein staining
D. Tear break-up time
E. Tear film osmolality
F. Tear lysozyme
G. Schirmer test without anesthesia
H. Impression cytology
I. Ocular ferning test
J. Tear lactoferrin

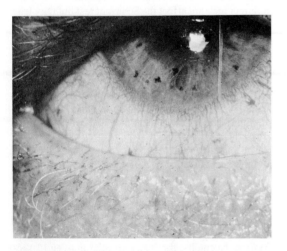

Figure 4–17. Rose bengal staining of corneal and conjunctival cells in a 54-year-old woman with keratoconjunctivitis sicca.

ing the lids open. The break-up time is shorter in eyes with aqueous tear deficiency and is always shorter than normal in eyes with mucin deficiency.

C. Ocular Ferning Test: A simple and inexpensive qualitative test for the study of conjunctival mucus is performed by drying conjunctival scrapings on a clean glass slide. Microscopic arborization (ferning) is observed in normal eyes. In patients with cicatrizing conjunctivitis (ocular pemphigoid, Stevens-Johnson syndrome, diffuse conjunctival cicatrization), ferning of the mucus is reduced or absent.

D. Impression Cytology: Impression cytology is a method by which goblet cell densities on the conjunctival surface can be counted. In normal persons, the goblet cell population is highest in the infranasal quadrant. Loss of goblet cells has been documented in cases of keratoconjunctivitis sicca, trachoma, cicatricial ocular pemphigoid, Stevens-Johnson syndrome, and avitaminosis A.

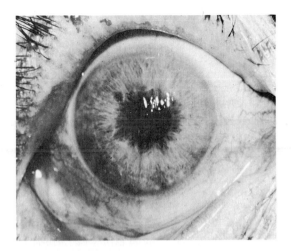

Figure 4–18. Corneal filaments in a 56-year-old patient with keratoconjunctivitis sicca.

E. Fluorescein Staining: Touching the conjunctiva with a dry strip of fluorescein is a good indicator of wetness, and the tear meniscus can be seen easily. Fluorescein will stain the eroded and denuded areas as well as microscopic defects of the corneal epithelium.

F. Rose Bengal Staining: Rose bengal is more sensitive than fluorescein. The dye will stain all desic-

cated nonvital epithelial cells of the cornea as well as conjunctiva.

G. Tear Lysozyme Assay: Reduction in tear lysozyme concentration usually occurs early in the course of Sjögren's syndrome and is helpful in the diagnosis of that disorder. Tears can be collected on Schirmer strips and assayed. The most common method is spectrophotometric assay.

H. Tear Osmolality: Hyperosmolality of tears has been documented in keratoconjunctivitis sicca and in contact lens wearers and is thought to be a consequence of decreased corneal sensitivity. Reports claim that hyperosmolality is the most specific test for keratoconjunctivitis sicca. It can occur even with normal A Schirmer test and normal rose bengal staining.

I. Lactoferrin: Tear fluid lactoferrin is low in patients with hyposecretion of the lacrimal gland. Testing kits are commercially available.

Complications

Early in the course of keratoconjunctivitis sicca, vision is slightly impaired. As the condition worsens, discomfort can become disabling. In advanced cases, corneal ulceration, corneal thinning, and perforation may develop. Secondary bacterial infection occasionally occurs, and corneal scarring and vascularization may result in marked reduction in vision. Early treatment may prevent these complications.

Treatment

The patient should understand that dry eyes is a chronic condition and complete relief is unlikely except in mild cases when the corneal and conjunctival epithelial changes are reversible. Artificial tears are the mainstay of treatment. Ointment is useful for prolonged lubrication, especially when sleeping. Additional relief can be achieved by using humidifiers, moisture chamber spectacles, or swim goggles.

The primary function of these measures is fluid replacement. Restoration of mucin is a more formidable task. In recent years, high-molecular-weight water-soluble polymers have been added to artificial tears in an attempt to improve and prolong surface wetting. Other mucomimetic agents include sodium hyaluronate and solutions of the patient's own serum as eye drops. If the mucus is tenacious, as in Sjögren's syndrome, mucolytic agents (eg, acetylcysteine 10%) are helpful.

Patients with excessive tear lipids require specific instructions for removal of lipid from the eyelid margin. Antibiotics topically or systemically may be necessary. Topical vitamin A may be useful in reversing ocular surface metaplasia.

All chemical preservatives in artificial tears induce a certain amount of corneal toxicity. Benzalkonium chloride is the most damaging of the commonly used preparations. Patients who require frequent drops fare

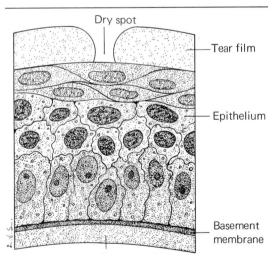

Figure 4–19. Baring of the corneal epithelium following formation of a dry spot in the tear film. (Modified and redrawn from Dohlman CH: The function of the corneal epithelium in health and disease. Invest Ophthalmol 1971;10:383.)

better with nonpreserved solutions. Preservatives can also cause idiosyncratic reactions. This is most common with thimerosal.

Patients with dry eyes from any cause are more likely to have concurrent infections. Chronic blepharitis is common and should be treated with hygiene and topical antibiotics. Acne rosacea is associated with keratoconjunctivitis sicca, and treatment with systemic tetracycline may be helpful.

Surgical treatment for dry eyes includes insertion of temporary (collagen) or extended (silicone) punctal plugs to retain lacrimal secretions. Permanent closure of the puncta and canaliculi can be done by thermal, electrocautery, or laser treatment.

REFERENCES

American Academy of Ophthalmology: Botulinum toxin therapy of eye muscle disorders: safety and effectiveness. Ophthalmology 1989;6(Suppl):37.

Anderson RL: Age of aponeurotic awareness. Ophthal Plast Reconstr Surg 1985;1:77.

Beard C: A new classification of blepharoptosis. Int Ophthalmol Clin 1989;29:214.

Beard C: Ptosis surgery past, present, future. Ophthal Plast Reconstr Surg 1985;1:69.

Bedford MA: Color Atlas of Ocular Tumors. Year Book, 1979.

Bullock JD, Goldberg SH: Lacrimal sac diverticula. Arch Ophthalmol 1989;107:753.

Callahan MA: Surgically mismanaged ptosis associated with double elevator palsy. Arch Ophthalmol 1981;99:108.

Callahan MA, Beard C: Beard's Ptosis, 4th ed. Aesculapius, 1990.

Char DH: Clinical Ocular Oncology. Churchill Livingstone, 1989.

Clarke JR, Spalton DJ: Treatment of senile entropion with botulinum toxin. Br J Ophthalmol 1988;72:361.

Collin JRO, O'Donnell BA: Adjustable sutures in eyelid surgery for ptosis and lid retraction. Br J Ophthalmol 1994;78:167.

Collin JRO, Rathbun JE: Involutional entropion. Arch Ophthalmol 1978;96:1058.

Custer PL, Tenzel RR, Kowalczyk AP: Blepharochalasis syndrome. Am J Ophthalmol 1985;99:424.

Doxanas MT, Green WR, Iliff CE: Factors in the successful surgical management of basal cell carcinoma of the eyelids. Am J Ophthalmol 1981;91:726.

Dutton J: Management of periocular basal cell carcinoma: Mohs' micrographic surgery versus radiotherapy. Surv Ophthalmol 1993;38:193.

Engstrom PF et al: Effectiveness of botulinum toxin therapy for essential blepharospasm. Ophthalmology 1987;94:971.

Frueh BR, Schoengarth LD: Evaluation and treatment of the patient with ectropion. Ophthalmology 1982;89:1049.

Garland PE, Patrinely JR, Anderson RL: Hemifacial spasm: Results of unilateral myectomy. Ophthalmology 1987; 94:288.

Goldberg RA, Shorr N: Complications of blepharopigmentation. Ophthalmic Surg 1989;20:420.

Johnson CC: Developmental abnormalities of the eyelids. Ophthalmic Plast Reconstr Surg 1986;2:2.

Jones LT: The lacrimal secretory system and its treatment. Am J Ophthalmol 1966;62:47.

Jones LT, Wobig JL: Surgery of the Eyelids and Lacrimal Apparatus. Aesculapius, 1976.

Jordan DR et al: Essential blepharospasm and related dystonias. Surv Ophthalmol 1989;34:123.

Kushner BJ: Congenital nasolacrimal system obstruction. Arch Ophthalmol 1982;100:597.

Lemp MA: Recent developments in dry eye management. Ophthalmology 1987;94:1299.

Lowery JC, Bartley GB: Complications of blepharoplasty. Surv Ophthalmol 1994;38:327.

Noda S, Hayasaka S, Setogawa T: Epiblepharon with inverted eyelashes in Japanese children. Br J Ophthalmol 1989;73:126.

Quickert MH: The eyelids. In: Modern Ophthalmology. Vols 3 and 4. Sorsby A (editor). Butterworths, 1972.

Rao NA et al: Sebaceous carcinomas of the ocular adnexa. Hum Pathol 1982;13:113.

Sevel D: Ptosis and underaction of the superior rectus muscle. Ophthalmology 1984;91:1080.

Shields CL et al: Clinicopathologic review of 142 cases of lacrimal gland lesions. Ophthalmology 1989;96:431.

Small RG, Sabates NR, Burrows D: The measurement and definition of ptosis. Ophthalmic Plast Reconstr Surg 1989;5:171.

Spencer WH (editor): Ophthalmic Pathology, 3rd ed. 3 vols. Saunders, 1985.

Stewart WB (editor): Surgery of the Eyelid, Orbit and Lacrimal System. American Academy of Ophthalmology, Manuals Program, 1993.

Sullivan JH, Beard C, Bullock JD: Cryosurgery for treatment of trichiasis. Am J Ophthalmol 1976;82:117.

Thygeson P: Complications of staphylococcic blepharitis. Am J Ophthalmol 1969;68:446.

Tucker SM, Linberg JV: Vascular anatomy of the eyelids. Ophthalmology 1994;101:1118.

Woog JJ, Metson R, Puliafito CA: Holmium:YAG endonasal laser dacryocystorhinostomy. Am J Ophthalmol 1993; 116:1.

Conjunctiva

5

Ivan R. Schwab, MD, & Chandler R. Dawson, MD

I. CONJUNCTIVITIS

Inflammation of the conjunctiva (conjunctivitis) is the most common eye disease worldwide. It varies in severity from a mild hyperemia with tearing to a severe conjunctivitis with copious purulent discharge. The cause is usually exogenous, but it may be endogenous.

CONJUNCTIVITIS DUE TO INFECTIOUS AGENTS

The types of conjunctivitis and their commonest causes are set forth in Tables 5–1 and 5–2.

Because of its location, the conjunctiva is exposed to many microorganisms and other stressful environmental factors. Several mechanisms protect the surface of the eye from external substances: In the tear film, the aqueous component dilutes infectious material, mucus traps debris, and a pumping action of the lids constantly flushes the tears to the tear duct; the tears contain antimicrobial substances, including lysozyme and antibodies (IgG and IgA).

Common pathogens that can cause conjunctivitis include *Streptococcus pneumoniae, Haemophilus influenzae, Staphylococcus aureus, Neisseria meningitidis,* most human adenovirus strains, herpes simplex virus type 1 and type 2, and two picornaviruses. Two sexually transmitted agents that cause conjunctivitis are *Chlamydia trachomatis* and *Neisseria gonorrhoeae.*

Cytology of Conjunctivitis

Damage to the conjunctival epithelium by a noxious agent may be followed by epithelial edema, cellular death and exfoliation, epithelial hypertrophy, or granuloma formation. There may also be edema of the conjunctival stroma (chemosis) and hypertrophy of the lymphoid layer of the stroma (follicle formation). Inflammatory cells, including neutrophils, eosinophils, basophils, lymphocytes, and plasma cells, may be seen and often indicate the nature of the damaging agent. The inflammatory cells migrate from the conjunctival stroma through the epithelium to the surface. They then combine with fibrin and mucus from the goblet cells to form the conjunctival exudate, which is responsible for the "mattering" on the lid margins (especially in the morning).

The inflammatory cells appear in the exudate or in scrapings taken with a sterile platinum spatula from the anesthetized conjunctival surface. The material is stained with Gram's stain (to identify the bacterial organisms) and with Giemsa's stain (to identify the cell types and morphology). A predominance of polymorphonuclear leukocytes is characteristic of bacterial conjunctivitis. Generally, a predominance of mononuclear cells—especially lymphocytes—is characteristic of viral conjunctivitis. If a pseudomembrane or true membrane is present (eg, epidemic keratoconjunctivitis or herpes simplex virus conjunctivitis), neutrophils then predominate because of coexistent necrosis. In chlamydial conjunctivitis, neutrophils and lymphocytes are usually present in equal numbers.

In allergic conjunctivitis, eosinophils and basophils are frequently present in conjunctival biopsies, but they are less common on conjunctival smears; eosinophils or eosinophilic granules are commonly found in vernal keratoconjunctivitis. Eosinophils and basophils are found in allergic conjunctivitis, and scattered eosinophilic granules and eosinophils are found in vernal keratoconjunctivitis. In all types of conjunctivitis, there are plasma cells in the conjunctival stroma. They do not migrate through the epithelium, however, and are therefore not seen in smears of exudate or of scrapings from the conjunctival surface unless the epithelium has become necrotic, as it may in trachoma; in this event, the rupturing of a follicle allows the plasma cells to reach the epithelial surface. Since the mature follicles of trachoma rupture easily, the finding of large, pale-staining lymphoblastic (germinal center) cells in scrapings strongly suggests trachoma.

Symptoms of Conjunctivitis

The important symptoms of conjunctivitis are a foreign body sensation, a scratching or burning sensation,

Table 5–1. Causes of conjunctivitis.

Bacterial
  Hyperacute (purulent)
    Neisseria gonorrhoeae
    Neisseria meningitidis
    Neisseria gonorrhoeae subsp *kochii*
  Acute (mucopurulent)
    Pneumococcus *(Streptococcus pneumoniae)* (temperate climates)
    Haemophilus aegyptius (Koch-Weeks bacillus) (tropical climates)
  Subacute
    Haemophilus influenzae (temperate climates)
  Chronic, including blepharoconjunctivitis
    Staphylococcus aureus
    Moraxella lacunata (diplobacillus of Morax-Axenfeld)
  Rare types (acute, subacute, chronic)
    Streptococci
    Moraxella catarrhalis
    Coliforms
    Proteus
    Corynebacterium diphtheriae
    Mycobacterium tuberculosis

Chlamydial
  Trachoma *(Chlamydia trachomatis* serotypes A–C)
  Inclusion conjunctivitis *(Chlamydia trachomatis* serotypes D–K)
  Lymphogranuloma venereum (LGV) *(Chlamydia trachomatis* serotypes L1–3)

Viral
  Acute viral follicular conjunctivitis
    Pharyngoconjunctival fever due to adenoviruses types 3 and 7 and other serotypes
    Epidemic keratoconjunctivitis due to adenovirus types 8 and 19
    Herpes simplex virus
    Acute hemorrhagic conjunctivitis due to enterovirus type 70; rarely, coxsackievirus type A24
  Chronic viral follicular conjunctivitis
    Molluscum contagiosum virus
  Viral blepharoconjunctivitis
    Varicella, herpes zoster due to varicella-zoster virus
    Measles virus

Rickettsial (rare)
  Nonpurulent conjunctivitis with hyperemia and minimal infiltration, often a feature of rickettsial diseases
    Typhus
    Murine typhus
    Scrub typhus
    Rocky Mountain spotted fever
    Mediterranean fever
    Q fever

Fungal (rare)
  Chronic exudative
    Candida
  Granulomatous
    Rhinosporidium seeberi
    Coccidioides immitis (San Joaquin Valley fever)
    Sporothrix schenckii

Parasitic (rare but important)
  Chronic conjunctivitis and blepharoconjunctivitis
    Onchocerca volvulus (Central America, Africa)
    Thelazia californiensis
    Loa loa
    Ascaris lumbricoides
    Trichinella spiralis
    Schistosoma haematobium (bladder fluke)
    Taenia solium (cysticercus)
    Pthirus pubis (*Pediculus pubis*, pubic louse)
    Fly larvae (*Oestrus ovis*, etc) (ocular myiasis)

Immunologic (allergic)
  Immediate (humoral) hypersensitivity reactions
    Hay fever conjunctivitis (pollens, grasses, animal danders, etc)
    Vernal keratoconjunctivitis

(continued)

Table 5–1. Causes of conjunctivitis. (continued)

Immunologic (allergic) (continued)
    Atopic keratoconjunctivitis
    Giant papillary conjunctivitis
   Delayed (cellular) hypersensitivity reactions
    Phlyctenulosis
    Mild conjunctivitis secondary to contact blepharitis
   Autoimmune disease
    Keratoconjunctivitis sicca associated with Sjögren's syndrome
    Cicatricial pemphigoid

Chemical or irritative
   Iatrogenic
    Miotics
    Idoxuridine
    Other topically applied drugs
    Contact lens solutions
   Occupational
    Acids
    Alkalies
    Smoke
    Wind
    Ultraviolet light
   Caterpillar hair

Etiology unknown
   Folliculosis
   Chronic follicular conjunctivitis (orphan's conjunctivitis, Axenfeld's conjunctivitis)
   Ocular rosacea
   Psoriasis
   Erythema multiforme major (Stevens-Johnson syndrome) and minor
   Dermatitis herpetiformis
   Epidermolysis bullosa
   Superior limbic keratoconjunctivitis
   Ligneous conjunctivitis
   Reiter's syndrome
   Mucocutaneous lymph node syndrome (Kawasaki disease)

Associated with systemic disease
   Thyroid disease (exposure, congestive)
   Gouty conjunctivitis
   Carcinoid conjunctivitis
   Sarcoidosis
   Tuberculosis
   Syphilis

Secondary to dacryocystitis or canaliculitis
   Conjunctivitis secondary to dacryocystitis
    Pneumococci or beta-hemolytic streptococci
   Conjunctivitis secondary to canaliculitis
    Actinomyces israelii, Candida spp, *Aspergillus* spp (rarely)

a sensation of fullness around the eyes, itching, and photophobia.

Foreign body sensation and a scratching or burning sensation are often associated with the swelling and papillary hypertrophy that normally accompany conjunctival hyperemia. If there is pain, the cornea is probably also affected. Pain of the iris or ciliary body is suggestive of corneal involvement.

Signs of Conjunctivitis (Table 5–2)

The important signs of conjunctivitis are hyperemia, tearing, exudation, pseudoptosis, papillary hypertrophy, chemosis, follicles, pseudomembranes and membranes, granulomas, and preauricular adenopathy.

Hyperemia is the most conspicuous clinical sign of acute conjunctivitis. The redness is most marked in the fornix and diminishes toward the limbus by virtue of the dilation of the posterior conjunctival vessels. (A perilimbal dilation or ciliary flush suggests inflammation of the cornea or deeper structures.) A brilliant red suggests bacterial conjunctivitis, and a milky appearance suggests allergic conjunctivitis. Hyperemia without cellular infiltration suggests irritation from physical causes such as wind, sun, smoke, etc, but may occur occasionally with diseases associated with vascular instability (eg, acne rosacea).

Tearing (epiphora) is often prominent in conjunctivitis, the tears resulting from the foreign body sensation, the burning or scratching sensation, or the itch-

Table 5–2. Differentiation of the common types of conjunctivitis.

Clinical Findings and Cytology	Viral	Bacterial	Chlamydial	Allergic
Itching	Minimal	Minimal	Minimal	Severe
Hyperemia	Generalized	Generalized	Generalized	Generalized
Tearing	Profuse	Moderate	Moderate	Moderate
Exudation	Minimal	Profuse	Profuse	Minimal
Preauricular adenopathy	Common	Uncommon	Common only in inclusion conjunctivitis	None
In stained scrapings and exudates	Monocytes	Bacteria, PMNs[1]	PMNs, plasma cells inclusion bodies	Eosinophils
Associated sore throat and fever	Occasionally	Occasionally	Never	Never

[1]Polymorphonuclear cells.

ing. Mild transudation also arises from the hyperemic vessels and adds to the tearing. An abnormally scant secretion of tears suggests keratoconjunctivitis sicca.

Exudation is a feature of all types of acute conjunctivitis. The exudate is flaky and amorphous in bacterial conjunctivitis and stringy in allergic conjunctivitis. "Mattering" of the eyelids occurs upon awakening in almost all types of conjunctivitis, and if the exudate is copious and the lids are firmly stuck together, the conjunctivitis is probably bacterial or chlamydial.

Pseudoptosis is a drooping of the upper lid secondary to infiltration of Müller's muscle. The condition is seen in several types of severe conjunctivitis, eg, trachoma and epidemic keratoconjunctivitis.

Papillary hypertrophy is a nonspecific conjunctival reaction that occurs because the conjunctiva is bound down to the underlying tarsus or limbus by fine fibrils. When the tuft of vessels that forms the substance of the papilla (along with cellular elements and exudates) reaches the basement membrane of the epithelium, it branches over the papilla like the spokes in the frame of an umbrella. An inflammatory exudate accumulates between the fibrils, heaping the conjunctiva into mounds. In necrotizing disease (eg, trachoma), the exudate may be replaced by granulation tissue or connective tissue.

When the papillae are small, the conjunctiva usually has a smooth, velvety appearance. A red papillary conjunctiva suggests bacterial or chlamydial disease (eg, a velvety red tarsal conjunctiva is characteristic of acute trachoma). With marked infiltration of the conjunctiva, giant papillae form which are flat-topped, polygonal, and milky-red in color. On the upper tarsus, they suggest vernal keratoconjunctivitis and giant papillary conjunctivitis with contact lens sensitivities; on the lower tarsus, they suggest atopic keratoconjunctivitis. Giant papillae may also occur at the limbus, especially in the area that is normally exposed when the eyes are open (between 2 and 4 o'clock and between 8 and 10 o'clock). Here they appear as gelatinous

mounds that may encroach on the cornea. Limbal papillae are characteristic of vernal keratoconjunctivitis but are rare in atopic keratoconjunctivitis.

Chemosis of the conjunctiva strongly suggests acute allergic conjunctivitis but may also occur in acute gonococcal or meningococcal conjunctivitis and especially in adenoviral conjunctivitis. Chemosis of the bulbar conjunctiva is seen in patients with trichinosis. Occasionally, chemosis may appear before there is any gross cellular infiltration or exudation.

Follicles are seen in most cases of viral conjunctivitis, in all cases of chlamydial conjunctivitis except neonatal inclusion conjunctivitis, in some cases of parasitic conjunctivitis, and in some cases of toxic conjunctivitis induced by topical medications such as idoxuridine, dipivefrin, and miotics. Follicles in the inferior fornix and at the tarsal margins have limited diagnostic value, but when they are located on the tarsi (especially the upper tarsus), chlamydial, viral, or toxic conjunctivitis (following topical medication) should be suspected.

The follicle consists of a focal lymphoid hyperplasia within the lymphoid layer of the conjunctiva and usually contains a germinal center. Clinically, it can be recognized as a rounded, avascular white or gray structure. On slitlamp examination, small vessels can be seen arising at the border of the follicle and encircling it.

Pseudomembranes and **membranes** are the result of an exudative process and differ only in degree. A pseudomembrane is a coagulum on the *surface* of the epithelium, and when it is removed the epithelium remains intact. A membrane is a coagulum involving the *entire* epithelium, and if it is removed a raw, bleeding surface remains. Pseudomembranes or membranes may accompany epidemic keratoconjunctivitis, primary herpes simplex virus conjunctivitis, streptococcal conjunctivitis, diphtheria, cicatricial pemphigoid, and erythema multiforme major. They may also be an aftermath of chemical burns, especially alkali burns.

Ligneous conjunctivitis is a peculiar form of recurring membranous conjunctivitis. It is bilateral, seen mainly in children, predominantly in females, and may be associated with other systemic findings, including nasopharyngitis and vulvovaginitis.

Granulomas of the conjunctiva always affect the stroma and most commonly are chalazia. Other endogenous causes include sarcoid, syphilis, cat-scratch disease, and, rarely, coccidioidomycosis. Parinaud's oculoglandular syndrome includes conjunctival granulomas and a prominent preauricular lymph node, and this group of diseases may require biopsy examination to secure diagnosis.

Phlyctenules represent a delayed hypersensitivity reaction to microbial antigen, eg, staphylococcal or mycobacterial antigens. Phlyctenules of the conjunctiva initially consist of a perivasculitis with lymphocytic cuffing of a vessel. When they progress to ulceration of the conjunctiva, the ulcer bed has many polymorphonuclear leukocytes.

Preauricular lymphadenopathy is an important sign of conjunctivitis. A grossly visible preauricular node is seen in Parinaud's oculoglandular syndrome and, rarely, in epidemic keratoconjunctivitis. A large or small preauricular node, sometimes slightly tender, occurs in primary herpes simplex conjunctivitis, epidemic keratoconjunctivitis, inclusion conjunctivitis, and trachoma. Small but nontender preauricular lymph nodes occur in pharyngoconjunctival fever and acute hemorrhagic conjunctivitis. Occasionally, preauricular lymphadenopathy may be observed in children with infections of the meibomian glands.

BACTERIAL CONJUNCTIVITIS

Two forms of bacterial conjunctivitis are recognized: acute (and subacute) and chronic. Acute bacterial conjunctivitis may be self-limited when caused by certain microorganisms such as *Haemophilus influenzae*. The course may take up to 2 weeks if proper treatment is not given.

Acute bacterial conjunctivitis may become chronic. Treatment with one of the many available antibacterial agents usually cures the condition in a few days. Purulent conjunctivitis caused by *Neisseria gonorrhoeae* or *Neisseria meningitidis* may lead to serious ocular complications if not treated early.

Clinical Findings

A. Symptoms and Signs: The organisms listed in Table 5–1 account for most cases of bacterial conjunctivitis. They produce bilateral irritation and injection, a purulent exudate with sticky lids on waking, and occasionally lid edema. The infection usually starts in one eye and is spread to the other by the hands. It may be spread from one person to another by fomites.

1. Hyperacute (and subacute) bacterial conjunctivitis–Purulent conjunctivitis (caused by *N gonorrhoeae, Neisseria kochii,* and *N meningitidis*) is marked by a profuse purulent exudate (Figure 5–1).

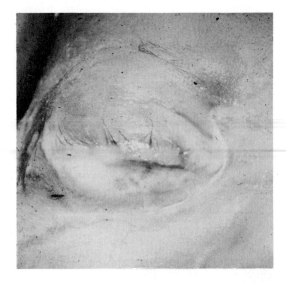

Figure 5–1. Gonorrheal conjunctivitis. Profuse purulent exudate. (Courtesy of P Thygeson.)

Meningococcal conjunctivitis may occasionally be seen in children. Any severe, profusely exudative conjunctivitis demands immediate laboratory investigation and immediate treatment. If there is any delay, there may be severe corneal damage or loss of the eye, or the conjunctiva could become the portal of entry for either *N gonorrhoeae* or *N meningitidis,* leading to septicemia or meningitis.

Acute mucopurulent (catarrhal) conjunctivitis often occurs in epidemic form and is called "pinkeye" by most laymen (Figure 5–2). It is characterized by an acute onset of conjunctival hyperemia and a moderate amount of mucopurulent discharge. The commonest causes are *Streptococcus pneumoniae* in temperate climates and *Haemophilus aegyptius* in warm climates. Less common causes are staphylococci and other

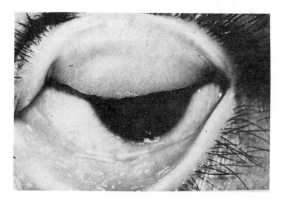

Figure 5–2. Acute catarrhal conjunctivitis caused by Koch-Weeks bacillus *(Haemophilus aegyptius).* (Courtesy of HB Ostler.)

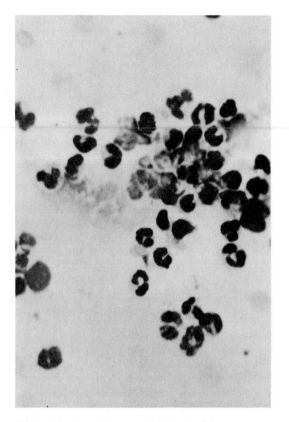

Figure 5–3. Polymorphonuclear reaction in Giemsa-stained scrapings from a patient with bacterial conjunctivitis. (Courtesy of M Okumoto.)

B. Laboratory Findings: In most cases of bacterial conjunctivitis, the organisms can be identified by the microscopic examination of conjunctival scrapings stained with Gram's stain or Giemsa's stain; this reveals numerous polymorphonuclear neutrophils (Figure 5–3). Conjunctival scrapings for microscopic examination and culture are recommended for all cases and are mandatory if the disease is purulent, membranous, or pseudomembranous. Antibiotic sensitivity studies are also desirable, but empirical antibiotic therapy should be started. When the results of antibiotic sensitivity tests become available, specific antibiotic therapy can then be instituted.

Complications & Sequelae

Chronic marginal blepharitis often accompanies staphylococcal conjunctivitis except in very young patients who are not subject to blepharitis. Conjunctival scarring may follow both pseudomembranous and membranous conjunctivitis, and in some cases corneal ulceration and perforation supervene.

Marginal corneal ulceration may follow infection with *N gonorrhoeae, N kochii, N meningitidis, H aegyptius, S aureus,* and *M catarrhalis*; if the toxic products of *N gonorrhoeae* diffuse through the cornea into the anterior chamber, they may cause toxic iritis.

Treatment

Specific therapy of bacterial conjunctivitis depends on identification of the microbiologic agent. While waiting for laboratory reports, the physician can start topical therapy with an antimicrobial drug. In any purulent conjunctivitis, an antibiotic suitable for treating *N gonorrhoeae* and *N meningitidis* infection should be selected, and both systemic and topical therapy should be started immediately after material for laboratory study has been collected.

In acute purulent and mucopurulent conjunctivitis, the conjunctival sac should be irrigated with saline solution as necessary to remove the conjunctival secretions. To prevent spread of the disease, the patient and family should be instructed to give special attention to personal hygiene.

Course & Prognosis

Acute bacterial conjunctivitis is almost always self-limited. Untreated, it may last 10–14 days; if properly treated, 1–3 days. The exceptions are staphylococcal conjunctivitis (which may progress to blepharoconjunctivitis and enter a chronic phase) and gonococcal conjunctivitis (which when untreated can lead to corneal perforation and endophthalmitis). Since the conjunctiva may be the portal of entry for the meningococcus to the bloodstream and meninges, septicemia and meningitis may be the end results of meningococcal conjunctivitis.

Chronic bacterial conjunctivitis may not be self-limited and may become a troublesome therapeutic problem.

streptococci. The conjunctivitis caused by *S pneumoniae* (Figure 5–3) and *H aegyptius* may be accompanied by subconjunctival hemorrhages. *H aegyptius* conjunctivitis in Brazil has been followed by a fatal purpuric fever produced by a plasmid-associated toxin of the bacteria.

Subacute conjunctivitis is caused most often by *H influenzae* and occasionally by *Escherichia coli* and *Proteus* spp. *H influenzae* infection is characterized by a thin, watery, or flocculent exudate.

2. Chronic bacterial conjunctivitis— Chronic bacterial conjunctivitis occurs in patients with nasolacrimal duct obstruction and chronic dacryocystitis, which are usually unilateral. It may also be associated with chronic bacterial blepharitis or meibomian gland dysfunction. Patients with floppy lid syndrome and ectropion may develop secondary bacterial conjunctivitis.

Rare bacterial conjunctivitides may be caused by *Corynebacterium diphtheriae* and *Streptococcus pyogenes.* Pseudomembranes or membranes caused by these organisms may form on the palpebral conjunctiva. The rare cases of chronic conjunctivitis produced by *Moraxella catarrhalis,* the coliform bacilli, *Proteus,* etc, are as a rule indistinguishable clinically.

CHLAMYDIAL CONJUNCTIVITIS

1. TRACHOMA

Trachoma is one of the most ancient of known diseases. It was recognized as a cause of trichiasis as early as the 27th century BC and affects all races. With 300–600 million of the world's population afflicted, it is one of the most common of all chronic diseases. Its regional variations in prevalence and severity can be explained on the basis of variations in the personal hygiene and standards of living of the world's peoples, the climatic conditions under which they live, the prevailing age at onset, and the frequency and type of the prevailing concomitant bacterial eye infections. Blinding trachoma occurs in many parts of Africa, some parts of Asia, among Australian aborigines, and in northern Brazil. Communities with milder nonblinding trachoma occur in the same regions and in some areas of Latin America and the Pacific Islands.

Trachoma is usually bilateral. It is spread by direct contact or fomites, usually from other family members (siblings, parents), who should also be examined for the disease. Insect vectors, especially flies and gnats, may play a role in transmission. The acute forms of the disease are more infectious than the cicatricial forms, and the larger the inoculum the more severe the disease. Spread is often associated with epidemics of bacterial conjunctivitis and with the dry seasons in tropical and semitropical countries.

Clinical Findings

A. Symptoms and Signs: Trachoma is initially a chronic follicular conjunctivitis of childhood that progresses to conjunctival scarring. In severe cases, inturned eyelashes occur in early adult life as a result of severe conjunctival scarring. The constant abrasion of inturned lashes and a defective tear film lead to corneal scarring, usually after the age of 50 years.

The incubation period of trachoma averages 7 days but varies from 5 to 14 days. In an infant or child, the onset is usually insidious, and the disease may resolve with minimal or no complications. In adults, the onset is often subacute or acute, and complications may develop early. At onset, trachoma often resembles bacterial conjunctivitis, the signs and symptoms usually consisting of tearing, photophobia, pain, exudation, edema of the eyelids, chemosis of the bulbar conjunctiva, hyperemia, papillary hypertrophy, tarsal and limbal follicles (Figure 5–4), superior keratitis, pannus formation, and a small, tender preauricular node.

In established trachoma, there may also be superior epithelial keratitis, subepithelial keratitis, pannus, superior limbal follicles, and ultimately the pathognomonic cicatricial remains of these follicles, known as **Herbert's pits**—small depressions in the connective tissue at the limbocorneal junction covered by epithelium. The associated pannus is a fibrovascular membrane arising from the limbus, with vascular loops ex-

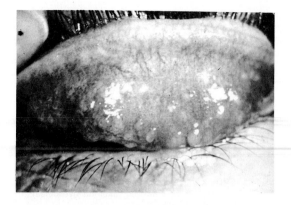

Figure 5–4. Trachoma. Papillae and follicles in upper tarsal conjunctiva. (Courtesy of P Thygeson.)

tending onto the cornea (Figure 5–5). All of the signs of trachoma are more severe in the upper than in the lower conjunctiva and cornea.

To establish the presence of endemic trachoma in a family or community, a substantial number of children must have at least two of the following signs:

(1) Five or more follicles on the flat tarsal conjunctiva lining the upper eye lid.

(2) Typical conjunctival scarring of the upper tarsal conjunctiva.

(3) Limbal follicles or their sequelae (Herbert's pits).

(4) An even extension of blood vessels onto the cornea, most marked at the upper limbus.

While occasional individuals will meet these criteria, it is the wide distribution of these signs in individ-

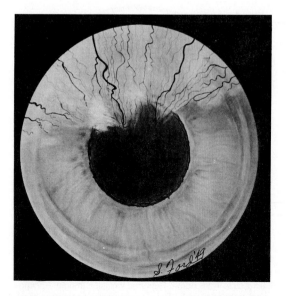

Figure 5–5. Trachomatous pannus. (Courtesy of P Thygeson.)

ual families and in a community that identify the presence of trachoma.

For control purposes, the World Health Organization has developed a simplified method to describe the disease. This includes the following signs:

TF:	Five or more follicles on the upper tarsal conjunctiva.
TI:	Diffuse infiltration and papillary hypertrophy of the upper tarsal conjunctiva obscuring at least 50% of the normal deep vessels.
TS:	Trachomatous conjunctival scarring.
TT:	Trichiasis or entropion (inturned eyelashes).
CO:	Corneal opacity.

The presence of TF and TI indicates active infectious trachoma and a need for treatment. TS is evidence of damage from the disease. TT is potentially blinding and is an indication for corrective lid surgery. CO is the final blinding lesion of trachoma.

B. Laboratory Findings: Chlamydial inclusions can be found in Giemsa-stained conjunctival scrapings, but they are not always present. Inclusions appear in the Giemsa-stained preparations as particulate, dark purple or blue cytoplasmic masses that cap the nucleus of the epithelial cell (Figure 5–6). Fluorescent antibody stains and enzyme immunoassay tests are available commercially and are widely used in clinical laboratories. These new tests have superseded Giemsa staining of conjunctival smears and isolation of chlamydial agent in cell culture.

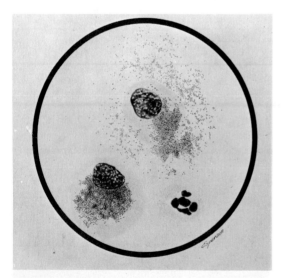

Figure 5–6. Cytoplasmic inclusion body in conjunctival epithelial cells in trachoma. Ruptured inclusion at right. Polymorphonuclear neutrophil (typical in conjunctival scrapings of trachoma) below. (Courtesy of P Thygeson and C Dawson.)

The agent of trachoma resembles the agent of inclusion conjunctivitis morphologically, but the two can be differentiated serologically by microimmunofluorescence. Trachoma is caused by *Chlamydia trachomatis* serotypes A, B, Ba, or C.

Differential Diagnosis

Epidemiologic and clinical factors to be considered in differentiating trachoma from other forms of follicular conjunctivitis can be summarized as follows:

(1) No history of exposure to endemic trachoma speaks against the diagnosis.

(2) Viral follicular conjunctivitis (due to infection with adenovirus, herpes simplex virus, picornavirus, and coxsackievirus) usually has an acute onset and is clearly resolving by 2–3 weeks.

(3) Infection with genitally transmitted chlamydial strains usually has an acute onset in sexually active individuals.

(4) Chronic follicular conjunctivitis with exogenous substances (molluscum nodules of the lids, topical eye medications) resolve slowly when the nodules are removed or the drug withdrawn.

(5) Parinaud's oculoglandular syndrome is manifested by massively enlarged preauricular or cervical lymph nodes, though the conjunctival lesion may be follicular.

(6) Young children often have some follicles (like hypertrophied tonsils), a condition known as folliculosis.

(7) The atopic conditions vernal conjunctivitis and atopic keratoconjunctivitis are associated with giant papillae that are elevated and often polygonal, with a milky-red appearance. Eosinophils are present in smears

(8) Look for a history of contact lens intolerance in patients with conjunctival scarring and pannus; giant papillae in some contact lens wearers can be confused with trachoma follicles.

Complications & Sequelae

Conjunctival scarring is a frequent complication of trachoma and can destroy the ductules of the accessory lacrimal glands and obliterate the orifices of the lacrimal gland. These effects may drastically reduce the aqueous component of the precorneal tear film, and the film's mucous components may be reduced by loss of goblet cells. The scars may also cause distortion of the upper lid with inward deviation of individual lashes (trichiasis) or of the whole lid margin (entropion), so that the lashes constantly abrade the cornea. This often leads to corneal ulceration, bacterial corneal infections, and corneal scarring (Figure 5–7).

Ptosis (Figure 5–8), nasolacrimal duct obstruction, and dacryocystitis are other common complications of trachoma.

Treatment

Striking clinical improvement can usually be achieved with tetracycline, 1–1.5 g/d orally in four di-

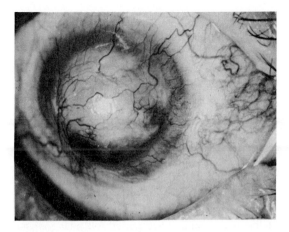

Figure 5–7. Advanced trachoma following corneal ulceration and scarring. (Courtesy of P Thygeson.)

vided doses for 3–4 weeks; doxycycline, 100 mg orally twice daily for 3 weeks; or erythromycin, 1 g/d orally in four divided doses for 3–4 weeks. Several courses are sometimes necessary for actual cure. Systemic tetracyclines should not be given to a child under 7 years of age or to a pregnant woman, since tetracycline binds to calcium in the developing teeth and in the growing bone and may lead to congenital yellowish discoloration of the permanent teeth and skeletal (eg, clavicular) abnormalities.

Topical ointments or drops, including preparations of sulfonamides, tetracyclines, erythromycin, and rifampin, used four times daily for 6 weeks, are equally effective.

From the time therapy is begun, its maximum effect is usually not achieved for 10–12 weeks. The persistence of follicles on the upper tarsus for some weeks after a course of therapy should therefore not be construed as evidence of therapeutic failure.

Surgical correction of inturned eyelashes is essential to prevent scarring from late trachoma in developing countries. Such surgery is sometimes done by non-

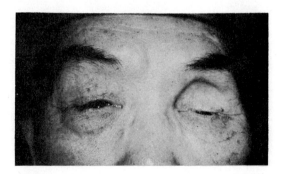

Figure 5–8. Ptosis with an S-shaped curve of lids associated with chronic trachoma. (Courtesy of P Thygeson.)

specialist physicians or specially trained auxiliary personnel.

Course & Prognosis

Characteristically, trachoma is a chronic disease of long duration. Under good hygienic conditions (specifically, face-washing of young children), the disease resolves or becomes milder so that severe sequelae are avoided. About 6–9 million people in the world today have major visual loss from trachoma.

2. INCLUSION CONJUNCTIVITIS (Inclusion Blennorrhea, Paratrachoma)

Inclusion conjunctivitis is often bilateral and usually occurs in sexually active young people. The chlamydial agent infects the urethra of the male and the cervix of the female. Transmission to the eyes of adults is usually by oral-genital sexual practices or hand to eye transmission. About one in 300 persons with genital chlamydial infection develops the eye disease. Indirect transmission has been reported to occur in inadequately chlorinated swimming pools. In newborns, the agent is transmitted during birth by direct contamination of the conjunctiva with cervical secretions. Credé prophylaxis gives only partial protection against inclusion conjunctivitis.

Clinical Findings

A. Symptoms and Signs: Inclusion conjunctivitis may have an acute or a subacute onset. The patient frequently complains of redness of the eyes, pseudoptosis, and discharge, especially in the mornings. Newborns have papillary conjunctivitis and a moderate amount of exudate, and in hyperacute cases pseudomembranes occasionally form and can lead to scarring. Since the newborn has no adenoid tissue in the stroma of the conjunctiva, there is no follicle formation; but if the conjunctivitis persists for 2–3 months, follicles appear and the conjunctival picture is like that in older children and adults. In the newborn, chlamydial infection may cause pharyngitis, otitis media, and interstitial pneumonitis.

In adults, the conjunctiva of both tarsi—especially the lower tarsus—have papillae and follicles (Figure 5–9). Since pseudomembranes do not usually form in the adult, scarring does not usually occur. Superficial keratitis may be noted superiorly and, less often, a small superior micropannus (< 1–2 mm). Subepithelial opacities, usually marginal, often develop. Otitis media may occur as a result of infection of the auditory tube.

B. Laboratory Findings: The same tests should be performed as for trachoma (above). In neonatal chlamydial ophthalmia, Giemsa-stained smears often have many inclusions. Inclusion conjunctivitis is caused by *C trachomatis* serotypes D–K with occa-

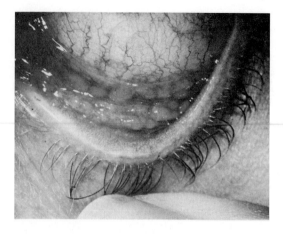

Figure 5–9. Acute follicular conjunctivitis caused by inclusion conjunctivitis in a 22-year-old man with urethritis. (Courtesy of K Tabbara.)

sional isolations of serotype B. Serologic determinations are not useful in the diagnosis of ocular infections, but measurement of IgM antibody levels is extremely valuable in the diagnosis of chlamydial pneumonitis in infants.

Differential Diagnosis

Inclusion conjunctivitis can be clinically differentiated from trachoma on the following grounds:

(1) Active, follicular trachoma occurs commonly in young children or others living in or exposed to a community with endemic trachoma; inclusion conjunctivitis occurs in sexually active adolescents or adults.

(2) Conjunctival scarring is very rare in adult inclusion conjunctivitis.

(3) Herbert's pits are a unique sign that trachoma was present at some time in the past.

Treatment

A. In Infants: Give oral erythromycin suspension, 40 mg/kg/d in four divided doses for at least 14 days. Oral medication is necessary because chlamydial infection also involves the respiratory and gastrointestinal tracts. Topical antibiotics (tetracyclines, erythromycin, sulfonamides) are not useful in newborns treated with oral erythromycin. Both parents should be treated with oral tetracyclines or erythromycin for their genital tract infection.

B. In Adults: Cure can be achieved with a 3-week course of oral tetracycline, 1–1.5 g/d; doxycycline, 100 mg orally twice daily; or erythromycin, 1 g/d. (Systemic tetracyclines should not be given to a pregnant woman or a child under 7 years of age, since they cause epiphysial problems in the fetus or staining of the young child's teeth.) The patient's sexual partners should be examined and treated.

When one of the standard therapeutic regimens is followed, recurrences are rare. If untreated, inclusion conjunctivitis runs a course of 3–9 months or longer. The average duration is 5 months.

3. CONJUNCTIVITIS CAUSED BY OTHER CHLAMYDIAL AGENTS

Lymphogranuloma venereum conjunctivitis is a rare sexually transmitted disease. Lymphogranuloma venereum causes a dramatic granulomatous conjunctival reaction with greatly enlarged preauricular nodes (Parinaud's syndrome). It is caused by *C trachomatis* serotypes L1, L2 or L3.

Chlamydia psittaci only rarely causes conjunctivitis in humans. Strains from parrots (psittacosis) and cats (feline pneumonitis) have caused follicular conjunctivitis in humans. The prototype strains of *Chlamydia pneumoniae* were isolated from the conjunctiva but have not been identified as a cause of eye disease.

VIRAL CONJUNCTIVITIS

Viral conjunctivitis, a common affliction, can be caused by a wide variety of viruses. Severity ranges from severe, disabling disease to mild, rapidly self-limited infection.

1. ACUTE VIRAL FOLLICULAR CONJUNCTIVITIS

Pharyngoconjunctival Fever

Pharyngoconjunctival fever is characterized by fever of 38.3–40 °C (101–104 °F), sore throat, and a follicular conjunctivitis in one or both eyes. The follicles are often very prominent on both the conjunctiva (Figure 5–10) and the pharyngeal mucosa. The disease can be either bilateral or unilateral. Injection and tearing often occur, and there may be transient superficial

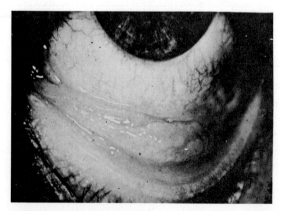

Figure 5–10. Acute follicular conjunctivitis due to adenovirus type 3. (Courtesy of P Thygeson.)

epithelial keratitis and occasionally some subepithelial opacities. Preauricular lymphadenopathy (nontender) is characteristic. The syndrome may be incomplete, consisting of only one or two of the cardinal signs (fever, pharyngitis, and conjunctivitis).

Pharyngoconjunctival fever is caused regularly by adenovirus type 3 and occasionally by types 4 and 7. The virus can be grown on HeLa cells and identified by neutralization tests. As the disease progresses, it can also be diagnosed serologically by a rising titer of neutralizing antibody to the virus. Clinical diagnosis is a simple matter, however, and clearly more practical.

Conjunctival scrapings contain predominantly mononuclear cells, and no bacteria grow in cultures. The condition is more common in children than in adults and can be transmitted poorly in chlorinated swimming pools. There is no specific treatment, but the conjunctivitis is self-limited, usually lasting about 10 days.

Epidemic Keratoconjunctivitis

Epidemic keratoconjunctivitis is usually bilateral. The onset is often in one eye only, however, and as a rule the first eye is more severely affected. At onset the patient notes injection, moderate pain, and tearing, followed in 5–14 days by photophobia, epithelial keratitis, and round subepithelial opacities. Corneal sensation is normal. A tender preauricular node is characteristic. Edema of the eyelids, chemosis, and conjunctival hyperemia mark the acute phase, with follicles and subconjunctival hemorrhages often appearing within 48 hours. Pseudomembranes (and occasionally true membranes) may occur and may be followed by flat scars or symblepharon formation (Figure 5–11).

The conjunctivitis lasts for 3–4 weeks at most. The subepithelial opacities are concentrated in the central cornea, usually sparing the periphery, and may persist for months but heal without scars.

Epidemic keratoconjunctivitis is caused by adeno-

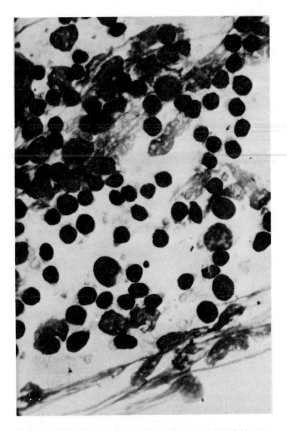

Figure 5–12. Mononuclear cell reaction in conjunctival scrapings of a patient with viral conjunctivitis caused by adenovirus type 8. (Courtesy of M Okumoto.)

virus types 8, 19, 29, and 37 (subgroup D of the human adenoviruses). They can be isolated in cell culture and identified by neutralization tests. Scrapings from the conjunctiva show a primarily mononuclear inflammatory reaction (Figure 5–12); when pseudomembranes occur, neutrophils may also be prominent. Epidemic keratoconjunctivitis in adults is confined to the external eye, but in children there may be such systemic symptoms of viral infection as fever, sore throat, otitis media, and diarrhea. Nosocomial transmission during eye examinations takes place all too often by way of the physician's fingers, use of improperly sterilized ophthalmic instruments, or use of contaminated solutions. Eye solutions, particularly topical anesthetics, can be contaminated when a dropper tip aspirates infected material from the conjunctiva or cilia. The virus can persist in the solution, which becomes a source of spread.

The danger of contaminated solution bottles can be avoided by the use of individual sterile droppers or unit-dose packages of eye drops. Regular hand washing between examinations and careful cleaning and sterilization of instruments that touch the eyes—especially tonometers—are also mandatory. Applanation

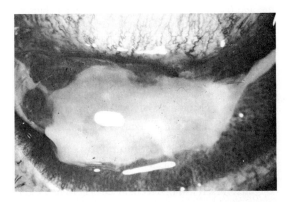

Figure 5–11. Epidemic keratoconjunctivitis. Thick white membrane in lower palpebral conjunctiva. (Courtesy of P Thygeson.)

tonometers should be cleaned by wiping with alcohol or hypochlorite, then rinsing with sterile water and carefully drying.

There is no specific therapy at present, but cold compresses will relieve some symptoms. Corticosteroids during acute conjunctivitis may prolong the late corneal involvement and so should be avoided. Antibacterial agents should be given if bacterial superinfection occurs.

Herpes Simplex Virus Conjunctivitis

Herpes simplex virus (HSV) conjunctivitis, usually a disease of young children, is an uncommon entity characterized by unilateral injection, irritation, mucoid discharge, pain, and mild photophobia. It occurs during primary infection with HSV or during recurrent episodes of ocular herpes (Figure 5–13). It is often associated with herpes simplex keratitis, in which the cornea shows discrete epithelial lesions that usually coalesce to form single or multiple branching epithelial (dendritic) ulcers. The conjunctivitis is follicular or, less often, pseudomembranous. (Patients receiving topical antivirals may develop follicular conjunctivitis that can be differentiated because the herpetic follicular conjunctivitis has an acute onset.) Herpetic vesicles may sometimes appear on the eyelids and lid margins, associated with severe edema of the eyelids. Typically, there is a small tender preauricular node.

No bacteria are found in scrapings or recovered in cultures. If the conjunctivitis is follicular, the predominant inflammatory reaction is mononuclear, but if it is pseudomembranous the predominant reaction is polymorphonuclear owing to the chemotaxis of necrosis. Intranuclear inclusions (because of the margination of the chromatin) can be seen in conjunctival and corneal cells if Bouin fixation and the Papanicolaou stain are used but not in Giemsa-stained smears. The finding of multinucleated giant epithelial cells has diagnostic value.

The virus can be readily isolated by gently rubbing

a dry cotton-tipped applicator over the conjunctiva and transferring the infected cells to a susceptible tissue culture.

HSV conjunctivitis may persist for 2–3 weeks, and if it is pseudomembranous it may leave fine linear or flat scars. Complications consist of corneal involvement (including dendrites) and vesicles on the skin. Although type 1 herpesvirus causes the overwhelming majority of ocular cases, type 2 is the usual cause in newborns and a rare cause in adults. In the newborn, there may be generalized disease with encephalitis, chorioretinitis, hepatitis, etc. Any HSV infection in the newborn must be treated with systemic antiviral therapy (acyclovir) and monitored in a hospital setting.

If the conjunctivitis occurs in a child over 1 year of age or in an adult, it is usually self-limited and may not require therapy. Topical or systemic antivirals should be given, however, to prevent corneal involvement. For corneal ulcers, corneal debridement may be performed by gently wiping the ulcer with a dry cotton swab, applying antiviral drops, and patching the eye for 24 hours. Topical antivirals alone should be applied for 7–10 days: trifluridine every 2 hours while awake, or vidarabine ointment five times a day, or idoxuridine 0.1%, 1 drop every hour while awake and 1 drop every 2 hours during the night. Herpetic keratitis may also be treated with 3% acyclovir ointment (not available in the USA) five times daily for 10 days or with oral acyclovir, 400 mg five times a day for 7 days.

For corneal ulcers, corneal debridement may be performed. Less commonly, vidarabine or idoxuridine may be used. Topical antivirals should be applied for 7–10 days. Herpetic keratitis may be treated with 3% acyclovir ointment (not available in the USA) five times daily for 10 days. The use of steroids is contraindicated, since they may aggravate herpes simplex infections and convert the disease from a short, self-limited process to a severe, greatly prolonged one.

Newcastle Disease Conjunctivitis

Newcastle disease conjunctivitis is a rare disorder characterized by burning, itching, pain, redness, tearing, and (rarely) blurring of vision. It often occurs in small epidemics among poultry workers handling infected birds or among veterinarians or laboratory helpers working with live vaccines or virus.

The conjunctivitis resembles that caused by other viral agents, with chemosis, a small preauricular node, and follicles on the upper and lower tarsus. No treatment is available or necessary for this self-limited disease.

Acute Hemorrhagic Conjunctivitis

All of the continents and most of the islands of the world have had major epidemics of acute hemorrhagic conjunctivitis. It was first recognized in Ghana in 1969. It is caused by enterovirus type 70 and occasionally by coxsackievirus A24.

Characteristically, the disease has a short incubation

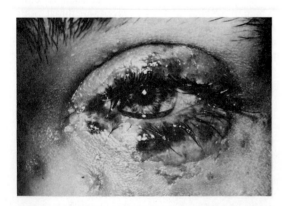

Figure 5–13. Primary ocular herpes. (Courtesy of HB Ostler.)

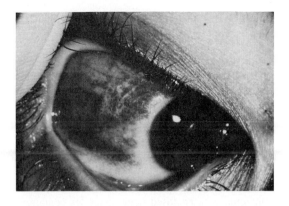

Figure 5–14. Acute hemorrhagic conjunctivitis. (Courtesy of K Tabbara.)

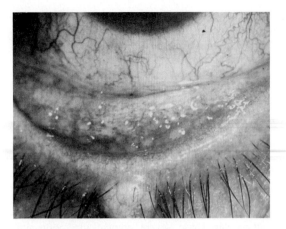

Figure 5–15. Molluscum contagiosum of lid margin with follicular conjunctivitis. (Courtesy of HB Ostler.)

period (8–48 hours) and course (5–7 days). The usual signs and symptoms are pain, photophobia, foreign body sensation, copious tearing, redness, lidedema, and subconjunctival hemorrhages (Figure 5–14). Chemosis sometimes also occurs. The subconjunctival hemorrhages are usually diffuse but may be punctate at onset, beginning in the upper bulbar conjunctiva and spreading to the lower. Most patients have preauricular lymphadenopathy, conjunctival follicles, and epithelial keratitis. Anterior uveitis has been reported; fever, malaise, and generalized myalgia have been observed in 25% of cases; and motor paralysis of the lower extremities has occurred in rare cases in India and Japan.

The virus is transmitted by close person-to-person contact and by such fomites as common linens, contaminated optical instruments, and water. Recovery occurs within 5–7 days, and there is no known treatment. In the USA, closing of schools has been done to stop epidemics.

2. CHRONIC VIRAL CONJUNCTIVITIS

Molluscum Contagiosum Blepharoconjunctivitis

A molluscum nodule on the lid margins or the skin of the lids and brow may produce unilateral chronic follicular conjunctivitis, superior keratitis, and superior pannus and may resemble trachoma. The inflammatory reaction is predominantly mononuclear (unlike the reaction in trachoma), and the round, waxy, pearly-white, noninflammatory lesion with an umbilicated center is typical of molluscum contagiosum (Figure 5–15). Biopsy shows eosinophilic cytoplasmic inclusions that fill the entire cytoplasm of the enlarged cell, pushing its nucleus to one side.

Excision, simple incision of the nodule to allow peripheral blood to permeate it, or cryotherapy cures the conjunctivitis. On very rare occasions (reports of only two cases have appeared in the literature), molluscum nodules have occurred on the conjunctiva. In these cases, excision of the nodule has also relieved the conjunctivitis.

Varicella-Zoster Blepharoconjunctivitis

Hyperemia and an infiltrative conjunctivitis—associated with the typical vesicular eruption along the dermatomal distribution of the ophthalmic branch of the trigeminal nerve—are characteristic of herpes zoster (preferably called simply zoster). The conjunctivitis is usually papillary, but follicles, pseudomembranes, and transitory vesicles that later ulcerate have all been noted. A tender preauricular lymph node occurs early in the disease. Scarring of the lid, entropion, and the misdirection of individual lashes are sequelae.

The lid lesions of varicella, which are like the skin lesions (pox) elsewhere, may appear on both the lid margins and the lids and often leave scars. A mild exudative conjunctivitis often occurs, but discrete conjunctival lesions (except at the limbus) are very rare. Limbal lesions resemble phlyctenules and may go through all the stages of vesicle, papule, and ulcer. The adjacent cornea becomes infiltrated and may vascularize.

In both zoster and varicella, scrapings from lid vesicles contain giant cells and a predominance of polymorphonuclear leukocytes; scrapings from the conjunctiva in varicella and from conjunctival vesicles in zoster may contain giant cells and monocytes. The virus can be recovered in tissue cultures of human embryo cells.

Oral acyclovir in high doses (800 mg orally five times daily for 10 days), if given early in the course of the disease, appears to limit the severity of the illness.

Measles Keratoconjunctivitis

The characteristic enanthem of measles frequently precedes the skin eruption. At this early stage, the conjunctiva may have a peculiar glassy appearance, followed within a few days by swelling of the semilunar fold (Meyer's sign). Several days before the skin eruption, an exudative conjunctivitis with a mucopurulent discharge develops, and at the time of the skin eruption, Koplik's spots appear on the conjunctiva and occasionally on the caruncle. At some time (early in children, late in adults), epithelial keratitis supervenes.

In the immunocompetent patient, measles keratoconjunctivitis has few or no sequelae, but in malnourished or otherwise immunoincompetent patients the ocular disease is frequently associated with a secondary HSV or bacterial infection due to *S pneumoniae, H influenzae,* and other organisms. These agents may lead to purulent conjunctivitis with associated corneal ulceration and severe visual loss. Herpes infection can cause severe corneal ulceration with corneal perforation and loss of vision in poorly nourished children in developing countries.

Conjunctival scrapings show a mononuclear cell reaction unless there are pseudomembranes or secondary infection. Giemsa-stained preparations contain giant cells. Since there is no specific therapy, only supportive measures are indicated unless there is secondary infection.

RICKETTSIAL CONJUNCTIVITIS

All rickettsiae recognized as pathogenic for humans may attack the conjunctiva, and the conjunctiva may be their portal of entry.

Q fever is associated with severe conjunctival hyperemia. Treatment with systemic tetracycline or chloramphenicol is curative.

Marseilles fever (boutonneuse fever) is often associated with ulcerative or granulomatous conjunctivitis and a grossly visible preauricular lymph node.

Endemic (murine) typhus, scrub typhus, Rocky Mountain spotted fever, and **epidemic typhus** have associated, variable, and usually mild conjunctival signs.

FUNGAL CONJUNCTIVITIS

Candidal Conjunctivitis

Conjunctivitis caused by *Candida* spp (usually *Candida albicans*) is a rare infection that usually appears as a white plaque. This may occur in diabetics or immunocompromised patients as an ulcerative or granulomatous conjunctivitis.

Scrapings show a polymorphonuclear cell inflammatory reaction. The organism grows readily on blood agar or Sabouraud's medium and can be readily identified as a budding yeast or, rarely, as pseudohyphae.

The infection responds to amphotericin B (3–8 mg/mL) in aqueous (not saline) solution or to applications of nystatin dermatologic cream (100,000 units/g) four to six times daily. The ointment must be applied

carefully to be sure that it reaches the conjunctival sac and does not just build up on the lid margins.

Other Fungal Conjunctivitides

Sporothrix schenckii may rarely involve the conjunctiva or the eyelids. It is a granulomatous disease associated with a visible preauricular node. Microscopic examination of a biopsy of the granuloma reveals gram-positive, cigar-shaped conidia (spores).

Rhinosporidium seeberi may rarely affect the conjunctiva, lacrimal sac, lids, canaliculi, and sclera. The typical lesion is a polypoid granuloma that bleeds after minimal trauma. Histologic examination shows a granuloma with enclosed large spherules containing myriads of endospores. Treatment is by simple excision and cauterization of the base.

Coccidioides immitis may rarely cause a granulomatous conjunctivitis associated with a grossly visible preauricular node (Parinaud's oculoglandular syndrome). This is not a primary disease but a manifestation of metastatic infection from a primary pulmonary infection (San Joaquin Valley fever). Disseminated disease suggests a poor prognosis.

PARASITIC CONJUNCTIVITIS*

Thelazia californiensis Infection

The natural habitat of this roundworm is the eye of the dog, but it can also infect the eyes of cats, sheep, black bears, horses, and deer. Accidental infection of the human conjunctival sac has occurred. The disease can be treated effectively by removing the worms from the conjunctival sac with forceps or a cotton-tipped applicator.

Loa loa Infection

L loa is the eye worm of Africa. It lives in the connective tissue of humans and monkeys, and the monkey may be its reservoir. The parasite is transmitted by the bite of the horse or mango fly. The mature worm may then migrate to the lid, the conjunctiva, or the orbit.

Infection with *L loa* is accompanied by a 60–80% eosinophilia, but diagnosis is made by identifying the worm on removal or by finding microfilariae in blood examined at midday.

Diethylcarbamazine is currently the drug of choice. Ivermectin is being evaluated.

Ascaris lumbricoides Infection (Butcher's Conjunctivitis)

Ascaris may cause a rare type of violent conjunctivitis. When butchers or persons performing postmortem examinations cut tissue containing *Ascaris,* the tissue juice of some of the organisms may hit them

---

*Onchocerciasis is discussed in Chapter 7.

in the eye. This can be followed by a violent and painful toxic conjunctivitis marked by extreme chemosis and lid edema. Treatment consists of rapid and thorough irrigation of the conjunctival sac.

Trichinella spiralis Infection

This parasite does not cause a true conjunctivitis, but in the course of its general dissemination there may be a doughy edema of the upper and lower eyelids, and over 50% of patients have chemosis—a pale, lemon-yellow swelling most marked over the lateral and medial rectus muscles and fading toward the limbus. The chemosis may last a week or more, and there is often pain on movement of the eyes.

Schistosoma haematobium Infection

Schistosomiasis (bilharziasis) is endemic in Egypt, especially in the region irrigated by the Nile. Granulomatous conjunctival lesions appearing as small, soft, smooth, pinkish-yellow tumors occur, especially in males. The symptoms are minimal. Diagnosis depends on microscopic examination of biopsy material, which shows a granuloma containing lymphocytes, plasma cells, giant cells, and eosinophils surrounding bilharzial ova in various stages of disintegration.

Treatment consists of excision of the conjunctival granuloma and systemic therapy with antimonials such as niridazole.

Taenia solium Infection

This parasite rarely causes conjunctivitis but more often invades the retina, choroid, or vitreous to produce ocular cysticercosis. As a rule, the affected conjunctiva shows a subconjunctival cyst in the form of a localized hemispherical swelling, usually at the inner angle of the lower fornix, which is adherent to the underlying sclera and painful on pressure. The conjunctiva and lid may be inflamed and edematous.

Diagnosis is based on a positive complement fixation or precipitin test or on demonstration of the organism in the gastrointestinal tract. Eosinophilia is a constant feature.

The best treatment is to excise the lesion. The intestinal condition can be treated by niclosamide.

Pthirus pubis Infection (Pubic Louse Infection)

P pubis may infest the cilia and margins of the eyelids. Because of its size, the pubic louse seems to require widely spaced hair. For this reason it has a predilection for the widely spaced cilia as well as for pubic hair. The parasites apparently release an irritating substance (probably feces) that produces a toxic follicular conjunctivitis in children and an irritating papillary conjunctivitis in adults. The lid margin is usually red, and the patient may complain of intense itching.

Finding the adult organism or the ova-shaped nits cemented to the eyelashes is diagnostic.

Lindane (Kwell) 1% or RID (pyrethrins), applied to the pubic area and lash margins after removal of the nits, is usually curative. Application of lindane or RID to the lid margins must be undertaken with great care to avoid contact with the eye. Any ointment applied to the lid margin tends to smother the adult organisms. The patient's family and close contacts should be examined and treated. All clothes and fomites should be washed.

Ophthalmomyiasis

Myiasis is infection with larvae of flies. Many different species of flies may produce myiasis. The ocular tissues may be injured by mechanical transmission of disease-producing organisms and by the parasitic activities of the larvae in the ocular tissues. The larvae are able to invade either necrotic or healthy tissue. Many become infected by accidental ingestion of the eggs or larvae or by contamination of external wounds or skin. Infants and young children, alcoholics, and debilitated unattended patients are common targets for infection with myiasis-producing flies.

These larvae may affect the ocular surface, the intraocular tissues, or the deeper orbital tissues.

Ocular surface involvement may be caused by *Musca domestica,* the housefly, *Fannia,* the latrine fly, and *Oestrus ovis,* the sheep botfly. These flies deposit their eggs at the lower lid margin or inner canthus, and the larvae may remain on the surface of the eye, causing irritation, pain, and conjunctival hyperemia.

Treatment of ocular surface myiasis is by mechanical removal of the larvae after topical anesthesia.

IMMUNOLOGIC (ALLERGIC) CONJUNCTIVITIS

IMMEDIATE HUMORAL HYPERSENSITIVITY REACTIONS

1. HAY FEVER CONJUNCTIVITIS

A mild, nonspecific conjunctival inflammation is commonly associated with hay fever (allergic rhinitis). There is usually a history of allergy to pollens, grasses, animal danders, etc. The patient complains of itching, tearing, and redness of the eyes and often states that the eyes seem to be "sinking into the surrounding tissue." There is mild injection of the palpebral and bulbar conjunctiva, and during acute attacks there is often severe chemosis (which no doubt accounts for the "sinking" description). There may be a small amount of ropy discharge, especially if the patient has been rubbing the eyes. Eosinophils are difficult to find in conjunctival scrapings. A papillary conjunctivitis can occur if the allergen persists.

Treatment consists of the instillation of local vasoconstrictors during the acute phase (epinephrine, 1:1000 solution applied topically, will relieve the chemosis and symptoms within 30 minutes). Cold compresses are helpful to relieve itching, and antihistamines by mouth are of some value. The immediate response to treatment is satisfactory, but recurrences are common unless the antigen is eliminated. Fortunately, the frequency of the attacks and the severity of the symptoms tend to moderate as the patient ages.

2. VERNAL KERATOCONJUNCTIVITIS

This disease, also known as "spring catarrh" and "seasonal conjunctivitis" or "warm weather conjunctivitis," is an uncommon bilateral allergic disease that usually begins in the prepubertal years and lasts for 5–10 years. It occurs much oftener in boys than in girls. The specific allergen or allergens are difficult to identify, but patients with vernal keratoconjunctivitis sometimes show other manifestations of allergy known to be related to grass pollen sensitivity. The disease is less common in temperate than in warm climates and is almost nonexistent in cold climates. It is almost always more severe during the spring, summer, and fall than in the winter.

The patient usually complains of extreme itching and a ropy discharge. There is often a family history of allergy (hay fever, eczema, etc) and sometimes in the young patient as well. The conjunctiva has a milky appearance, and there are many fine papillae in the lower tarsal conjunctiva. The upper palpebral conjunctiva often has giant papillae that give a cobblestone appearance (Figure 5–16). Each giant papilla is polygonal, has a flat top, and contains tufts of capillaries.

A stringy conjunctival discharge and a fine, fibrinous pseudomembrane (Maxwell-Lyons sign) may be noted. In some cases, especially in persons of black African ancestry, the most prominent lesions are located at the limbus, where gelatinous swellings (papil-

lae) are noted. A pseudogerontoxon (arcus) is often noted in the cornea adjacent to the limbal papillae. Tranta's dots are whitish dots seen at the limbus in some patients with vernal keratoconjunctivitis during the active phase of the disease. Many eosinophils and free eosinophilic granules are found in Giemsa-stained smears of the conjunctival exudate.

Micropannus is often seen in both palpebral and limbal vernal keratoconjunctivitis, but gross pannus is unusual. Conjunctival scarring usually does not occur unless the patient has been treated with cryotherapy, surgical removal of the papillae, irradiation, or other damaging procedure. Superficial corneal ("shield") ulcers (oval and located superiorly) may form and may be followed by mild corneal scarring. A characteristic diffuse epithelial keratitis frequently occurs. None of the corneal lesions respond well to standard treatment.

The disease may be associated with keratoconus.

Treatment

Since vernal keratoconjunctivitis is a self-limited disease, it must be recognized that the medication used to treat the symptoms may provide short-term benefit but long-term harm. Topical and systemic steroids, which relieve the itching, affect the corneal disease only minimally, and their side effects (glaucoma, cataract, and other complications) can be severely damaging. Topical cromolyn is a useful prophylactic agent in moderate to severe cases. Vasoconstrictors, cold compresses, and ice packs are helpful, and sleeping (if possible, also working) in cool, air-conditioned rooms can keep the patient reasonably comfortable. Probably the best remedy of all is to move to a cool, moist climate. Patients able to do so are benefited if not completely cured.

The severe symptoms of an extremely photophobic patient who is unable to function can often be relieved by a short course of topical or systemic steroids followed by vasoconstrictors, cold packs, and regular use of cromolyn eye drops. Newer nonsteroidal anti-inflammatory medications, including ketorolac and iodoxamide, may provide significant symptomatic relief. (See discussion in Chapter 3.) As has already been in-

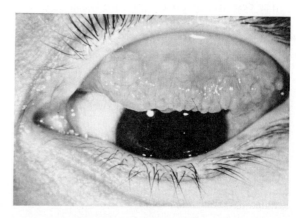

Figure 5–16. Vernal conjunctivitis. "Cobblestone" papillae in superior tarsal conjunctiva. (Courtesy of P Thygeson.)

dicated, the prolonged use of steroids must be avoided since it is all too often followed by herpes simplex keratitis, cataract, glaucoma, and fungal and other opportunistic corneal ulcers. Recent clinical studies have shown that topical 1% cyclosporine eye drops are effective in severe unresponsive cases.

Desensitization to grass pollens and other antigens has not been rewarding. Staphylococcal blepharitis and conjunctivitis are frequent complications and should be treated. Recurrences are the rule, particularly in the spring and summer; but after a number of recurrences the papillae disappear completely, leaving no scars.

3. ATOPIC KERATOCONJUNCTIVITIS

Patients with atopic dermatitis (eczema) often also have atopic keratoconjunctivitis. The symptoms and signs are a burning sensation, mucoid discharge, redness, and photophobia. The lid margins are erythematous, and the conjunctiva has a milky appearance. There are fine papillae, but giant papillae are less developed than in vernal keratoconjunctivitis and occur more frequently on the lower tarsus—unlike the giant papillae of vernal keratoconjunctivitis, which are on the upper tarsus. Severe corneal signs appear late in the disease after repeated exacerbations of the conjunctivitis. Superficial peripheral keratitis develops and is followed by vascularization. In severe cases, the entire cornea becomes hazy and vascularized, and visual acuity is reduced. The disease may be associated with keratoconus.

There is usually a history of allergy (hay fever, asthma, or eczema) in the patient or the patient's family. Most patients have had atopic dermatitis since infancy. Scarring of the flexure creases of the antecubital folds and of the wrists and knees is common. Like the dermatitis with which it is associated, atopic keratoconjunctivitis has a protracted course and is subject to exacerbations and remissions. Like vernal keratoconjunctivitis, it tends to become less active when the patient reaches the fifth decade.

Scrapings of the conjunctiva show eosinophils, though not nearly as many as are seen in vernal keratoconjunctivitis. Scarring of both the conjunctiva and cornea is often seen, and an atopic cataract, a posterior subcapsular plaque, or an anterior shield-like cataract may develop. Keratoconus, retinal detachment, and herpes simplex keratitis are all more than usually frequent in patients with atopic keratoconjunctivitis, and there are many cases of secondary bacterial blepharitis and conjunctivitis, usually staphylococcal.

The management of atopic keratoconjunctivitis is often discouraging. Any secondary infection must be treated. Environmental control should be considered. Oral antihistamines including terfenadine (60–120 mg twice daily), astemizole (10 mg four times daily), or hydroxyzine (50 mg at bedtime, increasing to 200 mg at bedtime) have been shown to be of value. Newer nonsteroidal anti-inflammatory medications, includ-

ing ketorolac and iodoxamide, show promise for symptomatic relief for these patients (see Chapter 3). A short course of topical steroids may relieve symptoms. In severe cases, plasmapheresis may be an adjunct to therapy. In advanced cases with severe corneal complications, corneal transplantation may be needed to improve the visual acuity.

4. GIANT PAPILLARY CONJUNCTIVITIS

Giant papillary conjunctivitis with signs and symptoms resembling those of vernal conjunctivitis may develop in patients wearing plastic artificial eyes or contact lenses. It is probably a basophil-rich delayed hypersensitivity disorder, perhaps with an IgE humoral component. Use of glass instead of plastic for prostheses and spectacle lenses instead of contact lenses is curative. If the goal is to maintain contact lens wear, additional therapy will be required. Careful contact lens care, including preservative-free agents, is essential. Hydrogen peroxide disinfection and enzymatic cleaning of contact lenses may also help. Changing to a different brand or style of contact lenses may be necessary if other measures fail. If these treatments are unsuccessful, contact lenses should be discontinued.

DELAYED HYPERSENSITIVITY REACTIONS

1. PHLYCTENULOSIS

Phlyctenular keratoconjunctivitis is a delayed hypersensitivity response to microbial proteins, including the proteins of the tubercle bacillus, *Staphylococcus* spp, *Candida albicans, Coccidioides immitis, Haemophilus aegyptius,* and *Chlamydia trachomatis* serotypes L1, L2, and L3. Until recently, by far the most frequent cause of phlyctenulosis in the USA was delayed hypersensitivity to the protein of the human tubercle bacillus. This is still the commonest cause in regions where tuberculosis is still prevalent. In the USA, however, most cases are now associated with delayed hypersensitivity to *S aureus*.

The conjunctival phlyctenule begins as a small lesion (usually 1–3 mm in diameter) that is hard, red, elevated, and surrounded by a zone of hyperemia. At the limbus it is often triangular in shape, with its apex toward the cornea. In this location it develops a grayish-white center that soon ulcerates and then subsides within 10–12 days. The patient's first phlyctenule and most of the recurrences develop at the limbus, but there may also be corneal, bulbar, and, very rarely, even tarsal phlyctenules.

Unlike the conjunctival phlyctenule, which leaves no scar, the corneal phlyctenule develops as an amorphous gray infiltrate and always leaves a scar. Consistent with this difference is the fact that scars form on the corneal side of the limbal lesion and not on the conjunctival side. The result is a triangular scar with its base at the limbus—a valuable sign of old phlyctenulosis when the limbus has been involved.

Conjunctival phlyctenules usually produce only irritation and tearing, but corneal and limbal phlyctenules are usually accompanied by intense photophobia. Phlyctenulosis is often triggered by active blepharitis, acute bacterial conjunctivitis, and dietary deficiencies. Phlyctenular scarring (Figure 5–17), which may be minimal or extensive, is often followed by Salzmann's nodular degeneration.

Histologically, the phlyctenule is a focal subepithelial and perivascular infiltration of small round cells, followed by a preponderance of polymorphonuclear cells when the overlying epithelium necrotizes and sloughs—a sequence of events characteristic of the delayed tuberculin type hypersensitivity reaction.

Phlyctenulosis induced by tuberculoprotein and the proteins of other systemic infections responds dramatically to topical corticosteroids. There is a major reduction of symptoms within 24 hours and disappearance of the lesion in another 24 hours. Phlyctenulosis produced by staphylococcal proteins responds somewhat more slowly. Topical antibiotics should be added for active staphylococcal blepharoconjunctivitis. Treatment should be aimed at the underlying disease, and the steroids, when effective, should be used only to control acute symptoms and persistent corneal scarring. Severe corneal scarring may call for corneal transplantation.

2. MILD CONJUNCTIVITIS SECONDARY TO CONTACT BLEPHARITIS

Contact blepharitis caused by atropine, neomycin, broad-spectrum antibiotics, and other topically applied medications is often followed by a mild infiltrative conjunctivitis that produces hyperemia, mild papillary hypertrophy, a mild mucoid discharge, and some irritation. Examination of Giemsa-stained scrapings often discloses only a few degenerated epithelial cells, a few polymorphonuclear and mononuclear cells, and no eosinophils.

Treatment should be directed toward finding the offending agent and eliminating it. The contact blepharitis may clear rapidly with topical corticosteroids, but their use should be limited. Long-term use of steroids on the lids may lead to steroid glaucoma and to skin atrophy with disfiguring telangiectasis.

CONJUNCTIVITIS DUE TO AUTOIMMUNE DISEASE

KERATOCONJUNCTIVITIS SICCA (Associated With Sjögren's Syndrome)

Sjögren's syndrome is a systemic disease characterized by a triad of disorders: keratoconjunctivitis sicca, xerostomia, and connective tissue dysfunction (arthritis). To establish the diagnosis of Sjögren's syndrome, at least two of the three disorders must be present. The disease is overwhelmingly more common in women at or beyond the menopause than in other groups, though men and younger women can also be affected. The lacrimal gland is infiltrated with lymphocytes and occasionally with plasma cells, and this leads to atrophy and destruction of the glandular structures.

Keratoconjunctivitis sicca is characterized by bulbar conjunctival hyperemia (especially in the palpebral aperture) and symptoms of irritation that are out of proportion to the mild inflammatory signs. It often begins as a mild conjunctivitis with a mucoid discharge. Blotchy epithelial lesions appear on the cornea, more prominently in its lower half, and filaments may be seen. Pain builds up in the afternoon and evening but is absent or only slight in the morning. The tear film is diminished and often contains shreds of mucus (Figure 5–18). Results of the Schirmer test are abnormal (see Chapter 4). Rose bengal staining in the palpebral aperture is a helpful diagnostic test.

The diagnosis is confirmed by demonstrating lymphocytic and plasma cell infiltration of the accessory salivary glands in a labial biopsy obtained by means of a simple surgical procedure (Figure 5–19).

Treatment should be directed toward preserving and replacing the tear film with artificial tears, with obliteration of the puncta, and with side shields, moisture chambers, and Buller shields. As a rule, the simpler measures should be tried first.

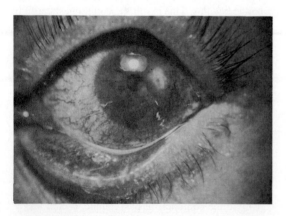

Figure 5–17. Postphlyctenulosis. Vascularized scar in temporal portion of left cornea.

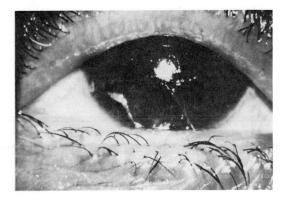

Figure 5–18. Keratoconjunctivitis sicca. (Courtesy of HB Ostler.)

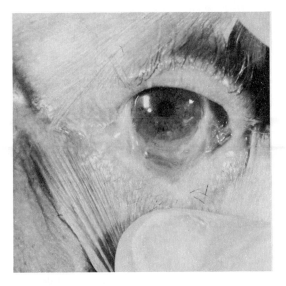

Figure 5–20. Cicatricial pemphigoid. (Courtesy of M Quickert.)

CICATRICIAL PEMPHIGOID

This disease usually begins as a nonspecific chronic conjunctivitis that is resistant to therapy. The conjunctiva may be affected alone or in combination with the mouth, nose, esophagus, vulva, and skin. The conjunctivitis leads to progressive scarring, obliteration of the fornices (especially the lower fornix) (Figure 5–20), and entropion with trichiasis. The patient complains of pain, irritation, and blurring of vision. The cornea is affected only secondarily as a result of trichiasis and lack of the precorneal tear film. The disease is more severe in women than in men. It is typically a disease of middle life, occurring very rarely before age 45. In women, it may progress to blindness in a year or less; in men, progress is slower, and spontaneous remission sometimes occurs.

Conjunctival biopsies may contain eosinophils, and the basement membrane will stain positively with certain immunofluorescent stains (IgG, IgM, IgA complement). Oral dapsone and immunosuppressive ther-

apy have been effective in some cases. Treatment must always be instituted at an early stage, prior to the onset of significant scarring. Generally, the course is long and the prognosis poor, with blindness due to complete symblepharon and corneal desiccation the usual outcome.

CHEMICAL OR IRRITATIVE CONJUNCTIVITIS

IATROGENIC CONJUNCTIVITIS FROM TOPICALLY APPLIED DRUGS

A toxic follicular conjunctivitis or an infiltrative, nonspecific conjunctivitis, followed by scarring, is often produced by the prolonged administration of dipivefrin, miotics, idoxuridine, neomycin, and other drugs prepared in toxic or irritating preservatives or vehicles. Silver nitrate instilled into the conjunctival sac at birth (Credé prophylaxis) is a frequent cause of mild chemical conjunctivitis. If tear production is reduced by continual irritation, the conjunctiva can be further damaged by the lack of dilution of the noxious agent as it is instilled into the conjunctival sac.

Conjunctival scrapings often contain keratinized epithelial cells, a few polymorphonuclear neutrophils, and an occasional oddly shaped cell. Treatment consists of stopping the offending agent and using bland drops

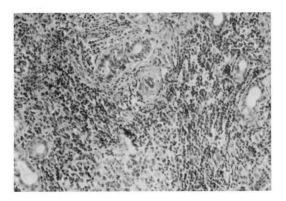

Figure 5–19. Mononuclear infiltration of the accessory salivary glands of a patient with Sjögren's syndrome. (Courtesy of K Tabbara.)

or none at all. Often the conjunctival reaction persists for weeks or months after its cause has been eliminated.

OCCUPATIONAL CONJUNCTIVITIS FROM CHEMICALS & IRRITANTS

Acids, alkalies, smoke, wind, and almost any irritating substance that enters the conjunctival sac may cause conjunctivitis. Some common irritants are fertilizers, soaps, deodorants, hair sprays, tobacco, makeup preparations (mascara, etc), and various acids and alkalies. In certain areas, smog has become the commonest cause of mild chemical conjunctivitis. The specific irritant in smog has not been positively identified, and treatment is nonspecific. There are no permanent ocular effects, but affected eyes are frequently chronically red and irritated.

In acid burns, the acids denature the tissue proteins and the effect is immediate. Alkalies do not denature the proteins but tend to penetrate the tissues deeply and rapidly and to linger in the conjunctival tissue. Here they continue to inflict damage for hours or days, depending on the molar concentration of the alkali and the amount introduced. Adhesion between the bulbar and palpebral conjunctiva (symblepharon) and corneal leukoma are more likely to occur if the offending agent is an alkali. In either event, pain, injection, photophobia, and blepharospasm are the principal symptoms of caustic burns. A history of the precipitating event can usually be elicited.

Immediate and profuse irrigation of the conjunctival sac with water or saline solution is of importance, and any solid material should be removed mechanically. Do not use chemical antidotes. General symptomatic measures include cold compresses for 20 minutes every hour, atropine 1% drops twice daily, and systemic analgesics as necessary. Bacterial conjunctivitis may be treated with appropriate antibacterial agents. Corneal scarring may require corneal transplantation, and symblephara may require a plastic operation on the conjunctiva. Severe conjunctival and corneal burns have a poor prognosis even with surgery, but if proper treatment is started immediately, scarring may be minimized and the prognosis improved.

CATERPILLAR HAIR CONJUNCTIVITIS (Ophthalmia Nodosum)

On rare occasions, caterpillar hairs are introduced into the conjunctival sac, where they produce one or many granulomas (ophthalmia nodosum). Under magnification, each granuloma is seen to contain a small foreign body.

Treatment by removal of each hair individually is effective. If a hair is retained, invasion of the sclera and uveal tract may occur.

CONJUNCTIVITIS OF UNKNOWN CAUSE

FOLLICULOSIS

Folliculosis is a widespread benign, bilateral noninflammatory conjunctival condition characterized by follicular hypertrophy. It is more common in children than in adults, and the symptoms are minimal. The follicles are more numerous in the lower than in the upper cul-de-sac and tarsal conjunctiva. There is no associated inflammation or papillary hypertrophy, and complications do not occur.

There is no treatment for folliculosis, which disappears spontaneously after a course of 2–3 years. The cause is unknown, but folliculosis may be only a manifestation of a generalized adenoidal hypertrophy.

CHRONIC FOLLICULAR CONJUNCTIVITIS (Orphan's Conjunctivitis, Axenfeld's Conjunctivitis)

Chronic follicular conjunctivitis is a bilateral transmissible disease of children characterized by numerous follicles in the upper and lower tarsal conjunctiva. There are minimal conjunctival exudates and minimal inflammation but no complications. Treatment is ineffective, but the disease is self-limited within 2 years.

OCULAR ROSACEA

Ocular rosacea is a common complication of acne rosacea and probably occurs more often in light-skinned people, especially of Irish descent, than in dark-skinned people. It is usually a blepharoconjunctivitis, but the cornea is sometimes also affected. The patient complains of mild injection and irritation. There is frequently an accompanying staphylococcal blepharitis. The blood vessels of the lid margins are dilated and the conjunctiva hyperemic, especially in the exposed interpalpebral region. Less often, there may be a nodular conjunctivitis with small gray nodules on the bulbar conjunctiva, especially near the limbus, which may ulcerate superficially. The lesions can be differentiated from phlyctenules by the fact that even after they subside, the large dilated vessels persist.

Microscopic examination of the nodules shows lymphocytes and epithelial cells. The peripheral cornea may ulcerate and vascularize, and the keratitis may have a narrow base at the limbus and a wider infiltrate centrally. The corneal pannus is often segmented or wedge-shaped inferiorly (Figures 5–21 and 5–22).

Treatment of ocular rosacea consists of the elimina-

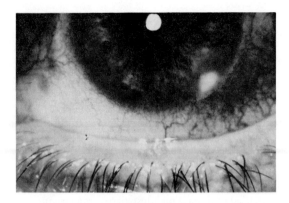

Figure 5–21. Conjunctivitis and corneal infiltrate in a patient with acne rosacea. (Courtesy of HB Ostler.)

tion of hot, spicy foods and of alcoholic beverages that cause dilation of the facial vessels. Any secondary staphylococcal infection should be treated. A course of oral tetracycline or doxycycline is often helpful, and a smaller maintenance dose may be needed to control the disease.

The disease is chronic, recurrences are common, and the response to treatment is usually poor. If the cornea is not affected, the visual prognosis is good; but corneal lesions tend to recur and progress, and the vision grows steadily worse over a period of years.

PSORIASIS

Psoriasis vulgaris usually affects the areas of the skin not exposed to the sun, but in about 10% of cases lesions appear on the skin of the eyelids, and the plaques may

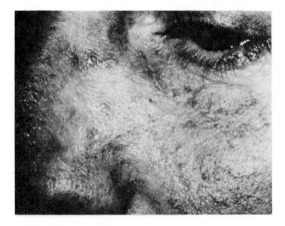

Figure 5–22. Skin lesions in acne rosacea. (Courtesy of HB Ostler.)

extend to the conjunctiva, where they cause irritation, a foreign body sensation, and tearing. Psoriasis can also cause nonspecific chronic conjunctivitis with considerable mucoid discharge. Rarely, the cornea may show marginal ulceration or a deep, vascularized opacity.

The conjunctival and corneal lesions wax and wane with the skin lesions and are not affected by specific treatment. In rare cases, conjunctival scarring (symblepharon, trichiasis), corneal scarring, and occlusion of the nasolacrimal duct have occurred.

ERYTHEMA MULTIFORME MAJOR (Stevens-Johnson Syndrome)

Erythema multiforme major is a disease of the mucous membranes and skin. The skin lesion is an erythematous, urticarial bullous eruption that appears suddenly and is often distributed symmetrically. Bilateral conjunctivitis, often membranous, is a common manifestation. The patient complains of pain, irritation, discharge, and photophobia. The cornea is affected secondarily, and vascularization and scarring may seriously reduce vision. Stevens-Johnson syndrome is typically a disease of young people, occurring only rarely after age 35.

Cultures are negative for bacteria; conjunctival scrapings show a preponderance of polymorphonuclear cells. Systemic steroids are thought to shorten the course of the systemic disease but have little or no effect on the eye lesions. Careful cleansing of the conjunctiva to remove the accumulated secretion is helpful, however, and tear replacement may be indicated. If trichiasis and entropion supervene, they should be corrected. Topical steroids probably have no beneficial effect, and their protracted use can cause corneal melting and perforation.

The acute episode of Stevens-Johnson syndrome usually lasts about 6 weeks, but the conjunctival scarring, loss of tears, and complications from entropion and trichiasis may result in prolonged morbidity and progressive corneal cicatrization (Figure 5–23). Recurrences are rare.

DERMATITIS HERPETIFORMIS

This is a rare skin disorder characterized by symmetrically grouped erythematous papulovesicular, vesicular, or bullous lesions. The disease has a predilection for the posterior axillary fold, the sacral region, the buttocks, and the forearms. Itching is often severe. Rarely, a pseudomembranous conjunctivitis occurs and may result in cicatrization resembling that seen in benign mucous membrane pemphigoid. The skin eruption and conjunctivitis usually respond readily to systemic sulfones or sulfapyridine.

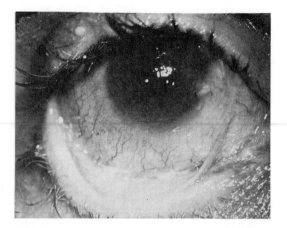

Figure 5–23. Late sequelae of Stevens-Johnson syndrome: conjunctival and corneal cicatrization and epidermalization. (Courtesy of P Thygeson.)

EPIDERMOLYSIS BULLOSA

This is a rare hereditary disease characterized by vesicles, bullae, and epidermal cysts. The lesions occur chiefly on the extensor surfaces of the joints and other areas exposed to trauma. The severe dystrophic type that leads to scarring may also produce conjunctival scars similar to those seen in dermatitis herpetiformis and benign mucous membrane pemphigoid. No known treatment is satisfactory.

SUPERIOR LIMBIC KERATOCONJUNCTIVITIS

Superior limbic keratoconjunctivitis is usually bilateral and limited to the upper tarsus and upper limbus. The principal complaints are irritation and hyperemia. The signs are papillary hypertrophy of the upper tarsus, redness of the superior bulbar conjunctiva, thickening and keratinization of the superior limbus, epithelial keratitis, recurrent superior filaments, and superior micropannus. Rose bengal staining is a helpful diagnostic test. The keratinized epithelial cells and mucous debris pick up the stain. Scrapings from the upper limbus show keratinizing epithelial cells.

In about 50% of cases, the condition has been associated with abnormal function of the thyroid gland. Applying 0.5% or 1% silver nitrate to the upper palpebral conjunctiva and allowing the tarsus to drop back onto the upper limbus usually result in shedding of the keratinizing cells and relief of symptoms for 4–6 weeks. This treatment can be repeated. There are no complications, and the disease usually runs a course of 2–4 years.

In severe cases, one may consider 5 mm resection of the perilimbal superior conjunctiva.

LIGNEOUS CONJUNCTIVITIS

This is a rare bilateral, chronic or recurrent, pseudomembranous or membranous conjunctivitis that arises early in life, predominantly in young girls, and often persists for many years. Granulomas are often associated with it, and the lids may feel very hard. Cyclosporine may be effective treatment, as suggested by recent reports.

REITER'S SYNDROME

A triad of disease manifestations—nonspecific urethritis, arthritis, and conjunctivitis or iritis—constitutes Reiter's syndrome. The disease occurs much more often in men than in women. The conjunctivitis is papillary in type and usually bilateral. Conjunctival scrapings contain polymorphonuclear cells. No bacteria grow in cultures. The arthritis usually affects the large weight-bearing joints. There is no satisfactory treatment, though nonsteroidal anti-inflammatory agents may be effective. Corticosteroids will help the iridocyclitis. The disease has been found in association with HLA-B27 antigen.

MUCOCUTANEOUS LYMPH NODE SYNDROME (Kawasaki Disease)

This disease of unknown cause was first described in Japan in 1967. Conjunctivitis is one of its six diagnostic features. The others are (1) fever that fails to respond to antibiotics; (2) changes in the lips and oral cavity; (3) such changes in the extremities as erythema of the palms and soles, indurative edema, and membranous desquamation of the fingertips; (4) polymorphous exanthem of the trunk; and (5) acute nonpurulent swelling of the cervical lymph nodes.

The disease occurs almost exclusively in prepubertal children and carries a 1–2% mortality rate from cardiac failure. The conjunctivitis has not been severe, and no corneal lesions have been reported.

Treatment is supportive only.

CONJUNCTIVITIS ASSOCIATED WITH SYSTEMIC DISEASE

CONJUNCTIVITIS IN THYROID DISEASE

In orbital Graves' disease, the conjunctiva may be red and chemotic and the patient may complain of copious tearing. As the disease progresses, the chemosis increases, and in advanced cases the chemotic conjunctiva may extrude between the lids.

Treatment is directed toward control of the thyroid disease, and every effort must be made to protect the conjunctiva and cornea by bland ointment, surgical lid adhesions (tarsorrhaphy) if necessary, or even orbital decompression if the lids do not close enough to cover the cornea and conjunctiva.

GOUTY CONJUNCTIVITIS

Patients with gout often complain of a "hot eye" during attacks. On examination, a mild conjunctivitis is found that is less severe than suggested by the symptoms. Gout may also be associated with episcleritis or scleritis, iridocyclitis, keratitis urica, vitreous opacities, and retinopathy. Treatment is aimed at controlling the gouty attack with colchicine and allopurinol.

CARCINOID CONJUNCTIVITIS

In carcinoid, the conjunctiva is sometimes congested and cyanotic as a result of the secretion of serotonin by the chromaffin cells of the gastrointestinal tract. The patient may complain of a "hot eye" during such attacks.

CONJUNCTIVITIS SECONDARY TO DACRYOCYSTITIS OR CANALICULITIS

CONJUNCTIVITIS SECONDARY TO DACRYOCYSTITIS

Both pneumococcal conjunctivitis (often unilateral and unresponsive to treatment) and beta-hemolytic streptococcal conjunctivitis (often hyperacute and purulent) may be secondary to chronic dacryocystitis. The nature and source of the conjunctivitis in both instances are often missed until the lacrimal system is investigated.

CONJUNCTIVITIS SECONDARY TO CANALICULITIS

Canaliculitis due to canalicular infection with *Actinomyces israelii* or *Candida* spp (or, very rarely, *Aspergillus* spp) may cause unilateral mucopurulent conjunctivitis, often chronic. The source of the condition is often missed unless the characteristic hyperemic, pouting punctum is noted. Expression of the canaliculus (upper or lower, whichever is involved) is curative provided the entire concretion is removed.

Conjunctival scrapings show a predominance of polymorphonuclear cells. Cultures (unless anaerobic) are usually negative. *Candida* grows readily on ordinary culture media, but almost all of the infections are caused by *A israelii,* which requires an anaerobic medium.

II. DEGENERATIVE DISEASES OF THE CONJUNCTIVA

PINGUECULA

Pingueculae are extremely common in adults. They appear as yellow nodules on both sides of the cornea (more commonly on the nasal side) in the area of the palpebral aperture. The nodules, consisting of hyaline and yellow elastic tissue, rarely increase in size, but inflammation is common. In general, no treatment is required, but in certain cases of pingueculitis, weak topical steroids (eg, prednisolone 0.12%) or topical nonsteroidal anti-inflammatory medications may be given (Figure 5–24).

PTERYGIUM

A pterygium is a fleshy, triangular encroachment of a pinguecula onto the cornea, usually on the nasal side bilaterally (Figure 5–25). It is thought to be an irritative phenomenon due to ultraviolet light, drying, and windy environments, since it is common in persons who spend much of their lives out of doors in sunny, dusty, or sandy, windblown surroundings. The pathologic findings in the conjunctiva are the same as those of pinguecula. In the cornea, there is replacement of Bowman's layer by hyaline and elastic tissue.

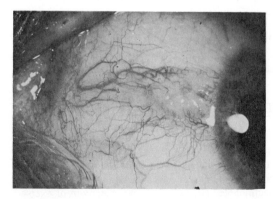

Figure 5–24. Pinguecula. (Courtesy of A Rosenberg.)

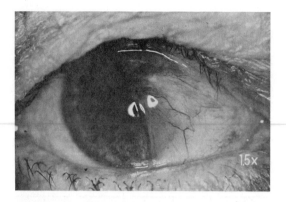

Figure 5–25. Pterygium encroaching on the cornea. (Courtesy of G Mintsioulis.)

If the pterygium is enlarging and encroaches on the pupillary area, it should be removed surgically along with a small portion of superficial clear cornea beyond the area of encroachment. To prevent recurrences, particularly in people who work out of doors, protective glasses should be worn.

CLIMATIC DROPLET KERATOPATHY (Bietti's Band-Shaped Nodular Dystrophy, Labrador Keratopathy, Spheroidal Degeneration, etc)

Climatic droplet keratopathy is an uncommon degenerative disorder of the cornea characterized by aggregates of yellowish-golden spherules that accumulate in the subepithelial layers. The cause is unknown, but certain factors such as exposure to ultraviolet light, aridity, and microtrauma are recognized predisposing factors. The deposits may result in elevation of the epithelium in a band-shaped configuration. The condition is more common in geographic regions with high levels of direct and reflected sunlight.

III. MISCELLANEOUS DISORDERS OF THE CONJUNCTIVA

LYMPHANGIECTASIS

Lymphangiectasis is characterized by localized small, clear, tortuous dilations in the conjunctiva. They are merely dilated lymph vessels, and no treatment is indicated unless they are irritating or cosmetically objectionable. They can then be cauterized or excised.

CONGENITAL CONJUNCTIVAL LYMPHEDEMA

This is a rare entity, unilateral or bilateral, and characterized by pinkish, fleshy edema of the bulbar conjunctiva. Usually observed as an isolated entity at birth, the condition is thought to be due to a congenital defect in the lymphatic drainage of the conjunctiva. It has been observed in chronic hereditary lymphedema of the lower extremities (Milroy's disease) and is thought to be an ocular manifestation of this disease rather than an associated anomaly.

CYSTINOSIS

Cystinosis is a rare congenital disorder of amino acid metabolism characterized by widespread intracellular deposition of cystine crystals in various body tissues, including the conjunctiva and cornea. Three types are recognized: childhood, adolescent, and adult. Life expectancy is reduced in the first two types.

SUBCONJUNCTIVAL HEMORRHAGE

This common disorder may occur spontaneously, usually in only one eye, in any age group. Its sudden onset and bright red appearance usually alarm the patient. The hemorrhage is caused by rupture of a small conjunctival vessel, sometimes preceded by a bout of severe coughing or sneezing.

The best treatment is reassurance. The hemorrhage usually absorbs in 2–3 weeks.

In rare instances the hemorrhages are bilateral or recurrent; the possibility of blood dyscrasias should then be ruled out.

OPHTHALMIA NEONATORUM

Ophthalmia neonatorum in its broad sense refers to any infection of the newborn conjunctiva. In its narrow and commonly used sense, however, it refers to a conjunctival infection, chiefly gonococcal, that follows contamination of the baby's eyes during its passage through the mother's cervix and vagina or during the postpartum period. Because gonococcal conjunctivitis can rapidly cause blindness, the etiology of all cases of ophthalmia neonatorum should be verified by examination of smears of exudate, epithelial scrapings, cultures, and rapid tests for gonococci.

Gonococcal neonatal conjunctivitis causes corneal ulceration and blindness if not treated immediately. Chlamydial neonatal conjunctivitis (inclusion blennorrhea) is less destructive but can last months if untreated and may be followed by pneumonia. Other causes include infections with staphylococci, pneumococci, *Haemophilus,* and herpes simplex virus and silver nitrate prophylaxis.

The time of onset is important in clinical diagnosis since the two principal types, gonorrheal ophthalmia and inclusion blennorrhea, have widely differing incubation periods: gonococcal disease 2–3 days and chlamydial disease 5–12 days. The third important birth canal infection (HSV-2 keratoconjunctivitis) has a 2- to 3-day incubation period and is potentially quite serious because of the possibility of systemic dissemination.

Treatment for neonatal gonococcal conjunctivitis is with ceftriaxone, 125 mg as a single intramuscular dose; a second choice is kanamycin, 75 mg intramuscularly. To treat chlamydial conjunctivitis in newborns, erythromycin oral suspension is effective at a dosage of 40 mg/kg/d in four divided doses for 2 weeks. In both gonococcal and chlamydial conjunctivitis, the parents need to be treated. Herpes simplex keratoconjunctivitis is treated with acyclovir, 30 mg/kg/d in three divided doses for 14 days. Other types of neonatal conjunctivitis are treated with erythromycin, gentamicin, or tobramycin ophthalmic ointment four times daily.

Credé 1% silver nitrate prophylaxis is effective for the prevention of gonorrheal ophthalmia but not inclusion blennorrhea or herpetic infection. The slight chemical conjunctivitis induced by silver nitrate is minor and of short duration. Accidents with concentrated solutions can be avoided by using wax ampules specially prepared for Credé prophylaxis. Tetracycline and erythromycin ointment are effective substitutes.

OCULOGLANDULAR DISEASE (Parinaud's Oculoglandular Syndrome)

This is a group of conjunctival diseases, usually unilateral, characterized by low-grade fever, grossly visible preauricular adenopathy, and one or more conjunctival granulomas (Figure 5–26). The commonest cause is cat-scratch disease, but there are many other causes, including *Mycobacterium tuberculosis, Treponema pallidum, Francisella tularensis, Pasteurella (Yersinia) pseudotuberculosis, Chlamydia trachomatis* serotypes L1, L2, and L3, and *Coccidioides immitis.*

Conjunctival Cat-Scratch Disease

This protracted but benign granulomatous conjunctivitis is found most commonly in children who have been in intimate contact with cats. The child often runs a low-grade fever and develops a reasonably enlarged preauricular node and one or more conjunctival granulomas. These may show focal necrosis and may sometimes ulcerate. The regional adenopathy does not suppurate. The clinical diagnosis is supported by a positive cat-scratch disease skin test.

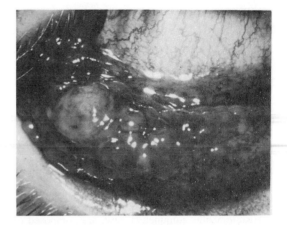

Figure 5–26. Conjunctival granuloma. (Courtesy of P Thygeson.)

The disease appears to be caused by a slender pleomorphic gram-negative bacillus (*Bartonella* [formerly *Rochalimaea*] henselae), which grows in the walls of blood vessels. With special stains, this organism can be seen in biopsies of conjunctival tissue. The organism closely resembles *Leptotrichia buccalis,* and the disease was previously known as leptotrichosis conjunctivae (Parinaud's conjunctivitis). The organism is commonly found in the mouth in humans and always in the mouth in cats. The eye may be contaminated by saliva on the child's fingers or by cat saliva on the child's pillow.

Afipia felis has been incriminated also and may still play a role.

The disease is self-limited (without corneal or other complications) and resolves in 2–3 months. The conjunctival nodule can be excised; in the case of a solitary granuloma, this may be curative. Systemic tetracyclines may shorten the course but should not be given to children under 7 years of age.

Conjunctivitis Secondary to Neoplasms (Masquerade Syndrome)

When examined superficially, a neoplasm of the conjunctiva or lid margin is often misdiagnosed as a chronic infectious conjunctivitis or keratoconjunctivitis. Since the underlying lesion is often not recognized, the condition has been referred to as masquerade syndrome. The masquerading neoplasms on record are conjunctival capillary carcinoma, conjunctival carcinoma in situ, infectious papilloma of the conjunctiva, sebaceous gland carcinoma, and verrucae. Verrucae and molluscum tumors of the lid margin may desquamate toxic tumor material that produces a chronic conjunctivitis, keratoconjunctivitis, or (rarely) keratitis alone.

IV. CONJUNCTIVAL TUMORS

J. Brooks Crawford, MD

PRIMARY BENIGN TUMORS OF THE CONJUNCTIVA

Nevus
(Figure 5–27)

One-third of melanocytic nevi of the conjunctiva lack pigment. Over half have cystic epithelial inclusions that can be seen clinically.

Histologically, conjunctival nevi are composed of nests or sheets of typical nevus cells. Conjunctival nevi, like other nevi, rarely become malignant. Many are excised because they are disfiguring.

Pigmented conjunctival nevi must be distinguished from primary acquired melanosis of the conjunctiva. The latter occurs later in life (after the third decade), is usually unilateral, tends to wax and wane in degree of pigmentation, and, depending on the degree of cellular atypia, has a risk of becoming malignant ranging from nil to 90%.

Papilloma

Conjunctival papillomas are not rare, occurring most frequently near the limbus, on the caruncle, or at the lid margins. Those on the caruncle and lid margin are usually soft and pedunculated, with irregular surfaces. They frequently recur after removal.

Granulomatous Inflammation

Granulomatous inflammation occurs around foreign bodies, around extravasated sebaceous material in chalazia, and in association with diseases such as coccidioidomycosis and sarcoidosis. These inflammatory foci may form elevated plaques or nodules in the skin or the conjunctiva of the eyelids.

Dermoid Tumor
(Figure 5–28)

This rare congenital tumor appears as a smooth, rounded, yellow elevated mass, frequently with hairs protruding. A dermoid tumor may remain quiescent, though it often increases in size. Removal is indicated only if cosmetic deformity is significant or if vision is impaired or threatened. Limbal dermoids and dermolipomas are part of the syndrome of oculoauriculovertebral dysplasia (Goldenhar's syndrome).

Dermolipoma

Dermolipoma is a common congenital tumor that usually appears as a smoothly rounded growth in the upper temporal quadrant of the bulbar conjunctiva near the lateral canthus. Treatment is usually not indicated, but at least partial removal may be indicated if the growth is enlarging or is cosmetically disfiguring. Posterior dissection must be undertaken with extreme care (if at all) since this lesion is frequently continuous with orbital fat; orbital derangement may cause scarring and complications far more serious than the original lesion.

Lymphoma & Lymphoid Hyperplasia

These are uncommon conjunctival lesions that may appear in adults without evidence of systemic disease or associated with systemic lymphosarcoma or various blood dyscrasias. Benign lymphoid hyperplasia can sometimes be distinguished by a pebbly appearance corresponding to follicle formation. However, the clinical appearance of benign lymphoid hyperplasia and malignant lymphoma can be similar; therefore, biopsy is essential to establish a diagnosis. Since many of these lymphoid tumors may involve the orbit, an MRI or CT scan may be required to determine the true extent of the tumor.

Treatment of both benign and malignant lesions is best accomplished with radiotherapy.

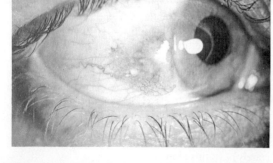

Figure 5–27. Conjunctival nevus. (Courtesy of A Irvine, Jr.)

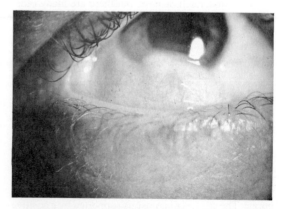

Figure 5–28. Dermoid tumor at the inferior limbus. (Courtesy of A Irvine, Jr.)

Angioma

Conjunctival angiomas may occur as isolated, circumscribed capillary hemangiomas or as more diffuse vascular tumors, often associated with a more extensive lid or orbital capillary or cavernous hemangioma. Hemangiomas should be distinguished from telangiectases involving conjunctival capillaries. Telangiectatic conjunctival vessels may occur as isolated lesions or may be associated with systemic vascular hamartomas in Rendu-Osler-Weber disease or in ataxia-telangiectasia (Louis-Bar syndrome).

Pyogenic granulomas are a variety of capillary hemangiomas. They frequently occur on the palpebral conjunctiva over chalazia or in an area of recent surgery.

In Kaposi's sarcoma associated with AIDS, red-blue vascular nodules ("malignant granulation tissue") may first become apparent in the conjunctiva.

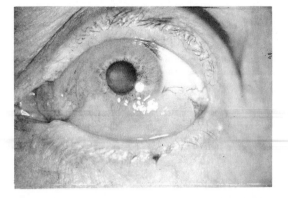

Figure 5–29. Intraepithelial epithelioma. (Courtesy of A Irvine, Jr.)

PRIMARY MALIGNANT TUMORS OF THE BULBAR CONJUNCTIVA

Carcinoma

Carcinoma of the conjunctiva (Figure 5–29) arises most frequently at the limbus in the area of the palpebral fissure and less often in nonexposed areas of the conjunctiva. Some of these tumors may resemble pterygia. Most have a gelatinous surface; sometimes, abnormal keratinization of the epithelium produces leukoplakia. Growth is slow, and deep invasion and metastases are extremely rare; therefore, complete excision is effective treatment. Recurrences are common if the lesion is incompletely excised; treatment consists of reexcision. The use of cryotherapy may help to prevent recurrences.

Conjunctival dysplasia, also called atypical epithelial dysplasia, is a benign condition that occurs as an isolated lesion or sometimes over pterygia and pingueculae and can resemble carcinoma in situ clinically and even histologically. The term **conjunctival intraepithelial neoplasia** (CIN) can be applied to lesions that have features intermediate between conjunctival dysplasia and obviously malignant carcinoma in situ.

Excisional biopsy will establish a diagnosis and result in cure of most of these lesions.

Malignant Melanoma

Malignant melanoma of the conjunctiva is rare. It may arise from a preexisting nevus, from an area of acquired melanosis, or de novo from formerly normal-appearing conjunctiva. Pigmentation may vary greatly, and the clinical course is often unpredictable.

Many tumors can be locally excised. More radical surgery (eg, exenteration of the orbit) does not usually improve the prognosis. The use of cryotherapy after excision of melanotic tumors may help to prevent recurrences.

Lymphosarcoma

Malignant lymphomas of the conjunctiva are much rarer than benign lymphoid hyperplasia. Many also involve the orbit, and a few are associated with systemic lymphoma. However, the conjunctival lesion may be the initial sign of a systemic problem.

REFERENCES

Al-Mutlaq F, Byrne-Rhodes KA, Tabbara KF: *Neisseria meningitidis* conjunctivitis in children. Am J Ophthalmol 1987;104:280.

Allansmith MR et al: Giant papillary conjunctivitis in contact lens wearers. Am J Ophthalmol 1977;83:697.

Bron AJ, Mengher LS: The ocular surface in keratoconjunctivitis sicca. Eye 1989;3:428.

Butrus SI, Abelson MB: Laboratory evaluation of ocular allergy. Int Ophthalmol Clin 1988;28:324.

Chandler JW: Controversies in ocular prophylaxis of newborns. Arch Ophthalmol 1989;107:814.

Courtright P et al: Trachoma and blindness in the Nile Delta: Current patterns and projections for the future in the rural Egyptian population. Br J Ophthalmol 1989;73:536.

Darougar S, Mohnickendam MA, Woodland RM: Management and prevention of ocular viral and chlamydial infections. CRC Critical Reviews in Microbiology 1989;16:369.

Dawson CR, Hanna L, Togni B: Adenovirus type 8 infections in the United States: IV. Observations on the pathogenesis of lesions in severe eye disease. Arch Ophthalmol 1972;87:258.

Dawson CR, Jones BR, Tarizzo ML: *Guide to Trachoma Control in Programmes for the Prevention of Blindness.* World Health Organization, 1981.

De Potter P et al: Clinical predictive factors for development of recurrence and metastasis in conjunctival melanoma: A review of 68 cases. Br J Ophthalmol 1993;77:624.

Duane TD (editor): *Clinical Ophthalmology,* 2nd ed. Harper & Row, 1990.

English CK et al: Cat-scratch disease: Isolation and culture of the bacterial agent. JAMA 1988;259:1347.

Fitch CP et al: Epidemiology and diagnosis of acute conjunctivitis at an inner city hospital. Ophthalmology 1989;96:1215.

Folberg R et al: Benign conjunctival melanocyte lesions: Clinicopathologic features. Ophthalmology 1989;96:436.

Ford E, Nelson KE, Warren D: Epidemiology of epidemic keratoconjunctivitis. Epidemiol Rev 1987;9:244.

Foster CS: Evaluation of topical cromolyn sodium in the treatment of vernal keratoconjunctivitis. Ophthalmology 1988;95:194.

Foster CS, Calonge M: Atopic keratoconjunctivitis. Ophthalmology 1990;97:992.

Heiligenhaus A et al: Long-term results of mucous membrane grafting in ocular cicatricial pemphigoid: Implications for patient selection and surgical considerations. Ophthalmology 1993;100:1283.

Hoang-Xuan T et al: Ocular rosacea. Ophthalmology 1990;97:1468.

Ishii K et al: Comparative studies on aetiology and epidemiology of viral conjunctivitis in three countries of East Asia: Japan, Taiwan and South Korea. Int J Epidemiol 1987; 16:98.

Jakobiec FA, Folberg R, Iwamoto T: Clinicopathologic characteristics of premalignant and malignant melanocytic lesions of the conjunctiva. Ophthalmology 1989;96:146.

Jakobiec FA, Knowles DM: An overview of ocular adnexal lymphoid tumors. Trans Am Ophthalmol Soc 1989;97:420.

Kersten RC, Shoukrey NM, Tabbara KF: Orbital myiasis. Ophthalmology 1986;93:1228.

Koehler JE et al: *Rochalimaea henselae* infection: A new zoonosis with the domestic cat as reservoir. JAMA 1994;271:531.

Krohn MA et al: The bacterial etiology of conjunctivitis in early infancy. Am J Epidemiol 1993;138:326.

Lemp MA, Mahmood MA, Weiler HH: Association of rosacea and keratoconjunctivitis sicca. Arch Ophthalmol 1984;102:556.

Moran JS, Zemilissian JM: Therapy for gonococcal infections: Options in 1989. Rev Inf Dis 1989;23(Suppl 6):33.

Paridaens ADA et al: Orbital exenteration in 95 cases of primary conjunctival malignant melanoma. Br J Ophthalmol 1994;78:520.

Paridaens ADA et al: Prognostic factors in primary malignant melanoma of the conjunctiva: A clinicopathological study of 256 cases. Br J Ophthalmol 1994;78:252.

Pfister RR: Chemical injuries of the eye. Ophthalmology 1983;90:1246.

Phillips G, Forsyth JS, Harper IA: Diagnosis of neonatal chlamydial conjunctivitis. Arch Dis Childhood 1990; 65:894.

Rice BA, Foster CS: Immunopathology of cicatricial pemphigoid affecting the conjunctiva. Ophthalmology 1990; 97:1476.

Savino DF, Margo CE: Conjunctival rhinosporidiosis: Light and electron microscopic study. Ophthalmology 1983; 90:1482.

Shuler JD, Engstrom RE Jr, Holland GN: External ocular disease and anterior segment disorders associated with AIDS. Int Ophthalmol Clin 1989;29:98.

Singer TR, Isenberg SJ, Apt L: Conjunctival anaerobic and aerobic bacterial flora in paediatric versus adult subjects. Br J Ophthalmol 1988;72:448.

Sjögren H: Keratoconjunctivitis sicca and the Sjögren syndrome. Surv Ophthalmol 1971;16:145.

Sommer A: Effects of vitamin A deficiency on the ocular surface. Ophthalmology 1983;90:592.

Spencer WH (editor): *Ophthalmic Pathology,* 3rd ed. 3 vols. Saunders, 1985.

Tabbara KF, Hyndiuk RA: *Infections of the Eye.* Little, Brown, 1986.

Tamesis RR, Foster CS: Ocular syphilis. Ophthalmology 1990;97:1281.

Thygeson P: Historical review of oculogenital disease. Am J Ophthalmol 1971;71:975.

Thygeson P: Observations on conjunctival neoplasms masquerading as chronic conjunctivitis or keratitis. Trans Am Acad Ophthalmol Otolaryngol 1969;73:969.

Thylefors B et al: A simple system for the assessment of trachoma and its complications Bull WHO 1987;65:477.

Wishart PK et al: Prevalence of acute conjunctivitis caused by *Chlamydia,* adenovirus, and herpes simplex virus in an ophthalmic casualty department. Br J Ophthalmol 1984; 68:653.

Cornea

6

Roderick Biswell, MD

PHYSIOLOGY

The cornea functions as a protective membrane and a "window" through which light rays pass to the retina. Its transparency is due to its uniform structure, avascularity, and deturgescence. Deturgescence, or the state of relative dehydration of the corneal tissue, is maintained by the active bicarbonate "pump" of the endothelium and the barrier function of the epithelium and endothelium. The endothelium is more important than the epithelium in the mechanism of dehydration, and chemical or physical damage to the endothelium is far more serious than damage to the epithelium. Destruction of the endothelial cells causes edema of the cornea and loss of transparency. On the other hand, damage to the epithelium causes only transient, localized edema of the corneal stroma that clears when the epithelial cells regenerate. Evaporation of water from the precorneal tear film produces hypertonicity of the film; that process and direct evaporation are factors that draw water from the superficial corneal stroma in order to maintain the state of dehydration.

Penetration of the intact cornea by drugs is biphasic. Fat-soluble substances can pass through intact epithelium, and water-soluble substances can pass through intact stroma. To pass through the cornea, drugs must therefore have both a lipid-soluble and a water-soluble phase.

CORNEAL RESISTANCE TO INFECTION

The epithelium is an efficient barrier to the entrance of microorganisms into the cornea. Once the epithelium is traumatized, however, the avascular stroma and Bowman's layer become susceptible to infection with a variety of organisms, including bacteria, amebas, and fungi. *Streptococcus pneumoniae* (the pneumococcus) is a true bacterial corneal pathogen; other pathogens require a heavy inoculum or a compromised host (eg, immune deficiency) to produce infection.

Moraxella liquefaciens, which occurs mainly in al-coholics (as a result of pyridoxine depletion), is a classic example of the bacterial opportunist, and in recent years a number of new corneal opportunists have been identified. Among them are *Serratia marcescens, Mycobacterium fortuitum-chelonei* complex, viridans streptococci, *Staphylococcus epidermidis,* and various coliform and *Proteus* organisms, along with viruses and fungi.

Local or systemic corticosteroids modify the host immune reaction in several ways and may allow opportunistic organisms to invade and flourish.

PHYSIOLOGY OF SYMPTOMS

Since the cornea has many pain fibers, most corneal lesions, superficial or deep (corneal foreign body, corneal abrasion, phlyctenule, interstitial keratitis), cause pain and photophobia. The pain is worsened by movement of the lids (particularly the upper lid) over the cornea and usually persists until healing occurs. Since the cornea serves as the window of the eye and refracts light rays, corneal lesions usually blur vision somewhat, especially if centrally located.

Photophobia in corneal disease is the result of painful contraction of an inflamed iris. Dilation of iris vessels is a reflex phenomenon caused by irritation of the corneal nerve endings. Photophobia, severe in most corneal disease, is minimal in herpetic keratitis because of the hypesthesia associated with the disease, which is also a valuable diagnostic sign.

Although tearing and photophobia commonly accompany corneal disease, there is usually no discharge except in purulent bacterial ulcers.

INVESTIGATION OF CORNEAL DISEASE

Symptoms & Signs

The physician examines the cornea by inspecting it under adequate illumination. Examination is often facilitated by instillation of a local anesthetic. Fluorescein staining can outline a superficial epithelial lesion that might otherwise be impossible to see. The biomicroscope (slitlamp) is essential in proper examination of the cornea; in its absence, a loupe and bright illumination can be used. One should follow the course of the light reflection while moving the light carefully over the entire cornea. Rough areas indicative of epithelial defects are demonstrated in this way.

The patient's history is important in corneal disease. A history of trauma can often be elicited—in fact, foreign bodies and abrasions are the two most common corneal lesions. A history of corneal disease may also be of value. The keratitis of herpes simplex infection is often recurrent, but since recurrent erosion is extremely painful and herpetic keratitis is not, these disorders can be differentiated by their symptoms. The patient's use of local medications should be investigated, since corticosteroids may have been used and may have predisposed to bacterial, fungal, or viral disease, especially herpes simplex keratitis. Immunosuppression also occurs with systemic diseases, such as diabetes, AIDS, and malignant disease, as well as with specific immunosuppressive therapy.

Laboratory Studies

To select the proper therapy for corneal infections, especially suppurating ulceration, laboratory aid is essential. Bacterial and fungal ulcers, for example, require completely different medications. Since a delay in identifying the organism may severely compromise the ultimate visual result, scrapings from the ulcer should be stained by both Gram's and Giemsa's stains and the infecting organism identified if possible while the patient waits. Cultures for bacteria and fungi must be done at the same time, since identification of the organism is critical. Appropriate therapy can then be instituted immediately. Therapy should not be withheld if an organism cannot be identified by smear and staining.

Morphologic Diagnosis of Corneal Lesions

A. Epithelial Keratitis: The corneal epithelium is involved in most types of conjunctivitis and keratitis and in rare cases may be the only tissue involved (eg, in superficial punctate keratitis). The epithelial changes vary widely from simple edema and vacuolation to minute erosions, filament formation, partial keratinization, etc. The lesions vary also in their location on the cornea. All of these variations have important diagnostic significance (Table 6–1), and biomicroscopic examination with and without fluorescein staining should be a part of every external eye examination.

B. Subepithelial Keratitis: There are a number of important types of discrete subepithelial lesions. These are often secondary to epithelial keratitis (eg, the subepithelial infiltrates of epidemic keratoconjunctivitis, caused by adenoviruses 8 and 19). They can usually be observed grossly but may also be recognized in the course of biomicroscopic examination of epithelial keratitis.

C. Stromal Keratitis: The responses of the corneal stroma to disease include infiltration, representing accumulation of inflammatory cells; edema manifested as corneal thickening, opacification, or scarring; thinning or melting, which may lead to perforation; and vascularization. The patterns of these responses are less specific for disease entities than those seen in epithelial keratitis, and the clinician often must rely on other clinical information and laboratory studies for clear identification of causes.

D. Endothelial Keratitis: Dysfunction of the corneal endothelium results in corneal edema, initially involving the stroma and later the epithelium. This contrasts with corneal edema due to raised intraocular pressure, in which the epithelium is affected before the stroma. As long as the cornea is not too edematous, it is often possible to visualize morphologic abnormalities of the corneal endothelium with the slitlamp. Inflammatory cells on the endothelium (keratic precipitates, or KPs) are not always an indication of endothelial disease because they are also a manifestation of anterior uveitis, which may or may not accompany stromal keratitis.

CORNEAL ULCERATION

Cicatrization due to corneal ulceration is a major cause of blindness and impaired vision throughout the world. Most of this visual loss is preventable, but only if an etiologic diagnosis is made early and appropriate therapy instituted. Central suppurative ulceration was once caused almost exclusively by *S pneumoniae*. In recent years, however, often as a result of the widespread use of compromising systemic and local medications (at least in the developed countries), opportunistic bacteria, fungi, and viruses have tended to cause more cases of corneal ulcer than *S pneumoniae*.

CENTRAL CORNEAL ULCERS

Central ulcers usually are infectious ulcers that follow epithelial damage. The lesion is situated centrally, away from the vascularized limbus. Hypopyon usually (not always) accompanies the ulcer. Hypopyon is a collection of inflammatory cells that appears as a pale layer in the inferior anterior chamber and is characteristic of both bacterial and fungal central corneal ulcers.

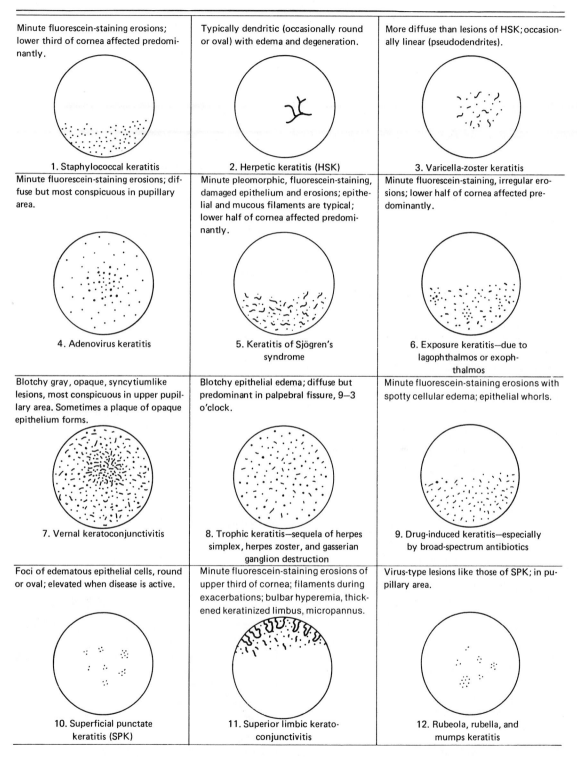

Minute fluorescein-staining erosions; lower third of cornea affected predominantly.

1. Staphylococcal keratitis

Typically dendritic (occasionally round or oval) with edema and degeneration.

2. Herpetic keratitis (HSK)

More diffuse than lesions of HSK; occasionally linear (pseudodendrites).

3. Varicella-zoster keratitis

Minute fluorescein-staining erosions; diffuse but most conspicuous in pupillary area.

4. Adenovirus keratitis

Minute pleomorphic, fluorescein-staining, damaged epithelium and erosions; epithelial and mucous filaments are typical; lower half of cornea affected predominantly.

5. Keratitis of Sjögren's syndrome

Minute fluorescein-staining, irregular erosions; lower half of cornea affected predominantly.

6. Exposure keratitis—due to lagophthalmos or exophthalmos

Blotchy gray, opaque, syncytiumlike lesions, most conspicuous in upper pupillary area. Sometimes a plaque of opaque epithelium forms.

7. Vernal keratoconjunctivitis

Blotchy epithelial edema; diffuse but predominant in palpebral fissure, 9–3 o'clock.

8. Trophic keratitis—sequela of herpes simplex, herpes zoster, and gasserian ganglion destruction

Minute fluorescein-staining erosions with spotty cellular edema; epithelial whorls.

9. Drug-induced keratitis—especially by broad-spectrum antibiotics

Foci of edematous epithelial cells, round or oval; elevated when disease is active.

10. Superficial punctate keratitis (SPK)

Minute fluorescein-staining erosions of upper third of cornea; filaments during exacerbations; bulbar hyperemia, thickened keratinized limbus, micropannus.

11. Superior limbic keratoconjunctivitis

Virus-type lesions like those of SPK; in pupillary area.

12. Rubeola, rubella, and mumps keratitis

continued

Table 6-1 (cont'd). Principal types of epithelial keratitis
(in order of frequency of occurrence).

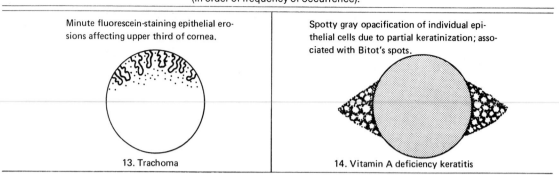

Minute fluorescein-staining epithelial erosions affecting upper third of cornea.	Spotty gray opacification of individual epithelial cells due to partial keratinization; associated with Bitot's spots.
13. Trachoma	14. Vitamin A deficiency keratitis

Although hypopyon is sterile in bacterial corneal ulcers unless there has been a rupture of Descemet's membrane, in fungal ulcers it may contain fungal elements.

1. BACTERIAL KERATITIS

Many types of bacterial corneal ulcers look alike and vary only in severity. This is especially true of ulcers caused by opportunistic bacteria (eg, alpha-hemolytic streptococci, *Staphylococcus aureus*, *Staphylococcus epidermidis*, *Nocardia*, and *M fortuitum-chelonei*), which cause indolent corneal ulcers that tend to spread slowly and superficially.

Pneumococcal Corneal Ulcer

S pneumoniae is still a common cause of bacterial corneal ulcer in many parts of the world. Before the popularization of dacryocystorhinostomy, pneumococcal ulcers often occurred in patients with obstructed nasolacrimal ducts.

Pneumococcal corneal ulcer usually occurs 24–48 hours after inoculation of an abraded cornea. It typically produces a gray, fairly well circumscribed ulcer that tends to spread erratically from the original site of infection toward the center of the cornea (Figure 6–1). The advancing border shows active ulceration and infiltration as the trailing border begins to heal. (This creeping effect suggested the term "acute serpiginous ulcer.") The superficial corneal layers become involved first and then the deep parenchyma. The cornea surrounding the ulcer is often clear. Hypopyon is common. Scrapings from the leading edge of a pneumococcal corneal ulcer contain gram-positive lancet-shaped diplococci. Drugs recommended for use in treatment are listed in Tables 6–2 and 6–3. Concurrent dacryocystitis should also be treated.

Pseudomonas Corneal Ulcer

Pseudomonas corneal ulcer begins as a gray or yellow infiltrate at the site of a break in the corneal epithelium (Figure 6–2). Severe pain usually accompanies it. The lesion tends to spread rapidly in all directions because of the proteolytic enzymes produced by the organisms. Although usually superficial at first, the ulcer may affect the entire cornea. There is often a large hypopyon that tends to increase in size as the ulcer progresses. The infiltrate and exudate may have a bluish-green color. This is due to a pigment produced by the organism and is pathognomonic of *P aeruginosa* infection.

Pseudomonas is a common cause of bacterial corneal ulcers. Cases of *Pseudomonas* corneal ulcer may follow minor corneal abrasion or the use of soft contact lenses—especially extended wear lenses. Corneal ulcers caused by this organism can vary from quite benign to devastating. The organism has been shown to adhere to the surface of soft contact lenses. Some cases have been reported following the use of contaminated fluorescein solution or eye drops. It is mandatory that the clinician use sterile medications and sterile technique when caring for patients with corneal injuries.

Scrapings from the ulcer contain long, thin gram-negative rods that are often few in number. Drugs recommended for use in treatment are listed in Tables 6–2 and 6–3.

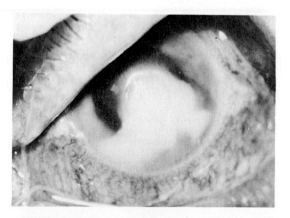

Figure 6–1. Pneumococcal corneal ulcer with hypopyon.

Table 6–2. Treatment of bacterial, fungal, and amebic keratitis.

Organisms	Drug Route[1]	First Choice	Second Choice	Third Choice
Gram-positive cocci: lancet-shaped with capsule = *S pneumoniae*[2]	Topical	Cefazolin	Penicillin G	Vancomycin or ceftazidime
	Subconjunctival	Cefazolin	Penicillin G	Methicillin
	Systemic	Cefazolin	Penicillin G	Oral: Erythromycin
Other gram-positive organisms: cocci and rods[3]	Topical	Cefazolin	Penicillin G	Vancomycin or ceftazidime
	Subconjunctival	Cefazolin	Methicillin	Vancomycin
Gram-negative cocci[4]	Topical	Penicillin G	Cefazolin	Vancomycin
	Subconjunctival	Penicillin G	Cefazolin	Vancomycin
	Systemic	Penicillin G	Cefazolin	Vancomycin
Gram-negative rods:[3] thin = *Pseudomonas*	Topical	Tobramycin	Gentamicin	Polymyxin B or carbenicillin
	Subconjunctival	Tobramycin	Gentamicin	Polymyxin B or carbenicillin
	Systemic	Tobramycin	Gentamicin	
Gram-negative rods: large, square-ended diplobacilli = *Moraxella*	Topical	Penicillin G	Gentamicin	Tobramycin
	Subconjunctival	Rarely necessary: Penicillin G	Gentamicin (rarely)	Tobramycin
	Systemic	...	...	...
Other gram-negative rods	Topical	Gentamicin	Tobramycin	Carbenicillin
	Subconjunctival	Gentamicin	Tobramycin	Carbenicillin
	Systemic	...	...	Carbenicillin
Gram-positive rods: slender and varying in length *Mycobacterium fortuitum*, *Nocardia* sp, *Actinomyces* sp	Topical	Amikacin	A fluoroquinolone[3]	...
	Subconjunctival	Amikacin	...	...
	Systemic	Amikacin	...	...
Yeast-like organisms = *Candida* sp[5]	Topical	Natamycin	Amphotericin B	Nystatin or micozole
	Subconjunctival	Natamycin	Miconazole	...
	Systemic	Oral: Flycytosine	Ketoconazole	...
Hyphae-like organisms = fungal ulcer	Topical	Natamycin	Amphotericin B	Miconazole or ketoconazole
	Subconjunctival	Amphotericin B	Miconazole	...
	Systemic	Fluconazole	Ketoconazole	...
Cysts, trophozoites = *Acanthamoeba*	Topical	Neomycin and propamidine	Paromomycin and dibrompropamidine	Clotrimazole or miconazole
	Subconjunctival	...	...	...
	Systemic	Ketoconazole (severe cases)	...	...
No organisms identified; ulcer suggestive of bacterial infection	Topical	Gentamicin and cefazolin	Tobramycin and bacitracin	Vancomycin and a fluoroquinolone[3]
	Subconjunctival	Gentamicin and cefazolin	Tobramycin and methicillin	Vancomycin and ceftazidime
	Systemic	Cefazolin	Penicillin G	...
No organisms identified; ulcer suggestive of fungal infection	Topical	Natamycin or amphotericin B	Amphotericin B	...
	Subconjunctival	Rarely necessary: Amphotericin B	Miconazole	...

[1]Systemic administration is intravenously unless orally is specified; systemic antimicrobials are seldom indicated in infectious keratitis.
[2]The fluoroquinolones are not recommended for treatment of streptococcal corneal disease.
[3]Topical fluoroquinolines (ciprofloxacin, norfloxacin, ofloxacin) are effective drugs in staphylococcal and pseudomonal infection.
[4]Ulcer associated with hyperacute conjunctivitis (eg, gonococcal conjunctivitis) should be treated with the same drug used to treat the conjunctivitis.
[5]Rarely, *Pityrosporum ovale* or *Pityrosporum orbiculare* may be confused with *Candida* spp.

Table 6–3. Drug concentrations and dosages for treatment of bacterial or fungal keratitis.

Drug	Topical[1]	Subconjunctival[2]	Systemic[3]
Amikacin	50–100 mg/mL	25 mg/0.5 mL/dose	10–15 mg/kg/d in 2 or 3 doses
Amphotericin B	1.5–3 mg/mL	0.5–1 mg	...
Ampicillin	...	...	150–200 mg/kg/d IV in 4 doses
Bacitracin	10,000 units/mL	...	...
Carbenicillin	4 mg/mL	125 mg/0.5 mL/dose	100–200 mg/kg/d IV in 4 doses
Cefazolin	50 mg/mL	100 mg/0.5 mL/dose	15 mg/kg/d IV in 4 doses
Ceftazidime	50 mg/mL	250 mg (0.5 mL)	1 g IV or IM every 8–12 hours (adult dose)
Chloramphenicol	5 mg/mL	...	...
Ciprofloxacin	0.3% solution	...	250–500 mg orally every 12 hours
Erythromycin	5 mg/g (ointment)	100 mg/0.5 mL/dose	1 g orally, then 0.5 g every 6 hours
Flucytosine	1% solution	...	50–150 mg/kg orally in 4 doses
Gentamicin	10–20 mg/mL	20 mg/0.5 mL/dose	...
Methicillin	...	100 mg/mL/dose	...
Miconazole	1% solution or 2% ointment	5–10 mg; 0.5–1 mL/dose	...
Nafcillin	...	...	1 g IV every 4–6 hours
Natamycin	5% suspension	...	...
Neomycin	20 mg/mL	...	...
Nystatin	50,000 units/mL or cream (100,000 units/g)	...	...
Paromomycin	10 mg/mL	...	...
Penicillin G	100,000 units/mL	1 million units/dose (painful)	40,000–50,000 units/kg IV in 4 doses; or continuously, 2–6 million units IV every 4–6 hours
Polymyxin B	1–2 mg/mL	10 mg/0.5 mL dose	...
Propamidine	0.1 mg/mL solution; 0.15% ointment	...	...
Rifampin	1% ointment	...	600 mg/d orally
Sodium sulfacetamide	10–15% solution	...	...
Tetracycline	5 mg/mL	...	Under 70 kg, 1.5 g/d orally in 4 doses; over 70 kg, 2 g/d orally in 4 doses
Tobramycin	10–20 mg/mL	20 mg/0.5 mL/dose	...
Vancomycin	50 mg/mL	25 mg/0.5 mL/dose	...
Zinc sulfate	0.5 mg/mL	...	...

[1]Topical: Every hour during the day and every 2 hours during the night for 5 days. The fortified preparations listed must be prepared by pharmacists with special training.
[2]Subconjunctival: One injection daily for 4 days unless otherwise stated; in exceptionally severe cases, initial dose sometimes repeated after 12 hours.
[3]Systemic: Intravenous or oral: One dose daily for 5 days (adult dosage).

Moraxella liquefaciens
Corneal Ulcer

M liquefaciens (diplobacillus of Petit) causes an indolent oval ulcer that usually affects the inferior cornea and progresses into the deep stroma over a period of days. There is usually no hypopyon or only a small one, and the surrounding cornea is usually clear. *M liquefaciens* ulcer almost always occurs in a patient with alcoholism, diabetes, or other immunosuppressing disease. Scrapings contain large, square-ended gram-negative diplobacilli. Drugs recommended for use in treatment are listed in Tables 6–2 and 6–3. Treatment can be difficult and prolonged.

Group A Streptococcus
Corneal Ulcer

Central corneal ulcers caused by beta-hemolytic streptococci have no identifying features. The surrounding corneal stroma is often infiltrated and edematous, and there is usually a moderately large hypopyon. Scrapings contain gram-positive cocci in

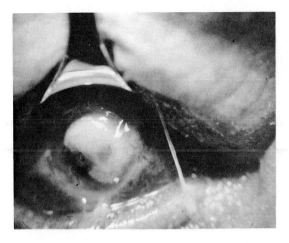

Figure 6–2. *Pseudomonas* corneal ulcer of right eye. Evisceration was done.

chains. Drugs recommended for use in treatment are listed in Tables 6–2 and 6–3.

Staphylococcus aureus, Staphylococcus epidermidis, & α-Hemolytic Streptococcus Corneal Ulcers

Central corneal ulcers caused by these organisms are now being seen more often than formerly, many of them in corneas compromised by topical corticosteroids. The ulcers are often indolent but may be associated with hypopyon and some surrounding corneal infiltration. They are often superficial, and the ulcer bed feels firm when scraped. Scrapings contain gram-positive cocci—singly, in pairs, or in chains. Infectious crystalline keratopathy (in which the cornea has a crystalline appearance) has been described in patients receiving long-term therapy with topical steroids; the disease is usually caused by α-hemolytic streptococci. Tables 6–2 and 6–3 show recommended drug regimens.

Mycobacterium fortuitum-chelonei & Nocardia Corneal Ulcers

Ulcers due to *M fortuitum-chelonei* and *Nocardia* are rare. They often follow trauma and are often associated with contact with soil. The ulcers are indolent, and the bed of the ulcer often has radiating lines that make it look like a cracked windshield. Hypopyon may or may not be present. Scrapings may contain acid-fast slender rods *(M fortuitum-chelonei)* or gram-positive filamentous, often branching organisms *(Nocardia).* See Tables 6–2 and 6–3 for recommended drug regimens.

2. FUNGAL KERATITIS

Fungal corneal ulcers, once seen most commonly in agricultural workers, have become more common in the urban population since the introduction of the corticosteroid drugs for use in ophthalmology. Before the corticosteroid era, fungal corneal ulcers occurred only if an overwhelming inoculum of organisms was introduced into the corneal stroma—an event that can still take place in an agricultural setting. The uncompromised cornea seems to be able to handle the small inocula to which urban residents are ordinarily subjected.

Fungal ulcers are indolent and have a gray infiltrate, often a hypopyon, marked inflammation of the globe, superficial ulceration, and satellite lesions (usually infiltrates at sites distant from the main area of ulceration) (Figure 6–3). The principal lesion—and often the satellite lesions as well—is an endothelial plaque with irregular edges underlying the principal corneal lesions, associated with a severe anterior chamber reaction and a corneal abscess.

Most fungal ulcers are caused by opportunists such as *Candida, Fusarium, Aspergillus, Penicillium, Cephalosporium,* and others. There are no identifying features that help to differentiate one type of fungal ulcer from another.

Scrapings from fungal corneal ulcers, except those caused by *Candida,* contain hyphal elements; scrapings from *Candida* ulcers usually contain pseudohyphae or yeast forms that show characteristic budding. Tables 6–2 and 6–3 list the drugs recommended for the treatment of fungal ulcers.

3. VIRAL KERATITIS

Herpes Simplex Keratitis

Herpes simplex keratitis occurs in two forms: primary and recurrent. It is the most common cause of corneal ulceration and the most common corneal cause of blindness in the USA. The epithelial form is the ocular counterpart of labial herpes, with which it shares immunologic and pathologic features as well as having a similar time course. The only difference is that the clinical course of the keratitis may be prolonged

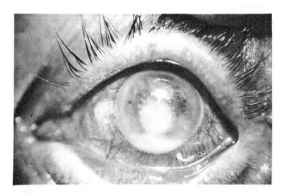

Figure 6–3. Corneal ulcer caused by *Candida albicans.* (Courtesy of P Thygeson.)

because of the avascularity of the corneal stroma, which retards the migration of lymphocytes and macrophages to the lesion. HSV ocular infection in the immunocompetent host is usually self-limited, but in the immunologically compromised host, including patients treated with topical corticosteroids, its course can be chronic and damaging. Stromal and endothelial disease has previously been thought to be a purely immunologic response to virus particles or virally induced cellular changes. However, there is increasing evidence that active viral infection can occur within stromal and possibly endothelial cells as well as in other tissues within the anterior segment such as the iris and trabecular endothelium. This highlights the need to assess the relative role of viral replication and host immune responses prior to and during therapy for herpetic disease. Topical corticosteroids may control damaging inflammatory responses but at the expense of facilitation of viral replication. Thus, whenever topical corticosteroids are to be used, antivirals are likely to be necessary. Any patient undergoing topical corticosteroid therapy for herpetic eye disease must be under the supervision of an ophthalmologist.

Serologic studies suggest that almost all adults have been exposed to the virus, though many do not recollect any episodes of clinical disease. Following primary infection, the virus establishes latency in the trigeminal ganglion. The factors influencing the development of recurrent disease, including its site, have yet to be unraveled. There is increasing evidence that the severity of disease is at least partly determined by the strain of virus involved. Most HSV infections of the cornea are still caused by HSV type 1 (the cause of labial herpes), but in both infants and adults a few cases caused by HSV type 2 (the cause of genital herpes) have been reported. The corneal lesions caused by the two types are indistinguishable.

Scrapings of the epithelial lesions of HSV keratitis and fluid from skin lesions contain multinucleated giant cells. The virus can be cultivated on the chorioallantoic membrane of embryonated hens' eggs and in many tissue cell lines—eg, HeLa cells, on which it produces characteristic plaques. In the majority of cases, however, diagnosis can be made clinically on the basis of characteristic dendritic or geographic ulcers and greatly reduced or absent corneal sensation.

A. Clinical Findings: Primary ocular herpes simplex is infrequently seen but is manifested as a vesicular blepharoconjunctivitis, occasionally with corneal involvement, and usually occurs in young children. It is generally self-limited, without causing significant ocular damage. Topical antiviral therapy may be used as prophylaxis against corneal involvement and as therapy for corneal disease.

Attacks of the common recurrent type of herpetic keratitis (Figure 6–4) are triggered by fever, overexposure to ultraviolet light, trauma, psychic stress, the onset of menstruation, or some other local or systemic source of immunosuppression. Unilaterality is the rule,

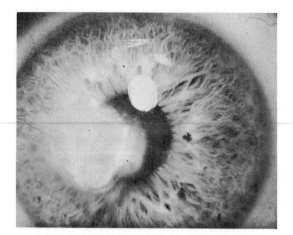

Figure 6–4. Corneal scar caused by recurrent herpes simplex keratitis. (Courtesy of A Rosenberg.)

but bilateral lesions develop in 4–6% of cases and are seen most often in atopic patients.

1. Symptoms—The first symptoms are usually irritation, photophobia, and tearing. When the central cornea is affected, there is also some reduction in vision. Since corneal anesthesia usually occurs early in the course of the infection, the symptoms may be minimal and the patient may not seek medical advice. There is often a history of fever blisters or other herpetic infection, but corneal ulceration can occasionally be the only sign of a recurrent herpetic infection.

2. Lesions—The most characteristic lesion is the **dendritic ulcer.** It occurs in the corneal epithelium, has a typical branching, linear pattern with feathery edges, and has terminal bulbs at its ends (Figure 6–5). Fluorescein staining makes the dendrite easy to identify, but unfortunately herpetic keratitis can also simulate many corneal infection and must be considered in the differential diagnosis of many corneal lesions.

Geographic ulceration is a form of chronic dendritic disease in which the delicate dendritic lesion takes a broader form. The edges of the ulcer lose their feathery quality. Corneal sensation, as with dendritic disease, is diminished. The clinician should always test for this sign.

Other corneal epithelial lesions that may be caused by HSV are a blotchy epithelial keratitis, stellate epithelial keratitis, and filamentary keratitis. All of these are usually transitory, however, and often become typical dendrites within a day or two.

Subepithelial opacities can be caused by HSV infection. A ghost-like image, corresponding in shape to the original epithelial defect but slightly larger, can be seen in the area immediately underlying the epithelial lesion. The "ghost" remains superficial but is often enhanced by the use of antiviral drugs, especially idoxuridine. As a rule, these subepithelial lesions do not persist for more than a year.

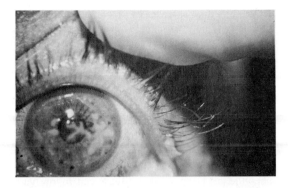

Figure 6–5. Dendritic figures seen in herpes simplex keratitis.

Disciform keratitis is the most common form of stromal disease in HSV infection. The stroma is edematous in a central, disk-shaped area, without significant infiltration and usually without vascularization. The edema may be sufficient to produce folds in Descemet's membrane. Keratic precipitates may lie directly under the disciform lesion but may also involve the entire endothelium because of the frequently associated anterior uveitis. The pathogenesis of disciform keratitis is generally regarded as an immunologic reaction to viral antigens in the stroma or endothelium, but active viral disease cannot be ruled out. Like most herpetic lesions in immunocompetent individuals, disciform keratitis is normally self-limited, lasting weeks to months. Edema is the most prominent sign, and healing can occur with minimal scarring and vascularization. A similar clinical appearance is seen with primary endothelial keratitis (endothelitis), which can be associated with anterior uveitis together with raised intraocular pressure and a focal inflammation of the iris. This is thought to be due to viral replication within the various anterior chamber structures.

Stromal HSV keratitis in the form of focal areas of infiltration and edema, often accompanied by vascularization, is likely to be predominantly due to viral replication. Corneal thinning and perforation may develop rapidly, particularly if topical corticosteroids are being used. If there is stromal disease in the presence of epithelial ulceration, it may be difficult to differentiate bacterial or fungal superinfection from herpetic disease. The features of the epithelial disease need to be carefully scrutinized for herpetic characteristics, but a bacterial or fungal component may be present and the patient must be managed accordingly. Stromal necrosis also may be caused by an acute immune reaction, again complicating the diagnosis with regard to active viral disease. Hypopyon may be seen with necrosis as well as secondary bacterial or fungal infection.

Peripheral lesions of the cornea can also be caused by HSV. They are usually linear and show a loss of epithelium before the underlying corneal stroma becomes infiltrated. (This is in contrast to the marginal ulcer associated with bacterial hypersensitivity—eg, to *S aureus* in staphylococcal blepharitis, in which the infiltration precedes the loss of the overlying epithelium.) Testing for corneal sensation is unreliable in peripheral herpetic disease. The patient is apt to be far less photophobic than patients with nonherpetic corneal infiltrates and ulceration usually are.

B. Treatment: The treatment of HSV keratitis should be directed at eliminating viral replication within the cornea, while minimizing the damaging effects of the inflammatory response.

1. Debridement—An effective way to treat dendritic keratitis is epithelial debridement, since the virus is located in the epithelium and debridement will also reduce the viral antigenic load to the corneal stroma. Healthy epithelium adheres tightly to the cornea, but infected epithelium is easy to remove. Debridement is accomplished with a tightly wound cotton-tipped applicator. Topical iodine or ether has no value and can cause chemical keratitis. A cycloplegic such as atropine 1% or homatropine 5% is then instilled into the conjunctival sac, and a pressure dressing is applied. The patient should be examined daily and the dressing changed until the corneal defect has healed—usually within 72 hours. Adjunctive therapy with a topical antiviral accelerates epithelial healing. Topical drug therapy without epithelial debridement for epithelial keratitis offers the advantage of not requiring patching but involves a hazard of drug toxicity.

2. Drug therapy—The topical antiviral agents used in herpetic keratitis are idoxuridine, trifluridine, vidarabine, and acyclovir. (Topical acyclovir for ophthalmic use is not available in the USA.) Trifluridine and acyclovir are much more effective in stromal disease than the others. Idoxuridine and trifluridine are frequently associated with toxic reactions. Oral acyclovir may be useful in the treatment of severe herpetic eye disease, particularly in atopic individuals who are susceptible to aggressive ocular and dermal (eczema herpeticum) herpetic disease. A multicenter study regarding the efficacy of acyclovir in the treatment of herpes simplex keratouveitis and in the prevention of recurrent disease is presently under way (Herpes Eye Disease Study).

Viral replication in the immunocompetent patient, particularly when confined to the corneal epithelium, usually is self-limited and scarring is minimal. It is then unnecessary and potentially highly damaging to use topical corticosteroids. Regrettably, the clinician sometimes immunosuppresses the patient by using corticosteroids to reduce local inflammation. This is based on the misconception that reducing inflammation reduces the disease. Even when the inflammatory response is thought to be purely immunologically driven, such as in disciform keratitis, topical corticosteroids are often best avoided if the episode is likely to be self-limited. Once topical corticosteroids have been used, this usually commits the patient to requiring the drug to control further episodes of keratitis, with the potential for uncontrolled viral replication and the other steroid-related side effects such as bacterial and fungal superinfection, glaucoma, and cataract. Topical corticosteroids may also accelerate corneal melting, thus increasing the risk of corneal perforation. If it becomes necessary to use topical corticosteroids because of the severity of the inflammatory response, it is absolutely essential that appropriate antiviral therapy be used to control viral replication.

3. Surgical treatment–Penetrating keratoplasty may be indicated for visual rehabilitation in patients with severe corneal scarring, but it should not be undertaken until the herpetic disease has been inactive for many months. Postoperatively, recurrent herpetic infection may occur as a result of the surgical trauma and the topical corticosteroids necessary to prevent corneal graft rejection. It may also be difficult to distinguish corneal graft rejection from recurrent stromal disease.

Corneal perforation due to progressive herpetic stromal disease or superinfection with bacteria or fungi may necessitate emergency penetrating keratoplasty. Cyanoacrylate tissue adhesives can be used effectively to seal small perforations, and lamellar "patch" grafts have been successful in selected cases. Lamellar keratoplasty has the advantage over penetrating keratoplasty of reduced potential for corneal graft rejection. A therapeutic soft contact lens or tarsorrhaphy may be required to heal epithelial defects associated with herpes simplex keratitis.

4. Control of trigger mechanisms that reactivate HSV infection–Recurrent HSV infections of the eye are common, occurring in about one-third of cases within 2 years after the first attack. A trigger mechanism can often be discovered by careful questioning of the patient. Once identified, the trigger can often be avoided. Aspirin can be used to avoid fever, excessive exposure to the sun or ultraviolet light can be avoided, situations that might cause psychic stress can be minimized, and aspirin can be taken just prior to the onset of menstruation.

Varicella-Zoster Viral Keratitis

Varicella-zoster virus (VZV) infection occurs in two forms: primary (varicella) and recurrent (zoster). Ocular manifestations are uncommon in varicella but common in ophthalmic zoster. In varicella (chickenpox), the usual eye lesions are pocks on the lids and lid margins. Rarely, keratitis occurs (typically a peripheral stromal lesion with vascularization), and still more rarely epithelial keratitis with or without pseudodendrites. Disciform keratitis, with uveitis of varying duration, has been reported.

In contrast to the rare and benign corneal lesions of varicella, the relatively frequent ophthalmic zoster is often accompanied by keratouveitis that varies in severity according to the immune status of the patient. Thus, although children with zoster keratouveitis usually have benign disease, the aged have severe and sometimes blinding disease. Corneal complications in ophthalmic zoster can be expected if there is a skin eruption in areas supplied by the branches of the nasociliary nerve.

Unlike recurrent HSV keratitis that usually affects only the epithelium, VZV keratitis affects the stroma and anterior uvea at onset. The epithelial lesions are blotchy and amorphous except for an occasional linear pseudodendrite that only vaguely resembles the true dendrites of HSV keratitis. Stromal opacities consist of edema and mild cellular infiltration and initially are subepithelial. Deep stromal disease can follow with necrosis and vascularization. A disciform keratitis sometimes develops and resembles HSV disciform keratitis. Loss of corneal sensation is always a prominent feature and often persists for months after the corneal lesion appears to have healed. The associated uveitis tends to persist for weeks or months, but with time it eventually heals. Scleritis (sclerokeratitis) can be a serious feature of VZV ocular disease.

Intravenous and oral acyclovir have been used successfully for the treatment of herpes zoster ophthalmicus, particularly in immunocompromised patients. The oral dosage is 800 mg five times daily for 10–14 days. Therapy needs to be started within 72 hours after appearance of the rash. The role of topical antivirals is less certain. Topical corticosteroids may be necessary to treat severe keratitis, uveitis, and secondary glaucoma. The use of systemic corticosteroids is controversial. They may be indicated in reducing the incidence and severity of postherpetic neuralgia, but the risk of steroid complications is significant. Unfortunately, systemic acyclovir has little influence on the development of postherpetic neuralgia. However, the condition is self-limited, and reassurance can be helpful as a supplement to analgesics.

4. *ACANTHAMOEBA* KERATITIS

Acanthamoeba is a free-living protozoan that thrives in polluted water containing bacteria and organic material. Corneal infection with *Acanthamoeba* is an increasingly recognized complication of soft contact lens wear, particularly when homemade saline solutions are used. It may also occur in non-contact lens wearers after exposure to contaminated water or soil.

The initial symptoms are pain out of proportion to the clinical findings, redness, and photophobia. The characteristic clinical signs are indolent corneal ulceration, a stromal ring, and perineural infiltrates. The earlier forms of the disease with changes confined to the corneal epithelium are being more frequently recognized. *Acanthamoeba* keratitis is commonly misdiagnosed initially as herpetic keratitis.

The diagnosis is confirmed by scrapings and by culturing on specially prepared media. Corneal biopsy may be required. Histopathologic sections reveal the presence of amebic forms (trophozoites or cysts). Contact lens cases and solutions should be cultured. Often the amebic forms can be identified in the contact lens case fluid.

The differential diagnosis includes fungal keratitis, herpetic keratitis, mycobacterial keratitis, and *Nocardia* infection of the cornea.

In the early stages of the disease, epithelial debridement may be beneficial. Medical treatment is usually started with intensive topical propamidine isethionate (1% solution) and fortified neomycin eye drops (Tables 6–2 and 6–3). Polyhexamethylene biguanide (0.01–0.02% solution), either in combination with the other drugs or as monotherapy, has gained support recently. Other agents that may be useful are paromomycin and various oral and topical imidazoles such as ketoconazole, miconazole, and itraconazole. *Acanthamoeba* spp may have variable drug sensitivities and may acquire drug resistance. Treatment is also hampered by the organisms' ability to encyst within the corneal stroma, necessitating prolonged treatment. Topical corticosteroids may be required to control the associated inflammatory reaction in the cornea.

Keratoplasty may be necessary in advanced disease to arrest progression of the infection or after resolution and scarring to restore vision. Once the organism has reached the sclera, medical and surgical treatment are usually fruitless.

PERIPHERAL CORNEAL ULCERS

1. MARGINAL INFILTRATES & ULCERS

The majority of marginal corneal ulcers are benign but extremely painful. They are secondary to acute or chronic bacterial conjunctivitis, particularly staphylococcal blepharoconjunctivitis and less often Koch-Weeks *(Haemophilus aegyptius)* conjunctivitis. They are not an infectious process, however, and scrapings do not contain the causal bacteria. They are the result of sensitization to bacterial products, antibody from the limbal vessels reacting with antigen that has diffused through the corneal epithelium.

Marginal infiltrates and ulcers (Figure 6–6) start as oval or linear infiltrates, separated from the limbus by a lucid interval, and only later may ulcerate and vascularize. They are self-limited, usually lasting from 7 to 10 days, but those associated with staphylococcal blepharoconjunctivitis usually recur. Treatment for blepharitis (shampoo scrubs, antimicrobials) usually will clear the problem; topical corticosteroids may be needed for severe cases. Topical corticosteroid preparations shorten their course and relieve symptoms, which are often severe, but treatment of the underlying blepharoconjunctivitis is essential if recurrences are to be prevented. Before starting corticosteroid therapy, great care must be taken to distinguish this entity, formerly known as "catarrhal corneal ulceration," from

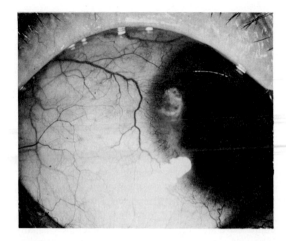

Figure 6–6. Marginal ulcer of temporal cornea, right eye. (Courtesy of P Thygeson.)

marginal herpetic keratitis. Since marginal herpetic keratitis is usually almost symptomless because of corneal anesthesia, differentiating it from the painful, hypersensitivity-type marginal ulcer is not difficult.

2. MOOREN'S ULCER (Figure 6–7)

The cause of Mooren's ulcer is still unknown, but an autoimmune origin is suspected. It is a marginal ulcer, unilateral in 60–80% of cases and characterized by painful, progressive excavation of the limbus and peripheral cornea that often leads to loss of the eye. It occurs most commonly in old age but does not seem to be related to any of the systemic diseases that most often afflict the aged. It is unresponsive to both antibiotics and corticosteroids. Surgical excision of the limbal conjunctiva in an effort to remove sensitizing substances has recently been advocated. Lamellar tectonic keratoplasty has been used with success in se-

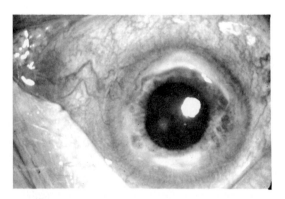

Figure 6–7. Mooren's ulcer. (Courtesy of M Hogan.)

lected cases. Systemic immunosuppressive therapy may be helpful in advanced disease.

3. PHLYCTENULAR KERATOCONJUNCTIVITIS

This hypersensitivity disease (due to delayed hypersensitivity to bacterial products, eg, the human tubercle bacillus) was formerly a major cause of visual loss in the USA, particularly among the Eskimos and Native Americans. Phlyctenules are localized accumulations of lymphocytes, monocytes, macrophages, and finally neutrophils. They appear first at the limbus, but in recurrent attacks they may involve the bulbar conjunctiva and cornea. Corneal phlyctenules, usually bilateral, cicatrize and vascularize, but conjunctival phlyctenules leave no trace.

Most cases of phlyctenular keratoconjunctivitis in the USA today are caused by delayed hypersensitivity to *S aureus*. The antigen is released locally from staphylococci that proliferate on the lid margin in staphylococcal blepharitis. Rare phlyctenules have occurred in San Joaquin Valley fever, a result of hypersensitivity to a primary infection with *Coccidioides immitis*. In this disease they are not visually important, however.

In the tuberculous type, the attack may be triggered by an acute bacterial conjunctivitis but is associated typically with a transient increase in the activity of a childhood tuberculosis. Untreated phlyctenules run a course to healing in 10–14 days, but topical therapy with corticosteroid preparations dramatically shortens the course to a day or two and often decreases scarring and vascularization. The corticosteroid response in the staphylococcal type is less dramatic, however, and treatment consists essentially of eliminating the causal bacterial infection.

4. MARGINAL KERATITIS IN AUTOIMMUNE DISEASE (Figure 6–8)

The corneal periphery receives its nourishment from the aqueous humor, the limbal capillaries, and the tear film. It is contiguous with the subconjunctival lymphoid tissue and the lymphatic arcades at the limbus. The perilimbal conjunctiva appears to play an important role in the pathogenesis of corneal lesions that arise both from local ocular disease and from systemic disorders, particularly those of autoimmune origin. There is a striking similarity between the limbal capillary network and the renal glomerular capillary network. On the endothelial basement membranes of the capillaries of both networks, immune complexes are deposited and immunologic disease results. Thus, the peripheral cornea often participates in such autoimmune diseases as rheumatoid arthritis, polyarteritis no-

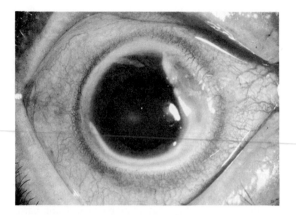

Figure 6–8. Marginal keratitis. (Courtesy of M Hogan.)

dosa, systemic lupus erythematosus, scleroderma, midline lethal and Wegener's granulomatosis, ulcerative colitis, Crohn's disease, and relapsing polychondritis. The corneal changes are secondary to scleral inflammation, with or without scleral vascular closure (see Chapter 7). The clinical signs include vascularization, infiltration and opacification, and peripheral guttering that may progress to perforation. Treatment is directed toward control of the associated systemic disease; topical therapy usually is ineffective, and systemic use of potent immunosuppressive drugs often is required. Corneal perforation may require keratoplasty.

5. CORNEAL ULCER DUE TO VITAMIN A DEFICIENCY

The typical corneal ulcer associated with avitaminosis A is centrally located and bilateral, gray and indolent, with a definite lack of corneal luster in the surrounding area (Figure 6–9). The cornea becomes soft and necrotic (hence the term, "keratomalacia"), and perforation is common. The epithelium of the conjunctiva is keratinized, as evidenced by the presence of a Bitot spot. This is a foamy, wedge-shaped area in the conjunctiva, usually on the temporal side, with the base of the wedge at the limbus and the apex extending toward the lateral canthus. Within the triangle the conjunctiva is furrowed concentrically with the limbus, and dry flaky material can be seen falling from the area into the inferior cul-de-sac. A stained conjunctival scraping from a Bitot spot will show many saprophytic xerosis bacilli (*Corynebacterium xerosis;* small curved rods) and keratinized epithelial cells.

Avitaminosis A corneal ulceration results from dietary lack of vitamin A or impaired absorption from the gastrointestinal tract and impaired utilization by the body. It may develop in an infant who has a feeding problem; in an adult who is on a restricted or generally

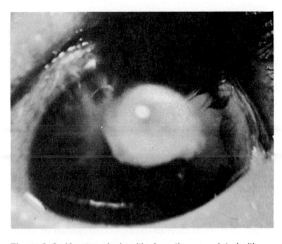

Figure 6–9. Keratomalacia with ulceration associated with xerophthalmia (dietary) in an infant. (Photo by Diane Beeston.)

inadequate diet; or in any person with a biliary obstruction since bile in the gastrointestinal tract is necessary for the absorption of vitamin A. Lack of vitamin A causes a generalized keratinization of the epithelium throughout the body. The conjunctival and corneal changes together are known as **xerophthalmia.** Since the epithelium of the air passages is affected, many patients, if not treated, will die of pneumonia. Avitaminosis A also causes a generalized retardation of osseous growth. This is extremely important in infants; for example, if the skull bones do not grow and the brain continues to grow, increased intracranial pressure and papilledema can result.

Mild vitamin A deficiency should be treatment in adults with a dose of 30,000 units/d for 1 week. Advanced cases will require much higher doses initially (20,000 units/kg/d). Sulfonamide or antibiotic ointment can be used locally in the eye to prevent secondary bacterial infection. The average daily requirement of vitamin A is 1500–5000 IU for children, according to age, and 5000 IU for adults.

6. NEUROTROPHIC KERATITIS

If the trigeminal nerve, which supplies the cornea, is interrupted by trauma, surgery, tumor, inflammation, or in any other way, the cornea loses its sensitivity and one of its best defenses against degeneration, ulceration, and infection—ie, a healthy blink reflex. In the early stages of a typical neurotrophic ulcer, fluorescein solution will produce punctate staining of the superficial epithelium. As this process progresses, patchy areas of denudation appear. Occasionally the epithelium may be absent from a large area of the cornea.

In the absence of corneal sensation, even a severe keratitis may produce little discomfort. Patients must

be warned to look out for redness of the eye, reduced vision, or increased conjunctival discharge and to seek ophthalmic care as soon as any of these develop.

Keeping the cornea moist with artificial tears and lubricant ointments may help to protect it. Once a keratitis develops, it must be treated promptly. The most effective management is to keep the eye closed either by careful horizontal taping of the eyelids, by tarsorrhaphy, or by means of ptosis induced with botulinum toxin A (Botox). Secondary corneal infection must be treated appropriately.

7. EXPOSURE KERATITIS

Exposure keratitis may develop in any situation in which the cornea is not properly moistened and covered by the eyelids. Examples include exophthalmos from any cause, ectropion, the floppy lid syndrome, the absence of part of an eyelid as a result of trauma, and inability to close the lids properly, as in Bell's palsy. The two factors at work are the drying of the cornea and its exposure to minor trauma. The uncovered cornea is particularly subject to drying during sleeping hours. If an ulcer develops it usually follows minor trauma and occurs in the inferior third of the cornea.

This type of keratitis will be sterile unless it is secondarily infected, and the therapeutic objective is to provide protection and moisture for the entire corneal surface. The treatment method depends upon the underlying condition: a plastic procedure on the eyelids, correction of exophthalmos, or use of the options mentioned above in the discussion of neurotrophic keratitis.

EPITHELIAL KERATITIS

CHLAMYDIAL KERATITIS

All five principal types of chlamydial conjunctivitis (trachoma, inclusion conjunctivitis, primary ocular lymphogranuloma venereum, parakeet or psittacosis conjunctivitis, and feline pneumonitis conjunctivitis) are accompanied by corneal lesions. Only in trachoma and lymphogranuloma venereum, however, have they been blinding or visually damaging. The corneal lesions of trachoma have been the most studied and are of great diagnostic importance. In order of appearance they consist of (1) epithelial microerosions affecting the upper third of the cornea; (2) micropannus; (3) subepithelial round opacities, commonly called trachoma pustules; (4) limbal follicles and their cicatricial remains, known as Herbert's peripheral pits; (5) gross pannus; and (6) extensive, diffuse, subepithelial cicatrization. Mild cases of trachoma may show only epithelial keratitis and micropannus and may heal without impairing vision.

The rare cases of lymphogranuloma venereum have shown fewer characteristic changes but are known to have caused blindness by diffuse corneal scarring and total pannus. The remaining types of chlamydial infection cause only micropannus, epithelial keratitis, and, rarely, subepithelial opacities which are not visually significant.

Chlamydial keratoconjunctivitis responds to systemic sulfonamides (except for the rare *C psittaci* infections, which are sulfonamide-resistant), tetracyclines, or erythromycin.

DRUG-INDUCED EPITHELIAL KERATITIS

Epithelial keratitis is not uncommonly seen in patients using antiviral medications (idoxuridine and trifluridine) and several of the broad-spectrum and medium-spectrum antibiotics such as neomycin, gentamicin, and tobramycin. It is usually a superficial keratitis affecting predominantly the lower half of the cornea and interpalpebral fissure.

KERATOCONJUNCTIVITIS SICCA (Sjögren's Syndrome)

Epithelial filaments in the lower quadrants of the cornea are the cardinal signs of this autoimmune disease in which secretion of the lacrimal and accessory lacrimal glands is diminished or eliminated. There is also a blotchy epithelial keratitis that affects mainly the lower quadrants. Severe cases show mucous pseudofilaments that stick to the corneal epithelium.

This keratitis of Sjögren's syndrome must be distinguished from the keratitis sicca of such cicatrizing diseases as trachoma and ocular pemphigoid, in which the goblet cells of the conjunctiva have been destroyed. Such cases sometimes still produce tears, but without mucus the corneal epithelium sheds the tears and continues to be dry.

Treatment of keratoconjunctivitis sicca calls for the frequent use of tear substitutes and lubricating ointments, of which there are many commercial preparations. When goblet cells have been destroyed, as in the cicatricial conjunctivitides, mucus substitutes must be used in addition to artificial tears. Topical vitamin A may help to reverse the epithelial keratinization. Moisture chambers or swim goggles may be required. Lacrimal punctal plugs and punctal occlusion are important in the management of advanced cases.

ADENOVIRUS KERATITIS

Keratitis usually accompanies all types of adenoviral conjunctivitis, reaching its peak 5–7 days after onset of the conjunctivitis. It is a fine epithelial keratitis best seen with the slit lamp after instillation of fluorescein. The minute lesions may group together to make up larger ones.

The epithelial keratitis is often followed by subepithelial opacities. In epidemic keratoconjunctivitis (EKC), which is due to adenovirus types 8 and 19, the subepithelial lesions are round and grossly visible. They appear 8–15 days after onset of the conjunctivitis and may persist for months or even (rarely) for several years. Similar lesions occur very exceptionally in other adenoviral infections, eg, those caused by types 3, 4, and 7, but tend to be transitory and mild, lasting a few weeks at most.

Although the corneal opacities of adenoviral keratoconjunctivitis tend to fade temporarily with the use of topical corticosteroids, and although the patient is often made temporarily more comfortable thereby, corticosteroid therapy may prolong the corneal disease and is therefore not recommended. No medication is needed.

OTHER VIRAL KERATITIDES

A fine epithelial keratitis may be seen in other viral infections such as measles (in which the central cornea is affected predominantly), rubella, mumps, infectious mononucleosis, acute hemorrhagic conjunctivitis, Newcastle disease conjunctivitis, and verruca of the lid margin. A superior epithelial keratitis and pannus often accompany molluscum contagiosum nodules on the lid margin.

DEGENERATIVE CORNEAL CONDITIONS

KERATOCONUS

Keratoconus is an uncommon degenerative bilateral disease that may be inherited as an autosomal recessive or autosomal dominant trait. Unilateral cases of unknown cause occur rarely. Symptoms appear in the second decade of life. The disease affects all races. Keratoconus has been associated with a number of diseases, including Down's syndrome, atopic dermatitis, retinitis pigmentosa, aniridia, vernal catarrh, Marfan's syndrome, Apert's syndrome, and Ehlers-Danlos syndrome. Pathologically, there are disruptive changes in Bowman's layer with keratocyte degeneration, ruptures in Descemet's membrane, and irregular, superficial linear scars at the apex of the cone that is formed.

Acute hydrops of the cornea may occur, in which there is sudden diminution of vision associated with central corneal edema. This arises as a consequence of rupture of Descemet's membrane and may be triggered by the patient rubbing the eye. The condition may be mistaken for extreme thinning with impending perforation. Acute hydrops usually clears gradually without treatment.

Blurred vision is the only symptom. Signs include cone-shaped cornea (Figure 6–10), indentation of the lower lid by the cornea when the patient looks down (Munson's sign), an irregular reflex on retinoscopy, and a distorted corneal reflection with Placido's disk or the keratoscope. Color-coded CT units are available at great expense which give more accurate information on corneal distortion. The fundi cannot be clearly seen because of corneal astigmatism.

Rigid contact lenses will markedly improve vision in the early stages by correcting irregular astigmatism. Keratoconus is one of the most common indications for penetrating keratoplasty. Surgery is indicated when a contact lens can no longer be effectively worn or when peripheral thinning will affect the surgery.

Keratoconus is often slowly progressive between the ages of 20 and 60, although an arrest in progression of the keratoconus may occur at any time. If a corneal transplant is done before extreme corneal thinning occurs, the prognosis is excellent; about 80–95% obtain reading vision.

CORNEAL DEGENERATION

The corneal degenerations are a rare group of slowly progressive, bilateral, degenerative disorders that usually appear in the second or third decades of life. Some are hereditary. Other cases follow ocular inflammatory disease, and some are of unknown cause.

Marginal Degeneration of the Cornea

A. Terrien's Disease: This is a rare bilateral symmetric degeneration characterized by marginal thinning of the upper nasal quadrants of the cornea. Males are more commonly affected than females, and the condition occurs more frequently in the third and fourth decades. There are no symptoms except for mild irritation during occasional inflammatory episodes, and the condition is slowly progressive. The clinical picture consists of marginal thinning, arcuate opacity distal to the thinned area simulating arcus senilis, and vascularization with lipid deposition. Perforation is a known complication, especially from trauma. Tectonic (structural) keratoplasty may be required. Histopathologic studies of affected corneas have revealed vascu-

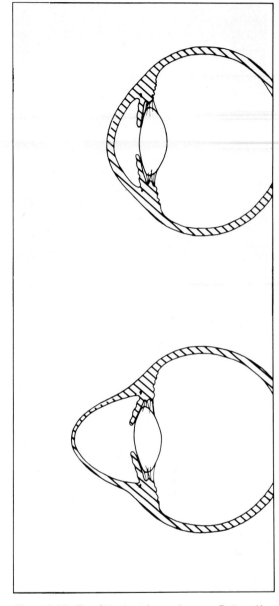

Figure 6–10. *Top:* Side view of normal cornea. *Bottom:* Keratoconus.

larized connective tissue with fibrillary degeneration and fatty infiltration of collagen fibers.

Because the course of progression is slow and the central cornea is spared, the prognosis is good.

B. Band (Calcific) Keratopathy: (Figure 6–11.) This disorder is characterized by the deposition of calcium salts in the anterior layers of the cornea. The keratopathy is usually limited to the interpalpebral area and appears as a band. The calcium deposits are noted in the basement membrane, Bowman's layer, and

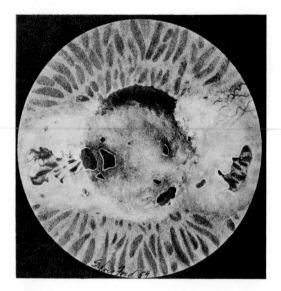

Figure 6–11. Calcific band keratopathy. (Courtesy of M Hogan.)

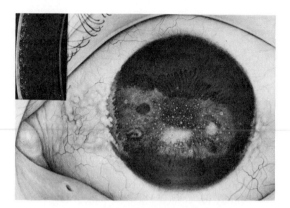

Figure 6–12. Climatic droplet keratopathy. Inset shows slit lamp view. (Courtesy of A Ahmad.)

anterior stromal lamellas. A clear margin separates the calcific band from the limbus, and clear holes may be seen in the band, giving the Swiss cheese appearance. Symptoms include irritation, injection, and blurring of vision.

Calcific band keratopathy has been described in a number of inflammatory, metabolic, and degenerative conditions. It is characteristically associated with juvenile rheumatoid arthritis. It has been described in long-standing inflammatory conditions of the eye, glaucoma, and chronic cyclitis. Band keratopathy may also be associated with hyperparathyroidism, vitamin D intoxication, sarcoidosis, and leprosy. Treatment consists of removal of the corneal epithelium by curettage under topical anesthesia followed by irrigation of the cornea with a sterile 0.01-molar solution of ethylenediaminetetraacetic acid (EDTA) or application of EDTA with a cotton applicator. The excimer laser has shown particular value in the treatment of band keratoplasty, or the band can be removed surgically.

Climatic Droplet Keratopathy (Pearl Diver's Keratopathy, Bietti's Keratopathy, Labrador Keratopathy, Spheroid Degeneration of the Cornea) (Figure 6–12)

Climatic droplet keratopathy affects mainly men who work out of doors. The corneal degeneration is thought to be caused by exposure to ultraviolet light and is characterized in the early stages by fine subepithelial yellow droplets in the peripheral cornea. As the disease advances, the droplets become central, with

subsequent corneal clouding causing blurred vision. Treatment in advanced cases is by corneal transplantation.

Salzmann's Nodular Degeneration

This disorder is always preceded by corneal inflammation, particularly phlyctenular keratoconjunctivitis or trachoma. Symptoms include redness, irritation, and blurring of vision. There is degeneration of the superficial cornea that involves the stroma, Bowman's layer, and epithelium with superficial whitish-gray elevated nodules sometimes occurring in chains.

Corneal transplantation is rarely required; superficial lamellar keratectomy can result in visual improvement.

Rigid contact lenses will significantly improve visual acuity in most cases.

ARCUS SENILIS (Corneal Annulus, Anterior Embryotoxon)

Arcus senilis is an extremely common, bilateral, benign peripheral corneal degeneration that may occur at any age but is far more common in elderly people as part of the aging process. Arcus senilis in people under age 50 is usually associated with hypercholesterolemia; blood lipid studies should be done.

Pathologically, lipid droplets involve the entire corneal thickness but are more concentrated in the superficial and deep layers, being relatively sparse in the corneal stroma.

There are no symptoms. Clinically, arcus senilis appears as a hazy gray ring about 2 mm in width and with a clear space between it and the limbus (Figure 6–13). No treatment is necessary, and there are no complications.

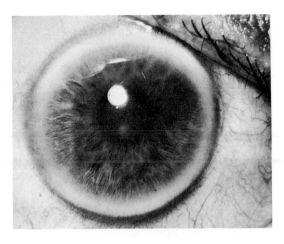

Figure 6–13. Arcus senilis. (Photo by Diane Beeston.)

HEREDITARY CORNEAL DYSTROPHIES

This is a group of rare hereditary disorders of the cornea of unknown cause characterized by bilateral abnormal deposition of substances and associated with alteration in the normal corneal architecture that may or may not interfere with vision. These corneal dystrophies usually manifest themselves during the first or second decade but sometimes later. They may be stationary or slowly progressive throughout life. Corneal transplantation, when indicated, improves vision in most patients with hereditary corneal dystrophy.

Anatomically, corneal dystrophies may be classified as epithelial, stromal, and posterior limiting membrane dystrophies.

Epithelial Corneal Dystrophies

A. Meesman's Dystrophy: This slowly progressive disorder is characterized by microcystic areas in the epithelium. The onset is in early childhood (first 1–2 years of life). The main symptom is slight irritation, and vision is slightly affected. The inheritance is autosomal dominant.

B. Anterior Membrane Dystrophies (Cogan's, Map-Dot-Fingerprint): Map or fingerprint patterns are seen at the level of the epithelial basement membrane. Debris, cysts, and dots also may be noted. Recurrent erosion is common. Vision usually is not significantly affected. In Cogan's dystrophy, intraepithelial opacities are seen in the pupillary area.

C. Recurrent Corneal Erosion: See below.

D. Others: Reis-Bücklers dystrophy is a dominantly inherited dystrophy affecting primarily Bowman's layer. The disease begins within the first decade of life with symptoms of recurrent erosion. Opacification of Bowman's layer gradually occurs and the epithelium is irregular. No vascularization is usually noted. Vision may be markedly reduced.

Vortex dystrophy, or cornea verticillata, is characterized by pigmented lines occurring in Bowman's layer or the underlying stroma and spreading over the entire corneal surface. Visual acuity is not markedly affected. Such a pattern of radiating pigmented lines may also be seen in patients treated with chlorpromazine, chloroquine, indomethacin, or amiodarone toxicity as well as Fabry's disease.

Stromal Corneal Dystrophies

There are three primary types of stromal corneal dystrophies:

A. Granular Dystrophy: This usually asymptomatic, slowly progressive corneal dystrophy most often begins in early childhood. The lesions consist of central, fine, whitish "granular" lesions in the stroma of the cornea. The epithelium and Bowman's layer may be affected late in the disease. Visual acuity is slightly reduced. Histologically, the cornea shows uniform deposition of hyaline material. Corneal transplant is not needed except in very severe and late cases. The inheritance is autosomal dominant.

B. Macular Dystrophy: This type of stromal corneal dystrophy is manifested by a dense gray central opacity that starts in Bowman's layer. The opacity tends to spread toward the periphery and later involves the deeper stromal layers. Recurrent corneal erosion may occur, and vision is severely impaired. Histologic examination shows deposition of acid mucopolysaccharide in the stroma and degeneration of Bowman's layer. Penetrating keratoplasty is often required.

The inheritance is autosomal recessive.

C. Lattice Dystrophy: Lattice dystrophy starts as fine, branching linear opacities in Bowman's layer in the central area and spreads to the periphery. The deep stroma may become involved, but the process does not reach Descemet's membrane. Recurrent erosion may occur. Histologic examination reveals amyloid deposits in the collagen fibers. Penetrating keratoplasty is common, as is recurrence of the dystrophy in the graft. The hereditary pattern for lattice dystrophy is autosomal dominant.

Posterior Limiting Membrane Corneal Dystrophies

A. Fuchs' Dystrophy: This disorder begins in the third or fourth decade and is slowly progressive throughout life. Women are more commonly affected than men. There are central wart-like deposits on Descemet's membrane, thickening of Descemet's membrane, and defects of size and shape in the endothelium. Decompensation of the endothelium occurs and leads to edema of the corneal stroma and epithelium, causing blurring of vision. The cornea becomes progressively more opaque. Glaucoma or iris atrophy may be associated with this disorder. Histologic examination of the cornea reveals the wart-like excrescences over Descemet's membrane that are secreted by the endothelial cells. Thinning and pigmentation of the endothelium and thickening of Descemet's membrane are characteristics. Penetrating keratoplasty, often combined with extracapsular lens extraction and a posterior lens implant, is often needed. Cataract surgery alone can trigger endothelial decompensation in advanced disease.

B. Posterior Polymorphous Dystrophy: This is a common disorder with onset in early childhood. Polymorphous plaques of calcium crystals are observed in the deep stromal layers. Vesicular lesions may be seen in the endothelium. Edema occurs in the deep stroma. The condition is asymptomatic in most cases, but in severe cases epithelial and total stromal edema may occur. The inheritance is autosomal dominant.

MISCELLANEOUS CORNEAL DISORDERS

THYGESON'S SUPERFICIAL PUNCTATE KERATITIS

Superficial punctate keratitis is an uncommon chronic and recurrent bilateral disorder without regard to sex or age. It is characterized by discrete and elevated oval epithelial opacities that show punctate staining with fluorescein, mainly in the pupillary area. The opacities are not visible grossly but can be easily seen with the slit lamp or loupe. Subepithelial opacities underlying the epithelial lesions (ghosts) are often observed as the epithelial disease resolves.

No causative organism has been identified, but a virus is suspected. A varicella-zoster virus has been isolated from the corneal scrapings of one case.

Mild irritation, slight blurring of vision, and photophobia are the only symptoms. The conjunctiva is not involved.

Epithelial keratitis secondary to staphylococcal blepharoconjunctivitis is differentiated from superficial punctate keratitis by its involvement of the lower third of the cornea. Epithelial keratitis in trachoma is ruled out by its location in the upper third of the cornea and the presence of pannus. Many other forms of keratitis involving the superficial cornea are unilateral or are eliminated by their histories.

Short-term instillation of corticosteroid drops will often cause disappearance of the opacities and subjective improvement, but recurrences are the rule. The ultimate prognosis is good since there is no scarring or vascularization of the cornea. Untreated, the disease runs a protracted course of 1–3 years. Long-term treatment with topical corticosteroids may prolong the course of the disease for many years and lead to

steroid-induced cataract and glaucoma. Therapeutic soft contact lenses have been used to control symptoms in especially bothersome cases.

RECURRENT CORNEAL EROSION

This is a fairly common and serious mechanical corneal disorder that presents some classic signs and symptoms but may be easily missed if the physician does not look for it specifically. The patient is usually awakened during the early morning hours by a pain in the affected eye. The pain is continuous, and the eye becomes red, irritated, and photophobic. When the patient attempts to open the eyes in the morning, the lid pulls off the loose epithelium, resulting in pain and redness.

Three types of recurrent corneal erosions can be recognized:

(1) Acquired recurrent erosion (traumatic): The patient usually gives a history of previous corneal injury. It is unilateral, occurs with equal frequency in males and females, and the family history is negative. The recurrent erosion occurs most frequently in the center below the pupil no matter where the site of the previous corneal injury was.

(2) Recurrent erosion associated with corneal disease: After corneal ulceration heals, the epithelium may break down in a recurrent fashion (as in HSV "metaherpetic" ulcer).

(3) Recurrent erosion associated with corneal dystrophies: (See above.) Recurrent erosions of the cornea may be observed in patients with Cogan's microcystic corneal dystrophy, fingerprint dystrophy, and Reis-Bücklers corneal dystrophy.

Recurrent corneal erosion is due to a defect in the basement membrane of the corneal epithelium. The hemidesmosomes of the basal layer of the corneal epithelium fail to adhere to the basement membrane, and the corneal epithelium remains loose over the basement membrane with very slight subepithelial edema. The loose epithelial layers are vulnerable to separation and erosion.

Instillation of a local anesthetic relieves the symptoms immediately, and fluorescein staining will show the eroded area. This is typically a small area in the lower central cornea.

Treatment consists of a pressure bandage on the eye to promote healing. Mechanical denuding of the loose corneal epithelium may be necessary. The other eye should be kept closed most of the time to minimize movement of the lid over the affected eye. Bed rest is desirable for 24 hours. The cornea usually heals in 2–3 days. To prevent recurrence and to promote continued healing, it is important for these patients to use a bland ointment (eg, boric acid or other ocular lubricant) at bedtime for several months. In more severe cases, artificial tears are instilled during the day. The use of hypertonic ointment (glucose 40%) or 5% saline drops

(Adsorbonac 5%) is often of value. Therapeutic soft contact lenses and needle micropuncture of Bowman's layer have been useful in cases that do not respond to more conservative management.

Rare instances of bilateral atraumatic dystrophic recurrent corneal erosion with a poor prognosis have also been reported.

INTERSTITIAL KERATITIS DUE TO CONGENITAL SYPHILIS

This self-limited inflammatory disease of the cornea is a late manifestation of congenital syphilis. There has been a sharp decrease in the incidence of the disease in recent years—almost to the point of extinction in some parts of the USA. It occasionally starts unilaterally but almost always becomes bilateral weeks to months later. It affects all races and is more common in females than males. Symptoms appear between the ages of 5 and 20. Pathologic findings include edema, lymphocytic infiltration, and vascularization of the corneal stroma.

Interstitial keratitis may be immune in nature since *Treponema pallidum* is not found in the cornea during the acute phase. It has been postulated that these organisms enter the cornea at birth and that later in life there is a violent allergic reaction in the cornea to the organisms circulating in the bloodstream.

Clinical Findings

A. Symptoms and Signs: Other signs of congenital syphilis may be present, such as saddle nose and Hutchinson's triad (interstitial keratitis, deafness, and notched upper central incisors). The patient complains of pain, photophobia, and blurring of vision. Physical signs include conjunctival injection, corneal edema, vascularization of the deeper corneal layers, and miosis. There is an associated severe anterior granulomatous uveitis and blepharospasm due to photophobia. The grayish-pink appearance of the cornea (due to edema and vascularization) that occurs in the acute phase is sometimes referred to as a "salmon patch."

B. Laboratory Findings: Serologic tests for syphilis are positive.

Complications & Sequelae

Corneal scarring occurs if the process has been particularly severe and prolonged. Secondary glaucoma may result from the uveitis.

Treatment

There are no specific measures. Treatment is aimed at preventing the development of posterior synechiae, which will occur if the pupil is not dilated.

Both eyes should be dilated with frequent instillation of 2% atropine solution. Corticosteroid drops often relieve the symptoms dramatically but must be continued for long periods to prevent recurrence of symptoms. Dark glasses and a darkened room may be necessary if photophobia is severe. Treatment should be given for systemic syphilis, even though this usually has little effect on the ocular condition.

Corneal scarring may necessitate corneal transplant, and glaucoma, if present, may be difficult to control.

Course & Prognosis

The corneal disease process itself is not affected by treatment, which is aimed at prevention of complications. The inflammatory phase lasts 3 or 4 weeks. The corneas then gradually clear, leaving ghost vessels and scars in the corneal stroma.

INTERSTITIAL KERATITIS DUE TO OTHER CAUSES

Although congenital syphilis is no longer a common cause of interstitial keratitis, the disease still occurs as a complication of other granulomatous diseases, eg, tuberculosis and leprosy. Certain viruses (eg, cytomegalovirus, measles virus, mumps virus) as well as the spirochete of Lyme disease have been described as causing a type of interstitial keratitis. Treatment is usually symptomatic, but it is important to establish the cause.

Cogan's syndrome is a rare disorder generally believed to be a vascular hypersensitivity reaction of unknown origin. It is a disease of young adults and is characterized by nonsyphilitic interstitial keratitis and a vestibuloauditory difficulty. Corticosteroids are reputed to be of value, but some degree of visual impairment and complete nerve deafness, with unresponsive labyrinths, usually supervene.

CORNEAL PIGMENTATION

Pigmentation of the cornea may occur with or without ocular or systemic disease. There are several distinct varieties.

Krukenberg's Spindle

In this disorder, brown uveal pigment is deposited bilaterally upon the central endothelial surface in a vertical spindle-shaped fashion. It occurs in a small percentage of people over age 20, usually in myopic women. It can be seen grossly but is best observed with the loupe or slit lamp. The visual acuity is only slightly affected, and the progression is extremely slow. Pigmentary glaucoma must be ruled out by yearly intraocular pressure measurements.

Blood Staining

This disorder occurs occasionally as a complication of traumatic hyphema and is due to hemosiderin in the corneal stroma. The cornea is golden brown, and vision is blurred. In most cases the cornea gradually clears in 1–2 years.

Kayser-Fleischer Ring

This is a pigmented ring whose color varies widely from ruby red to bright green, blue, yellow, or brown. The ring is 1–3 mm is diameter and located just inside the limbus posteriorly. In exceptional cases there is a second ring. The pigment is composed of fine granules immediately below the endothelium. It involves Descemet's membrane, rarely the stroma. Electron microscopic studies suggest that the pigment is a copper compound. The intensity of the pigmentation can be reduced markedly by the use of chelating agents.

These rings, which were long considered to be pathognomonic of hepatolenticular degeneration (Wilson's disease), have recently been described in three nonwilsonian patients with chronic hepatobiliary disease and in one patient with chronic cholestatic jaundice. Recognition of the Kayser-Fleischer rings, however, remains important, since they call attention to the possibility that the patient has Wilson's disease. Specific medical treatment with the copper chelating agent penicillamine may dramatically improve a disease that would otherwise inevitably be fatal.

Iron Lines
(Hudson-Stähli Line, Fleischer's Ring, Stocker's Line, Ferry's Line)

Localized deposits of iron within the corneal epithelium may occur in sufficient quantity to become visible clinically. The Hudson-Stähli line is a horizontal line at the junction of the middle and lower thirds of the cornea, corresponding to the line of lid closure, in otherwise normal elderly patients. Fleischer's ring surrounds the base of the cone in keratoconus. Stocker's line is a vertical line associated with pterygia, and Ferry's line develops adjacent to limbal filtering blebs. Similar iron deposits are seen at the site of corneal scars.

CONTACT LENSES

Glass contact lenses were first described in 1888 by Adolf Fick and were then used for the treatment of keratoconus by Eugene Kalt. Poor results were achieved until 1945, when Kevin Tuohy of Los Angeles produced a plastic precorneal lens with a diameter of 11 mm. Since that time, advances in contact lens technology have produced several different varieties of lenses, which are broadly divided into two types: rigid and soft lenses. The basic requirement for success of contact lenses is to overcome the effect on respiration of the cornea from wearing an occlusive lens. The optical features of contact lenses are discussed in Chapter 21.

Rigid (Hard) Lenses:
A. Standard Hard Lenses: These direct descendants of Tuohy's lens are made of polymethylmethacrylate (PMMA, Perspex), are impervious to oxygen, and thus rely on pumping of tears into the space between the lens and the cornea during blinking to provide respiration for the cornea. They are smaller than the corneal diameter. Always for daily wear, these lenses are easy to care for, are relatively inexpensive, and correct vision efficiently, particularly if there is significant astigmatism. Unfortunately, many persons cannot tolerate them. Corneal edema due to corneal hypoxia and spectacle blur (poor vision with spectacle correction after a period of contact lens wear) are common complaints.

B. Gas-Permeable Hard Lenses: These are rigid lenses made from cellulose acetate butyrate, silicone acrylate, or silicone combined with polymethylmethacrylate. They have the advantage of high oxygen permeability, thus improving corneal metabolism, and greater comfort, while retaining the optical properties of rigid lenses. They are generally used on a daily wear basis but can be used on an extended-wear (24-hour) basis in exceptional circumstances. In keratoconus, the gas-permeable lens has become the lens of first choice.

Soft Lenses
A. Cosmetic Soft Lenses: Hydrogel lenses, based on hydroxymethyl methacrylate (HEMA), are considerably more comfortable than rigid lenses but are flexible and thus conform to the surface of the cornea. Regular astigmatism can be partially corrected by incorporating cylinder into the soft lens; irregular astigmatism is poorly corrected. The oxygen permeability and water content values vary among different types of hydrogel lens. They are more difficult to care for and more expensive than rigid lenses. Complications are also much more common and include ulcerative keratitis, (particularly if the lenses are worn overnight), immune corneal reactions to deposits on the lenses, giant papillary conjunctivitis, reactions to lens care solutions (especially those containing the preservative thimerosal), corneal edema, and corneal vascularization.

Cosmetic soft contact lenses are usually worn on a daily wear basis. For aphakic correction, it is occasionally necessary to resort to extended wear because of the patient's inability to insert and remove the lenses themselves. Extended wear increases the risks associated with use of contact lenses.

B. Disposable Soft Lenses: These recently introduced lenses are designed to be discarded after extended wear for 1 week, thus eliminating the use of contact lens solutions and theoretically reducing the risk of ulcerative keratitis by minimizing corneal trauma due to manipulation of the lenses and by limiting the adherence of bacteria to the lenses. However, ulcerative keratitis appears to be a major risk with these lenses, as with other extended-wear lenses. It would appear that it is the overnight wear of contact lenses, even for one night, that generates the risk of ulcerative keratitis and that cleanliness of the lenses plays only a small role. Disposable contact lenses are expensive.

C. Therapeutic Soft Lenses: For the past 20 years, the use of therapeutic soft contact lenses has become an indispensable part of the ophthalmologist's management of external eye disease. The lenses can form a soft barrier between the outside and the cornea, providing protection against trichiasis or lid disorders. Lenses with high water content can act as a "stent" for epithelial healing, such as in the treatment of recurrent erosions. Patients with pain due to epithelial disease, such as in bullous keratopathy, particularly benefit from therapeutic soft contact lenses. Lenses with low water content can be used to seal small corneal perforations or wound leaks. In all cases of therapeutic contact lens wear, infection must be anticipated. Antimicrobial coverage may be indicated if epithelial defects exist.

Contact Lens Care

It is essential that all contact lens wearers be made aware of the risks associated with contact lens wear—particularly those patients choosing the high-risk varieties such as extended-wear or disposable soft lenses for cosmetic optical correction purely on the grounds of convenience. All wearers must be under the regular care of a contact lens practitioner. Many of the chronic complications of contact lens wear are asymptomatic in their early and easily treated stages. Any contact lens should be removed immediately if the eye becomes uncomfortable or inflamed, and ophthalmic attention must be sought straightaway if symptoms do not rapidly resolve.

Contact lenses require regular cleaning and disinfecting, and in the case of soft and gas-permeable lenses removal of protein deposits is required. Disinfection regimens include heat, chemical soaking, and hydrogen peroxide systems. All are effective if used according to the manufacturer's instructions, though heat systems may be preferable for combating resistant organisms such as *Acanthamoeba*. Soft and gas-permeable lenses are much less durable than hard lenses; contact lenses vary in tolerance to disinfection.

There is a significant trend among soft lens wearers toward the use of nonpreserved contact lens care systems because of the development of preservative-related hypersensitivity reactions. It is important that such individuals be aware of the ability of organisms such as *Pseudomonas* and *Acanthamoeba* to survive in nonpreserved saline solutions, such as may be found in their contact lens storage cases. The use of nonpreserved contact lens solutions requires much greater vigilance in the regular disinfection of lenses and lens storage cases.

CORNEAL TRANSPLANTATION

Corneal transplantation (keratoplasty) is indicated for a number of serious corneal conditions, eg, scarring, edema, thinning, and distortion. The term penetrating keratoplasty denotes full-thickness corneal replacement; lamellar keratoplasty denotes a partial-thickness procedure.

Younger donors are preferred for penetrating keratoplasties; there is a direct relationship between age and the health and number of the endothelial cells. Because of the rapid endothelial cell death rate, the eyes should be enucleated soon after death and refrigerated immediately. Whole eyes should be used within 48 hours, preferably within 24 hours. Modern storage media allow for longer storage. Corneoscleral caps stored in nutrient media may be used up to 6 days after donor death, and preservation in tissue culture media allows storage for as long as 6 weeks.

For lamellar keratoplasty, corneas can be frozen, dehydrated, or refrigerated for several weeks; the endothelial cells are not important in this partial-thickness procedure.

Technique

The recipient eye is prepared by a partial-thickness cutting of a circle of diseased cornea with a suction trephine (cookie cutter action) and full-thickness removal with scissors or partial-thickness removal with dissection.

The donor eye is prepared in two ways. For penetrating keratoplasty, the corneoscleral cap is placed endothelium up on a Teflon block; the trephine (Figure 6–14) is pressed down into the cornea, and a full-thickness button is punched out. In lamellar keratoplasty, a partial-thickness trephine incision is made in the cornea of a whole globe and the lamellar button is dissected free. Certain refinements in technique, such as free hand grafts, may be necessary.

In recent years, refined sutures (Figure 6–15) and instruments and sophisticated operating microscopes and illuminating systems have significantly improved the prognosis in all patients requiring corneal trans-

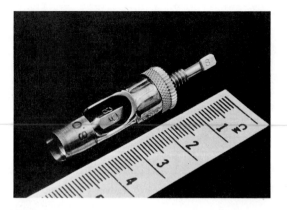

Figure 6–14. Eight-millimeter Castroviejo disposable trephine. (Courtesy of R Biswell and T King.)

plants. Their is no significant value to blood type matching in corneal transplant surgery.

Corneal graft rejection continues to be a major management problem (see Chapter 16), as does the difficulty in controlling postgraft astigmatism.

REFRACTIVE CORNEAL SURGERY

The inconvenience of spectacles to many wearers and the complications associated with contact lenses have resulted in a search for surgical solutions to the problem of refractive error.

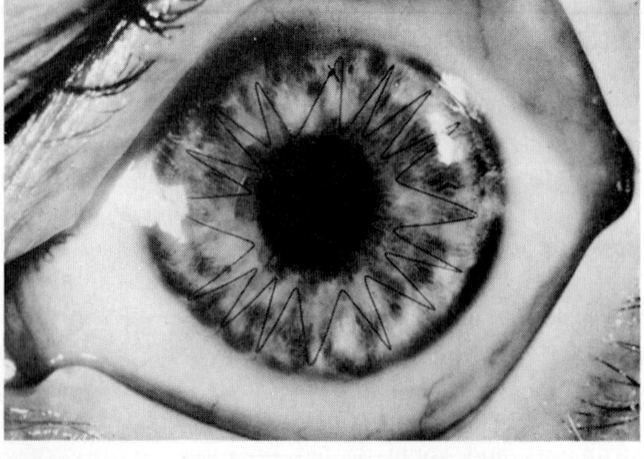

Figure 6–15. Penetrating keratoplasty with 10-0 nylon running suture, 3 months after operation. (Courtesy of R Biswell.)

Radial Keratotomy

In the late 1940s, Sato of Japan created anterior and posterior corneal incisions to alter the curvature of the cornea. Results were poor, and endothelial decompensation with corneal edema occurred frequently. In 1972, Fyodorov of the USSR began to use anterior corneal cuts only. Currently, the operation consists of radial incisions involving 90% of the corneal thickness and extending from a clear optical zone (usually the central 3 mm or more of the cornea) toward but not reaching the limbus. The amount of correction achieved is modified by the size of the optical zone and the number and depth of the incisions. Various formulas and computer programs are used to determine the value of these parameters in each case.

There is general agreement that radial keratotomy does reduce the degree of myopia and is most effective for myopia in the lower range (–2 to –4 diopters). There is a significant degree of unpredictability in the final result, with under- or overcorrection or even progressive hyperopia. Glare and fluctuations of vision during the day are commonly reported side effects. Delayed healing of corneal incisions, with corneal infections occurring up to 2 years after the procedure, have been reported. Endophthalmitis, traumatic cataract, and endothelial cell loss are rare but have been reported. Agreement on whether the procedure should be done at all has not been reached.

Keratomileusis

In 1961, Barraquer of Colombia reported on the technique of myopic keratomileusis for the correction of high degrees of myopia. The procedure has been performed in other countries but by relatively few surgeons. A deep lamellar corneal autograft is cut; the tissue is frozen and then reshaped with a cryolathe to obtain a flatter curvature after thawing; and the autograft is then sutured back into position. Expensive cryolathe and microkeratome equipment is required. The procedure has also been used for hyperopia. Automated lamellar keratoplasty (ALK) is a new form of this procedure.

Complications of keratomileusis include improper depth of the lamellar bed, delayed epithelialization over the resutured tissue, interface epithelial growth and opacity, and irregular astigmatism.

Keratophakia

In keratophakia, a cryolathe is used to shape a donor cornea into a lens, which is then inserted into a lamellar bed. The outer disk of the recipient cornea, which was removed prior to placement of the donor lenticule, is sutured back into position, thus thickening and steepening the cornea. Up to +15 diopters can be corrected. The procedure has been recommended for young aphakic patients who cannot tolerate contact lenses and are poor candidates for secondary lens implantation. The operation has also been performed at the time of cataract extraction. Complications have included interface opacities and astigmatism, both of which may take many months to stabilize or may never do so.

Epikeratophakia

In epikeratophakia, an epigraft of homologous tissue is sutured to a peripheral circular groove formed in the superficial corneal stroma, following removal of the host corneal epithelium. The donor lens is precut on a cryolathe and lyophilized. The procedure has been described by Kaufman and others as useful for myopia, hypermetropia, keratoconus, and even astigmatism (toric epigraft). Epikeratophakia has been used in adult aphakia when contact lenses have failed and a secondary lens implant is contraindicated. Childhood aphakia has been mentioned prominently as an indication, since contact lenses are difficult for children to use and intraocular lens implants may result in long-term complications in children. Epikeratophakia has also been used on scarred corneas and on corneas affected with endothelial dystrophy. It has been described as having few complications because the graft can be removed at any time; the procedure has not gained general acceptance.

Operation to Correct Astigmatism

Various patterns of keratotomy have been described to correct corneal astigmatism. These cuts can be used alone or with radial keratotomy. Irregular astigmatism continues to be a serious problem following most corneal operations, including radial keratotomy and penetrating keratoplasty, and after cataract surgery. Troutman and others have described relaxing incisions, compression sutures, and wedge resections for postkeratoplasty astigmatism, utilizing a surgical keratometer. Various techniques for cataract incision, such as scleral tunnel incisions and clear corneal incisions, have been reported as useful in preventing postoperative astigmatism after cataract surgery.

Alloplastic Corneal Implants

Disks of many different materials have been inserted into corneal stromal pockets, initially to control corneal edema but more recently to correct refractive errors. In most cases, the corneal tissue anterior to the implant undergoes necrosis. Hydrogel and polysulfone lenses have been more successful than other types of lenses tried so far. Use of alloplastic corneal implants would remove the need to rely on autologous or homologous material in refractive surgery. A plastic ring meant to be implanted intrastromally is under investigation as a refractive surgery procedure.

Clear Lens Removal

A few surgeons around the world have advocated the removal of clear lenses in high degrees of myopia, suggesting that the risk of doing so is minimal owing to the safety of extracapsular lens extraction. The procedure is controversial because of a significant risk of retinal detachment in high myopes.

Lasers

An exciting approach to refractive corneal surgery involves the use of lasers (see Chapter 24). The excimer laser has received the most publicity, but other machines such as the solid-state neodymium:YAG laser and "minilasers" have been shown to be effective also. Laser photorefractive keratectomy (PRK) produces precisely controlled flattening of the anterior cornea to reduce myopia. The procedure can be done for astigmatism and hyperopia. Like radial keratotomy, it is most successful for myopia in the lower range. Anterior stromal haze, irregular astigmatism, and regression have been observed after PRK. In the USA, the FDA has given conditional approval for PRK to one laser company; the procedure has been done in many other countries for years.

REFERENCES

Adams AP et al: Fuchs' endothelial dystrophy of the cornea. Surv Ophthalmol 1993;38:149.

Aswand MI et al: Bacterial adherence to extended wear soft contact lenses. Ophthalmology 1990;97:296.

Bacon AS et al: Acanthamoeba keratitis: The value of early diagnosis. Ophthalmology 1993;100:1238.

Baum J, Barza M: *Pseudomonas* keratitis and extended-wear contact lenses. (Editorial.) Arch Ophthalmol 1990; 108:663.

Berger ST et al: Successful medical management of *Acanthamoeba* keratitis. Am J Ophthalmol 1990; 110:395.

Boger WP III et al: Keratoconus and acute hydrops. Am J Ophthalmol 1981;91:231.

Boisjoly HM et al: Superinfections in herpes simplex keratitis. Am J Ophthalmol 1983;96:354.

Boyd BF: Does refractive surgery have a significant future? Highlights of Ophthalmology 1985;13(12):1. [Entire issue.]

Breebart AC et al: Toxic endothelial cell destruction of the cornea after routine extracapsular cataract surgery. Arch Ophthalmol 1990;108:1121.

Buehler PO et al: The increased risk of ulcerative keratitis among disposable soft contact lens users. Arch Ophthalmol 1992;110:1555.

Clinch TE et al: Microbial keratitis in children. Am J Ophthalmol 1994;117:65.

Cobo LM et al: Oral acyclovir in the treatment of acute herpes zoster ophthalmicus. Ophthalmology 1986;93: 763.

Dawson CR, Jones BR, Tarizzo M: Guide to trachoma control in programmes for the prevention of blindness. World Health Organization, 1982.

DeLuise VP, Tabbara KF: *Peripheral Corneal Disorders.* Little, Brown, 1986.

Erie JC et al: Incidence of ulcerative keratitis in a defined population from 1950 through 1988. Arch Ophthalmol 1993;111:1665.

Falcon MG: Rational acyclovir therapy in herpetic eye disease. Br J Ophthalmol 1987;71:102.

Ficker L et al: *Acanthamoeba* keratitis: Resistance to medical therapy. Eye 1991;4:835.

Foster A, Sommer A: Corneal ulceration, measles, and childhood blindness in Tanzania. Br J Ophthalmol 1987; 71:331.

Gartry D, Kerr Muir M, Marshal J: Excimer laser treatment of corneal surface pathology: A laboratory and clinical study. Br J Ophthalmol 1991;75:258.

Hay J et al: Drug resistance and *Acanthamoeba* keratitis: The quest for alternative antiprotozoal chemotherapy. Eye 1994;8:555.

Heidemann DG et al: *Acanthamoeba* keratitis associated with disposable contact lenses. Am J Ophthalmol 1990; 110:630.

Hope-Ross MW et al: Oral tetracycline in the treatment of recurrent corneal erosions. Eye 1994;8:384.

Hope-Ross MW et al: Recurrent corneal erosions: Clinical features. Eye 1994;8:373.

Hwang DG, Biswell R: Ciprofloxacin therapy of *Mycobacterium chelonae* [sic] keratitis. Am J Ophthalmol 1993;115:114.

Johns KJ, O'Day DM: Pharmacologic management of keratomycoses. Surv Ophthalmol 1988;33:178.

Larkin DFP: Corneal allograft rejection. Br J Ophthalmol 1994;78:649.

Lindquist TD, Sher NA, Doughman DJ: Clinical signs and medical therapy of early *Acanthamoeba* keratitis. Arch Ophthalmol 1988;106:73.

Maguire MG et al: Risk factors for corneal graft failure and rejection in the Collaborative Corneal Transplantation Studies. Ophthalmology 1994;101:1536.

Malbran ES: Corneal dystrophies: A clinical, pathological, and surgical approach: The 28th Edward Jackson Memorial Lecture. Am J Ophthalmol 1972;74:771.

Margolis TP, Ostler HB: Treatment of ocular disease in eczema herpeticum. Am J Ophthalmol 1990;110:274.

Matoba AY et al: Infectious crystalline keratopathy due to *Streptococcus pneumoniae:* Possible association with serotype. Ophthalmology 1994;101:1000.

Matsuda M et al: Corneal endothelial changes associated with aphakic extended contact lens wear. Arch Ophthalmol 1988;106:70.

McDonnell PJ et al: Community care of corneal ulcers. Am J Ophthalmol 1992;114:531.

Meisler DM, Friedlander MH, Okumoto M: *Mycobacterium chelonei* keratitis. Am J Ophthalmol 1982;92:398.

Mondino BJ: Inflammatory diseases of the peripheral cornea. Ophthalmology 1988;95:463.

Murray PI, Rahi AHS: Pathogenesis of Mooren's ulcer: Some new concepts. *Br J Ophthalmol* 1984;68:182.

O'Brart DPS, Kerr Muir MG, Marshal J: Phototherapeutic keratectomy for recurrent corneal erosions. Eye 1994; 8:378.

O'Brart DPS et al: Disturbances in night vision after excimer laser photorefractive keratectomy. Eye 1994;8:46.

O'Brart DPS et al: Treatment of band keratopathy by excimer laser phototherapeutic keratectomy: Surgical techniques and long term follow up. Br J Ophthalmol 1993;77:702.

Pepose JS: Herpes simplex keratitis: Role of viral infection versus immune response. Surv Ophthalmol 1991;35:345.

Poggio EC et al: The incidence of ulcerative keratitis among users of daily wear and extended wear soft contact lenses. New Engl J Med 1989;321:779.

Price FW Jr et al: Five-year corneal graft survival: A large, single-center patient cohort. Arch Ophthalmol 1993; 111:799.

Remeijer L et al: Deep corneal stromal opacities in long-term contact lens wear. Ophthalmology 1990;97:281.

Roper-Hall MJ: Anterior segment surgery. (Review.) Br J Ophthalmol 1990;74:368.

Rosa RH, Miller D, Alfonso EC: The changing spectrum of fungal keratitis in south Florida. Ophthalmology 1994; 101:1005.

Schein OD et al: The impact of overnight wear on the risk of contact lens-associated ulcerative keratitis. Arch Ophthalmol 1994;112:186.

Schein OD et al: Microbial keratitis associated with contaminated ocular medications. Am J Ophthalmol 1988; 105:361.

Schein OD et al: The relative risk of ulcerative keratitis among users of daily-wear and extended-wear soft contact lenses: A case-control study. New Engl J Med 1989; 321:773.

Schwab IR: Oral acyclovir in the management of herpes simplex ocular infections. Ophthalmology 1988;95:423.

Seiler T et al: Excimer laser keratectomy for correction of astigmatism. Am J Ophthalmol 1988;105:117.

Smolin G, Thoft RA: *The Cornea,* 2nd ed. Little, Brown, 1987.

Sommer A: Effects of vitamin A deficiency on the ocular surface. Ophthalmology 1983;90:592.

Spencer WH (editor): *Ophthalmic Pathology,* 3rd ed. 3 vols. Saunders, 1985.

Tabbara KF et al: Thygeson's superficial punctate keratitis. Ophthalmology 1981;88:75.

Thygeson P, Okumoto M: Keratomycosis: A preventable disease. Trans Am Acad Ophthalmol Otolaryngol 1974; 78:433.

Vail A et al: Corneal graft survival and visual outcome: A multicenter study. Ophthalmology 1994;101:120.

Waltman SR: Combined corneal disease and cataract. Arch Ophthalmol 1990;108:926.

Waring GO: The 50-year epidemic of pseudophakic corneal edema. (Editorial.) Arch Ophthalmol 1989;107:657.

Uveal Tract & Sclera

7

William G. Hodge, MD, FRCS(C)

I. UVEAL TRACT

PHYSIOLOGY OF SYMPTOMS

Symptoms of uveal tract disorders depend upon the site of the disease process. For example, since there are pain fibers in the iris, the patient with iritis will complain of moderate pain and photophobia. Inflammation of the iris itself does not cause blurring of vision unless the process is severe or advanced enough to cause clouding of the aqueous humor, cornea, or lens. Choroidal disease itself does not cause pain or blurred vision. Because of the close contact of the choroid with the retina, choroidal disease almost always affects the retina (eg, chorioretinitis). If the macular area of the retina is involved, central vision will be impaired.

The vitreous may also become cloudy as a result of infiltration by cells from inflamed portions of the choroid and retina. The impairment of vision is in proportion to the density of vitreous opacity and is reversible as the inflammation subsides.

The physician examines for disease of the anterior uveal tract with the flashlight and loupe or slitlamp, and disease of the posterior uveal tract with the ophthalmoscope. The principal diseases that affect the uveal tract consist of inflammations and tumors.

UVEITIS

Inflammation of the uveal tract has many causes and may involve one or all three portions simultaneously, as in sarcoidosis. The most frequent form of uveitis is acute anterior uveitis (iritis), usually unilateral and characterized by a history of pain, photophobia, and blurring of vision; a red eye (circumcorneal flush) without purulent discharge; and a small or irregular pupil. It is important to make the diagnosis early and to dilate the pupil to prevent the formation of permanent posterior synechiae.

Inflammatory disorders of the uveal tract, usually unilateral, are common principally in the young and middle age groups. In most cases the cause is not known. In posterior uveitis the retina is almost always secondarily affected. This is known as chorioretinitis.

Two major types of uveitis may be distinguished upon pathologic grounds: nongranulomatous (more common) and granulomatous (Table 7–1). Because pathogenic organisms have not generally been found in the nongranulomatous type and because it responds to corticosteroid therapy, it is thought to be a hypersensitivity phenomenon. Granulomatous uveitis usually follows active microbial invasion of the tissues by the causative organism (eg, *Mycobacterium tuberculosis* or *Toxoplasma gondii*). However, these pathogens are rarely recovered, and a definite etiologic diagnosis is seldom possible. The possibilities can often be narrowed down by clinical and laboratory examination.

Nongranulomatous uveitis occurs mainly in the anterior portion of the tract, ie, the iris and ciliary body. There is an inflammatory reaction, as evidenced by the cellular infiltration of lymphocytes and plasma cells in significant numbers and an occasional mononuclear cell. In severe cases, a large fibrin clot or a hypopyon may form in the anterior chamber.

Granulomatous uveitis may involve any portion of the uveal tract but has a predilection for the posterior uvea. Nodular collections of epithelioid cells and giant cells surrounded by lymphocytes are present in the affected areas. Inflammatory deposits on the posterior surface of the cornea are composed mainly of macrophages and epithelioid cells. It is possible to make a specific etiologic diagnosis histologically in an enucleated eye by identifying the cysts of *Toxoplasma,* the acid-fast bacillus of tuberculosis, the spirochete of syphilis, the distinctive granulomatous appearance of sarcoidosis or sympathetic ophthalmia, and a few other rare specific causes.

Although an attempt has been made to categorize all forms of uveitis by location and morphology, it should be realized that there may be considerable overlap. Thus, sarcoidosis may present distinct noncaseating tubercles, or it may appear as a diffuse uveitis.

Table 7–1. Differentiation of granulomatous and nongranulomatous uveitis.

	Nongranulomatous	Granulomatous
Onset	Acute	Insidious
Pain	Marked	None or minimal
Photophobia	Marked	Slight
Blurred vision	Moderate	Marked
Circumcorneal flush	Marked	Slight
Keratic precipitates	Fine white	Large gray ("mutton fat")
Pupil	Small and irregular	Small and irregular (variable)
Posterior synechiae	Sometimes	Sometimes
Iris nodules	Sometimes	Sometimes
Site	Anterior uvea	Posterior and anterior uvea
Course	Acute	Chronic
Recurrence	Common	Sometimes

Clinical Findings

A. Symptoms and Signs: In the nongranulomatous form, the onset is characteristically acute, with pain, injection, photophobia, and blurred vision. There is a circumcorneal flush caused by dilated limbal blood vessels. Fine white deposits (keratic precipitates, "KPs") on the posterior surface of the cornea can be seen with the slitlamp or with a loupe. The pupil is small, and there may be a collection of fibrin with cells in the anterior chamber. If posterior synechiae are present, the pupil will be irregular in shape (Figures 7–1 to 7–4).

The patient should be asked about previous episodes

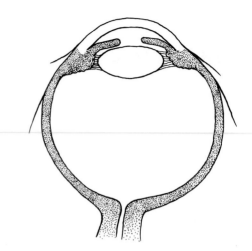

Figure 7–2. Anterior synechiae (adhesions). The peripheral iris adheres to the cornea.

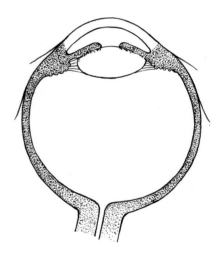

Figure 7–3. Posterior synechiae. The iris adheres to the lens.

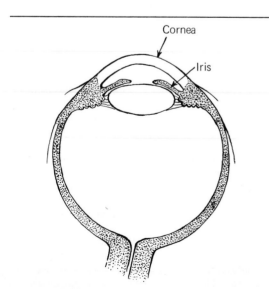

Cornea

Iris

Figure 7–1. Normal anterior chamber.

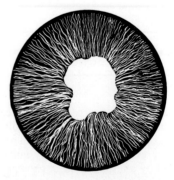

Figure 7–4. Posterior synechiae (anterior view). The iris is adherent to the lens in several places as a result of previous inflammation, causing an irregular fixed pupil.

of arthritis and possible exposure to toxoplasmosis, histoplasmosis, tuberculosis, and syphilis. The remote possibility of a focus of infection elsewhere in the body should also be investigated.

In granulomatous uveitis (which may cause anterior uveitis, posterior uveitis, or both), the onset is usually insidious. Vision gradually becomes blurred, and the affected eye becomes diffusely red with circumcorneal flush. Pain is minimal, and photophobia is less marked than in the nongranulomatous form. The pupil is often constricted and becomes irregular as posterior synechiae form. Large "mutton fat" KPs on the posterior surface of the cornea may be seen with the slit-lamp. Flare and cells are seen in the anterior chamber, and nodules consisting of clusters of white cells are seen on the pupillary margin of the iris (Koeppe nodules). These nodules are the equivalent of mutton fat KPs. Similar nodules found throughout the iris stroma are termed Busacca nodules.

Fresh active lesions of the choroid and retina appear as yellowish-white patches seen hazily with the ophthalmoscope through the cloudy vitreous body. Such posterior cases are generally classified as granulomatous disease. Because of the intimate relationship of the choroid and retina, the retina is nearly always involved (chorioretinitis). As healing progresses, the vitreous haze lessens, and pigmentation occurs gradually at the edges of the yellowish-white spots. In the healed stage, there is usually considerable pigment deposition. If the macula has not been involved, recovery of central vision is usually complete. The patient is usually not aware of the scotoma in the peripheral field corresponding to the scarred area.

B. Laboratory Findings: Extensive laboratory investigation is usually not indicated in anterior uveitis, particularly if it is nongranulomatous or is readily responsive to nonspecific treatment. In persistent nonresponsive anterior or posterior uveitis, an attempt should be made to arrive at an etiologic diagnosis. Skin tests for tuberculosis and histoplasmosis may be helpful, as well as antibodies against toxoplasmosis. On the basis of these tests and the clinical appearance, it is often possible to make an etiologic diagnosis.

Differential Diagnosis

In conjunctivitis, vision is not blurred, pupillary responses are normal, a discharge is present, and there is usually no pain, photophobia, or ciliary injection.

In keratitis or keratoconjunctivitis, vision may be blurred and pain and photophobia may be present. Some causes of keratitis such as herpes simplex and herpes zoster may be associated with a true anterior uveitis.

In acute glaucoma the pupil is dilated, there are no posterior synechiae, and the cornea is steamy.

After repeated attacks, nongranulomatous uveitis may acquire the characteristics of granulomatous uveitis. In recent years there has been less emphasis on this differentiation, and some authorities are disregarding it completely. Nevertheless, the differentiation is still of value as a guide to treatment and prognosis.

Complications & Sequelae

Anterior uveitis may produce peripheral anterior synechiae (Figure 7–2), which impede aqueous outflow at the anterior chamber angle and cause glaucoma. Posterior synechiae can cause glaucoma by allowing aqueous to accumulate behind the iris, bringing about a forward bulging of the iris. Early and constant pupillary dilatation lessens the likelihood of posterior synechiae. Interference with lens metabolism may cause cataract. Retinal detachment occasionally occurs as a result of traction on the retina by vitreous strands. Cystoid macular edema and degeneration can result from long-standing anterior uveitis.

Treatment

A. Nongranulomatous Uveitis: Systemic analgesics as necessary for pain, and dark glasses for photophobia. The pupil must be kept dilated. Atropine is unrivaled in its ability to relieve ciliary spasm. Once relief has been achieved, short-acting dilators such as cyclopentolate should be used to prevent spasm and posterior synechia formation. Local steroid drops are usually quite effective for their anti-inflammatory action. In severe and unresponsive cases, a periocular steroid injection and rarely even systemic steroids can be given.

B. Granulomatous Uveitis: If the process includes the anterior segment, pupillary dilatation with atropine, 2%, is indicated. Since it is often possible to make a tentative or likely diagnosis of the cause, an attempt at specific therapy is indicated as outlined in Table 7–2.

C. Treatment of Complications: Glaucoma is a common complication. Treatment of the uveitis is of primary importance, particularly dilating the pupil with atropine (not constricting the pupil, as with all forms of primary glaucoma). Topical beta-blockers are frequently useful, and occasionally the beta-agonist dipivefrin can provide some help. In severe cases, systemic carbonic anhydrase inhibitors are very helpful. They act by decreasing aqueous production.

Cataract frequently develops in chronic uveitis. The prognosis of cataract surgery in these cases depends upon the cause of the uveitis as well as the surgeon's ability to control the intraocular inflammation preoperatively. The same can be said about retinal detachment surgery.

Course & Prognosis

With treatment, an attack of nongranulomatous uveitis usually lasts a few days to weeks. Recurrences are common. Granulomatous uveitis lasts months to years, sometimes with remissions and exacerbations, and may cause permanent damage with marked visual loss despite the best treatment. The prognosis for a focal peripheral chorioretinal lesion is considerably better, often healing well with no significant visual loss.

Table 7–2. Treatment of granulomatous uveitis.

	Anti-Infective Chemotherapy	Use of Corticosteroids
Toxoplasmosis	If central vision is threatened, give pyrimethamine, 75 mg orally as a loading dose for 2 days followed by 25 mg once daily for 4 weeks, in combination with trisulfapyrimidines (sulfadiazine, sulfamerazine, and sulfamethazine, 0.167 g of each per tablet), 2 g orally as loading dose followed by 0.5 g 4 times daily for 4 weeks. If a fall in the white or platelet count occurs during therapy, give folinic acid (leucovorin), 1 mL IM twice weekly or 3 mg orally 3 times a week. Alternative chemotherapeutic approach for ocular toxoplasmosis: Clindamycin, 300 mg orally 4 times a day with sulfonamides (as above), or minocycline, 100 mg orally daily for 3–4 weeks.	If the response is not favorable after 2 weeks, continue anti-infective therapy and give systemic corticosteroids, eg, prednisolone, 20–25 mg 4 times a day for 1 week, followed by 60–120 mg every other day thereafter,[1] to protect the macula. Corticosteroids may activate the organisms of toxoplasmosis and tuberculosis but are given as a calculated risk to control the inflammatory response when it threatens vision.
Tuberculosis	Isoniazid, 300 mg orally daily; ethambutol, 400 mg orally twice daily; pyridoxine, 50 mg orally daily. Continue treatment for 9 months.	If a favorable response does not occur in 6 weeks, continue antimycobacterial therapy and give systemic corticosteroids, eg, prednisolone, 40–80 mg every other day for 2 months.[1]
Sarcoidosis	Treat with local corticosteroids and mydriatics and, during active stages, with systemic corticosteroids such as prednisolone, 40–80 mg every other day.[1] Give supplemental potassium chloride, 2 g 3 times daily. The usual contraindications to systemic corticosteroid therapy apply.	
Sympathetic ophthalmia	Treat with local corticosteroids and mydriatics and systemic corticosteroids in high doses, eg, prednisone, 40–120 mg every other day.[1] The usual contraindications to systemic corticosteroid therapy apply, and the drugs may be needed in higher doses and for a longer time. Therefore, management of the side effects is often more difficult. Azathioprine may be helpful in reducing the required dose of corticosteroids. In severe cases that fail to respond to corticosteroids, treatment with cytotoxic agents such as chlorambucil and cyclophosphamide or other immunosuppressants such as cyclosporine has met with some success. *Caution:* White blood counts and platelets must be monitored very carefully in these patients, and these drugs should not be used without careful consideration.	

[1]Administration every other day has been advocated to minimize the effects of adrenal suppression and make drug withdrawal easier and safer.

ANTERIOR UVEITIS
(Table 7–3)

1. UVEITIS ASSOCIATED WITH JOINT DISEASE

About 20% of children with the pauciarticular form of **juvenile rheumatoid arthritis** develop a chronic bilateral nongranulomatous iridocyclitis. Females are far more commonly affected than males (4:1). The average age at which the uveitis is detected is 5½ years. In most cases the onset is insidious, the disease being discovered only when the child is noted to have a difference in the color of the two eyes, a difference in the size or shape of the pupil, or the onset of strabismus. There is no correlation between the onset of the arthritis and that of the uveitis. The uveitis may precede the arthritis by 3–10 years. The knee is the most common joint involved. The cardinal signs of the disease are cells and flare in the anterior chamber, small to medium-sized white KPs with or without flecks of fibrin on the endothelium, posterior synechiae, often progressing to seclusion of the pupil, complicated cataract, variable secondary glaucoma, macular edema,and calcific band keratopathy late in the course of the disease.

Treatment of this disorder is challenging. Topical corticosteroids, nonsteroidal anti-inflammatory agents, and mydriatics are of value. In resistant cases, systemic immunosuppression may be needed, and weekly methotrexate has been used successfully by some experts. The prognosis for cataract surgery is guarded.

Iridocyclitis occurring in association with adult peripheral rheumatoid arthritis is strictly coincidental. The adult group is more likely to develop scleritis and sclero-uveitis. It is unfortunate that the associated cells and flare in the aqueous humor that accompany the scleritis have been misinterpreted as "iridocyclitis." About 10–60% of patients with **Marie-Strümpell ankylosing spondylitis** develop an anterior uveitis. There is a marked preponderance in males. The uveitis presents as a mild to fairly severe nongranulomatous type of iridocyclitis with moderate to severe ciliary injection, pain, blurred vision, and photophobia. It is usually recurrent and eventually may lead to permanent damage if not adequately treated. Histocompatibility antigen HLA-B27 is present in approximately 90% of patients with ankylosing spondylitis.

Ocular examination shows ciliary injection, moderate cells and flare in the anterior chamber, and fine white keratic precipitates located mostly on the inferior cornea (Arlt's triangle). Posterior synechiae, peripheral anterior synechiae, cataracts, and glaucoma are common complications after hyperacute attacks of inflammation. Macular edema occurs in 1% of cases

Table 7–3. Causes of anterior uveitis.

Autoimmune
  Juvenile rheumatoid arthritis
  Ankylosing spondylitis
  Reiter's syndrome
  Ulcerative colitis
  Lens-induced uveitis
  Sarcoidosis
  Crohn's disease
  Psoriasis
Infections
  Syphilis
  Tuberculosis
  Leprosy (Hansen's disease)
  Herpes zoster
  Herpes simplex
  Onchocerciasis
  Adenovirus
Malignancy
  Masquerade syndrome
    Retinoblastoma
    Leukemia
    Lymphoma
    Malignant melanoma
Other
  Idiopathic
  Traumatic uveitis, including penetrating injuries
  Retinal detachment
  Fuchs' heterochromic iridocyclitis
  Gout
  Glaucomatocyclitic crisis

with severe anterior iridocyclitis. Persistent edema leads to cystoid degeneration and loss of central vision.

Confirmation of the diagnosis is by x-rays of the sacroiliac joints. In about 50% of patients, clinical signs and symptoms of spinal disease be absent so that the diagnosis may be made only by the radiologist.

The erythrocyte sedimentation rate, although nonspecific and sometimes normal in mild cases, is elevated in most patients, indicating active disease. The rheumatoid factor test is not useful.

2. HETEROCHROMIC UVEITIS (Fuchs' Heterochromic Iridocyclitis)

This disease of unknown cause accounts for about 3% of all cases of uveitis. It is essentially a quiet cyclitis associated with depigmentation of the iris in the affected eye. Pathologically, the iris and ciliary body show moderate atrophy, patchy depigmentation of the pigment layer, and diffuse infiltration of lymphocytes and plasma cells. Involvement is typically unilateral but may be bilateral, and the irides assume different colors. Early in the course of the disease, the difference in color may not be readily apparent and is best noted in daylight.

The onset is insidious in the third or fourth decade, with no redness, pain, or photophobia; the patient is of-ten unaware of the disorder until cataract formation results in blurred vision.

With the slitlamp (or loupe), one sees fine, white, evenly distributed deposits on the posterior corneal surface. These stellate keratic precipitates are characteristic of this disease. Flare and cells in the anterior chamber and a slightly atrophic iris can be seen as well. Anterior floaters may be evident with the ophthalmoscope or slitlamp. Telangiectatic blood vessels may be seen in the chamber angle on gonioscopy.

Cataract develops within a few years in about 15% of cases. Glaucoma occurs in 10–15% of cases. It is usually not necessary to dilate the pupil, as this is one type of uveitis in which posterior synechiae rarely form. The disease does not subside spontaneously, but the visual prognosis is good since the cataract can usually be removed safely despite the low-grade active uveitis.

3. LENS-INDUCED UVEITIS

There are no data at present to substantiate the implication that lens material per se is toxic, so that the term phacotoxic uveitis should no longer be used to describe lens-induced uveitis. The terms phacogenic or lens-induced uveitis are more appropriate when referring to an autoimmune disease secondary to lens antigen. The classic case of lens-induced uveitis occurs when the lens develops a hypermature cataract. The lens capsule leaks and lens material passes into the posterior and anterior chambers, causing an inflammatory reaction characterized by the accumulation of plasma cells, mononuclear phagocytes, and a few polymorphonuclear cells. The eye becomes red and moderately painful; the pupil is small; and vision is markedly reduced (at times to light perception only). Lens-induced uveitis may also occur following traumatic cataracts.

Endophthalmitis phaco-anaphylactica, the term used for the more severe form of lens-induced uveitis, occurs following an extracapsular lens extraction when the same operation has already been performed on the fellow eye and the patient has been sensitized to his or her own lens material. Many polymorphonuclear leukocytes and mononuclear phagocytes appear in the anterior chamber. The eye becomes red and painful, and vision is blurred. Since most of the lens material has already been removed, treatment is conservative, consisting of corticosteroids locally and systemically plus atropine drops to keep the pupil dilated. If this is ineffective, the cataract incision must be opened and the anterior chamber irrigated.

Glaucoma (phacolytic glaucoma) is a common complication of lens-induced uveitis. Treatment consists of lens extraction after intraocular pressure has been brought under control. If this is done, both the uveitis and the glaucoma are cured, and the visual prognosis is good if the process has not been present for more than 1–2 weeks.

INTERMEDIATE UVEITIS
(Pars Planitis, Chronic Cyclitis)

Intermediate uveitis is a form of inflammation that affects neither the anterior nor the posterior uvea directly. Rather, it affects an intermediate zone of the eye. It is seen mainly among young adults whose chief complaint is "floating spots" in the field of vision. In most cases, both eyes are affected. The sex distribution is equal. Pain, redness, and photophobia do not occur. The patient may be unaware of any ocular problem, but the physician detects vitreous opacities, often overlying the inferior pars plana, with the ophthalmoscope.

There are few, if any, signs of anterior uveitis. A few cells may occasionally be seen in the anterior chamber; very rarely, anterior or posterior synechiae occur. Inflammatory cells are more likely to be seen in the retrolental space or in the anterior vitreous on slitlamp examination. Posterior subcapsular cataract occurs frequently. Indirect ophthalmoscopy often reveals soft, round, white opacities over the peripheral retina. These cellular exudates may be confluent, often overlying the pars plana. Some of these patients may also have vasculitis, as shown by perivascular sheathing of retinal vessels.

In most patients, the disease remains stationary or gradually improves over a 5- to 10-year period. Some patients develop cystoid macular edema and permanent macular scarring as well as posterior subcapsular cataracts. In severe cases, cyclitic membranes and retinal detachments may occur. Secondary glaucoma is a rare complication.

The cause is unknown. Corticosteroids constitute the only helpful treatment but should only be used in more severe cases, especially when there is decreased vision secondary to macular edema. Topical corticosteroids are used first; if they fail, sub-Tenon or retrobulbar injections of corticosteroids may be effective. Such treatment increases the risk of cataract development. Fortunately, these patients do well following cataract surgery.

POSTERIOR UVEITIS
(Table 7–4)

The retina and choroid are affected by a variety of infectious and noninfectious disorders. Table 7–4 lists disorders that might involve the posterior segment of the eye.

Most cases of posterior uveitis are associated with some form of systemic disease. The cause of posterior uveitis can often be established on the basis of (1) the morphology of the lesions, (2) the mode of onset and course of the disease, or (3) the association with systemic disease. Other considerations are the age of the patient and whether involvement is unilateral or bilateral. Laboratory tests are of help in confirmation.

Lesions of the posterior segment of the eye can be fo-

Table 7–4. Causes of posterior uveitis.

Infectious disorders
  Viruses
    CMV, herpes simplex, herpes zoster, rubella, rubeola, human immune deficiency virus, Epstein-Barr virus, coxsackie virus. Acute retinal necrosis.
  Bacteria
    Mycobacterium tuberculosis, brucellosis, sporadic and endemic syphilis, *Nocardia, Neisseria meningitidis, Mycobacterium avium-intracellulare, Yersinia,* and *Borrelia* (cause of Lyme disease).
  Fungi
    Candida, Histoplasma, Cryptococcus, and *Aspergillus.*
  Parasites
    Toxoplasma, Toxocara, Cysticercus, and *Onchocerca.*
Noninfectious disorders
  Autoimmune
    Behçet's disease
    Vogt-Koyanagi-Harada syndrome
    Polyarteritis nodosa
    Sympathetic ophthalmia
    Retinal vasculitis
  Malignancy
    Reticulum cell sarcoma
    Malignant melanoma
    Leukemia
    Metastatic lesions
  Unknown etiology
    Sarcoidosis
    Geographic choroiditis
    Acute multifocal placoid pigment epitheliopathy
    Birdshot retinopathy
    Retinal pigment epitheliopathy

cal, geographic, or diffuse. Those that cause clouding of the overlying vitreous should be differentiated from those that never give rise to vitreous cells. The type and distribution of vitreous opacities must be described.

Inflammatory lesions of the posterior segment are generally insidious in onset, but some may be accompanied by abrupt development of vitreous clouding and visual loss. Such diseases are usually accompanied by anterior uveitis, which in turn is sometimes associated with a form of secondary glaucoma.

In the United States, the most common causes of posterior uveitis are cytomegalovirus retinitis, toxoplasmosis, Behçet's disease, and Vogt-Koyanagi-Harada disease.

Diagnosis & Clinical Features

In the following paragraphs, clues to the diagnosis and some characteristic clinical features of posterior uveitis are described.

A. Age of the Patient: Posterior uveitis in patients up to 3 years of age may be caused by a "masquerade syndrome," such as retinoblastoma or leukemia. Infectious causes of posterior uveitis in this age group include cytomegalovirus infection, toxoplasmosis, syphilis, herpetic retinitis, and rubella infection.

In the age group from 4 to 15 years, the causes of posterior uveitis may include toxocariasis, toxoplasmosis, intermediate uveitis, cytomegalovirus infection, masquerade syndrome, subacute sclerosing panencephalitis, and, less frequently, bacterial or fungal infections of the posterior segment.

In the age group from 16 to 40 years, the differential diagnosis includes toxoplasmosis, Behçet's disease, Vogt-Koyanagi-Harada syndrome, syphilis, candidal endophthalmitis, and, less frequently, endogenous bacterial infection, eg, meningococcal meningitis.

Patients who present with posterior uveitis and are over age 40 years may have acute retinal necrosis syndrome, toxoplasmosis, cytomegalovirus infection, retinitis, reticulum cell sarcoma, or cryptococcosis.

B. Laterality: Unilateral involvement favors a diagnosis of uveitis due to toxoplasmosis, candidiasis, toxocariasis, acute retinal necrosis syndrome, or endogenous bacterial infection.

C. Symptoms:

1. Reduced vision–Reduced visual acuity may be present in all types of posterior uveitis and so is not useful in differential diagnosis.

2. Ocular injection–Redness of the eye is absent in conditions that affect only the posterior segment. Thus, it is rare in toxoplasmosis and absent in histoplasmosis.

3. Pain–Pain occurs in patients with acute retinal necrosis syndrome, syphilis, endogenous bacterial infection, and posterior scleritis and in conditions involving the optic nerve. Patients with toxoplasmosis, toxocariasis, and cytomegalovirus retinitis who do not have evidence of glaucoma usually present with no pain in the eye. Other noninfectious posterior segment diseases typically not associated with pain include acute multifocal placoid pigment epitheliopathy, geographic choroiditis, and Vogt-Koyanagi-Harada syndrome.

D. Signs: Signs important in the diagnosis of posterior uveitis include hypopyon, granuloma formation, glaucoma, vitritis, morphology of the lesions, vasculitis, retinal hemorrhages, and old scars.

1. Hypopyon–Disorders of the posterior segment that may present with inflammatory changes in the anterior uvea associated with hypopyon include leukemia, Behçet's disease, syphilis, toxocariasis, and endogenous bacterial infections.

2. Type of uveitis–Anterior granulomatous uveitis may be associated with conditions that affect the posterior retina and choroid. Sarcoidosis, tuberculosis, toxoplasmosis, syphilis, Vogt-Koyanagi-Harada syndrome, and sympathetic ophthalmia may lead to inflammatory changes in the posterior segment of the eye and are usually associated with "mutton fat" KPs. On the other hand, nongranulomatous anterior uveitis may be associated with Behçet's disease, acute multifocal placoid pigment epitheliopathy, brucellosis, reticulum cell sarcoma, and acute retinal necrosis syndrome.

3. Glaucoma–Secondary glaucoma may be observed in patients with acute retinal necrosis syndrome, toxoplasmosis, tuberculosis, or sarcoidosis.

4. Vitritis–Inflammation of the vitreous body may be associated with posterior uveitis. The inflammatory changes in the vitreous are due to spillover from inflammatory foci in the posterior segment of the eye. Inflammatory changes in the vitreous are not observed in patients with geographic choroiditis or histoplasmosis. Minimal inflammatory cells in the vitreous may be observed in patients with reticulum cell sarcoma, cytomegalovirus infection, and rubella and in some cases of toxoplasmosis in which small foci of infection are seen in the retina. On the other hand, severe inflammatory changes in the vitreous associated with many cells and large exudates may be seen in tuberculosis, toxocariasis, syphilis, Behçet's disease, nocardiosis, and toxoplasmosis and in patients with endogenous candidal or bacterial endophthalmitis.

5. Morphology and location of lesions–

a. Retina–The retina is the primary target of many types of infectious agents. Toxoplasmosis is a typical example, causing chiefly retinitis with inflammation of subjacent choroid. Furthermore, infections with cytomegalovirus, herpesviruses, rubella virus, and rubeola virus usually involve the retina primarily and cause more retinitis than choroiditis (see Chapter 15).

Each of these known entities affects the retina more prominently than any other structure in the posterior segment of the eye, and the clinical pictures are fairly characteristic. The active lesion of toxoplasmosis is generally seen in the company of old healed scars of retinochoroiditis that may be heavily pigmented. The lesions may appear in a juxtapapillary location and often give rise to retinal vasculitis. The vitreous is generally clouded when large lesions are present. The lesions of cytomegalovirus infection affect the retina of immunologically compromised hosts, notably those with AIDS. On the other hand, the choroid (see below) is the primary target of insults by a variety of other disorders.

b. Choroid–In patients with tuberculosis, the choroid is the primary target of a granulomatous process also affecting the retina. Patients with tuberculosis may present with geographic choroiditis. By contrast, patients with presumed ocular histoplasmosis syndrome have multiple small coin-like lesions that never cloud the overlying vitreous. There is often evidence of peripapillary scarring and of macular lesions leading to subretinal neovascular nets. In general, there are no signs of systemic disease in patients with presumed ocular histoplasmosis syndrome; but x-rays of the chest may show evidence of dissemination and calcific changes in the periphery of the lung fields. Patients with geographic choroiditis develop predominant involvement of the choroid with little or no affection of the retina and have no systemic disease. The choroid, on the other hand, is primarily involved in sympathetic ophthalmia and Lyme disease.

c. Morphologic features–Active lesions in the various disorders causing posterior uveitis may vary in shape-some geographic and others punctate or nummular. Geographic lesions are seen in cytomegalovirus retinitis, tuberculosis, toxocariasis, geographic choroiditis, and acute retinal necrosis syndrome. Nummular or punctate lesions are seen in patients with Epstein-Barr viral infection, rubella, rubeola, Behçet's disease, acute multifocal placoid pigment epitheliopathy (AMPPE), and toxoplasmosis. In Vogt-Koyanagi-Harada syndrome and sympathetic ophthalmia, Dalen-Fuchs nodules are seen. Sarcoidosis affects any tissue in the eye and may show geographic lesions, retinal vasculitis, and "candle wax drippings," peculiar exudates along retinal vessels. In patients with cytomegalovirus infection, herpes simplex, rubella, rubeola, and acute retinal necrosis syndrome, the lesions are strictly retinal, with minimal or no inflammatory changes in the subjacent tissue. In patients with Epstein-Barr viral infection, histoplasmosis, tuberculosis, syphilis, nonendemic syphilis, and cryptococcosis, the inflammatory lesions are choroidal and multifocal. On the other hand, in patients with Vogt-Koyanagi-Harada syndrome and AMPPE, the lesions are at the level of the retinal pigment epithelium. Elevated necrotic whitish lesions are seen in patients with candidal retinitis and toxoplasmosis. In addition, patients with candidal retinitis may also show the "string of pearls" appearance in the vitreous as well as snowball-like opacities floating in the vitreous. Exudative retinal detachment is typically seen in patients with Vogt-Koyanagi-Harada syndrome and Lyme disease. Diffuse choroiditis is seen in Vogt-Koyanagi-Harada syndrome, sympathetic ophthalmia, leukemia, and Lyme disease.

E. Trauma: A history of trauma is important to rule out intraocular foreign body or sympathetic ophthalmia in patients with uveitis. Surgical trauma, including routine operations such as cataract extraction, may introduce microorganisms into the eye. Severe infections such as staphylococcal endophthalmitis, if left untreated, may destroy all of the internal structures of the eye.

F. Mode of Onset: The onset of posterior uveitis may be acute and sudden or slow and insidious. Diseases of the posterior segment of the eye that may present with sudden onset include toxoplasmic retinitis, acute retinal necrosis, and bacterial infections. Most other causes of posterior uveitis have an insidious onset.

1. OCULAR TOXOPLASMOSIS

Toxoplasmosis is caused by *Toxoplasma gondii,* an obligate intracellular protozoan. The ocular lesions may be acquired in utero or may occur following an episode of acute systemic infection. Clinical manifestations range from subclinical to generalized disease with fatal outcome. Toxoplasmosis is the most common current cause of retinochoroiditis in humans and accounts for 28% of cases of posterior uveitis.

The domestic cat and other feline species serve as definitive hosts for the parasite. Susceptible women who acquire the disease during pregnancy may trans-

mit the disease to the fetus. Sources of human infection include oocysts in soil or airborne in dust, undercooked meat containing bradyzoites (encysted forms of the parasite), and tachyzoites (proliferative form) via transplacental transmission.

Clinical Findings
(Figure 7–5)

A. Symptoms and Signs: Patients with toxoplasmic retinochoroiditis present with a history of seeing floaters, blurring of vision, or photophobia. The ocular lesions consist of fluffy-white areas of necrotic focal retinochoroiditis that may be small or large and single or multiple. Active lesions may be adjacent to healed punched-out retinal scars surrounded by retinal edema. Retinal vasculitis may occur, leading to retinal hemorrhages. The inflammation gives rise to vitreous cells and exudations. Cystoid macular edema may occur.

Iridocyclitis is frequently seen in patients with toxoplasmic retinochoroiditis. Intraocular pressure is variable, but it is important to note that this is one of the few uveitis entities that may present with increased intraocular pressure. Healing of retinochoroiditis is associated with decrease in the inflammatory reactions of the iris, ciliary body, and vitreous. The retinal lesion develops sharp borders with pigment proliferations.

B. Laboratory Findings: *Toxoplasma* antibodies can be detected in the serum by the Sabin-Feldman dye test, the indirect immunofluorescent antibody test, the hemagglutination test, or ELISA. A finding of a positive serologic test for *Toxoplasma* with consistent clinical signs is considered diagnostically significant. No increase in antibody titer is detected during the recurrences of retinochoroiditis. New diagnostic techniques using the polymerase chain reaction are now being tested.

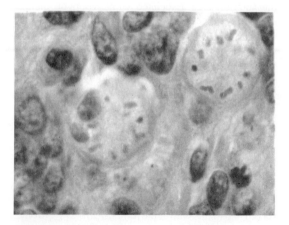

Figure 7–5. *Toxoplasma* cysts in the retina. (Courtesy of K Tabbara.)

Treatment

Small lesions in the periphery of the retina that are not associated with significant vitreous cells may be left without treatment. Treatment of toxoplasmic retinochoroiditis can be initiated by the simultaneous administration of pyrimethamine, 25 mg orally daily, and sulfadiazine, 0.5–1 g orally four times daily for 4 weeks. A loading dose of 75 mg of pyrimethamine and 2 g of sulfadiazine may be given at initiation of therapy. In addition, patients are given 3 mg of leucovorin calcium orally twice weekly, and the urine should be kept alkaline by daily intake of 1 tsp of sodium bicarbonate. Because pyrimethamine may cause bone marrow depression, hematopoietic function must be monitored (Table 7–2).

An alternative approach for ocular toxoplasmosis consists of administration of clindamycin, 300 mg orally four times daily, with trisulfapyrimidines, 0.5–1 g orally four times daily. Clindamycin may cause pseudomembranous colitis in 10–15% of patients. Minocycline has been shown to be effective in the treatment of experimental ocular toxoplasmosis.

Other antibiotics that have been shown to be effective in ocular toxoplasmosis include spiramycin and minocycline. The former drug may be particularly useful during pregnancy. Photocoagulation and cryotherapy have been advocated, but these ablative procedures may lead to complications such as retinal hemorrhages or retinal detachment. Certain retinal neovascular membranes caused by toxoplasmosis may be treated by photocoagulation.

Anterior uveitis associated with ocular toxoplasmosis may be treated with 1% prednisolone eye drops three or four times daily and 5% homatropine eye drops twice daily. Timolol maleate (0.25% eye drops) may be added if intraocular pressure is increased. Periocular steroid injections are contraindicated. Systemic corticosteroids in conjunction with antimicrobial therapy may be administered for vision-threatening inflammatory lesions. Corticosteroids should not be given without appropriate antimicrobial coverage.

2. HISTOPLASMOSIS

In some areas of the USA where histoplasmosis is endemic (the Ohio and Mississippi River Valley areas), the diagnosis of choroiditis presumably due to histoplasmosis is being made with increasing frequency. The patient usually has a positive skin test to histoplasmin and demonstrates "punched-out" spots in the peripheral fundus. These spots are small, irregularly round or oval, depigmented areas, sometimes with a fine pigmented border. They are smaller and have less pigment than the usual healed chorioretinal lesion. Peripapillary atrophy and hyperpigmentation are usually present. Macular lesions that begin as small edematous areas and may progress to hemorrhagic detach-

ments are the most visually threatening feature of the disease. *Vitreous haze does not occur.*

It has been postulated that in areas where histoplasmosis is endemic, many persons develop a benign form of asymptomatic peripheral chorioretinitis. These lesions soon heal, leaving "histo" spots. This exposure sensitizes the choroid. A later antigenic insult to the choroid results in the observed macular changes. This hypothesis has not been verified, but it has stood the test of time since first postulated by Woods in 1959. Many types of treatment have been advocated, including systemic corticosteroids, amphotericin B, antihistamines, and intradermal desensitization with histoplasmin. The results have been questionable in all cases, and treatment with amphotericin B is now contraindicated.

Blue-green argon laser photocoagulation has been shown to be effective in the treatment of those paramacular lesions that cause leaks demonstrable by fluorescein angiography.

3. OCULAR TOXOCARIASIS

Toxocariasis is infection with *Toxocara cati* (an intestinal parasite of cats) or *Toxocara canis* (of dogs). Visceral larva migrans is a disseminated systemic infection occurring in a young child (Table 7–5). Ocular involvement rarely occurs in visceral larva migrans.

Ocular toxocariasis may occur without systemic manifestations. Children acquire the disease by close association with pets and by eating dirt contaminated with *Toxocara* ova. The ingested ova form larvae that penetrate the intestinal mucosa and gain access to the

Table 7–5. Comparison between visceral and ocular larva migrans.

	Visceral Larva Migrans	Ocular Larva Migrans[1]
Average age at onset	2 years	7 years
Fever	+	−
Abdominal symptoms (pain, nausea, diarrhea)	+	−
Nonspecific pulmonary disease	+	−
Hepatosplenomegaly	+	−
Eosinophilia	+	−
Hypergammaglobulinemia	+	−
ELISA (serum anti-*Toxocara* antibodies)	+	±
ELISA (aqueous anti-*Toxocara* antibodies)	−	+
Ocular findings[1]	−	+

[1]Ocular findings of ocular larva migrans: diffuse chronic panuveitis, posterior pole granuloma, or peripheral granuloma.

systemic circulation and finally to the eye. The parasite does not infect the intestinal tract of humans.

Clinical Findings

A. Symptoms and Signs: The disease is usually unilateral. *Toxocara* larvae lodge in the retina and die, leading to a marked inflammatory reaction and local production of *Toxocara* antibodies. Children are brought to the ophthalmologist because of redness, blurred vision, or a whitish pupil or after failing a screening vision test at school.

Three clinical presentations are recognized. Chronic endophthalmitis is the most common presentation in the very young (2–9 years). Localized posterior granuloma and peripheral granuloma with intermediate uveitis are the other two presentations and may affect any age group.

B. Laboratory Findings: The enzyme-linked immunosorbent assay (ELISA) for *T canis* antibody has helped in the diagnosis of toxocariasis. The presence of any serum antibody titer may be significant. The antibody titer of the ocular fluids of patients with ocular toxocariasis is elevated and is higher than that in serum, suggesting local antibody production. Aqueous and vitreous specimens subjected to ELISA are therefore helpful in the diagnosis of ocular toxocariasis.

Treatment

Systemic or periocular injections of corticosteroids should be given when there is evidence of an intraocular inflammatory reaction. Vitrectomy may have to be considered in patients with marked vitreous fibrosis. No anthelmintic has been shown to be effective in ocular toxocariasis, and the intraocular inflammation is aggravated by the death and disintegration of the parasite. Corticosteroids help to prevent ocular damage from the inflammatory reactions.

4. ACQUIRED IMMUNODEFICIENCY SYNDROME

Posterior uveitis may be seen in patients with AIDS. Ophthalmic manifestations in this disease are frequent and may have both prognostic and diagnostic significance. Clinical and histopathologic studies have led to a better understanding of ophthalmic disorders associated with AIDS. Ocular manifestations include cotton-wool spots, retinal hemorrhages, Kaposi's sarcoma of the ocular surface and adnexa, and neuro-ophthalmologic abnormalities associated with intracranial disease.

In addition, patients with AIDS frequently develop infections by opportunistic organisms. Cytomegalovirus retinopathy is a blinding disease and is the most common ocular infection in patients with AIDS. Other pathogens that may cause ocular manifestations in patients with AIDS include *Pneumocystis carinii, Candida*

species, *Toxoplasma gondii, Mycobacterium avium-intracellulare,* and *Cryptococcus.* (See Chapter 15.)

DIFFUSE UVEITIS
(Table 7–6)

The term "diffuse uveitis" denotes a condition in which there is more or less uniform cellular infiltration of all elements of the uveal tract. Specific morphologic features such as geographic infiltrates are characteristically absent.

1. SYMPATHETIC OPHTHALMIA (Sympathetic Uveitis)

Sympathetic ophthalmia is a rare but devastating granulomatous bilateral uveitis that comes on 10 days to many years following a perforating eye injury in the region of the ciliary body, or following retained foreign body. Ninety percent of cases occur within 1 year after injury. The cause is not known, but the disease is probably related to hypersensitivity to some element of the pigment-bearing cells in the uvea. It very rarely occurs following uncomplicated intraocular surgery for cataract or glaucoma.

The injured (exciting) eye becomes inflamed first and the fellow (sympathizing) eye second. Pathologically, there is a diffuse granulomatous uveitis. The epithelioid cells, together with giant cells and lymphocytes (Figure 7–6), form noncaseating tubercles. From the uveal tract the inflammatory process spreads to the optic nerve and to the pia and arachnoid surrounding the optic nerve.

The patient complains of photophobia, redness, and blurring of vision. If a history of trauma is obtained, look for a scar representing the wound of entry in the exciting eye. With the slitlamp or loupe one sees KPs and flare in the anterior chamber of both eyes. Iris nodules may be present. Vitreous cells and soft yellow-white exudates in the deep layer of the retina (Dalen-Fuchs nodules) are seen in the posterior segment.

Sympathetic ophthalmia may be differentiated from other granulomatous uveitides by the history of trauma

Table 7–6. Causes of diffuse uveitis.

Sarcoidosis
Tuberculosis
Syphilis
Onchocerciasis
Brucellosis
Sympathetic ophthalmia
Behçet's disease
Cysticercosis
Vogt-Koyanagi-Harada syndrome
Masquerade syndrome: Retinoblastoma, leukemia
Retained intraocular foreign body

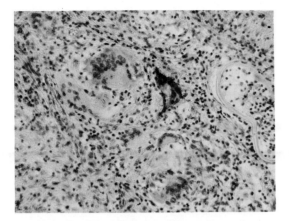

Figure 7–6. Microscopic section of giant cells and lymphocytes in sympathetic ophthalmia involving the choroid. (Courtesy of R Carriker.)

or ocular surgery and by the fact that it is bilateral, diffuse, and (usually) acute rather than unilateral, localized, and chronic.

The recommended treatment of a severely injured sightless eye (eg, a penetrating injury through the sclera, ciliary body, and lens, with loss of vitreous) is immediate enucleation to prevent sympathetic ophthalmia, and every effort must be made to procure the patient's informed consent to the operation. If enucleation can be performed within 10 days after injury, there is almost no chance that sympathetic ophthalmia will develop. However, when the inflammation in the sympathizing eye is advanced, it is generally unwise to enucleate the injured eye, since it may eventually prove to be the better of two very bad eyes.

If inflammation appears in the sympathizing eye, treat at once with local corticosteroids and atropine. Systemic corticosteroids or cytotoxic drugs may be required. Cyclosporine has also proved useful in intractable cases. (See Table 7–2.)

Without treatment, the disease progresses slowly but relentlessly over a period of months or years to complete bilateral blindness.

2. TUBERCULOUS UVEITIS

Tuberculosis causes a granulomatous type of uveitis. Tuberculous uveitis is diagnosed clinically far more often than the disease can be proved by positive identification of tubercle bacilli in the tissues. Although the infection is said to be transmitted from a primary focus elsewhere in the body, uveal tuberculosis is rare in patients with active pulmonary tuberculosis (see Chapter 15).

Tuberculous uveitis may be diffuse but is character-

istically localized in the form of a severe necrotizing granulomatous chorioretinitis. The tubercle itself consists of giant cells and epithelioid cells. Caseation necrosis commonly occurs.

The patient complains of blurred vision, and the eye is moderately injected. If the anterior segment is involved, iris nodules and "mutton fat" KPs are visible on slitlamp examination. If the choroid and retina are primarily affected, one can see a localized yellowish mass partially obscured by a hazy vitreous.

The nodules and the localized nature of tuberculous uveitis help to make a clinical differentiation from sympathetic ophthalmia, and the caseation necrosis differentiates it pathologically from sympathetic ophthalmia and Boeck's sarcoid.

The pupil should be kept dilated with atropine 1%, 1 drop two or three times daily. Antituberculosis drugs should be prescribed systemically if a reasonably certain clinical diagnosis can be made. (See Table 7–2.)

After a prolonged course of several months, the disease usually resolves, leaving permanently damaged tissue and blurred vision because of scarring of the retina.

3. SARCOIDOSIS

Sarcoidosis is a chronic granulomatous disease of unknown cause characterized by multiple cutaneous and subcutaneous nodules, with similar invasions in the viscera and bones, and periodic exacerbations and remissions. The onset is usually in the third decade. The tissue reaction is much less severe than in tuberculous uveitis, and caseation does not occur. The tuberculin skin test is usually negative or only faintly positive. When the parotid glands are involved, the disease is called uveoparotid fever (Heerfordt's disease); when the lacrimal glands are involved, it is called Mikulicz' syndrome.

Thirty percent of cases are complicated by chronic bilateral anterior uveitis, whereas posterior uveitis is far less common. Anterior uveitis is nodular, and in prolonged cases it may lead to severe visual impairment due to cataract and secondary glaucoma. Posterior uveitis is characterized by multiple whitish-yellow retinal exudates ("candle wax drippings") along with perivasculitis. Cystoid macular edema is common.

Diagnosis should be supported by biopsy of the cutaneous nodules. In a small number of cases, typical nodules were also found on the tarsal or bulbar conjunctiva. Chest x-ray may show prominent hilar adenopathy, and serum angiotensin converting enzyme or serum lysozyme concentrations may be elevated. Finally, adjusted serum calcium may be increased, and skin testing with common antigens may show anergy.

Corticosteroid therapy (Table 7–2) given early in the disease may be effective, but recurrences are common and the long-term visual prognosis is poor.

4. ONCHOCERCIASIS

Onchocerciasis is caused by *Onchocerca volvulus.* The disease afflicts about 30 million people in Africa and Central America and is a major cause of blindness. It is transmitted by *Simulium damnosum,* a black fly that breeds in areas of rapidly flowing streams—thus the term "river blindness." Microfilariae picked up from the skin by the fly mature into larvae that become adult worms in 1 year. The adult parasite produces cutaneous nodules 5–25 mm in diameter on the trunk, thighs, arms, head, and shoulders. Microfilariae cause itching, and healing of skin lesions may lead to loss of skin elasticity and areas of depigmentation.

Clinical Findings

A. Symptoms and Signs: Skin nodules may be seen. The cornea reveals nummular keratitis and sclerosing keratitis. Microfilariae swimming actively in the anterior chamber look like silver threads. Death of the microfilariae causes an intense inflammatory reaction and severe uveitis, vitritis, and retinitis. Focal retinochoroiditis may be seen. Optic atrophy may develop secondary to glaucoma.

B. Laboratory Findings: The diagnosis of onchocerciasis is made by a snip skin biopsy and microscopic examination looking for live microfilariae.

Treatment

The preferred treatment for onchocerciasis is with nodulectomy and ivermectin. Diethylcarbamazine and suramin have significant toxicity and should be used only when ivermectin is not available.

The great advantage of ivermectin over diethylcarbamazine is that a single oral dose of 100 or 200 μg/kg reduces the worm burden in the skin and anterior chamber more slowly and therefore with a significant reduction in systemic and ocular reactions. The reduction also persists longer.

The minimum effective dose remains to be determined. A dose of 100 μg/kg may be as effective as 200 μg/kg and is associated with fewer of the mild and transient side effects: fever, headache, etc. Treatment is repeated at 6 or 12 months.

Ivermectin is not marketed in the USA, but the drug is available on a compassionate basis from the manufacturer, Merck Sharp & Dohme.

Topical therapy with corticosteroids and cycloplegics is helpful for uveitis.

5. CYSTICERCOSIS

Cysticercosis is a common cause of serious ocular morbidity. The disease is endemic in Mexico and other Central and South American countries, with ocular involvement occurring in about one-third of patients. It is caused either by the ingestion of eggs of *Taenia solium* or by reverse peristalsis in cases of intestinal obstruction caused by adult tape worms. Eggs mature and embryos penetrate intestinal mucosa, thus gaining access to the circulation. The larva *(Cysticercus cellulosae)* is the most common tapeworm that invades the human eye.

Clinical Findings

The larvae may reach the subretinal space, producing acute retinitis with retinal edema and subretinal exudates; or the vitreous cavity, where a translucent cyst with a dense white spot formed by the invaginated scolex develops. Larvae may live in the eye for as long as 2 years. Death of the larvae inside the eye leads to a severe inflammatory reaction.

Movements of larvae within the ocular tissue may stimulate a chronic inflammatory reaction and fibrosis.

In rare instances, the larva may be seen in the anterior chamber. Involvement of the brain is a cause of seizures. Calcification may be seen in the subcutaneous tissue by x-ray.

Treatment

Treatment of cysticercosis is by surgical removal. Subretinal cysticerci can be removed by localized sclerotomy or destroyed by photocoagulation. Intravitreal larvae are removed by pars plana vitrectomy.

TUMORS INVOLVING THE UVEAL TRACT

J. Brooks Crawford, MD

Several important tumors that may be first identified during ophthalmoscopic examination are discussed below.

Nevus

Nevi (Figures 7–7 and 7–8) are usually flat lesions with or without pigment lying in the stroma of the tissue. On the anterior surface of the iris, they may be noted as iris "freckles." Posteriorly in the choroid, one may see flat pigmented areas. Large choroidal nevi are difficult to differentiate from malignant melanomas. Their flat appearance and especially their lack of growth on repeat serial examinations are important in the differential diagnosis from malignant melanoma.

Because of the difficulties in differentiation from malignant melanomas, fundus photographs or careful line drawings should be made of all suspicious lesions. Observations should be made periodically for changes.

Hemangioma of the Choroid

Choroidal hemangiomas occur as isolated localized tumors or as diffuse hamartomas associated with

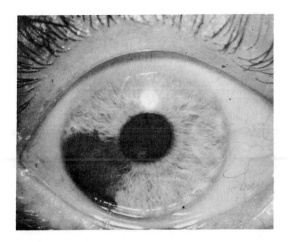

Figure 7–7. Nevus of the iris. (Courtesy of A Rosenberg.)

Sturge-Weber syndrome. Both types can be capillary, cavernous, or mixed hemangiomas. The retinal pigment epithelium over these tumors is often hyperplastic, producing a dark surface instead of the usual pink-orange color and adding to the problem of differentiating this tumor form choroidal melanoma. Ultrasonography can help in the differential diagnosis. Visual loss is the result of secondary retinal detachment, degenerative changes in the retinal pigment epithelium or sensory retina, and secondary glaucoma.

Occasionally, choroidal hemangiomas can be treated with photocoagulation to limit the extent and degree of associated serous detachment of the retina. Enucleation may be necessary for tumors associated with intractable, painful glaucoma.

Medulloepitheliomas ("Diktyoma") of the Ciliary Body

Benign and malignant medulloepitheliomas are rare tumors that may arise from the ciliary body epithelium.

Those with one or more heteroplastic elements, such as hyaline cartilage, brain tissue, or rhabdomyoblasts, are called teratoid medulloepitheliomas. Those that arise soon after birth may infiltrate the area around the lens and produce a white pupillary reflex similar to that seen in eyes with retinoblastoma.

Malignant Melanoma

It has been estimated that intraocular malignant melanoma occurs in 0.02–0.06% of the total eye patient population in the USA. It is seen only in the uveal tract and is the most common intraocular malignant tumor in the white population. It is almost always unilateral. Eighty-five percent appear in the choroid (Figure 7–9), 9% in the ciliary body, and 6% in the iris.

This tumor may be seen in its early stages only accidentally during routine ophthalmoscopic examination or because of blurring due to macular invasion. Blood-borne metastases may occur at any time. Glaucoma may be a late manifestation.

Histologically, these tumors are composed of spindle-shaped cells, with or without prominent nucleoli, and large epithelioid tumor cells. Tumors composed of the former have a good prognosis; tumors with the latter a poorer prognosis.

Intraocular malignant melanomas may extend into adjacent intraocular tissues or outside the eye through the scleral canals or by intravascular invasion.

Clinical manifestations are usually absent unless the macula is involved. In the later stages, growth of the tumor may lead to retinal detachment with loss of visual field. A tumor located in the iris may be large

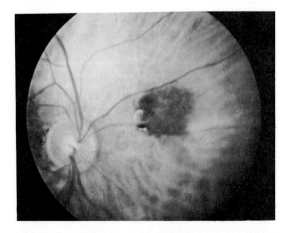

Figure 7–8. Nevus of the choroid. (Photo by Diane Beeston.)

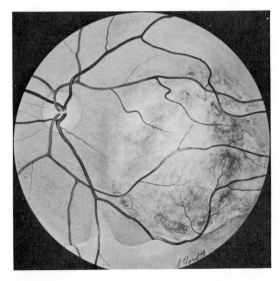

Figure 7–9. Malignant melanoma of the choroid, macular area, left eye (drawing). (Courtesy of F Cordes.)

enough to change the color of the iris or deform the pupil. Pain does not occur in the absence of glaucoma or inflammation.

The first step in diagnosis is to suspect the lesion. Most intraocular malignant melanomas can be seen ophthalmoscopically. Always suspect the presence of a tumor in eyes with nonrhegmatogenous retinal detachment. A significant incidence of intraocular melanomas has been found in blind, painful eyes; ultrasonography will help detect these.

Enucleation of an eye with a choroidal melanoma has been the traditional treatment. Recently, other forms of therapy, particularly local resection or radiotherapy with charged particles such as helium ions and protons or with plaques of radioactive isotopes sutured to the sclera, have been used for eyes with small tumors and useful vision. Very small melanomas (< 10 mm in diameter) have an excellent prognosis and are often impossible to differentiate from benign nevi; therefore, many authorities advocate not treating these tumors until unequivocal growth can be documented (usually with serial photographs or ultrasound measurements). In patients with metastatic disease, the median survival time is less than 1 year, the value of chemotherapy is limited, and treatment to the affected eye is for symptomatic relief only.

Small melanomas of the iris that have not invaded the iris root can be safely observed until growth is documented; then they can be removed by iridectomy. Lesions that invade the iris root and ciliary body can sometimes be treated with iridocyclectomy. Iris melanomas have an excellent prognosis; the mortality rate is less than 1%. Many pigmented iris tumors are actually large nevi rather than malignant melanomas.

Choroidal Metastases

Because of its rich blood supply, the choroid is an important site for blood-borne metastases. In females, carcinoma of the breast is much the most common source. In males, lung, genitourinary, and gastrointestinal malignancies are the usual primaries. Metastasis to the choroid usually becomes apparent within 2 years after diagnosis of the primary malignancy, but occasionally it does not become manifest until many years later.

The usual presenting symptoms of choroidal metastasis are decreased vision and photopsia. The tumor appears as a pale, non-pigmented elevation of the choroid, often associated with serous retinal detachment. There may be multiple lesions involving one or both eyes, in which case the diagnosis is relatively easily made. A solitary metastasis may be mistaken for an amelanotic choroidal malignant melanoma. Ultrasonography and fine-needle biopsy may aid in differentiation.

Chemotherapy for concurrent metastatic disease is usually effective against the choroidal component. In the absence of other metastases, local radiotherapy is the treatment of choice.

II. SCLERA
FRCOphth

Paul Riordan-Eva, FRCS, FRCOphth

DISEASES & DISORDERS OF THE SCLERA

BLUE SCLERAS

The normal sclera is white and opaque, so that the underlying uveal structures are not visible. Structural changes of the scleral collagen fibers and thinning of the sclera may allow the underlying uveal pigment to be seen, giving the sclera a bluish discoloration. Blue sclera occurs in several disorders that lead to disturbances in the connective tissues, particularly the collagen fibers. Blue scleras are part of the clinical picture in osteogenesis imperfecta, Ehlers-Danlos syndrome, pseudoxanthoma elasticum, Marfan's syndrome (all of these conditions are discussed further in Chapter 15), and pseudohypoparathyroidism and may occur with prolonged use of corticosteroids. Blue scleras are sometimes noted in normal newborn infants, in keratoconus, and in keratoglobus.

SCLERAL ECTASIA

Prolonged elevation of intraocular pressure early in infancy, such as occurs in cases of congenital glaucoma, may lead to stretching and thinning of the sclera. Scleral ectasia may occur also as a congenital anomaly surrounding the disk or occasionally in the macular area. It may also follow inflammation or injury of the sclera.

STAPHYLOMA

Staphyloma results from bulging of the uvea into ectatic sclera. It may be anterior, equatorial, or posterior. Anterior staphylomas are generally located over the ciliary body (ciliary staphyloma) (Figure 7–10) or between the ciliary body and the limbus (intercalary staphyloma). Equatorial staphylomas are located at the equator and posterior staphylomas posterior to the equator. Posterior staphylomas are most commonly seen at the optic nerve head. Patients are generally poorly sighted and extremely myopic, although cases of congenital peripapillary staphylomas in patients with normal or nearly normal vision have been reported. Posterior staphyloma is usually associated with areas of pronounced choroidal atrophy.

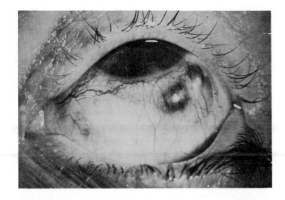

Figure 7–10. Ciliary staphyloma. (Courtesy of P Thygeson.)

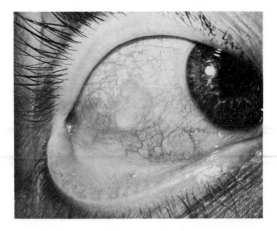

Figure 7–11. Nodular scleritis, right eye. (Photo by Diane Beeston.)

Staphyloma must be differentiated from extreme myopia and central coloboma of the optic nerve head.

INTRASCLERAL NERVE LOOPS OF AXENFELD

The intrascleral nerve loops are sites of branches of the long ciliary nerves. They enter the sclera close to the ciliary body and about 3.5 mm from the limbus. They are more commonly seen nasally. They may be pigmented and are usually accompanied by the small anterior ciliary artery in its inward course.

INFLAMMATION OF THE SCLERA & EPISCLERA

Inflammation involving the episclera, the thin layer of vascular elastic tissue overlying the sclera, is referred to as **episcleritis. Scleritis** is inflammation of the sclera itself. The two diseases are considered distinct clinical entities and will be considered separately.

Episcleritis

This is a relatively common localized inflammation of the episclera. It is unilateral in about two-thirds of cases, and the sex incidence is equal. It may recur at the same or adjacent sites in the palpebral fissure.

The cause is not known, but hypersensitivity reactions may play a role. Certain systemic diseases such as rheumatoid arthritis, Sjögren's syndrome, coccidioidomycosis, syphilis, herpes zoster, and tuberculosis have been associated with episcleritis. Hyperuricemia and gout are the most significant associations.

Symptoms of episcleritis include redness, pain, photophobia, tenderness, and lacrimation. Ocular examination reveals localized hyperemia that gives the eyeball a pink or purple color. There is also infiltration, congestion, and edema of the episclera, the overlying conjunctiva, and the underlying Tenon's capsule. Two types of episcleritis are recognized: simple and nodular (Figure 7–11). The sclera itself is not involved. About 15% of patients with episcleritis develop mild iritis.

Conjunctivitis is ruled out by the localized nature of episcleritis and the lack of palpebral conjunctival involvement.

The condition is benign, and the course is generally self-limited in 1–2 weeks. However, recurrences may torment the patient for years. Topical therapy with corticosteroids (dexamethasone 0.1%) resolves the inflammatory changes in 3 or 4 days. Corticosteroids are more effective in simple episcleritis than in nodular episcleritis. Oral nonsteroidal anti-inflammatory agents (flurbiprofen, 300 mg daily, reducing to 150 mg daily once symptoms are controlled, or indomethacin 25 mg three times a day) may be helpful in both forms of episcleritis, particularly in recurrent cases. Gout should be specifically treated.

Scleritis

Scleritis is a chronic granulomatous disorder characterized by destruction of collagen, cellular infiltration, and vascular changes indicative of vasculitis. In many cases, these changes are purely immunologically mediated, with both type IV (delayed hypersensitivity) and type III (immune complex) reactions, occurring in association with systemic disease. In a few cases, there may be direct microbial invasion, and in a number of cases immunologically mediated processes appear to be triggered by local events, such as cataract surgery (Table 7–7). Laboratory studies are often helpful in identifying associated systemic diseases or in establishing the nature of the immunologic reaction (Table 7–8). Scleritis is an uncommon disorder. It may be unilateral or bilateral, of sudden or insidious onset, and may occur as a single episode or may be recurrent.

Table 7–7. Causes of scleritis.

Autoimmune diseases
   Ankylosing spondylitis
   Rheumatoid arthritis
   Polyarteritis nodosa
   Relapsing polychondritis
   Wegener's granulomatosis
   Systemic lupus erythematosus
   Pyoderma gangrenosum
   Ulcerative colitis
   IgA nephropathy
   Psoriatic arthritis
Granulomatous diseases
   Tuberculosis
   Syphilis
   Sarcoidosis
   Leprosy
   Vogt-Koyanagi-Harada syndrome (rare)
Metabolic disorders: Gout, thyrotoxicosis, active rheumatic
   heart disease
Infections: Onchocerciasis, toxoplasmosis, herpes zoster,
   herpes simplex, infections with *Pseudomonas, Aspergillus,*
   Streptococcus, Staphylococcus
Others
   Physical (irradiation, thermal burns)
   Chemical (alkali or acid burns)
   Mechanical (penetrating injuries)
   Lymphoma
   Rosacea
   Post cataract extraction
Unknown

Women are more commonly affected than men. Patients with scleritis almost always complain of pain, typically of a constant, boring nature, that may prevent them from sleeping. Visual acuity is often slightly reduced. More marked visual loss occurs when there is associated anterior chamber inflammation, anterior scleritis due to direct microbial invasion, and in posterior scleritis. The globe is frequently tender. A key clinical sign is deep violaceous discoloration of the globe due to dilatation of the deep vascular plexus of the sclera and episclera. Together with the deep scleral injection, there is injection of the overlying episclera and conjunctiva. Examination in daylight rather than artificial illumination and instillation of epinephrine 1:1000 or phenylephrine 10% drops—which constrict the conjunctival and superficial episcleral vascular

Table 7–8. Laboratory workup for scleritis.

Complete blood count and sedimentation rate
Serum complement (C3) level
Serum immune complexes
Serum rheumatoid factor
Serum antinuclear antibodies
PPD, chest x-ray
Serum FTA-ABS, VDRL
X-ray of the orbit to rule out foreign body, especially in
   patients with nodular scleritis
X-ray of the sinuses
Serum levels of uric acid
Urinalysis

plexuses—help in the detection of the deep scleral involvement and differentiation from episcleritis, conjunctivitis, and ciliary injection. The sclera is also swollen, with edema in the overlying episclera and Tenon's capsule. Slitlamp examination helps in assessing the depth and nature of the scleral and episcleral inflammation and in identifying associated corneal disease. Use of a green filter in the slitlamp highlights the vascular changes. Areas of avascularity suggest occlusive vasculitis and a poor prognosis. The clinician must be wary of the relatively white eye because this may be due to ischemia and necrosis rather than a low level of inflammation. Areas of scleral translucency are good indicators of previous scleritis.

Posterior scleritis may present with periorbital edema, proptosis, limitation of ocular movements, and visual loss. There is often little pain or anterior scleral inflammation, and the eye may therefore not appear inflamed on external inspection. Posterior segment signs include vitritis, disk swelling, macular edema, and exudative retinal detachment. Diagnosis is based on detection of thickening of the posterior sclera and choroid on ultrasonography or CT scan. Localized thickening may be mistaken on ultrasonography for malignant melanoma. Many patients have had the diagnosis of posterior scleritis made only after enucleation for this and other presumed diagnoses.

Scleritis is classified according to its clinical and pathologic features. Two major types are recognized: anterior and posterior. Anterior scleritis is subdivided into diffuse, nodular (Figure 7–12), and necrotizing, of which the latter is further subdivided according to whether there is or is not associated inflammation. Necrotizing anterior scleritis and posterior scleritis are much less common than diffuse and nodular anterior scleritis. All forms of scleritis show reduced vascular perfusion on anterior segment angiography. (In episcleritis, there is increased blood flow.) In **necrotizing scleritis,** there is also vascular closure, particularly in the subgroup without inflammation when arteriolar occlusion is a major feature. Necrotizing scleritis is also associated with loss of scleral tissue ("scleral melt-

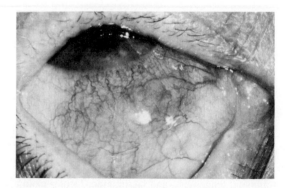

Figure 7–12. Nodular scleritis, left eye, associated with rheumatoid arthritis. (Courtesy of GR O'Connor.)

ing"), leading to staphyloma formation. These areas rarely perforate unless there is associated glaucoma or direct trauma, including surgery.

All forms of **anterior scleritis** tend to have a progressive course, usually by circumferential advancement from previously affected areas. The major distinction between the simpler nodular and diffuse forms of anterior scleritis and the necrotizing forms is the time scale of this progression. In necrotizing scleritis with inflammation, it may be only a few weeks before the eye is virtually destroyed, and thus urgent investigation and treatment must be carried out. In necrotizing scleritis without inflammation (scleromalacia perforans), patients often present with extensive established disease.

An associated systemic disease is found in about 40% of all patients with scleritis and 60% of those with necrotizing disease. Identification of the systemic disease is important because it tends to be one of the more severe forms of connective tissue disease, which in itself is a threat to the patient's life, and its presence indicates that the scleritis is likely to be severe. The nature of the associated systemic disease is also helpful in determining appropriate immunosuppressive therapy. Scleromalacia perforans is particularly associated with severe rheumatoid arthritis. A 360-degree uniform peripheral shallow corneal guttering ("contact lens cornea") is peculiar to scleritis associated with long-standing rheumatoid arthritis. Acute anterior scleritis associated with a deep peripheral corneal gutter that crosses the limbus, is characteristic of polyarteritis nodosa and Wegener's granulomatosis. Failure to control the disease is likely to be followed by corneal perforation. In scleritis due to direct bacterial or fungal invasion, which most commonly occurs after ocular surgery, there is usually a nodular anterior scleritis with marked local tissue destruction and secondary intraocular inflammation.

The complications of scleritis include keratitis, uveitis, and glaucoma. Keratitis is manifested as peripheral guttering, superficial vascularization, or deep vascularization with or without opacification. Uveitis is an ominous sign because of its frequent failure to respond to treatment. It is often associated with visual loss due to macular edema. Both open-angle and angle-closure glaucoma occur. Steroid-induced glaucoma may also develop.

The initial treatment of scleritis is with systemic non-steroidal anti-inflammatory agents. Either indomethacin, 100 mg daily, or ibuprofen, 300 mg daily, is the agent of choice. In most cases, there is a virtually immediate reduction in pain and subsequent resolution of inflammation. If there is no response in 1–2 weeks—or as soon as vascular closure becomes apparent—high-dose systemic steroid therapy should be started. This is usually given orally, starting with prednisolone, 80 mg daily, and reducing rapidly over 2 weeks to a maintenance dose of about 10 mg daily. Occasionally, severe disease necessitates intravenous pulse therapy with methylprednisolone, 1 g weekly. Other immunosuppressive agents can also be used. Cyclophosphamide is particularly valuable if there is a high level of circulating immune complexes. Topical steroid therapy is not effective on its own but may be useful as an adjunct to systemic therapy. Specific therapy should be given if an infectious cause is identified. The role of systemic steroid therapy will then be determined by the nature of the disease process, ie, whether it is a hypersensitivity response or an effect of direct microbial invasion. Surgery is rarely required except for repair of scleral or corneal perforations. This is most likely to be needed when there has been severe destruction from direct microbial invasion, or in Wegener's granulomatosis or polyarteritis nodosa complicated by corneal perforation. The scleral thinning of purely inflammatory scleritis rarely leads to perforation unless there is coexistent glaucoma or direct trauma—particularly attempts to obtain a biopsy specimen. Scleral grafting has been used prophylactically in the treatment of necrotizing scleritis, but such grafts infrequently melt away unless concomitant chemotherapy is being administered.

Scleromalacia perforans is not amenable to treatment unless it is started in the very early stages of the disease. Since presentation rarely occurs at this stage, most cases are not treated unless there are complications.

HYALINE DEGENERATION

Hyaline degeneration is a fairly frequent finding in the scleras of persons over age 60. It is manifested by small, round, translucent gray areas that are usually about 2–3 mm in diameter and located anterior to the insertion of the rectus muscles. These lesions cause no symptoms or complications.

REFERENCES

Diseases of the Uveal Tract

Bialasiewicz AA et al: Bilateral diffuse choroiditis and exudative retinal detachments with evidence of Lyme disease. Am J Ophthalmol 1988;105:419.

Cristina N et al: Detection of *Toxoplasma gondii* in AIDS patients by the polymerase chain reaction. Infection 1993; 21:150.

de Souza EC et al: Unusual central chorioretinitis as the first manifestation of early secondary syphilis. Am J Ophthalmol 1988;105:271.

Foster CS, Barrett F: Cataract development and cataract surgery in patients with juvenile rheumatoid arthritis-associated iridocyclitis. Ophthalmology 1993;100:809.

Foulds WS: The choroidal circulation and retinal metabolism: An overview. Eye 1990;4:243.

Froebel KS et al: An investigation of the general immune status and specific immune responsiveness to retinal-(S)-antigen in patients with chronic posterior uveitis. Eye 1989;3:263.

Hawkins BS, Ganley P: Risk of visual impairment attributable to ocular histoplasmosis. Arch Ophthalmol 1994;112:655.

Howe LJ et al: The efficacy of systemic corticosteroids in sight-threatening retinal vasculitis. Eye 1994;8:443.

Hylkema HA et al: Circulating immune complexes in uveitis patients. Int Ophthalmol 1989;13:253.

Jacquier P et al: Immunodiagnosis of toxocarosis in humans: Evaluation of a new enzyme-linked immunosorbent assay kit. J Clin Microbiol 1991;29:1831.

Kanski JJ: Juvenile arthritis and uveitis. Surv Ophthalmol 1990;34:253.

Klok et al: Antibodies against ocular and oral antigens in Behçet's disease associated with uveitis. Curr Eye Res 1989;8:957.

Kraus-Mackiw E, O'Connor GR: *Uveitis: Pathophysiology and Therapy.* Thieme-Stratton, 1983.

Margolis TP et al: Varicella-zoster virus retinitis in patients with the acquired immunodeficiency syndrome. Am J Ophthalmol 1991;112:119.

Nussenblat RB, Palestine AG: Uveitis: *Fundamentals and Clinical Practice.* Year Book, 1989.

O'Connor GR: Factors related to the initiation and recurrence of uveitis. Am J Ophthalmol 1983;96:577.

Passo MS, Rosenbaum JT: Ocular syphilis in patients with human immunodeficiency virus infection. Am J Ophthalmol 1988;106:1.

Rosenbaum JT: An algorithm for the systemic evaluation of patients with uveitis: Guidelines for the consultant. Semin Arthritis Rheum 1990;19:248.

Rothova A et al: Clinical features of acute anterior uveitis. Am J Ophthalmol 1987;103:137.

Tabbara KF: Ocular toxoplasmosis. In: *Clinical Ophthalmology.* Duane TD (editor). Harper & Row, 1987.

Tabbara KF, Al-Kassimi H: Ocular brucellosis. Br J Ophthalmol 1990;74:249.

Tiedman JS: Epstein-Barr viral antibodies in multifocal choroiditis and panuveitis. Am J Ophthalmol 1987;103:659.

Wilson CA, Choromokos EA, Sheppard R: Acute posterior multifocal placoid pigment epitheliopathy and cerebral vasculitis. Arch Ophthalmol 1988;106:796.

Tumors Involving the Uveal Tract

Char DH: *Clinical Ocular Oncology.* Churchill Livingstone, 1989.

Char DH et al: Cytomorphometry of uveal melanomas: fine-needle aspiration versus standard histology. Trans Am Ophthalmol Soc 1990;87:197.

Char DH et al: Uveal melanoma radiation: I^{125} brachytherapy versus helium ion irradiation. Ophthalmology 1989;96:1708.

Damato BE, Paul J, Foulds WS: Predictive factors of visual outcome after local resection of choroidal melanoma. Br J Ophthalmol 1993;77:616.

Kath R et al: Prognosis and treatment of disseminated uveal melanoma. Cancer 1993;72:2219.

Lee KJ, Peyman GA, Raichand S: Internal eye wall resection for posterior uveal melanoma. Jpn J Ophthalmol 1993;37:287.

Minatel E et al: The efficacy of radiotherapy in the treatment of intraocular metastases. Br J Radiol 1993;66:699.

Spencer WH (editor): *Ophthalmic Pathology,* 3rd ed. 3 vols. Saunders, 1985.

Sclera

Calthorpe CM, Watson PG, McCartney ACE: Posterior scleritis: A clinical and histological survey. Eye 1988;2:267.

Foster CS, Forstot SL, Wilson LA: Mortality rate in rheumatoid arthritis patients developing necrotizing scleritis or peripheral ulcerative keratitis: Effects of systemic immunosuppression. Ophthalmology 1984;91:1253.

Meyer PAR et al: "Pulsed" immunosuppressive therapy in the treatment of immunologically induced corneal and scleral disease. Eye 1987;1:487.

Mondino BJ, Phinney RB: Treatment of scleritis with combined oral prednisolone and indomethacin therapy. Am J Ophthalmol 1988;106:473.

Pheng Fong LP et al: Immunopathology of scleritis. Ophthalmology 1991;98:472.

Sainz de la Mata M, Jabbur NS, Foster CS: An analysis of therapeutic decision for scleritis. Ophthalmology 1993;100:1372.

Sainz de la Maza M, Jabbur NS, Foster CS: Severity of scleritis and episcleritis. Ophthalmology 1994; 101:389.

Sainz de la Maza M, Tauber J, Foster CS: Scleral grafting for necrotizing scleritis. Ophthalmology 1989;96:306.

Tuft SJ, Watson PG: Progression of scleral disease. Ophthalmology 1991;98:467.

Watson PG, Bovey E: Anterior segment fluorescein angiography in the diagnosis of scleral inflammation. Ophthalmology 1985;92:1.

Lens

8

John P. Shock, MD, & Richard A. Harper, MD

The primary function of the lens is to focus light rays upon the retina. In order to focus light from a distant object, the ciliary muscle relaxes, tautening the zonular fibers and reducing the anteroposterior diameter of the lens to its minimal dimension; in this position the refractive power of the lens is minimized, and parallel rays are thus focused upon the retina. In order to focus light from a near object, the ciliary muscle contracts, releasing the tension on the zonules. The elastic lens capsule then molds the lens into a more spherical body with correspondingly greater refractive power. The physiologic interplay of the ciliary body, zonule, and lens that results in focusing near objects upon the retina is known as **accommodation.** As the lens ages, its accommodative power is gradually reduced.

PHYSIOLOGY OF SYMPTOMS

Disorders of the lens include opacification, distortion, dislocation, and geometric anomalies. Patients with these conditions have blurred vision without pain. Examination for diseases of the lens is by visual acuity testing and by viewing the lens with a slitlamp, ophthalmoscope, hand flashlight, or loupe, preferably through a dilated pupil.

CATARACT

A cataract is a lens opacity. Cataracts vary markedly in degree of density and may be due to a variety of causes but are usually associated with aging. Cross-sectional studies have identified cataracts in about 10% of all Americans, and this prevalence increases to about 50% for those between the ages of 65 and 74 and to about 70% for those over 75. Most are bilateral, although the rate of progression in each eye is seldom equal. Traumatic cataract, congenital cataract, and other types are less common.

Cataractous lenses are characterized by lens edema,

protein alteration, increasing proliferation, and disruption of the normal continuity of the lens fibers. In general, lens edema varies directly with the stage of cataract development. The immature (incipient) cataract is only slightly opaque. A completely opaque mature (moderately advanced) cataractous lens is somewhat edematous. If the water content is maximal and the lens capsule is stretched, the cataract is called intumescent (swollen). In the hypermature (far-advanced) cataract, water has escaped from the lens, leaving a relatively dehydrated, very opaque lens and a wrinkled capsule.

In congenital cataracts, the principal changes occur either in the nucleus of the lens—the fetal nucleus or the embryonic nucleus, depending on the timing of the cataractogenic stimulus—or at the anterior or posterior pole of the lens if the abnormality is in the lens capsule. In age-related cataracts, changes may involve chiefly the nucleus (nuclear sclerosis), the cortex (coronary or cuneiform opacities [Figure 8–1]), or the posterior subcapsular region. Cataracts associated with uveitis and systemic steroid therapy are also commonly of the posterior subcapsular type. Blue dot lens opacities are commonly seen in Down's syndrome. Anterior shield-shaped subcapsular opacity is characteristic of atopic dermatitis, and polychromatic "Christmas tree" opacities of myotonic dystrophy. Cortical and anterior polar cataracts often produce little change in visual function even when they are quite marked. Posterior subcapsular and posterior polar opacities cause marked visual symptoms even when they are relatively mild. Nuclear sclerosis frequently leads to increasing myopia.

Most cataracts are not visible to the casual observer until they become dense enough (mature or hypermature) to cause blindness. However, a cataract in its earliest stages of development can be observed through a well-dilated pupil with an ophthalmoscope, loupe, or slitlamp.

The ocular fundus becomes increasingly more difficult to visualize as the lens opacity becomes denser, until the fundus reflection is completely absent. At this stage the cataract is usually mature and the pupil may be white.

The clinical degree of cataract formation, assuming

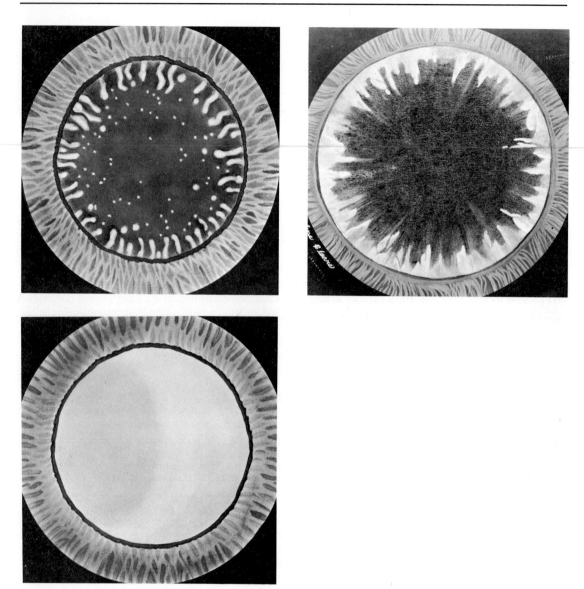

Figure 8–1. Cataract types. ***Above, left:*** senile cataract, "coronary" type: club-shaped peripheral opacities with clear central lens; slowly progressive. ***Above, right:*** Senile cataract, "cuneiform" type: peripheral spicules and central clear lens; slowly progressive. ***Left:*** Senile cataract, "morgagnian" type (hypermature lens); the entire lens is opaque, and the lens nucleus has fallen inferiorly. (Reproduced, with permission, from Cordes FC: *Cataract Types,* 3rd ed. American Academy of Ophthalmology and Otolaryngology, 1954.)

that no other eye disease is present, is judged primarily by the Snellen visual acuity test. Generally speaking, the decrease in visual acuity is directly proportionate to the density of the cataract. However, some individuals who have clinically significant cataracts when examined with the ophthalmoscope or slitlamp see well enough to carry on with their normal activities. Others have a decrease in visual acuity out of proportion to the degree of lens opacification. This is due to distortion of the image by the partially opaque lens. The Cataract Management Guideline Panel recom-

mends reliance on clinical judgment combined with Snellen acuity as the best guide to the appropriateness of surgery but recognizes the need for flexibility with due regard to a patient's particular functional and visual needs, the environment, and other risks—all of which may vary widely.

Cataract formation is characterized chemically by a reduction in oxygen uptake and an initial increase in water content followed by dehydration. Sodium and calcium content is increased; potassium, ascorbic acid, and protein content is decreased. Glutathione is not present in cataractous lenses. Attempts to accelerate or retard these chemical changes by medical treatment have not yet been successful.

During the past few years, there has been increasing evidence implicating ultraviolet radiation as a significant factor in the occurrence of senile cataracts. Epidemiologic investigations have shown that there is an increased incidence of cortical and posterior subcapsular cataracts in geographic areas where there are long periods of strong sunlight. Further investigation of the effects of ultraviolet light on the lens is being undertaken.

AGE-RELATED CATARACT
(Senile Cataract)

Age-related cataract (Figures 8–1 to 8–3) is by far the most common type of cataract. Increasingly blurred vision and visual distortion are the only symptoms. Paradoxically, although distant vision is blurred in the incipient stage of cataract formation, near vision may improve slightly, so the patient will read better without glasses ("second sight"). This artificial myopia is due to the greater refractive index of the lens in the incipient stage.

There is no medical treatment for cataract. Lens extraction (see Cataract Surgery, below) is indicated when visual impairment interferes with the patient's normal activities. If glaucoma secondary to lens swelling (intumescent lens) occurs, surgical extraction of the lens is indicated.

Glaucoma and lens-induced uveitis are uncommon complications. Lens-induced uveitis requires surgical extraction of the lens to remove the source of the offending lens products.

Senile cataract is usually slowly progressive over years, and death may occur before surgery becomes necessary. If surgery is indicated, lens extraction definitely improves visual acuity in well over 90% of cases. The remainder of patients either have preexisting retinal damage or develop serious postsurgical complications such as glaucoma, retinal detachment, vitreous hemorrhage, infection, or epithelial downgrowth into the anterior chamber, which prevent significant visual improvement. Intraocular lenses and corneal contact lenses have made adjustment following cataract operation much easier than was the rule when only thick cataract glasses were available.

CHILDHOOD CATARACT
(Figures 8–4 and 8–5)

Childhood cataracts are divided into two groups: congenital (infantile) cataracts, which are present at birth or appear shortly thereafter; and acquired cataracts, which occur later and are usually related to a specific cause. Either type may be unilateral or bilateral and partial or complete. Many congenital cataracts are of unknown cause though probably genetically determined; others are secondary to metabolic or infectious diseases or associated with a variety of syndromes. A search for a cause is appropriate, but in most cases none can be identified. Acquired cataracts arise most commonly from trauma, either blunt or penetrating. Other causes include uveitis, acquired ocular infections, diabetes, and drugs.

Clinical Findings

A. Congenital Cataract: Congenital lens opacities are common and often visually insignificant. A partial opacification or one out of the visual axis—or not dense enough to interfere significantly with light transmission—requires no treatment other than observation for progression. Dense central congenital cataracts require surgery.

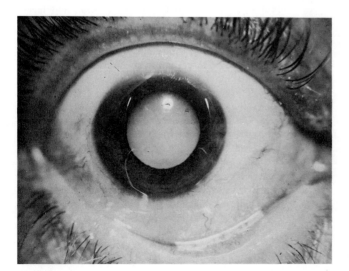

Figure 8–2. Mature senile cataract viewed through a dilated pupil. (Courtesy of A Rosenberg.)

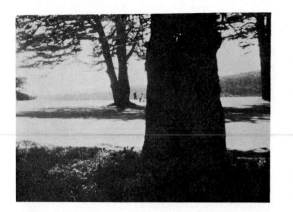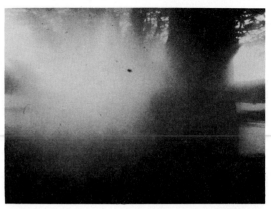

Figure 8–3. Senile cataract. In the photo at right the scene shown at left is reproduced as if seen by a person with a moderately advanced senile cataract (opacity denser centrally). (Courtesy of E Goodner.)

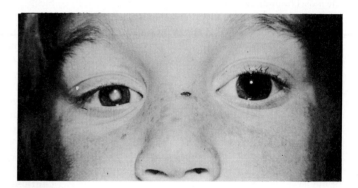

Figure 8–4. Congenital cataract.

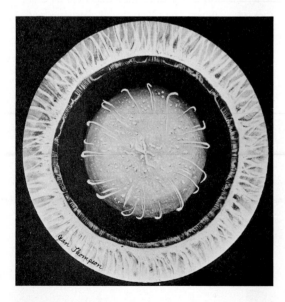

Figure 8–5. Congenital cataract, zonular type. One zone of lens involved. The cortex is relatively clear.

[Figures 8–5 to 8–10 are reproduced, with permission, from Cordes FC: *Cataract Types,* 3rd ed. American Academy of Ophthalmology and Otolaryngology, 1954.]

Congenital cataracts that cause significant visual loss must be detected early—preferably in the newborn nursery by the pediatrician or family physician. Large, dense white cataracts may present as leukocoria noticeable by the parents, but many dense cataracts cannot be seen by the parents. Unilateral infantile cataracts that are dense, central, and larger than 2 mm in diameter will cause permanent deprivation amblyopia if not treated within the first 2 months of life and thus may require surgical management on an urgent basis. Symmetric bilateral cataracts demand less urgent management, but bilateral deprivation amblyopia can result from unwarranted delay.

B. Acquired Cataract: Acquired cataracts do not require the same urgent care (aimed at preventing amblyopia) as infantile cataracts, because the children are older and the visual system more mature. Surgical assessment is based on the location, size, and density of the cataract, but a period of observation along with subjective visual acuity testing can be part of the decision process. Because unilateral cataracts in children will not produce any symptoms or signs parents would routinely notice, screening programs are important for case finding.

Treatment

Surgical treatment of infantile and early childhood cataracts involves lens extraction through a 3-mm limbal incision utilizing a mechanical irrigation-aspiration handpiece. Phacoemulsification is rarely required, because the lens nucleus is soft. In contrast to adult lens extraction, the posterior capsule and anterior vitreous are removed by most surgeons using a mechanical vitreous suction-cutting instrument. This prevents formation of secondary capsular opacification, or after-cataract. Primary removal of the posterior capsule therefore avoids the necessity for secondary surgery and enhances early optical correction.

Using today's sophisticated surgical techniques, operative and postoperative complications are similar to those reported with adult cataract procedures. With experience, the childhood cataract surgeon can expect good technical results in well over 90% of cases. Optical correction is crucial in infants and requires much time and effort by the surgeon and the parents. It can consist of spectacles in older bilaterally aphakic children, but most childhood cataract operations should be followed by contact lens correction. Epikeratophakia has shown some promise for correction of aphakia in the pediatric patient unable to tolerate contact lenses.

Prognosis

The visual prognosis for childhood cataract patients requiring surgery is not as good as that for patients with senile cataract. The associated amblyopia and occasional anomalies of the optic nerve or retina limit the degree of useful vision that can be achieved in this group of patients. The prognosis for improvement of visual acuity is worst following surgery for unilateral congenital cataracts and best for incomplete bilateral congenital cataracts that are slowly progressive.

TRAUMATIC CATARACT

Traumatic cataract (Figures 8–6 to 8–8) is most commonly due to a foreign body injury to the lens or blunt trauma to the eyeball. BB shot is a frequent cause; less frequent causes include arrows, rocks, contusions, overexposure to heat ("glassblower's cataract"), x-rays, and radioactive materials. Most traumatic cataracts are preventable. In industry, the best safety measure is a good pair of safety goggles.

The lens becomes white soon after the entry of the foreign body, since the interruption of the lens capsule allows aqueous and sometimes vitreous to penetrate into the lens structure. The patient is often an industrial worker who gives a history of striking steel upon steel. A minute fragment of a steel hammer, for example, may pass through the cornea and lens at a tremendous rate of speed and lodge in the vitreous,

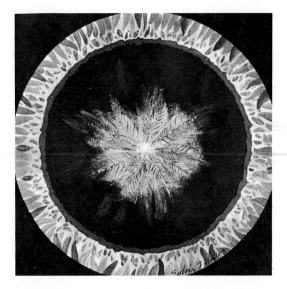

Figure 8–6. Traumatic "star-shaped" cataract in the posterior lens. This is usually due to ocular contusion and is only detectable through a well-dilated pupil.

where it can usually be seen with the ophthalmoscope.

The patient complains immediately of blurred vision. The eye becomes red, the lens opaque, and there may be an intraocular hemorrhage. If aqueous or vitreous escapes from the eye, the eye becomes extremely soft. Complications include infection, uveitis, retinal detachment, and glaucoma.

A magnetic intraocular foreign body should be removed without delay.

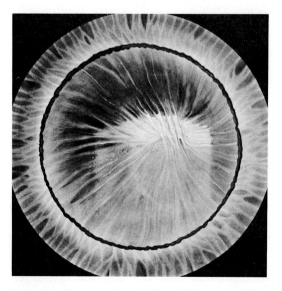

Figure 8–7. Traumatic cataract with wrinkled anterior capsule.

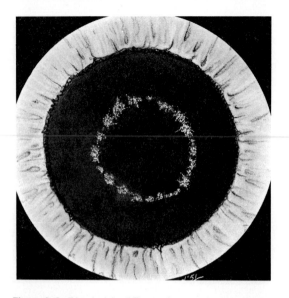

Figure 8–8. "Vossius' ring." Traumatic cataract caused by the imprint of the iris pigment on the anterior surface of the lens. The remainder of the lens is clear, and vision is not impaired.

Systemic and topical antibiotics and topical corticosteroids should be given over a period of several days to minimize the chance of infection and uveitis. Atropine sulfate, 1%, 1 drop three times daily, is recommended to keep the pupil dilated and to prevent the formation of posterior synechiae.

The cataract can be removed at the same time the foreign body is removed or after the inflammation subsides. If glaucoma occurs during the waiting period, cataract surgery should not be delayed even though inflammation is still present. Some time after cataract surgery, a thin opaque membrane may occur, in which case discission with the neodymium:YAG laser (see After-Cataract) or a knife may be necessary to improve vision. The same techniques utilized for removal of congenital cataracts are generally used for the removal of traumatic cataracts, especially in patients under 30 years of age.

CATARACT SECONDARY TO INTRAOCULAR DISEASE ("Complicated Cataract")

Cataract may develop as a direct effect of intraocular disease upon the physiology of the lens (eg, severe recurrent uveitis). The cataract usually begins in the posterior subcapsular area and eventually involves the entire lens structure. Intraocular diseases commonly associated with the development of cataracts are chronic or recurrent uveitis, glaucoma, retinitis pigmentosa, and retinal detachment.

These cataracts are usually unilateral. The visual prognosis is not as good as in ordinary senile cataract.

CATARACT ASSOCIATED WITH SYSTEMIC DISEASE

Bilateral cataracts may occur in association with the following systemic disorders: diabetes mellitus (Figure 8–9), hypoparathyroidism, myotonic dystrophy, atopic dermatitis, galactosemia, and Lowe's, Werner's, and Down's syndromes. (These entities are discussed in Chapters 15 and 18.)

TOXIC CATARACT

Toxic cataract is uncommon. Many cases appeared in the 1930s as a result of ingestion of dinitrophenol, a drug taken to suppress appetite. Corticosteroids administered over a long period of time, either systemically or in drop form, can cause lens opacities. It has been suggested that echothiophate iodide, a strong miotic used in the treatment of glaucoma, may cause cataracts.

AFTER-CATARACT (Secondary Membrane)

After-cataract (Figure 8–10) denotes opacification of the posterior capsule due to partially absorbed traumatic cataract or following extracapsular cataract extraction.

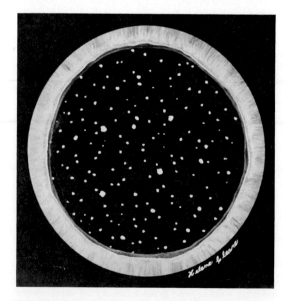

Figure 8–9. Punctate dot cataract. This type of cataract is sometimes seen as an ocular complication of diabetes mellitus. It may also be congenital.

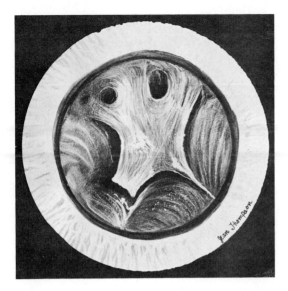

Figure 8–10. After-cataract.

Persistent subcapsular lens epithelium may attempt regeneration of lens fibers, giving the posterior capsule a "fish egg" appearance (Elschnig's pearls). The proliferating epithelium may produce multiple layers, leading to frank opacification. These cells may also undergo myofibroblastic differentiation. Their contraction produces numerous tiny wrinkles in the posterior capsule, resulting in visual distortion. All of these factors may lead to reduced visual acuity following extracapsular cataract extraction.

After-cataract is a significant problem in almost all pediatric patients unless the posterior capsule and anterior vitreous are removed at the time of surgery. Up to one-half of all adult patients develop an opaque secondary membrane after extracapsular cataract extraction. Before the neodymium:YAG laser came into use, this condition was treated by performing a small capsulotomy with a needle knife or barbed 27-gauge needle, either at the time of the original operation or as a secondary procedure.

In recent years, the neodymium:YAG laser has gained popularity as a noninvasive method for discission of the posterior capsule (see Chapter 24). Pulses of laser energy cause small "explosions" in target tissue, creating a small hole in the posterior capsule in the pupillary axis. Complications of this technique include a transient rise in intraocular pressure, damage to the intraocular lens, and rupture of the anterior hyaloid face with forward displacement of vitreous into the anterior chamber. The rise in intraocular pressure is usually detectable within 3 hours posttreatment and resolves within a few days with treatment. Rarely, the pressure may not return to normal for several weeks. Small pits or cracks may occur on the intraocular lens, but they usually have no ef-

fect on visual acuity. In the aphakic eye, rupture of the vitreous face with anterior displacement of vitreous may predispose to development of rhegmatogenous retinal detachment or cystoid macular edema. Current studies indicate that no significant damage is done to corneal endothelium with the neodymium:YAG laser.

CATARACT SURGERY

Cataract surgery has changed dramatically over the past 20 years, principally as a result of introduction of the operating microscope, better instrumentation, improved suture material, and refinement of the intraocular lens. In cataract surgery, the lens is removed from the eye (lens extraction) by an intracapsular or extracapsular procedure.

Intracapsular extraction, which is performed infrequently today, consists of removing the lens in toto, ie, within its capsule, through a 140- to 160-degree superior limbal incision. In **extracapsular extraction,** a superior limbal incision is also made; the anterior portion of the capsule is cut and removed; the nucleus is extracted; and the lens cortex is removed from the eye by irrigation with or without aspiration, leaving the posterior capsule behind (Figure 8–11).

Some patients develop secondary opacity of the posterior capsule that requires discission using the neodymium:YAG laser (see After-Cataract, above).

Phacofragmentation and **phacoemulsification** with irrigation or aspiration (or both) are extracapsular techniques that utilize ultrasonic vibrations to remove the nucleus and cortex through a small limbal incision (2–5 mm), thus facilitating postoperative wound healing. These techniques are useful in congenital, traumatic, and most senile cataracts. They are less effective with dense senile cataracts, and the advantage of a small limbal incision is somewhat negated if an intraocular lens is to be inserted, although flexible intraocular lenses that can be inserted through such small incisions are currently being used more often.

Over the past few years, extracapsular operations have replaced intracapsular procedures by a large percentage as the most common type of cataract surgery. The principal reason is that an intact posterior capsule allows the surgeon to insert a posterior chamber intraocular lens. The incidence of postoperative complications, such as retinal detachment and cystoid macular edema, is less when the posterior capsule is intact.

Intraocular Lens

Over 90% of all cataract operations in the USA—or over 1 million per year—involve intraocular lens implantation. Refinements in surgical technique and improved lens implants have played major roles in this

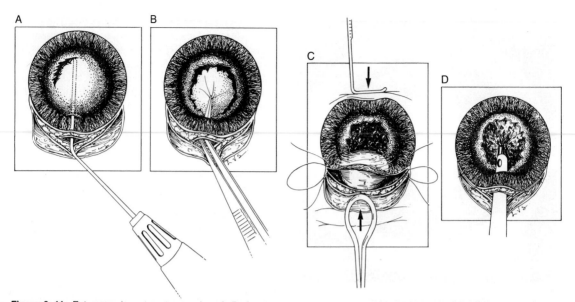

Figure 8–11. Extracapsular cataract extraction. **A:** Performing a circular anterior capsulotomy. **B:** Removal of the excised anterior capsule of the cataract. **C:** Expression of the nucleus of the cataract. **D:** Removal of the remaining cortical material by irrigation and aspiration. (Reproduced, with permission, from Way LW (editor): *Current Surgical Diagnosis & Treatment,* 9th ed. Appleton & Lange, 1991.)

advance. However, the major stimulus has been the inherent disadvantages of aphakic spectacles, including image magnification, spherical aberrations, limited visual field, and no chance of binocular vision if the other eye is phakic.

About 90% of implants are in the posterior chamber and 10% in the anterior chamber. There are many styles of lenses, but all consist of two basic parts: a spherical optic, usually made of polymethylmethacrylate; and footplates or haptics to maintain the optic in position.

Posterior chamber lenses are generally used in extracapsular procedures. This combination is preferred over anterior chamber lenses because of a lower incidence of sight-threatening complications such as hyphema, secondary glaucoma, macular edema, and pupillary block. There is also a lower incidence of corneal endothelial damage and subsequent pseudophakic bullous keratopathy in patients with posterior chamber lenses. However, newer anterior chamber lens styles have reduced the incidence of these complications. Anterior chamber lenses are used for patients undergoing intracapsular surgery or when the posterior capsule has been inadvertently ruptured in extracapsular surgery.

Contraindications to intraocular lens implantation include recurrent uveitis, proliferative diabetic retinopathy, rubeosis iridis, and neovascular glaucoma. Patients with open-angle glaucoma and ocular hypertension may receive an intraocular lens, but posterior chamber lenses are preferred. Age is considered

by many to be a relative contraindication, but younger and younger patients are receiving intraocular lenses each year.

An alternative to the intraocular lens is the contact lens, but many elderly patients are unable to tolerate them or insert them easily. In rare situations where an intraocular lens or contact lens cannot be used, aphakic eyeglasses are prescribed.

Postoperative Care (Senile Cataract)

If a small-incision technique is used, the postoperative recovery period is usually shortened. The patient may be ambulatory on the day of surgery but is advised to move cautiously and avoid straining or heavy lifting for about a month. The eye can be bandaged for a few days, but if the eye is comfortable, the bandage can be removed on the first postoperative day and the eye protected by spectacles or by a shield during the day. Protection at night by a metal shield is required for several weeks. Temporary glasses can be used a few days after surgery, but usually the patient sees well enough through the intraocular lens to wait for permanent glasses (usually provided 6–8 weeks after surgery).

In the USA, cataract surgery has been an outpatient procedure (by federal regulatory decisions) since 1984. This change in procedure emphasizes the need for home care by an experienced ophthalmic nurse in the immediate postoperative period.

DISLOCATED LENS
(Ectopia Lentis)

Partial or complete lens dislocation (Figure 8–12) may be hereditary or may result from trauma.

Hereditary Lens Dislocation

Hereditary lens dislocation is usually bilateral and may be associated with coloboma of the lens, homocystinuria, Marfan's syndrome, and Marchesani's syndrome (see Chapter 15). The vision is blurred, particularly if the lens is dislocated out of the line of vision. If dislocation is partial, the edge of the lens and the zonular fibers holding it in place can be seen in the pupil. If the lens is completely dislocated into the vitreous, it can be seen with the ophthalmoscope.

A partially dislocated lens is often complicated by cataract formation. If so, the cataract may have to be removed, but this should be delayed as long as possible because vitreous loss, predisposing to subsequent retinal detachment, is possible during surgery. If the lens is free in the vitreous, it may lead in later life to the development of glaucoma of a type that responds poorly to treatment.

If dislocation is partial and the lens is clear, the visual prognosis is good.

Traumatic Lens Dislocation

Partial or complete traumatic lens dislocation may occur following a contusion injury such as a

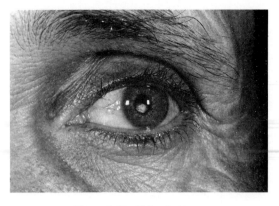

Figure 8–12. Dislocated lens.

blow to the eye with a fist. If the dislocation is partial, there may be no symptoms; but if the lens is floating in the vitreous, the patient has blurred vision and usually a red eye. **Iridodonesis,** a quivering of the iris when the patient moves the eye, is a common sign of lens dislocation and is due to the lack of lens support. This is present both in partially and completely dislocated lenses but is more marked in the latter.

Iritis, uveitis, and glaucoma are common complications of dislocated lens, particularly if dislocation is complete.

If there are no complications, dislocated lenses are best left untreated. If uveitis or uncontrollable glaucoma occurs, lens extraction must be done despite the poor results possible from this operation.

REFERENCES

Adamsons I et al: Prevalence of lens opacities in surgical and general populations. Arch Ophthalmol 1991;109:993.

Andley U: Photooxidative stress. In: *Principles and Practice of Ophthalmology: Clinical Practice,* vol 1. Albert DM, Jakobiec FA (editors). Saunders, 1994.

Apple DJ et al: Posterior capsule opacification. Surv Ophthalmol 1992;37:73.

Arkin M, Axar D, Fraioli A: Infantile cataracts. Int Ophthalmol Clin 1992;32:107.

Bourne WM, Nelson LR, Hodge DO: Continued endothelial cell loss ten years after lens implantation. Ophthalmology 1994;101:1014.

Canner JK, Javitt JC, McBean AM: National Outcomes of Cataract Extraction: III. Corneal edema and transplant following inpatient surgery. Arch Ophthalmol 1992; 110:1137.

Cataract Management Guideline Panel: *Cataract in Adults: Management of Functional Impairment.* Clinical Practice Guideline No. 4. U.S. Department of Health and Human Services, Public Health Service, Agency for Health Care Policy and Research. AHCPR Pub. No. 93-0542, February 1993.

Christen WG et al: A prospective study of cigarette smoking and risk of cataract in men. JAMA 1992;268:989.

Dutton JJ et al: Visual rehabilitation of aphakic children. Surv Ophthalmol 1990;34:365.

Hakin KN et al: Management of the subluxed crystalline lens. Ophthalmology 1992;99:542.

Harding JJ: Pharmacological treatment strategies in age-related cataracts. Drugs Aging 1992;2:287.

Hardten DR, Lindstrom RL: Complications of cataract surgery. Int Ophthalmol Clin 1992;32:131.

Holland GN et al: Results of inpatient and outpatient cataract surgery: A historical cohort comparison. Ophthalmology 1992;99:845.

Javitt JC et al: National Outcomes of Cataract Extraction: Increased risk of retinal complications associated with Nd:YAG laser capsulotomy. Ophthalmology 1992; 99:1487.

Javitt JC et al: National Outcomes of Cataract Extraction:

Retinal detachment and endophthalmitis after outpatient cataract surgery. Ophthalmology 1994;101:100.

Leske MC, Chylack LT, Suh-Yuh MA: The Lens Opacities Case-Control Study: Risk factors for cataract. Arch Ophthalmol 1991;109:244.

Mares-Perlman JA et al: Relation between lens opacities and vitamin and mineral supplement use. Ophthalmology 1994;101:315.

Plager DA et al: Surgical treatment of subluxated lenses in children. Ophthalmology 1992;99:1018.

Powe NR et al: Synthesis of the literature on visual acuity and complications following cataract extraction with intraocular lens implantation. Arch Ophthalmol 1994;112:239.

Schein OD et al: Variation in cataract surgery practice and clinical outcomes. Ophthalmology 1994;102:1142.

West SK: Who develops cataracts? (Editorial.) Arch Ophthalmol 1991;109:196.

Wright KW, Christensen LE, Noguchi BA: Results of late surgery for presumed congenital cataracts. Am J Ophthalmol 1992;114:409.

Vitreous

Conor O'Malley, MD

EXAMINATION OF THE VITREOUS

Slitlamp Examination

Normal vitreous is not visible by either direct or indirect ophthalmoscopy. The numerous ophthalmoscopically visible features are anomalies attributable either to structural changes, such as the floaters of syneresis and the ring-like form associated with posterior vitreous detachment (Figure 9–1), or to invasive elements, such as blood, white blood cell masses, or fibrovascular proliferations from adjacent tissues. Normal vitreous in situ and many important anomalies (eg, the retraction, condensation, and shrinkage of vitreous characteristic of diabetes or injury) can be viewed only with a slitlamp. The slitlamp (biomicroscope) is a microscope with a specialized illuminating system that make transparent and near-transparent ocular fluids and tissues visible. Although slitlamp examination of the vitreous is quite easy to learn and plays an important role in the management of vitreous disease, too few ophthalmologists make optimal use of this instrument.

Contact Lenses as Aid in Vitreous Examination

The anterior central vitreous is the only part of the inner eye (behind the lens) that can be seen with the slitlamp alone. In order to view other areas, special contact lenses must be placed in the patient's eye (1) to modify the light-focusing power of the aqueous lens and the lens lens and (2) to expand the limited range through which the illumination beam of the slitlamp can be angulated with respect to the visual axis of the eyeball.

A relatively thin contact lens with a flat front surface will neutralize the light-bending property of the eye, so that tissues *on and near the visual axis of the eye*—the optic disk, the posterior retina and choroid, and the axial vitreous—can be illuminated in three-dimensional detail. Much thicker contact lenses with built-in mirrors and a flat front surface can be used to displace the illumination and viewing pathways of the slitlamp with respect to the visual axis of the eyeball, so that much of the nonaxial retina and vitreous can be seen.

These special contact lenses are also used in therapeutic procedures. Fundus contact lenses with built-in mirrors are widely used in laser surgery for panretinal photocoagulation of the peripheral retina. This prevents vitreous hemorrhage that may result from the retinal neovascularizations of diabetic retinopathy, retinal vein occlusions, and (more rarely) sickle cell anemia. The thinner contact lenses are sometimes used in ablation of macular lesions associated with age-related macular degeneration and histoplasmosis.

Use of special contact lenses, whether for diagnostic or therapeutic procedures, requires maximum dilation of the pupil with a combination of mydriatic and cycloplegic solutions; use of a topical anesthetic to make the patient more comfortable; and use of a clear viscous solution of methylcellulose to prevent air from entering the lens-cornea interface.

B-Scan Ultrasonography

B-scan ultrasonography is an important diagnostic and prognostic tool used in many posterior segment problems associated with gross vitreous opacification (Figure 9–2). Where light-dependent ophthalmoscopes and slitlamps are of limited value, skillful use of B-scan ultrasonography can provide much information about the vitreous and adjacent structures. For example, it is possible to identify and locate vitreous membranes (Figure 9–3), vitreoretinal relationships and retinal de-

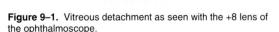

Figure 9–1. Vitreous detachment as seen with the +8 lens of the ophthalmoscope.

175

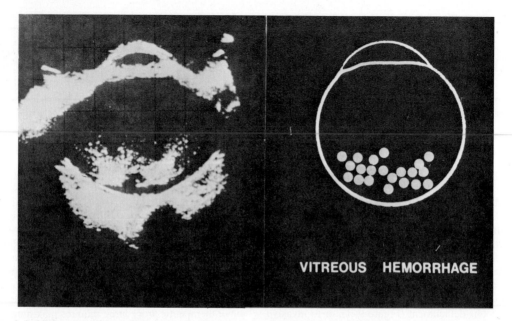

Figure 9–2. Vitreous hemorrhage limited to posterior vitreous region in aphakic eye. (Reproduced, with permission, from Coleman DJ: Ultrasound in vitreous surgery. Trans Am Acad Ophthalmol Otolaryngol 1972;76:469.)

tachments greater than 1 mm in depth (Figures 9–3 to 9–5), scleral ruptures, and intraocular foreign bodies (even nonlucent plastic and glass).

DISORDERS OF THE VITREOUS

"FLASHING LIGHTS"

"Flashing lights" are a common symptom of an abnormal relationship between the retina and the vitreous. The patient is aware of a localized "light," "glow," "streak of light," or "flashing" (as of a neon tube) in the field of vision in the absence of a corresponding light source in the environment. The patient can usually point to the area of the disturbance and often describes an arc-shaped flicker in the periphery of one or two quadrants. The light seldom persists for more than a fraction of a second. It frequently recurs at short intervals for a few minutes and then disappears for hours, days, or even weeks. It is most readily identified on moving the eye and when illumination is dim or absent. Bilateral episodes may occur simultaneously but more commonly are separated by an interval of days to many years.

The light represents a cerebral awareness of the initial physical traction on and excitation of the sensory retina by abnormal vitreous. It is most commonly associated with recent collapse and detachment of the vitreous due to syneresis with focal vitreous traction on vitreoretinal lesions such as lattice degeneration, meridional folds, congenital rosettes, and other visually subclinical vitreoretinal adhesions. A careful history will readily distinguish the light from the scintillating scotoma of migraine, which is characterized by a symmetric quivering scotoma usually in both eyes, of predictable configuration and progression, accompanied by variable nausea or headache.

The vitreoretinal traction may require no treatment. However, as it can induce retinal tears, retinal detachment (Figure 9–6), or vitreous hemorrhage, every new case requires a survey of the vitreoretinal relationship, especially in the periphery.

VITREOUS FLOATERS

Vitreous floaters are by far the most common symptom of abnormal vitreous. A given floater represents the patient's awareness of the shadow of a mobile vitreous opacity cast upon the retina. The mind projects the corresponding dark form onto the appropriate area of the visual field.

The term "vitreous floaters" denotes a common, po-

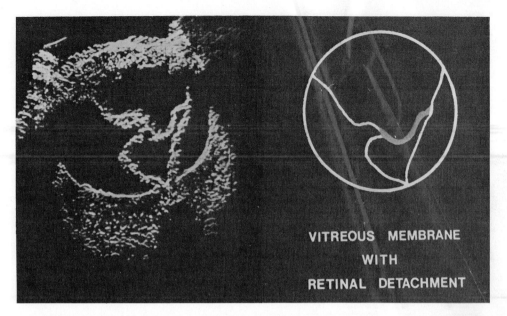

Figure 9–3. Total retinal detachment viewed horizontally below iris plane. A vitreous membrane connecting 2 leaves of retina is clearly demonstrated. (Reproduced, with permission, from Coleman DJ: Ultrasound in vitreous surgery. Trans Am Acad Ophthalmol Otolaryngol 1972;76:469.)

tentially serious symptom that was formerly called *muscae volitantes*—Latin for flies that flit, flutter, or fly to and fro.

The onset may be either insidious or acute and unilateral or bilateral. The patient is aware of one or more (or even many) fine, dark forms in the field of vision. Their configuration is usually so pronounced that the patient spontaneously classifies them as "spots," "soot," "particles," "spiders," "cobwebs," "threads," "worms," "dark streaks," "a ring," etc. Combinations are often reported. The objects continue to migrate after the eye comes to rest—hence the name "floaters."

Central, relatively immobile floaters are visually annoying and may even be disabling. Peripheral ones are

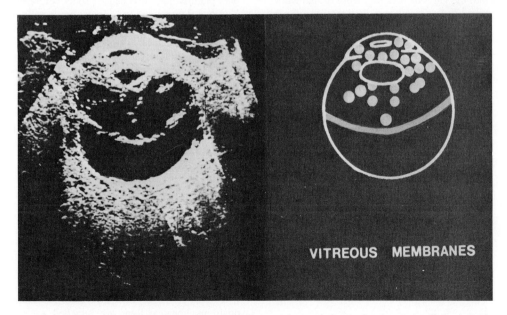

Figure 9–4. Vitreous membrane extending along posterior limiting membrane of vitreous from ora to ora. Retina is in place. (Reproduced, with permission, from Coleman DJ: Ultrasound in vitreous surgery. Trans Am Acad Ophthalmol Otolaryngol 1972;76:469.)

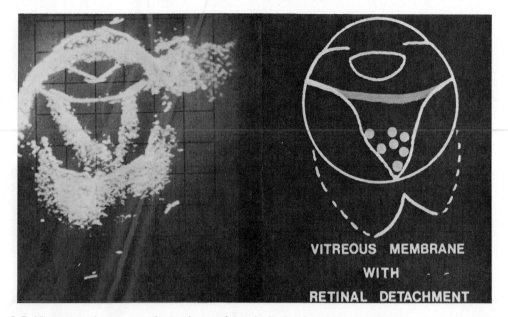

Figure 9–5. Vitreous membrane connecting two leaves of detached retina. Lens is normal. (Reproduced, with permission, from Coleman DJ: Ultrasound in vitreous surgery. Trans Am Acad Ophthalmol Otolaryngol 1972;76:469.)

readily overlooked, as they are intermittent and require large eye motion or special positions merely to be seen. Unlike "flashing lights," they are most readily seen against bright lights or a uniform light background. They are extremely common in myopes and people with syneresis.

Floaters are commonly caused by small hemorrhages into the vitreous resulting from retinal tears or hemorrhagic diseases such as diabetic retinopathy, hy-

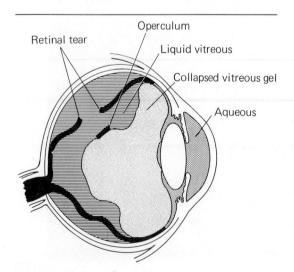

Figure 9–6. Schematic representation of vitreous collapse causing the retina to tear and detach.

pertension, leukemia, old retinal branch vein occlusions, Eales' disease, Coats' disease, and subacute infective endocarditis. Individual red cells are seen as small round black spots. Recent hemorrhages are often seen as black streaks or cobwebs that later break up into small round spots.

White cell invasion of the vitreous gel associated with pars planitis may also cause "spots before the eyes." Vitreous floaters due to pigment are usually a consequence of long-standing tear-induced detachment of the retina that has not yet reached the macula.

Vitreous floaters should never be dismissed as harmless or imaginary. A careful survey of the vitreous and retina is always indicated in order to identify the nature and origin of floaters and to decide on management. Failure to make such an examination not infrequently leads to missed diagnosis. In the absence of a serious causative pathologic process, the patient may be reassured that the condition is harmless.

ASTEROID HYALOSIS

Asteroid hyalosis is an uncommon condition that occurs in otherwise healthy eyes in elderly people. Unilateral cases are three times as common as bilateral cases. Hundreds of small yellow spheres consisting of calcium soaps are seen in the vitreous. These move when the eyes move but always return to their original positions because they are attached to interlacing fibers. There are no related ocular or systemic diseases. The opacities have little or no effect upon vision but reflect the examiner's light very strongly. If there are enough asteroid bodies, the fundus is not viewable by ophthalmoscopy.

ACUTE VITREOUS COLLAPSE

The vitreous cavity is bounded by the retina, optic disk, pars plana, zonule, and crystalline lens. Normal vitreous fills this cavity and remains firmly attached to the retina and pars plana near the ora serrata.

All types of gels, whether vitreous or gelatin, become increasingly susceptible with the passage of time to a degenerative process known as **syneresis,** involving the drawing together of particles of the dispersed medium, separation of the medium, and shrinkage of the gel. Syneresis affects at least 65% of persons over 60 years of age. Myopes are especially susceptible, even in childhood.

With age, the center of the vitreous may undergo syneresis and become filled with liquid breakdown products of the degenerated gel (Figure 9–7). The liquid contents of the cavity can migrate into the preretinal space. The more solid, heavier vitreous gel collapses downward and forward to create a posterior vitreous detachment (Figure 9–8). The dynamic forces that accompany this collapse can rupture the last vestiges of the adhesions that once connected the vitreous to the disk, blood vessels, and sensory retina in childhood.

The patient and examiner can often see portions of the adhesions that remain attached to the collapsed vitreous as opacities. If they arise from the disk margin, the patient and examiner may note a ring-shaped opacity on the back of the vitreous.

Since the front of the vitreous is attached to the globe and the back of the vitreous is collapsed in on itself, abrupt motions of the eye transmit a whip-like force to the back of the vitreous. The vitreous tends to fill out toward its normal configuration; liquid vitreous is drawn into the syneretic cavity, and the posterior separation tends to disappear (Figure 9–9).

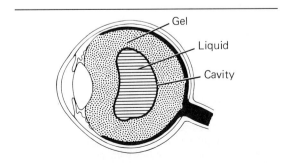

Figure 9–7. Large intravitreal cavity filled with liquid breakdown products of syneresis.

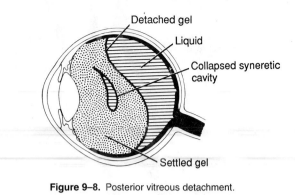

Figure 9–8. Posterior vitreous detachment.

The whip-like motions of the vitreous can give rise to **photopsia** (an appearance of sparks or flashes) by causing stimulation of the vitreoretinal juncture and may cause a characteristic floating motion of posterior vitreous opacities, or floaters. The floaters move with the eye and float to a resting position after the eye comes to rest.

Since acute vitreous collapse can also cause asymptomatic retinal tears or detachment, *it should be assumed that patients with new floaters or photopsia have retinal tears or detachment until proved otherwise by thorough examination of the peripheral retina with an indirect ophthalmoscope.*

RETINAL TEARS
(See also Chapter 10.)

While retinal tears can be caused by trauma, vitreous shrinkage, or proliferative vitreoretinopathy, most are caused by acute vitreous collapse. Tears following acute vitreous collapse are the result of a dynamic interaction between a focal vitreoretinal adhesion, collapsed mobile vitreous, and normal eye movement (Figure 9–10).

Since the gel and liquid components of the collapsed vitreous are structurally relatively independent of the retina, they do not move synchronously with the retina. When the eye (and hence the retina) moves, the gel and liquid tend to lag behind the retina, and when the eye stops moving, the gel and liquid tend to continue in motion. The vitreous gel and liquid are said to exhibit inertial lag with respect to the retina. Inertial lag of the gel can cause the vitreous to tear the friable sensory retina at the point where they adhere to each other (Figure 9–11). With the ophthalmoscope, the torn retina is seen to be pulled inward as a flap or a detached operculum (Figure 9–12). If retinal vessels are broken, they bleed briefly. A variable amount of blood accumulates in the vitreous cavity.

Some patients are not aware of the onset of retinal tears but often complain of photopsia and floaters.

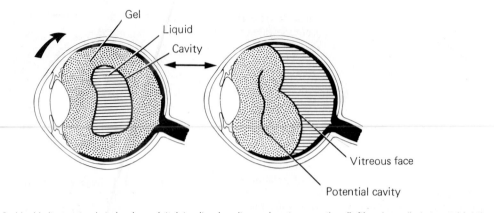

Figure 9–9. Liquid vitreous tends to be drawn into intravitreal cavity on abrupt eye motion *(left)* and expelled at rest *(right)*.

Some present with gross vitreous hemorrhage. Many retinal tears never lead to retinal detachment, but recent symptomatic tears, especially those with symptomatic vitreous hemorrhage, have a strong tendency to cause retinal detachment. Patients with symptoms of acute vitreous collapse or vitreous hemorrhage should therefore undergo careful examination of the retina from the optic disk to the ora serrata to rule out one or more tears. Management of tears by prophylactic laser therapy or cryopexy is relatively simple and very effective compared to the performance of silicone buckling once retinal detachment has occurred.

Retinal tears are usually located anterior to the equator and are more often in the upper quadrants (Figure 9–12 left).

VITREOUS HEMORRHAGE

Vitreous hemorrhage can occur whenever the sensory retina is torn. Retinitis proliferans, central vein occlusion, branch vein occlusion, and hypertension are also frequent causes of vitreous hemorrhage. Acute collapse of the vitreous with posterior vitreous detachment will sometimes cause bleeding without tear formation. The patient often complains of floaters that

suggest red blood cells, a sudden shower of small black dots, or even tiny ring-like forms with clear centers. Visual loss ranges from imperceptible to gross.

The appearance of the retina and its visibility vary with the cause and amount of bleeding in the vitreous cavity (see Chapter 10). Fresh blood is red and tends to be located behind the vitreous gel or within a syneretic cavity (Figure 9–13). Within weeks to months, the blood tends to break down, becomes a pale color, and migrates into the gel (Figure 9–14).

Vitrectomy may be indicated to facilitate surgical reattachment of the retina. For example, vitreous hemorrhage following recent retinal detachment (diagnosed possibly by ultrasonography) may be extensive enough to hamper retinal surgery, which may need to be performed promptly to prevent irreversible macular atrophy.

Vitrectomy is not indicated for 3–6 months if treatment of the underlying cause can wait, as the vitreous may clear adequately without surgery.

RETINAL DETACHMENT
(See also Chapter 11.)

In the normal eye, the intact sensory retina is kept opposed to the pigment epithelium by the suction the latter exerts on the watertight space between them. If a retinal tear is present, rapid eye motions and sudden rotation of the globe can readily generate enough inertial force to initiate retinal detachment (Figure 9–15). The space between the two layers of the retina fills with liquid vitreous, and eddy currents develop in this space, further accelerating the detachment process (Figure 9–16). Almost invariably, detachment continues until it is total.

Surgery with cryopexy and silicone buckling is required (1) to close the hole in the retina, reestablishing a watertight intraretinal space; (2) to restrict the inertial lag of the liquid and gel with respect to the retina; and (3) to approximate and seal together the two layers of the retina around the tear to counter the effects of eddy currents in the vitreous cavity. (See also Chapter 11.)

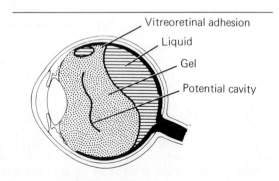

Figure 9–10. Local vitreoretinal adhesion.

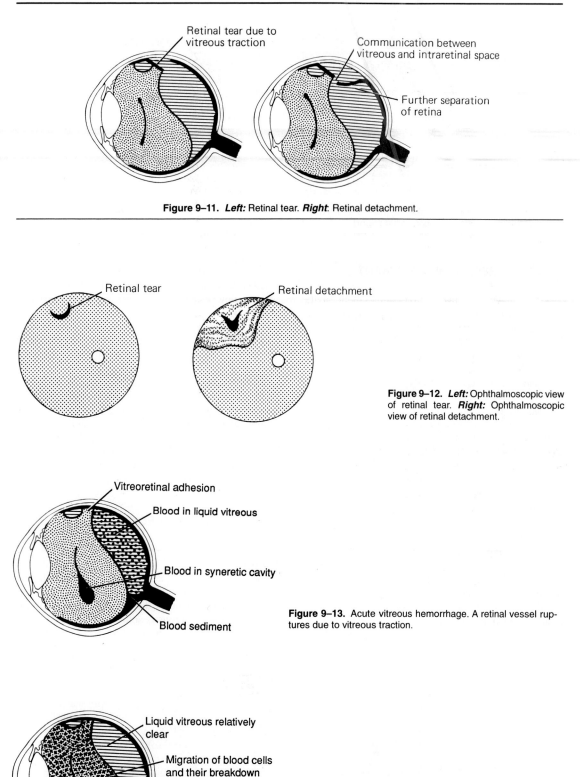

Figure 9–11. *Left:* Retinal tear. *Right:* Retinal detachment.

Figure 9–12. *Left:* Ophthalmoscopic view of retinal tear. *Right:* Ophthalmoscopic view of retinal detachment.

Figure 9–13. Acute vitreous hemorrhage. A retinal vessel ruptures due to vitreous traction.

Figure 9–14. Chronic vitreous hemorrhage.

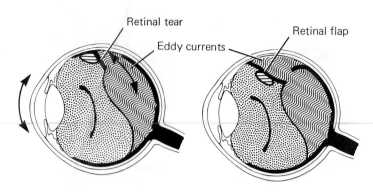

Figure 9–15. Abrupt rotation of globe generates eddy currents in liquid vitreous, a result of inertial lag *(left)*, that tends to lift the retinal flap and surrounding sensory retina *(right)*.

TRACTION RETINAL DETACHMENT

Traction retinal detachment is detachment of the sensory retina without retinal tears. The most common cause is long-standing diabetes. The detachment is typically found posterior to the equator and is due to vitreous traction on an area of retinitis proliferans (Figure 9–17).

Reattachment by vitrectomy is indicated only if there is clear-cut recent extension of the detachment into the macula.

PROLIFERATIVE VITREORETINOPATHY

A number of abnormal conditions of the vitreous and retina are characterized by contractile membranes arising metaplastically from abnormally located retinal pigment epithelial cells and retinal glial cells. The membranes can occur on either the inner or outer surface of the sensory retina or on several vitreous surfaces. The membranes may be weak and subtle or strong, easily seen, and capable of causing great distortion of the host tissues.

The causal retinal pigment epithelial cells and retinal glial cells are pluripotential cells, with great metaplastic potential. They may proliferate at remote sites and take on the characteristics of myofibroblasts. These myofibroblast-like cells readily form contractile membranes that may deform the inner and outer surfaces of the retina and the posterior vitreous surfaces (Figure 9–18).

The basic process, or its outcome, is known as massive vitreous retraction, preretinal traction, preretinal vitreous membrane, subretinal fibrosis, macular pucker, or surface wrinkling retinopathy.

Proliferative vitreoretinopathy requires no treatment unless it causes surface wrinkling retinopathy of the macula (also known as macular pucker) or unduly complicates therapy for retinal detachment. While research holds some promise for an antiproliferative pharmaceutical agent, current treatment involves a special surgical procedure that employs distention, severing, or removal of vitreous tissue (see below).

INJURY TO THE VITREOUS

Contusion

Because the vitreous is inelastic compared with the adjacent tissues, contusions that abruptly though briefly alter the shape of the eye are apt to cause injuries where the vitreous is adherent.

Disinsertion of the vitreous base is not uncommon.

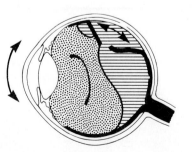

Figure 9–16. Enlargement of retinal detachment due to inertial lag of liquid vitreous within the retina.

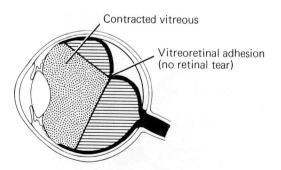

Figure 9–17. Traction detachment of retina.

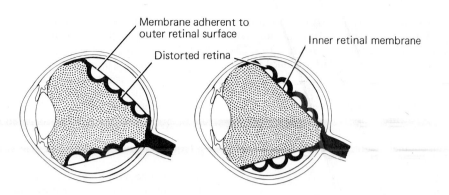

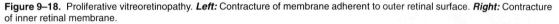

Figure 9–18. Proliferative vitreoretinopathy. *Left:* Contracture of membrane adherent to outer retinal surface. *Right:* Contracture of inner retinal membrane.

It is frequently associated with tearing of the pars plana or retina, vitreous hemorrhage, or detachment of the retina—as long as 20 years later.

Less commonly, "flashing lights," vitreous floaters, and even vitreous hemorrhage or detachment of the retina may result from stress behind the vitreous base. The affected sites may be previously subclinical anomalous vitreoretinal adhesions (eg, lattice degeneration) or areas of frank vitreoretinal disease such as diabetic retinopathy.

Rupture of the Globe

Rupture of the globe is always a serious injury that may result in early or late blindness or even loss of the eyeball. Prolapse of the vitreous through the wound is a severe complication often associated with acute secondary tearing or detachment of the retina. A seemingly uncomplicated prolapse may be followed by late retinal detachment with or without tears due to fibrous ingrowth from the orbit and subsequent contraction. The latter may be visible as membranes or bands in the vitreous. Various forms of vitreous surgery are used to prevent or treat such complications.

Penetration of the Globe

An almost endless variety of material may accidentally penetrate the globe. Common examples are needles, BB shot, and small particles of metal, stone, or plastic that fly into the eye at high velocity.

Prolapse of the vitreous may occur at the site of entry or exit or both. The part traversed by the foreign body is permanently damaged and is often marked by visible condensation, shrinkage, or fibrous elements. Vitreous surgery is increasingly used to prevent or treat complications such as retinal detachment with or without tears.

Vitreous Loss

Vitreous loss is an iatrogenic complication. The vitreous gel prolapses through a surgical wound, usually at (but not limited to) the corneal limbus during the course of operating on the lens, iris, or cornea.

Fibrous tissue invasion and contraction are frequent sequels that are prone to cause traction complications involving the retina. Corneal edema and iris displacement (eg, "updrawn pupil") may also occur. An acute prolapse can be effectively excised. An old prolapse may require surgery for release of vitreous traction.

VITREOUS INFLAMMATION

Vitreous inflammation includes a wide spectrum of disorders ranging from a few scattered white cells to abscess formation. Most commonly, one or more focal inflammatory lesions in the choroid or retina—as in chorioretinitis or retinitis—are responsible for a secondary cellular invasion of the liquid vitreous or relatively resistant gel. There may be a mild localized blurring of the fundus landmarks and lesions that provoke little or no visual complaint except for a possible vitreous floater effect. With greater infiltration, vision is decreased and the fundus is invisible or almost so. The condition may be so marked that the red reflection is lost and the vitreous appears opaque and white. Since these conditions spare the anterior segment, there is no pain and the external eye appears normal. The prognosis and treatment depend upon the underlying condition. The vitreous usually clears when the primary defect is quiescent. Vitreous surgery is used to remove gross residual opacities that show no sign of clearing spontaneously.

Vitreous Abscess (Endophthalmitis)*

Vitreous abscess may occur following penetrating ocular trauma, including ocular surgery. The vitreous is an excellent culture medium; following bacterial invasion, it undergoes liquefaction and abscess formation.

---

*If all three coats of the eye as well as the vitreous are involved by an inflammatory process, the condition is known as panophthalmitis. The line of demarcation between endophthalmitis and panophthalmitis is usually obscure.

The diagnosis of vitreous abscess is confirmed by aspirating 0.5–1 mL of vitreous under local anesthesia through a pars plana sclerotomy using a 20- to 23-gauge needle. The aspirate should be examined microscopically.

Once the organism is identified, immediate medical treatment is indicated (see Table 3–1).

In some cases, vitrectomy is indicated to drain the abscess and allow better visualization of the fundus.

Even with optimal treatment, vitreous abscess carries a grave prognosis.

VITREOUS SURGERY

Vitreous surgery is useful for a broad spectrum of intraocular disorders. Airtight and watertight incisions measuring 1–4 mm are made in the pars plana and sclera (Figure 9–19). One incision is used for an indwelling gravity-fed infusion terminal, which maintains the desired tension and configuration of the globe. Surgical gases and medications are also instilled through this terminal. Another incision is used for a hand-held endoilluminator, which illuminates the contents and all of the walls of the vitreous cavity. The illuminated structures are viewed microscopically through the pupil with the aid of a corneal contact lens that neutralizes the light-focusing power of the eye. The remaining incision is used to allow for instrumentation (severing or removal of tissue), diathermy, and laser photocoagulation (Figure 9–19).

Vitreous surgery provides access to virtually all of the intraocular tissues between the endothelium of the cornea and the retinal pigment epithelium. Surgery is most commonly done (1) to remove vitreous opacified by blood (Figure 9–20 top), (2) to remove shrunken vitreous causing traction retinal detachment (Figure 9–20 middle), (3) to treat vitreous contracture complicating retinal detachment (Figure 9–20 bottom) (see preretinal membranes), (4) to remove metaplastic membranes that deform or detach the sensory retina (Figures 9–18 and 9–19), (5) to create an optical opening in recalcitrant pupillary membranes, and (6) to remove infected vitreous in endophthalmitis (so as to dilute the organismal toxins and reduce the population of causal organisms and to instill therapeutic solutions). Vitreous surgery is frequently combined with scleral buckling for retinal detachment.

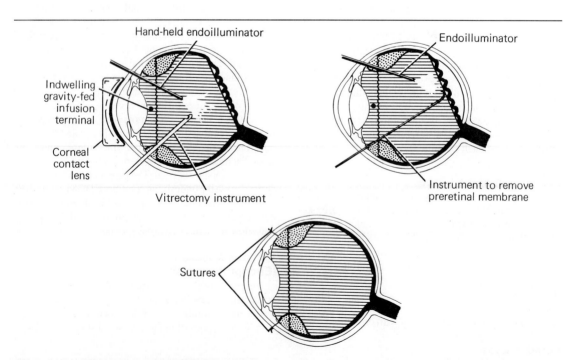

Figure 9–19. Vitreous surgery. **Top left:** Position of corneal contact lens and intraocular devices. **Top right:** Removal of preretinal membrane. **Bottom:** Placement of sutures at completion of procedure.

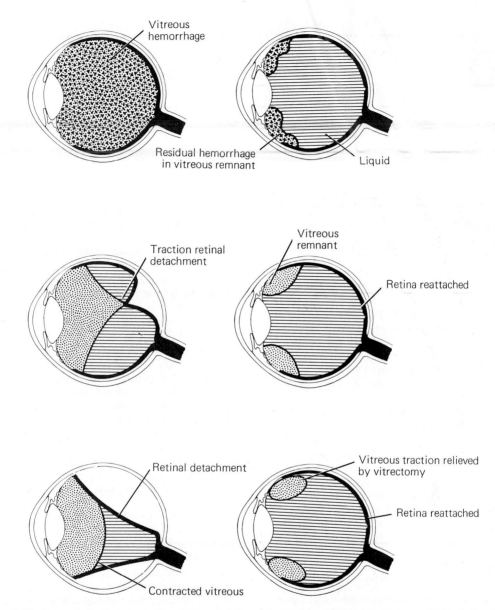

Figure 9–20. Scope of vitreous surgery. ***Top:*** Removal of vitreous hemorrhage. Residual hemorrhage will clear in time from vitreous remnants. ***Middle:*** Reattachment of traction retinal detachment following vitrectomy. ***Bottom:*** Vitreous contracture complicating retinal detachment. Removal of vitreous and repair of retinal detachment.

REFERENCES

Bacon AS et al: Infective endophthalmitis following vitreoretinal surgery. Eye 1993;7:529.

Lewis H, Ryan SJ (editors): *Medical and Surgical Retina: Advances, Controversies and Management.* Mosby, 1994.

McCormack P et al: Is surgery for proliferative vitreoretinopathy justifiable? Eye 1994;8:75.

O'Malley C et al: Closed eye intraocular microsurgery. In: *Highlights of Ophthalmology,* vol 1. Boyd B (editor). Highlights of Ophthalmology Press, 1981.

Snead MP et al: Vitreous detachment and the posterior hyaloid membrane: A clinicopathological study. Eye 1994;8:204.

Thompson JT et al: Infectious endophthalmitis after penetrating injuries with retained intraocular foreign bodies. Ophthalmology 1993;100:1468.

10

Retina & Intraocular Tumors

Robert A. Hardy, MD

I. RETINA

The human retina is a highly organized structure, consisting of alternate layers of cell bodies and synaptic processes. Despite its compact size and apparent simplicity when compared with nervous structures such as the cerebral cortex, the retina has a remarkably sophisticated level of processing power. Visual processing of the retina is elaborated upon by the brain, and the perception of color, contrast, depth, and form occurs in the cortex.

The anatomy of the retina is presented in Chapter 1. Figure 1–17 shows the major cell types and identifies the layers of this tissue. Division of the retina into layers composed of groups of similar cells permits the clinician to localize a function or functional disturbance to a single layer or group of cells. Processing of retinal information proceeds from the photoreceptor layer through the ganglion cell axon to the optic nerve and brain.

PHYSIOLOGY

The retina is the most complex of the ocular tissues. In order to see, the eye must perform as an optical instrument, as a complex receptor, and as an effective transducer. Rod and cone cells in the photoreceptor layer are capable of transforming light stimulus into a nerve impulse that is conducted by the nerve fiber layer of the retina through the optic nerve and ultimately to the occipital visual cortex. The macula is responsible for the best visual acuity and for color vision, and most of its photoreceptor cells are cones. In the central fovea, there is a nearly 1:1 relationship between the cone photoreceptor, its ganglion cell, and the emerging nerve fiber, and this ensures the most acute vision. In the peripheral retina, many photoreceptors are coupled to the same ganglion cell, and a more complex system of relays is necessary. The result of such an arrangement is that the macula is used primarily for central and color vision (photopic vision) while the re-

maining retina, which is populated mostly by rod photoreceptors, is utilized primarily for peripheral and night (scotopic) vision.

The rod and cone photoreceptors are located in the avascular outermost layer of the sensory retina and are the site of the chemical reaction initiating the visual process. Each rod photoreceptor cell contains rhodopsin, which is a photosensitive visual pigment formed when opsin protein molecules combine with 11-*cis* retinal. As a photon of light is absorbed by rhodopsin, 11-*cis* retinal is immediately isomerized to its all-*trans* form. Rhodopsin is a membrane-bound glycolipid that is partially embedded in the double membrane disks of the photoreceptor outer segment. Peak light absorption by rhodopsin occurs at approximately 500 nm, which is the blue-green region of the light spectrum. Spectral sensitivity studies of cone photopigments have shown peak wavelength absorption at 430, 540, and 575 nm for blue-, green-, and red-sensitive cones, respectively. The cone photopigments are composed of 11-*cis*retinal bound to a variety of opsin proteins.

Scotopic vision is mediated entirely by the rod photoreceptors. With this dark-adapted form of vision, varying shades of gray are seen, but colors cannot be distinguished. As the retina becomes fully light-adapted, the spectral sensitivity of the retina shifts from a rhodopsin-dominated peak of 500 nm to approximately 560 nm, and color sensation becomes evident. An object takes on color when it contains photopigments that absorb specific wavelengths and selectively reflect or transmit certain wavelengths of light within the visible spectrum (400–700 nm). Daylight vision is mediated primarily by cone photoreceptors, twilight by a combination of cones and rods, and night vision by the rod photoreceptors.

EXAMINATION

The examination of the retina is described in Chapter 2 and depicted in Figures 2–13 to 2–19. The retina can be examined with a direct or indirect ophthalmoscope or with a slitlamp (biomicroscope) and contact or handheld biconvex lens. With these instruments, the skilled observer is clinically able to dissect the layers of the retina in order to determine the type, level, and extent of retinal disease. Fundus photography and fluorescein angiography (Figures 2–28 to 2–31) are useful adjuncts to the clinical examination; photography allows pictorial documentation for future comparison, and angiography provides the vascular detail needed for laser treatment of retinal diseases.

The clinical application of visual electrophysiologic and psychophysical tests is described in Chapter 2. Such tests may be helpful in establishing the diagnosis of certain disease entities.

DISEASES OF THE MACULA

AGE-RELATED MACULAR DEGENERATION

Age-related macular degeneration is the leading cause of permanent blindness in the elderly. The exact cause is unknown, but the incidence increases with each decade over age 50. Other associations besides age include race (usually Caucasian), sex (slight female predominance), family history, and a history of cigarette smoking. The disease includes a broad spectrum of clinical and pathologic findings that can be classified into two groups: nonexudative ("dry") and exudative ("wet"). Although both types are progressive and usually bilateral, they differ in their manifestations, prognosis, and management. The more severe exudative form accounts for approximately 90% of all cases of legal blindness due to age-related macular degeneration.

1. NONEXUDATIVE MACULAR DEGENERATION

Nonexudative age-related macular degeneration is characterized by variable degrees of atrophy and degeneration of the outer retina, retinal pigment epithelium, Bruch's membrane and choriocapillaris. Of the ophthalmoscopically visible changes in the retinal pigment epithelium and Bruch's membrane, drusen the most typical (Figure 10–1). **Drusen** are discrete, round, yellow-white deposits of variable size beneath the pigment epithelium and are scattered throughout the macula and posterior pole. With time, they may enlarge, coalesce, calcify, and increase in number. Histopathologically, most drusen consist of focal collections of eosinophilic material lying between the pigment epithelium and Bruch's membrane; they therefore represent focal detachment of the pigment epithelium. In addition to drusen, clumps of pigment irregularly dispersed within depigmented areas of at-

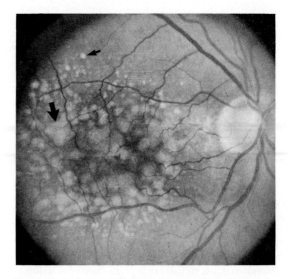

Figure 10–1. Age-related macular degeneration with discrete (small arrow) and large confluent (large arrow) macular drusen.

rophy may progressively appear throughout the macula. The level of associated visual impairment is variable and may be minimal. Fluorescein angiography demonstrates irregular patterns of retinal pigment epithelial hyperplasia and atrophy. Electrophysiologic testing in most patients is normal.

There is no generally accepted treatment or means of prevention of this type of macular degeneration. The concept that antioxidants decrease the risk of vision loss is being tested in a randomized clinical trial. Most patients with macular drusen never experience significant loss of central vision; the atrophic changes may stabilize or progress slowly. However, the exudative stage may develop suddenly at any time, and in addition to regular ophthalmic examinations, patients are given an Amsler grid (Figure 2–23) to help monitor and report any symptomatic changes.

2. EXUDATIVE MACULAR DEGENERATION

Although patients with age-related macular degeneration usually manifest nonexudative changes only, the majority of patients who experience severe vision loss from this disease do so from the development of subretinal neovascularization and related exudative maculopathy. Serous fluid from the underlying choroid can leak through small defects in Bruch's membrane, causing focal detachment of the pigment epithelium. Additional fluid may lead to further separation of the overlying sensory retina, and vision usually decreases if the fovea is involved. Retinal pigment epithelial detachments may spontaneously flatten, with variable visual results, and leave a geographic area of depigmentation at the involved site.

The ingrowth of new vessels extending from the choroid into the subretinal space may occur and is the most important histopathologic change that predisposes patients with drusen to macular detachment and irreversible loss of central vision. These new vessels grow in a flat cartwheel or sea-fan configuration away from their site of entry into the subretinal space. The clinical changes of early subretinal neovascularization are subtle and may be easily overlooked; during this occult stage of new vessel formation, the patient is asymptomatic, and the new vessels may not be apparent either ophthalmoscopically or angiographically.

The ophthalmologist must maintain a high index of suspicion that subretinal neovascularization is present whenever a patient with evidence of age-related macular degeneration has sudden or recent central vision loss, including blurred vision, distortion, or a new scotoma. If the fundus examination reveals subretinal blood, exudate, or a grayish-green choroidal lesion in the macula, there is great likelihood that neovascularization is present, and a fluorescein or indocyanine green angiogram should be obtained promptly to determine if a treatable lesion can be identified.

Although some subretinal neovascular membranes may spontaneously regress, the natural course of subretinal neovascularization in age-related macular degeneration is toward irreversible loss of central vision over a variable period of time. The sensory retina may be damaged by long-standing edema, detachment, or underlying hemorrhage. Furthermore, a hemorrhagic detachment of the retina may undergo fibrous metaplasia, resulting in an elevated subretinal mass called a disciform scar. This elevated fibrovascular mound of variable size represents the cicatricial end stage of exudative age-related macular degeneration. It is usually centrally located and results in permanent loss of central vision.

Treatment

In the absence of subretinal neovascularization, no medical or surgical treatment of serous retinal pigment epithelial detachment is of proved benefit. The use of parenteral alpha interferon, for example, has not been effective for this disease. However, if a well-defined extrafoveal ($\geq$ 200 μm from the center of the foveal avascular zone) subretinal neovascular membrane is present, laser photocoagulation is indicated. Angiography defines the precise location and borders of the neovascular membrane, which is then completely ablated by heavy confluent laser burns. Photocoagulation destroys the overlying retina as well but is worthwhile if the subretinal membrane can be halted short of the fovea (see Chapter 24).

Krypton laser photocoagulation of juxtafoveal (< 200 μm from the center of the foveal avascular zone) subretinal neovascularization is recommended in nonhypertensive patients. The Macular Photocoagulation Study Group has refined its treatment recommendations for subfoveal disease and shown that selected patients may benefit from laser photocoagulation. The ability to determine the probable rate and direction of growth of a subretinal neovascular membrane would facilitate clinical decisions about if and when to treat a given membrane in cases where treatment indications are unclear.

Following successful photocoagulation of a subretinal neovascular membrane, recurrent neovascularization either contiguous with or remote from the laser scar may occur in one-half of cases by 2 years. Recurrence is often accompanied by severe vision loss, so that careful monitoring with Amsler grids, ophthalmoscopy, and angiography is essential. Patients with impaired central vision in both eyes may benefit from a variety of low vision aids.

CENTRAL SEROUS CHORIORETINOPATHY

Central serous chorioretinopathy is characterized by serous detachment of the sensory retina as a consequence of focal leakage of fluid from the choriocapillaris through a defect in the retinal pigment epithelium (Figures 10–2 and 10–3). This disease typically affects young to middle-aged men and may be related to life stress events. Most patients present with the sudden onset of blurred vision, micropsia, metamorphopsia, and central scotoma. Visual acuity is often only moderately decreased and may be improved to near-normal with a small hyperopic correction.

The diagnosis is made by slitlamp examination of the fundus; the presence of serous detachment of the sensory retina in the absence of ocular inflammation, subretinal neovascularization, an optic pit, or a choroidal tumor is diagnostic. The retinal pigment ep-

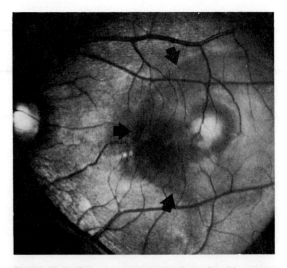

Figure 10–2. Central serous chorioretinopathy with sensory retinal detachment (arrows) extending into the fovea.

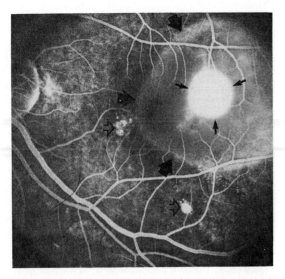

Figure 10–3. Fluorescein angiogram of central serous chorioretinopathy shows active disease with both a retinal pigment epithelial detachment (small arrows) and a sensory retinal detachment (large arrows). Two foci of inactive disease (open arrows) are also present.

ithelial lesion appears as a small, round or oval, yellowish-gray spot that is variable in size and may be difficult to detect without the aid of fluorescein angiography. Fluorescein dye leaking from the choriocapillaris may accumulate below the pigment epithelium or sensory retina, resulting in a variety of patterns including the well-recognized smokestack configuration.

Approximately 80% of eyes with central serous chorioretinopathy undergo spontaneous resorption of subretinal fluid and recovery of normal visual acuity within 6 months after the onset of symptoms. Despite normal acuity, however, many patients have a mild permanent visual defect, such as a decrease in color sensitivity, micropsia, or relative scotoma. Twenty to 30 percent of patients will have one or more recurrences of the disease, and complications—including subretinal neovascularization and chronic cystoid macular edema—have been described in patients with frequent and prolonged serous detachments.

The cause of central serous chorioretinopathy is unknown; there is no convincing evidence that the disease is either infectious or due to retinal pigment epithelial dystrophy. Argon laser photocoagulation directed to the active leak significantly shortens the duration of the sensory detachment and hastens the recovery of central vision, but there is no evidence that prompt photocoagulation reduces the chance of permanent loss of visual function. Although the complications of retinal laser photocoagulation are few, it is probably not advisable to recommend immediate photocoagulation treatment in all patients with central serous chorioretinopathy. The duration and location of

disease, the condition of the fellow eye, and occupational visual requirements are all considerations upon which treatment decisions are based.

MACULAR EDEMA

Retinal edema involving the macula may be associated with a variety of intraocular inflammatory diseases, retinal vascular diseases, intraocular surgery, inherited or acquired retinal degenerations, medications, macular membranes, or unknown causes. Macular edema may be diffuse, with nonlocalized intraretinal fluid causing thickening of the macula. When edema fluid accumulates in honeycomb-like spaces of the outer plexiform and inner nuclear layers, it is called **cystoid macular edema.** On fluorescein angiography, fluorescein dye leaks from the perifoveal retinal capillaries and accumulates in a flower-petal pattern about the fovea (Figure 10–4).

The most widely recognized association with cystoid macular edema is intraocular surgery. Approximately 50% of eyes undergoing uneventful intracapsular cataract extraction and 20% of eyes undergoing extracapsular cataract extraction develop angiographic cystoid macular edema. Clinically significant edema usually occurs within 4–12 weeks postoperatively, but in some instances its onset may be delayed for months or years. Many patients with cystoid macular edema of less than 6 months' duration have self-limited leakage that will resolve without treatment. Topical or local (or both) anti-inflammatory therapy may be of value in restoring visual acuity in some patients with chronic postoperative macular edema. YAG laser vitreolysis (see Chapter 24) and surgical vitrectomy may be of benefit when the macular edema is associated with vit-

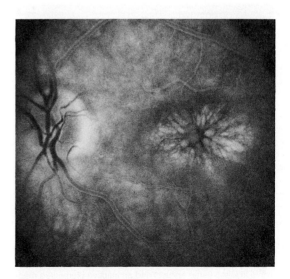

Figure 10–4. Flower-petal pattern of fluorescein dye in a patient with cystoid macular edema after cataract surgery.

reous tissue incarcerated in the cataract wound. When an intraocular lens implant is the cause of postoperative macular edema due to its design, positioning, or inadequate fixation, removal of the lens implant can be considered.

INFLAMMATORY DISORDERS INVOLVING THE MACULA

Presumed Ocular Histoplasmosis Syndrome (Figures 10–5 to 10–7)

In this disease, serous and hemorrhagic detachments of the macula are associated with multiple peripheral atrophic chorioretinal scars and peripapillary chorioretinal scarring (see Chapter 7). The syndrome usually occurs in healthy patients between the third and sixth decades of life, and the scars are probably caused by an antecedent subclinical systemic infection with *Histoplasma capsulatum*. The macular detachments are due to subretinal neovascularization, and the visual prognosis depends on the proximity of the neovascular membrane to the center of the fovea. If the membrane extends inside the foveal avascular zone, only 15% of eyes will retain 20/40 vision. A macular scar may change over time, and 10% of patients with normal maculae will develop new atrophic scars in this region. The relative risk of developing macular subretinal neovascularization in the second eye of an affected patient is significant, and these patients should be instructed in the frequent use of the Amsler grid and the importance of prompt examination when changes are detected.

Argon laser photocoagulation of a subretinal neo-

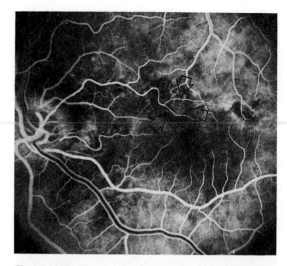

Figure 10–6. The early fluorescein angiogram shows an inactive hypofluorescent scar (small arrow) and the characteristic lacy hyperfluorescence of subretinal neovascularization (open arrows).

vascular membrane outside the foveal avascular zone in symptomatic patients is of value in preventing severe vision loss.

Acute Multifocal Posterior Placoid Pigment Epitheliopathy (AMPPPE)

AMPPPE typically affects healthy young patients who develop rapidly progressive bilateral vision loss in association with ophthalmoscopically visible multifocal flat gray-white subretinal lesions involving the

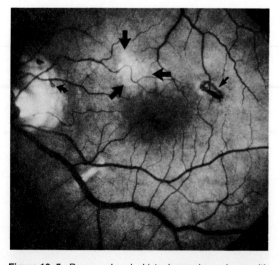

Figure 10–5. Presumed ocular histoplasmosis syndrome with active disease (large arrows) and an inactive pigmented macular scar (small arrow). Peripapillary pigmentation (curved arrow) is also present.

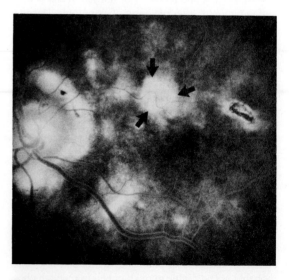

Figure 10–7. Late fluorescein leakage from macular subretinal neovascularization in a patient with presumed ocular histoplasmosis syndrome.

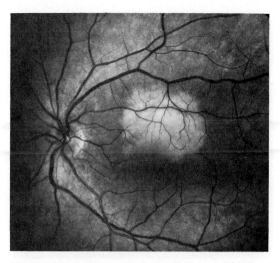

Figure 10–8. Typical macular lesion of acute multifocal posterior placoid pigment epitheliopathy.

pigment epithelium (Figure 10–8). The cause of this disease, which in many instances is associated with evidence of an influenza-like illness, is unknown; the course and nature of the illness suggests the possibility of viral infection. The characteristic feature of the disease is the rapid resolution of the fundus lesions and a delayed return of visual acuity to near-normal levels. Although the prognosis for visual recovery in this acute self-limited disease is good, many patients will identify small residual paracentral scotomas when carefully tested. Extensive pigmentary changes remaining during the late stages of AMPPPE may mimic widespread retinal degeneration; the clinical history and normal electrophysiologic findings aid in this differential diagnosis.

Geographic Helicoid Peripapillary Choroidopathy

This is a chronic progressive and recurrent multifocal inflammatory disease of the retinal pigment epithelium, choriocapillaris, and choroid. It characteristically involves the juxtapapillary retina and extends radially to involve the macula and peripheral retina. The active stage manifests itself as sharply demarcated gray-yellow lesions with irregular borders that appear to involve the pigment epithelium and choriocapillaris. Vitritis, anterior uveitis, and subretinal neovascularization have been associated with this disorder. Involvement is usually bilateral, and the cause is unknown. The natural history of this indolent inflammatory disease is variable and may correlate with the presence of disease in the fellow eye. Local or systemic corticosteroid treatment may be of benefit when active inflammation is present; laser photocoagulation is administered as indicated for the complication of subretinal neovascularization.

Vitiliginous Chorioretinitis (Birdshot Retinochoroidopathy)

This is a syndrome characterized by diffuse cream-colored patches at the level of the pigment epithelium and choroid, retinal vasculitis associated with cystoid macular edema, and vitritis. The associations with HLA-A29 and with retinal S-antigen suggest that this disease has a genetic predisposition and that retinal autoimmunity plays a role in its manifestations. In many cases, electroretinography, electro-oculography, and dark adaptation studies are abnormal. The course of the disease is that of exacerbation and remission with variable visual outcomes; visual loss has been attributed to chronic cystoid macular edema, optic atrophy, macular scarring, or subretinal neovascularization. Corticosteroid therapy has not proved effective against this disease.

Acute Macular Neuroretinopathy

Acute macular neuroretinopathy is characterized by the acute onset of paracentral scotomas and mild visual acuity loss accompanied by wedge-shaped parafoveal retinal lesions in the deep sensory retina of one or both eyes. The macular lesions are subtle, reddish-brown, and best seen with a red-free light. The patients are usually young adults with a history of acute viral illness. While the retinal lesions may fade, the scotomas tend to persist and remain symptomatic.

Multiple Evanescent White Dot Syndrome

This is an acute and self-limited unilateral disease that affects mainly young women and is characterized clinically by multiple white dots at the level of the pigment epithelium, vitreal cells, and transient electroretinographic abnormalities. The cause is unknown. There is no evidence of associated systemic disease. The retinal lesions gradually regress in a matter of weeks, leaving only minor retinal pigment epithelial defects.

ANGIOID STREAKS

Angioid streaks appear as irregular, jagged tapering lines that radiate from the peripapillary retina into the macula and peripheral fundus (Figure 10–9). The streaks represent linear crack-like dehiscences in Bruch's membrane. The lesions are rarely noted in children and probably develop in the second or third decade of life. Early in the disease the streaks are sharply outlined and red-orange or brown. Subsequent fibrovascular tissue growth may partially or totally obscure the streak margins.

Nearly 50% of patients with angioid streaks have an associated systemic disease. Pseudoxanthoma elasticum, Paget's disease of bone, Ehlers-Danlos syndrome, and several hemoglobinopathies and hemolytic disorders have been associated with this retinal disease,

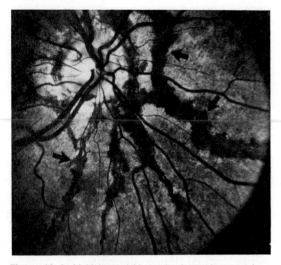

Figure 10–9. Multiple angioid streaks (arrows) extend from the optic nerve. (Courtesy of University of California, San Francisco.)

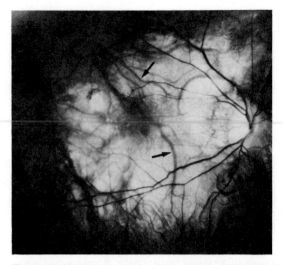

Figure 10–10. Myopic macular degeneration with choroidal vessels (arrows) visible through atrophic retinal pigment epithelium.

but the most common association is with age-related degeneration of Bruch's membrane. Patients with angioid streaks should be warned of the potential risk of choroidal rupture from even relatively mild eye trauma. Older patients with the disease are at risk of developing serous and hemorrhagic detachments of the retina as a consequence of subretinal neovascularization.

Laser treatment may be used to photocoagulate extrafoveal neovascular membranes; however, other neovascular membranes are likely to occur. Prophylactic treatment of angioid streaks before subretinal neovascularization develops is not recommended.

MYOPIC MACULAR DEGENERATION

Pathologic myopia is one of the leading causes of blindness in the United States and is characterized by progressive elongation of the eye with subsequent thinning and atrophy of the choroid and pigment epithelium in the macula. Peripapillary chorioretinal atrophy and linear breaks in Bruch's membrane ("lacquer cracks") are characteristic findings on ophthalmoscopy (Figure 10–10). The degenerative changes of the macular pigment epithelium resemble those found in the older patient with age-related macular degeneration. A characteristic lesion of this disease is a raised, circular, pigmented macular lesion called a Fuchs spot. Most patients are in the fifth decade when the degenerative macular changes cause a slowly progressive loss of vision; rapid loss of visual acuity is usually caused by serous and hemorrhagic macular degeneration overlying a subretinal neovascular membrane.

Fluorescein angiography in patients with pathologic myopia may show delayed filling of choroidal and reti-

nal blood vessels. Angiography is helpful in identifying and locating the site of subretinal neovascularization in patients who develop serous or hemorrhagic detachments of the macula. Because of the frequent close proximity of the subretinal neovascular membrane to the foveola in these patients, laser photocoagulation may not be possible. As subretinal neovascular membranes tend to remain small and because photocoagulation-associated chorioretinal atrophy tends to progress in patients with pathologic myopia, retinal laser treatment is not as beneficial as in other diseases associated with macular subretinal neovascularization.

The chorioretinal changes of pathologic myopia predispose the retina to breaks and thus to retinal detachment. Peripheral retinal findings may include paving stone degeneration, pigmentary degeneration, and lattice degeneration. Retinal breaks usually occur in areas involved with chorioretinal lesions, but they also arise in areas of apparently normal retina. Some of these breaks, particularly those of the "horseshoe" and round retinal tear type, will progress to rhegmatogenous retinal detachment.

Macular Hole

A macular hole is a partial or full-thickness absence of the sensory retina in the macula. This disorder occurs most often in elderly women, and although sometimes bilateral, it rarely comes on simultaneously in the two eyes. The typical finding on biomicroscopy of the symptomatic eye is a full-thickness, round or oval, sharply defined hole measuring one-third disk diameter in the center of the macula, which may be surrounded by a ring detachment of the sensory retina (Figure 10–11). With a full-thickness macular hole, visual acuity is impaired and metamorphopsia, as well as a central scotoma, are present on the Amsler grid. An

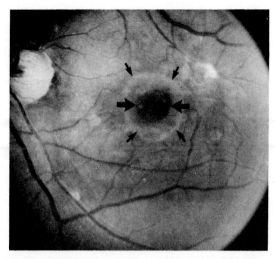

Figure 10–11. Macular hole (large arrows) with surrounding sensory retinal detachment (small arrows).

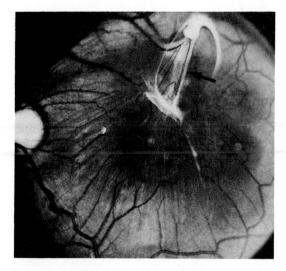

Figure 10–12. Epiretinal macular membrane elevates retinal vessels (arrow) and produces retinal striae.

operculum of retinal tissue may overlie the macular hole. Tangential traction from epiretinal vitreous cortex plays an important role in the pathogenesis of macular hole. Early stages of macular hole formation, such as a deep foveal yellow spot or ring, may be reversible as the posterior vitreous cortex spontaneously separates from the retina. Therapy for macular hole disease involves reattaching and potentially restoring function to the retina overlying the cuff of subretinal fluid surrounding the hole. An ongoing study comparing vitrectomy surgery to observation will assess the clinical value of the procedure.

EPIRETINAL MACULAR MEMBRANES

Fibrocellular membranes may proliferate on the surface of the retina, either in the macula or peripheral retina. Contraction or shrinkage of these epiretinal membranes may cause varying degrees of visual distortion, intraretinal edema, and degeneration of the underlying retina. Biomicroscopy usually shows retinal wrinkles and vessel tortuosity and may rarely also show retinal hemorrhages, cotton-wool spots, serous retinal detachment, and macular hole; a posterior vitreous detachment is nearly always present (Figure 10–12). Disorders associated with epiretinal membranes include retinal tears with or without rhegmatogenous retinal detachment, vitreous inflammatory diseases, trauma, and a variety of retinal vascular diseases.

Patients with macular distortion and vision loss caused by epiretinal membrane contraction are usually left with stable visual acuity, suggesting that membrane contraction is a short-lived and self-limited process. Surgical peeling of severe epiretinal membranes can be performed successfully, but regrowth of epiretinal tissues occurs in some cases. There is no role

for photocoagulation in the treatment of epiretinal macular membrane disease.

TRAUMATIC MACULOPATHY

Blunt trauma to the anterior segment of the eye may cause a contrecoup injury to the retina called **commotio retinae.** The retina develops a gray-white color that affects primarily the outer retina and may be confined to the macular area (Berlin's edema) or may involve extensive areas of the peripheral retina. The retinal whitening in the macular area may clear completely, or impairment of central vision may be permanent and associated with a pigmented retinal scar (Figure 10–13) or a macu-

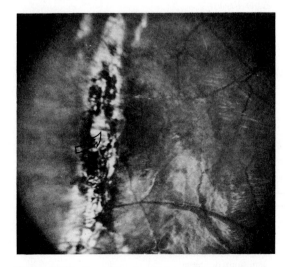

Figure 10–13. Traumatic choroidal rupture resulting in pigmented scar. A choroidal vessel (arrow) is visible through the scar.

lar hole. Trauma similar to that which causes Berlin's edema may also cause choroidal rupture with subretinal hemorrhage and permanent central vision loss.

In addition to blunt trauma, several other traumatic injuries involving the macula are of importance. **Purtscher's retinopathy** is characterized by multiple patches of superficial retinal whitening and retinal hemorrhages in each eye of a patient after severe compression injury to the head or trunk. **Terson's syndrome** is seen in approximately 20% of patients after traumatic (or spontaneous) subarachnoid or subdural hemorrhage and is characterized by vitreous and superficial macular hemorrhage. **Solar retinopathy** refers to a specific foveolar lesion that occurs after sungazing and is best described as a usually bilateral sharply circumscribed and often irregularly shaped partial-thickness hole or depression in the center of the fovea.

MACULAR DYSTROPHIES

Macular dystrophies differ from degenerations in that the former are inherited, are not necessarily evident at birth, and are not associated with systemic diseases. Most often the disorder is restricted to the macula; it may be symmetric or asymmetric, but eventually both eyes are affected. In the early stages of some of these disorders the visual acuity may be reduced while the macular changes are subtle or absent on ophthalmoscopy, and the patient's complaint may be dismissed as spurious. Conversely, in other macular dystrophies, the ophthalmoscopic changes may be very striking at a time when the patient is free of visual symptoms. One method of classifying the more common macular dystrophies is to consider the presumptive anatomic layer or layers of the retina involved (Table 10–1).

X-Linked Juvenile Retinoschisis

This is a congenital disease of males characterized by a macular lesion called "foveal schisis." On slitlamp examination, foveal schisis appears as small superficial retinal cysts arranged in a stellate pattern accom-

panied by radial striae centered in the foveal area (Figure 10–14). Visual acuity is usually between 20/40 and 20/200; peripheral visual field abnormalities are present in the 50% of patients with associated peripheral retinoschisis. The posterior pole appears normal on fluorescein angiography, and this may be helpful in the clinical differentiation from cystoid macular edema. B wave abnormalities on the electroretinogram are consistent with the histopathologic finding of intraretinal splitting in the nerve fiber layer.

Cone-Rod Dystrophies

The cone-rod dystrophies constitute a relatively rare group of disorders that may be regarded as a single entity showing variable expressivity. Most cases are sporadic, but familial cases are usually transmitted by an autosomal dominant inheritance pattern. Cone-rod dystrophy is characterized by predominant involvement of the cone photoreceptors with progressive color vision defects and associated loss of visual acuity. A bilateral and symmetric bulls-eye pattern of depigmentation and a corresponding zone of hyperfluorescence surrounding a central nonfluorescent spot (similar to that seen in chloroquine retinopathy) are the most commonly described biomicroscopic and angiographic changes in these patients (Figure 10–15). As the disease progresses, the electroretinogram shows marked loss of cone function associated with a slight to moderate loss of rod function. Histopathologic study shows absence of macular and paramacular photoreceptors, and there is associated pigment epithelium degeneration.

Fundus Albipunctatus

Fundus albipunctatus is an autosomal recessive nonprogressive dystrophy characterized by a myriad of

Table 10–1. Anatomic classification of macular dystrophies.

Nerve fiber layer
   X-linked juvenile retinoschisis
Photoreceptor cells
   Cone-rod dystrophy
Retinal pigment epithelium
   Fundus albipunctus
   Fundus flavimaculatus
   Vitelliform dystrophy
    (Best's disease)

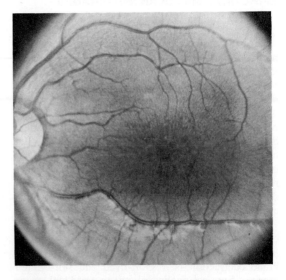

Figure 10–14. X-linked juvenile retinoschisis with typical superficial retinal cysts in the fovea.

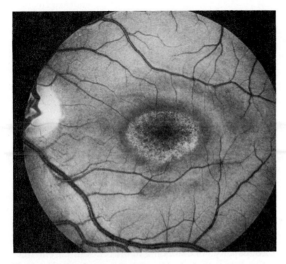

Figure 10–15. Cone dystrophy with depigmentation and a bull's-eye pattern to the macula.

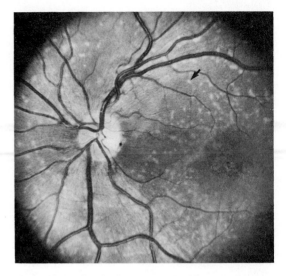

Figure 10–16. Fundus flavimaculatus with multiple irregular fleck lesions (arrow) involving the macula.

discrete small white dots at the level of the pigment epithelium sprinkled about the posterior pole and midperiphery of the retina. Patients are night-blind with normal visual acuity, normal visual fields, and normal color vision. While the electroretinogram and electro-oculogram are usually normal, dark adaptation thresholds are markedly elevated. **Retinitis punctata albescens** is the less common progressive variant of this dystrophy.

Fundus Flavimaculatus (Stargardt's Disease)

This is a bilateral and symmetric autosomal recessive disorder characterized by multiple yellow-white fleck lesions of variable size and shape confined to the retinal pigment epithelium (Figure 10–16). Many patients suffer central visual loss in childhood; however, macular involvement and the ultimate visual outcome are variable. Fluorescein angiography is important in differentiating flecks from drusen; the former are usually hypofluorescent. The electroretinogram and electro-oculogram are usually normal. Histopathologic abnormalities are confined to the pigment epithelium; the yellow flecks seen clinically are dense accumulations of lipofuscin within engorged pigment epithelial cells.

Vitelliform Dystrophy (Best's Disease)

Vitelliform dystrophy is an autosomal dominant disorder with variable penetrance and expressivity with onset usually in childhood. The ophthalmoscopic appearance is variable and ranges from a mild pigmentary disturbance within the fovea to the typical vitelliform or "egg yoke" lesion located within the central

macula (Figure 10–17). This characteristic cyst-like lesion is generally quite round and well demarcated and contains homogeneous opaque yellow material lying at the apparent level of the retinal pigment epithelium. The "egg yoke" may degenerate and be associated with subretinal neovascularization, subretinal hemorrhage, and extensive macular scarring. Visual acuity often remains good, and the electroretinogram is normal; the distinctly abnormal electro-oculogram is the hallmark of this disease.

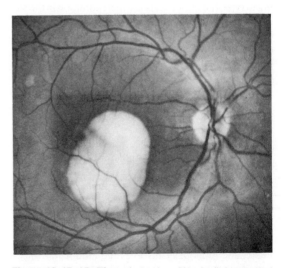

Figure 10–17. Vitelliform dystrophy with a well-demarcated cyst-like macular lesion.

DISEASES OF THE PERIPHERAL RETINA

RETINAL DETACHMENT

The term "retinal detachment" denotes separation of the sensory retina, ie, the photoreceptors and inner tissue layers, from the underlying retinal pigment epithelium. There are three main types: rhegmatogenous detachment, traction detachment, and serous or hemorrhagic detachment.

1. RHEGMATOGENOUS RETINAL DETACHMENT

The most common of the three major types of retinal detachments is **rhegmatogenous retinal detachment.** The characteristics of a rhegmatogenous detachment are a full-thickness break (a "rhegma") in the sensory retina, variable degrees of vitreous traction, and passage of liquefied vitreous through the sensory retinal defect into the subretinal space. A spontaneous rhegmatogenous retinal detachment is usually preceded or accompanied by a posterior vitreous detachment. Myopia, aphakia, lattice degeneration, and ocular trauma are associated with this type of retinal detachment. Binocular indirect ophthalmoscopy with scleral depression (Figures 2–17 and 2–19) reveals elevation of the translucent detached sensory retina. A careful search usually reveals one or more full-thickness sensory retinal breaks such as a horseshoe tear, round atrophic hole, or anterior circumferential tear (retinal dialysis). The location of retinal breaks varies according to type; horseshoe tears are most common in the superotemporal quadrant, atrophic holes in the temporal quadrants, and retinal dialysis in the inferotemporal quadrant. When multiple retinal breaks are present, the defects are usually within 90 degrees of one another.

Treatment

Scleral buckling or pneumatic retinopexy are the two most popular and effective surgical techniques for the repair of rhegmatogenous retinal detachment. Each procedure requires careful localization of the retinal break and treatment with diathermy, cryotherapy, or laser in order to create an adhesion between the pigment epithelium and the sensory retina. With scleral buckling surgery, the retinal break is mounted on sclera indented by an explant. The scleral indentation can be achieved by a variety of techniques and materials, each of which has inherent advantages and disadvantages. Pneumatic retinopexy involves the intraocular injection of air or an expandable gas in order to tamponade the retinal break while the chorioretinal adhesion forms. An overall reattachment rate of 90% is reported;

however, the visual results are dependent on the preoperative status of the macula. If the macula is involved in rhegmatogenous retinal detachment, the prognosis for complete visual recovery is less optimistic.

2. TRACTION RETINAL DETACHMENT

Traction retinal detachment is the second most common type and is most commonly due to proliferative diabetic retinopathy, proliferative vitreoretinopathy, retinopathy of prematurity, or ocular trauma. In contrast to the convex appearance of rhegmatogenous retinal detachment, the typical traction retinal detachment has a more concave surface and is likely to be more localized, usually not extending to the ora serrata. The tractional forces that actively pull the sensory retina away from the underlying pigment epithelium are caused by a clinically apparent vitreal, epiretinal, or subretinal membrane consisting of fibroblasts and of glial and retinal pigment epithelial cells. In diabetic traction retinal detachment, vitreous contraction draws the fibrovascular tissue and underlying retina anteriorly toward the vitreous base. Initially the detachment may be localized along the vascular arcades, but progression may spread to involve the midperipheral retina and the macula. Proliferative vitreoretinopathy is a complication of rhegmatogenous retinal detachment and is the most common cause of failure of surgical repair in these eyes.

The basic pathologic process in eyes with proliferative vitreoretinopathy is growth and contraction of cellular membranes on both sides of the retina and on the posterior vitreous surface. Focal traction from cellular membranes can produce a retinal tear and lead to combined tractional-rhegmatogenous retinal detachment.

Treatment

The primary treatment of traction retinal detachment is vitreoretinal surgery and may involve vitrectomy, membrane removal, scleral buckling, and injection of intraocular gas.

3. SEROUS & HEMORRHAGIC RETINAL DETACHMENT

Serous and hemorrhagic retinal detachment can occur in the absence of either retinal break or vitreoretinal traction. These detachments are the result of a collection of fluid beneath the sensory retina and are caused primarily by diseases of the retinal pigment epithelium and choroid. Degenerative, inflammatory, and infectious diseases limited to the macula, including the multiple causes of subretinal neovascularization, may be associated with this third type of retinal detachment and are described in an earlier section of the this chapter. This type of detachment may also be associated with systemic vascular and inflammatory disease as described in Chapters 7 and 15.

RETINOPATHY OF PREMATURITY

Retinopathy of prematurity is a vasoproliferative retinopathy that is the leading cause of childhood blindness in the United States and a major cause of blindness throughout the developed world. An international classification of this disease divides the retina into three zones and characterizes the extent of disease by the number of clock hours involved; the retinal changes are divided into five stages described in Table 10–2.

The demarcation line is a narrow white band that marks the junction of vascular and avascular retina in stage 1; it is the first definite ophthalmoscopic sign of retinopathy of prematurity. As this band increases in height, width, and volume and rises up from the plane of the retina, the ridge of stage 2 is seen. Neovascular proliferation along the posterior aspect of the ridge and extending into the vitreous defines stage 3. Stage 4 is characterized by subtotal retinal detachment, and the clinical sign of stage 5 is a funnel-shaped total retinal detachment.

Treatment

The treatment of retinopathy of prematurity is based on the classification and stage of the disease. It is important to note that a significant number of patients with retinopathy of prematurity undergo spontaneous regression. Peripheral retinal changes of regressed retinopathy of prematurity include avascular retina, peripheral folds, and retinal breaks; associated changes in the posterior pole may include straightening of the temporal vessels, temporal stretching of the macula, and retinal tissue that appears to be dragged over the disk (Figure 10–18). Other ocular findings of regressed retinopathy of prematurity include myopia (which may be asymmetric), strabismus, cataract, and angle-closure glaucoma.

While stage 1 and stage 2 disease require nothing more than observation, transscleral cryotherapy or laser photocoagulation to the avascular retina should be considered in eyes with stage 3 disease. Vitreoretinal surgery as described above in the section on traction retinal detachment may be appropriate for eyes with stage 4 or stage 5 disease. The etiology and treatment of retinopathy of prematurity as well as the

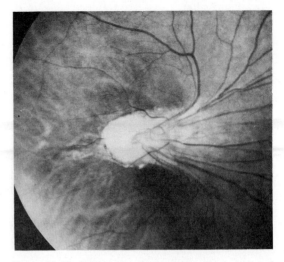

Figure 10–18. Retinopathy of prematurity with stretching of the macula and straightening of retinal vessels.

recommended screening protocols are discussed in Chapter 8.

RETINAL DEGENERATIONS

This group of disorders encompasses a number of diseases with various ocular and, in some instances, systemic manifestations. In this section, several specific disorders will be used as prototypes with which to understand the major characteristics of retinal degenerations.

Retinitis Pigmentosa

Retinitis pigmentosa is a group of hereditary retinal degenerations characterized by progressive dysfunction of the photoreceptors and associated with progressive cell loss and eventual atrophy of several retinal layers. The typical form of this disease can be inherited as an autosomal recessive, autosomal dominant, or X-linked recessive trait; one-third of cases will have a negative family history. The hallmark symptoms of retinitis pigmentosa are night blindness (nyctalopia) and gradually progressive peripheral visual field loss. The most characteristic ophthalmoscopic findings are narrowing of the retinal arterioles, mottling of the retinal pigment epithelium, and peripheral retinal pigment clumping, referred to as "bone-spicule formation" (Figure 10–19). While retinitis pigmentosa is a generalized photoreceptor disorder, in most cases rod function is more severely affected, leading to subjective sensations associated with poor scotopic function. The electroretinogram usually shows either markedly reduced or absent retinal function; the electrooculogram lacks the usual light rise. The fundus appearance of retinitis pigmentosa may be mimicked by

Table 10–2. Stages of retinopathy of prematurity.

Stage	Clinical Findings
1	Demarcation line
2	Intraretinal ridge
3	Ridge with extraretinal fibrovascular proliferation
4	Subtotal retinal detachment
5	Total retinal detachment

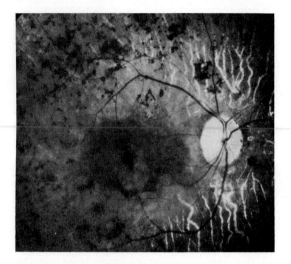

Figure 10–19. Retinitis pigmentosa with arteriolar narrowing and peripheral retinal pigment clumping.

several disorders, including chorioretinitis, trauma, vascular occlusion, and remote retinal detachment.

The effects of supplemental vitamins on the progression of retinitis pigmentosa require further study before treatment recommendations can be made. Patients with the disease benefit from genetic counseling and appropriate referral to agencies that provide services to the visually impaired.

Leber's Congenital Amaurosis

Leber's congenital amaurosis is a group of disorders characterized by severe visual impairment or blindness from infancy with no discernible cause. The disorders are usually inherited in an autosomal recessive manner and may be associated with mental retardation, seizures, and renal or muscular abnormalities. The ophthalmoscopic findings are variable; most patients show either a normal fundus appearance or only subtle retinal pigment epithelial granularity and mild vessel attenuation. A markedly reduced or absent electroretinogram indicates generalized photoreceptor dysfunction, and in infants this test is the only method by which an absolute diagnosis can be made.

Gyrate Atrophy

Gyrate atrophy is an autosomal recessive disorder caused by reduced activity of ornithine aminotransferase, a mitochondrial matrix enzyme that catalyzes several amino acid pathways. The incidence of this disorder is relatively high in Finland, and the ophthalmologic features are the most prominent manifestations of the disease. Patients usually develop nyctalopia within the first decade of life, and progressive peripheral visual field loss follows. Characteristic sharply demarcated circular areas of chorioretinal atrophy develop in the midperiphery of the fundus during the teenage years and become confluent with mac-

ular involvement late in the course of the disease. The electroretinogram is decreased or absent, and the electro-oculogram is reduced.

Treatment approaches to this disease have included pyridoxine supplementation, restriction of dietary arginine, and supplemental dietary lysine.

Peripheral Chorioretinal Atrophy

Peripheral chorioretinal atrophy (paving stone degeneration) is a common chorioretinal degeneration found in nearly one-third of adult eyes. Ophthalmoscopically, the lesions appear as isolated or grouped, small, discrete, yellow-white areas with prominent underlying choroidal vessels and pigmented borders. Choroidal vascular insufficiency is thought to be the cause of this benign disorder because the pathologic changes are limited to that portion of the retina supplied by the choriocapillaris. Paving stone degeneration is not of great pathologic significance, though it may be a sign of peripheral vascular disease.

Lattice Degeneration

Lattice degeneration is the most common of the inherited vitreoretinal degenerations, with an estimated incidence of 7% of the general population. Lattice degeneration is more commonly found in myopic eyes and is frequently associated with retinal detachment, occurring in nearly one-third of retinal detachment patients. The ophthalmoscopic appearance may be that of localized round, oval, or linear retinal thinning, with pigmentation, branching white lines, and whitish-yellow flecks; the hallmarks of the disease are the thinned retina punctuated by sharp borders with firm vitreoretinal adhesions at the margins. The mere presence of lattice degeneration is not cause enough for prophylactic therapy. A strong family history of retinal detachments, retinal detachment in the fellow eye, high myopia, and aphakia are risk factors for retinal detachment in eyes with lattice degeneration, and prophylactic treatment with cryosurgery or laser photocoagulation may be warranted.

RETINOSCHISIS

Degenerative retinoschisis, unlike X-linked juvenile retinoschisis described above, is a common acquired peripheral retinal disorder that is believed to develop from preexisting peripheral cystoid degeneration. The cystic changes of peripheral cystoid degeneration are seen to some degree in virtually all adults. This cystoid degeneration is characterized by intraretinal microcysts that often coalesce, giving the appearance of lobulated, irregularly branching, tortuous channels. Peripheral cystoid degeneration may develop into either of two degenerative forms of retinoschisis, each of which is characterized by sharply demarcated and absolute visual field defects.

Typical degenerative retinoschisis occurs in 1% of

adults and is a bilateral disease in one-third of affected patients. On clinical examination, the disorder appears as a round or ovoid area of retinal splitting with fusiform elevation of the inner layer and an optically empty schisis cavity. The retinal splitting occurs at the outer plexiform layer. Complications such as hole formation and marked posterior extension are very uncommon and rarely require treatment.

Reticular degenerative retinoschisis is characterized by round or oval areas of retinal splitting in which a bullous elevation of an extremely thin inner layer occurs, most commonly in the lower temporal quadrant. In this form of the disease, the splitting usually occurs in the nerve fiber layer, and typical peripheral cystoid degeneration is usually present anterior to the lesion. When retinal breaks are present in both the inner and the outer layers, progressive rhegmatogenous retinal detachment may develop and threaten the macula, thus requiring treatment.

RETINAL VASCULAR DISEASES

DIABETIC RETINOPATHY

Diabetic retinopathy is one of the leading causes of blindness in the Western world. The view that chronic hyperglycemia of diabetes mellitus is the major determinant of diabetic retinopathy is supported by the observation that retinopathy in young people with type I (insulin-dependent) diabetes does not occur for at least 3–5 years after the onset of this systemic disease. Similar results have been obtained for type II (non-insulin-dependent) diabetes, but in such patients the time of onset and therefore the duration of disease are more difficult to determine precisely. It is recommended that patients with type I diabetes mellitus be referred for ophthalmologic examination within 3 years after diagnosis and reexamined on at least an annual basis. Type II diabetic patients should be referred for ophthalmologic examination at the time of diagnosis and reexamined at least annually. As diabetic retinopathy can become particularly aggressive during pregnancy, any diabetic woman who becomes pregnant should be examined by an ophthalmologist in the first trimester and at least every 3 months thereafter until parturition.

In terms of both prognosis and treatment, it is useful to divide diabetic retinopathy into nonproliferative and proliferative categories. The prevalence of proliferative retinopathy in type I diabetics with 15 years of systemic disease is 50%. While the prevalence of proliferative disease at 15 years is much less in type II diabetics, the prevalence of macular edema as a function of the duration of systemic disease is the same in both groups.

1. NONPROLIFERATIVE DIABETIC RETINOPATHY

Diabetic retinopathy is a progressive microangiopathy characterized by small vessel damage and occlusion. The earliest pathologic changes are thickening of the capillary endothelial basement membrane and reduction of the number of pericytes. **Nonproliferative diabetic retinopathy** is a clinical reflection of the hyperpermeability and incompetence of involved vessels. The capillaries develop tiny dot-like outpouchings called microaneurysms, while the retinal veins become dilated and tortuous (Figure 10–20).

Multiple hemorrhages may appear throughout different levels of the retina. Flame-shaped hemorrhages are so shaped because of their location within the horizontally oriented nerve fiber layer, while dot and blot hemorrhages are in the deeper retina, where cells and axons are vertically oriented.

Macular edema is the most frequent cause of visual loss among patients with nonproliferative diabetic retinopathy. The edema is caused primarily by a breakdown of the inner blood-retinal barrier at the level of the retinal capillary endothelium, allowing leakage of fluid and plasma constituents into the surrounding retina. The edema may be focal or diffuse and appears clinically as thickened, cloudy retina with associated microaneurysms and intraretinal exudate. Circinate zones of yellow, lipid-rich exudate may form around clusters of microaneurysms and are most frequently centered in the temporal portion of the macula. While the prevalence of macular edema is 10% in the diabetic population as a whole, there is a dramatic increase in prevalence in eyes with more severe retinopathy.

With progressive microvascular occlusion, signs of

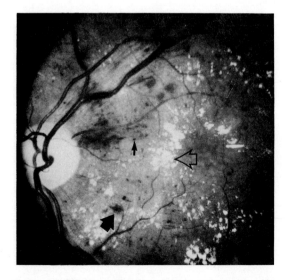

Figure 10–20. Nonproliferative diabetic retinopathy with abundant macular exudate (open arrow), microaneurysms (small arrows), and intraretinal hemorrhage (large arrow).

increasing ischemia may be superimposed on the picture of background retinopathy and produce the clinical picture of **preproliferative diabetic retinopathy.** The most typical findings here are multiple cotton-wool spots, beading of the retinal veins, and irregular segmental dilation of the retinal capillary bed (intraretinal microvascular abnormalities). Closure of retinal capillaries surrounding the foveal avascular zone may cause significant ischemia, manifest clinically by the presence of large dark retinal hemorrhages and small thread-like macular arterioles. Eyes with macular edema and significant ischemia have a poorer visual prognosis—with or without laser treatment—than eyes with edema and relatively good perfusion.

The visual and electrophysiologic dysfunctions associated with diabetes probably result from the local vascular abnormalities and the systemic metabolic effects of the disease to which the retina is subjected. A characteristic blue-yellow color vision abnormality develops, and hue discrimination may be impaired. Contrast sensitivity may be reduced in patients, even in the presence of normal visual acuity. Visual field testing may show relative scotomas corresponding to areas of retinal edema and nonperfusion, and abnormalities in dark adaptation have also been described. Electroretinographic abnormalities bear a relationship to the severity of retinopathy and may aid in predicting progression of retinopathy. Fluorescein angiography is invaluable in defining the microvascular abnormalities of diabetic retinopathy (Figures 10–21 and 10–22). Large filling defects of capillary beds—"capillary nonperfusion"—show the extent of retinal ischemia (Figure 10–23) and are usually most prominent in the midperiphery. The fluorescein leakage associated with retinal edema may assume the petaloid configuration of cystoid macular edema or may be diffuse. Other flu-

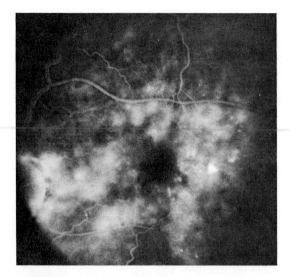

Figure 10–22. Late phase fluorescein angiogram shows hyperfluorescence typical of noncystoid diabetic macular edema.

orescein abnormalities include vascular loops and intraretinal shunts. The focus of treatment in patients with nonproliferative diabetic retinopathy and no macular edema is treatment of hyperglycemia and intercurrent systemic disease. A controlled clinical trial has shown that aldose reductase inhibitor therapy does not prevent progression of diabetic retinopathy. Several recent clinical trials provide compelling evidence that focal argon laser treatment of discrete points of retinal leakage in patients with clinically significant macular edema reduces the risk of visual loss and increases the likelihood of visual improvement (see Chapter 24). Eyes with diabetic macular edema that is not clinically

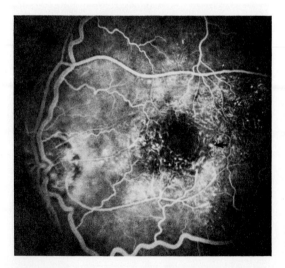

Figure 10–21. Fluorescein angiogram in nonproliferative diabetic retinopathy shows microaneurysms (arrow) and perifoveal retinal vascular changes.

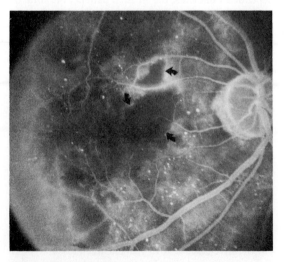

Figure 10–23. Fluorescein angiogram shows hypofluorescence from capillary drop-out (arrows) typical of ischemic diabetic maculopathy.

significant should usually be monitored closely without laser treatment. As macular edema may be present with little or no change in visual acuity, primary health care providers should recognize the importance of prompt and early referral of diabetic patients to the ophthalmologist.

2. PROLIFERATIVE DIABETIC RETINOPATHY

The most severe ocular complications of diabetes mellitus are associated with proliferative diabetic retinopathy. Progressive retinal ischemia eventually stimulates the formation of delicate new vessels that leak serum proteins (and fluorescein) profusely. Neovascularization is frequently located on the surface of the disk and at the posterior edge of the peripheral zones of "nonperfusion" (Figures 10–24 and 10–25). Iris neovascularization, or rubeosis iridis, can also result.

The fragile new vessels proliferate onto the posterior face of the vitreous and become elevated once the vitreous starts to contract away from the retina. If the vessels bleed (Figure 10–26), massive vitreous hemorrhage may cause sudden visual loss. Eyes in which posterior vitreous detachment is complete are at less risk of developing neovascularization and vitreous hemorrhage. In eyes with proliferative diabetic retinopathy and persistent vitreoretinal adhesions, elevated neovascular fronds may undergo fibrous change and form tight fibrovascular bands that tug on the retina and exert continued vitreous contraction. This can cause either a progressive traction retinal detachment or, if a retinal tear is produced, rhegmatogenous retinal detachment. The retinal detachment may be heralded or

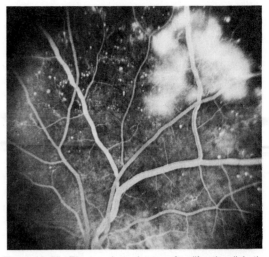

Figure 10–25. Fluorescein angiogram of proliferative diabetic retinopathy shows leakage from the neovascular tissue. The pinpoint areas of hyperfluorescence are microaneurysms.

concealed by vitreous hemorrhage. When vitreous contraction is complete in these eyes, proliferative retinopathy tends to enter the burned-out or "involutional" stage.

Treatment

Argon laser panretinal photocoagulation is usually indicated in proliferative diabetic retinopathy. Patients at greatest risk of significant visual loss are those with preretinal or vitreous hemorrhage or neovascularization of the disk. Panretinal photocoagulation can significantly reduce the chance of massive vitreous hemorrhage and retinal detachment in these patients by

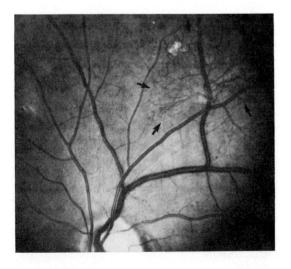

Figure 10–24. A frond of neovascular tissue (arrows) is seen along the superotemporal vascular arcade in this eye with proliferative diabetic retinopathy.

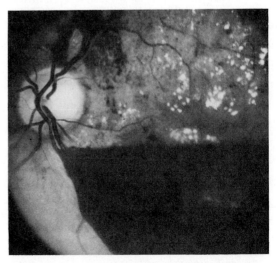

Figure 10–26. Proliferative diabetic retinopathy with preretinal hemorrhage obscuring the inferior macula. Macular exudate, microaneurysms, and intraretinal hemorrhages are also present.

causing the regression and, in some cases, the disappearance of new vessels. The technique involves scattering up to several thousand regularly spaced laser burns throughout the retina, sparing the central region bordered by the disk and the major temporal vascular arcades (Chapter 24). Although the mechanism is not precisely understood, panretinal photocoagulation presumably works by reducing the angiogenic stimulus from ischemic retina.

The role of vitreoretinal surgery in proliferative diabetic eye disease continues to evolve. Conservative management of monocular vision impairing diabetic vitreous hemorrhage in the binocular patient had been to allow spontaneous resolution over the course of several months. The results of a 4-year study designed to assess the role of early vitrectomy for severe vitreous hemorrhage and proliferative diabetic retinopathy support this surgery as a means by which good vision may be restored or maintained. The role of vitreoretinal surgery in the treatment of diabetic traction retinal detachment is described elsewhere in this chapter.

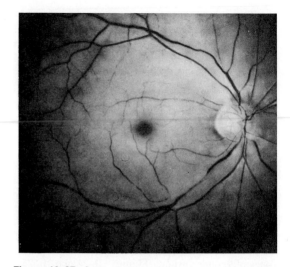

Figure 10–27. Acute central retinal artery occlusion with opaque white retina and attenuated vessels. (Courtesy of University of California, San Francisco.)

CENTRAL RETINAL ARTERY OCCLUSION

The patient with central retinal artery occlusion routinely relates a history of painless catastrophic visual loss occurring over a period of seconds; antecedent transient visual loss (amaurosis fugax) may be reported. The visual acuity ranges between counting fingers and light perception in 90% of eyes at the time of initial examination. An afferent pupillary defect can appear within seconds after retinal arterial obstruction, preceding the fundus abnormalities by an hour.

Ophthalmoscopically, the superficial retina becomes opacified except in the foveola, where a cherry-red spot is evident (Figure 10–27). The cherry-red spot is pigment of the choroid and retinal pigment epithelium viewed through the extremely thin overlying foveolar retina and contrasted with the thicker and translucent perifoveolar retina. Twenty-five percent of eyes with central retinal artery occlusion have cilioretinal arteries that spare macular retina and may preserve some central visual acuity. Clinically, the retinal opacification resolves within 4–6 weeks, leaving a pale optic disk as the major ocular finding. In older patients, giant cell arteritis must be excluded and if necessary treated immediately with high doses of systemic corticosteroids. Other causes of central retinal artery occlusion are arteriosclerosis and emboli from carotid or cardiac sources. These are discussed further in Chapter 15.

Treatment
Currently, there is no satisfactory treatment by which to improve the visual outcome of patients who have central retinal artery occlusion. As irreversible retinal damage has been shown to occur after 90 minutes of complete central retinal artery occlusion in the subhuman primate model, precious little time is available in which to begin therapy. Anterior chamber paracentesis can be employed in order to decrease intraocular pressure and increase retinal perfusion. Intravenous acetazolamide has been used to decrease intraocular pressure, and an inhaled oxygen-carbon dioxide mixture has been employed to induce retinal vasodilation and increase the PO_2 at the retinal surface. Systemic anticoagulants are generally not employed.

BRANCH RETINAL ARTERY OCCLUSION

Branch retinal artery occlusion usually presents with sudden loss of visual field and with reduction in visual acuity if the fovea is involved. Fundus signs of retinal edema with associated cotton-wool spots are limited to the area of retina supplied by the occluded vessel. Embolic causes are proportionately more common than in central retinal artery occlusion, and emboli are frequently identified on clinical examination (see Chapter 15). Migraine, oral contraceptive use, and vasculitis must also be considered.

CENTRAL RETINAL VEIN OCCLUSION

Central retinal vein occlusion is a common and easily diagnosed retinal vascular disorder with potentially

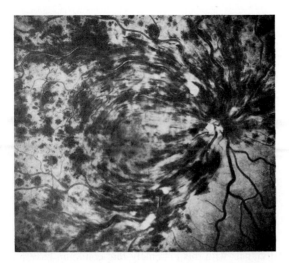

Figure 10–28. Central retinal vein occlusion with extensive superficial retinal hemorrhage obscuring macular and optic nerve detail.

blinding complications. The patient presents with sudden painless loss of vision. The clinical appearance varies from a few small scattered retinal hemorrhages and cotton-wool spots (Figure 10–28) to a marked hemorrhagic appearance with both deep and superficial retinal hemorrhage, which may rarely break through into the vitreous cavity. Most patients who develop the disease are over 50 years of age, and more than half have associated cardiovascular disease. Predisposing factors and their investigation are discussed in Chapter 15. Chronic open-angle glaucoma should always be excluded (see Chapter 11).

The two major complications associated with central retinal vein occlusion are reduced vision from macular edema and neovascular glaucoma secondary to iris neovascularization. Macular dysfunction occurs in almost all eyes with central vein occlusion. Although some eyes will show spontaneous improvement, most eyes will have persistent decreased central vision as a result of chronic macular edema. Nearly one-third of eyes with central retinal vein occlusion show significant retinal capillary nonperfusion on fluorescein angiography; one-half of these eyes will develop neovascular glaucoma.

Treatment

Panretinal laser photocoagulation is effective in prevention and treatment of neovascular glaucoma in eyes with ischemic central retinal vein occlusion. No treatment for macular edema resulting from central retinal vein occlusion has been proved effective to date; however, macular grid pattern laser photocoagulation may have a role in the treatment of this disease.

BRANCH RETINAL VEIN OCCLUSION

Branch retinal vein occlusion presents as sudden unilateral vision loss with segmentally distributed intraretinal hemorrhage. The vein occlusion always occurs at the site of an arteriovenous crossing (Figure 10–29), and retinal neovascularization may develop if the occlusion produces an area of retinal capillary nonperfusion that is more than 5 disk diameters in area. Sight-threatening complications of the disease are macular edema, macular ischemia, and vitreous hemorrhage from retinal neovascularization.

Treatment
Retinal laser photocoagulation has an important role in the treatment of this disease. When peripheral neovascularization is confirmed by fluorescein angiography, laser treatment can reduce the risk of vitreous hemorrhage by one-half. When vision loss due to macular edema persists for several months without spontaneous improvement, grid pattern argon laser macular photocoagulation is usually indicated. Anticoagulant therapy has not been shown to be beneficial in either the prevention or the management of branch retinal vein occlusion. Investigation for an underlying systemic cause is discussed in Chapter 15. Important associated ocular diseases are chronic open-angle glaucoma and uveitis secondary to Behçet's syndrome.

RETINAL ARTERIAL MACROANEURYSM

Retinal macroaneurysms are fusiform or round dilations of the retinal arterioles occurring within the first

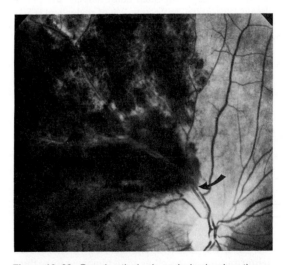

Figure 10–29. Branch retinal vein occlusion involves the superotemporal vein. The point of obstruction (arrow) is at an arteriovenous crossing.

three orders of arteriolar bifurcation. Most cases are unilateral, and the superotemporal artery is the most commonly involved vessel. Two-thirds of patients have associated systemic arterial hypertension.

The most common clinical symptom is loss of central vision as a result of retinal edema, exudation, or hemorrhage. Macroaneurysms may bleed into the subretinal space, into the retina, beneath the internal limiting membrane, or into the vitreous; the "hourglass" hemorrhage is typical and is due to bleeding beneath and anterior to the retina.

Although no clear indication for treatment with laser photocoagulation has been established, laser treatment of the macroaneurysm should be considered if lipid exudate coming from it threatens the fovea.

COLOR VISION DEFECTS

The perception of color is a cortical response to specific physical stimuli received by the retina. A narrow band of the electromagnetic spectrum, wavelengths between 400 and 700 nm, is capable of being absorbed by visual pigments contained in the outer segments of cone photoreceptors. As described above, spectral sensitivity studies of cone photopigments have identified blue, green, and red cone photoreceptors. A minimal requirement for color discrimination is the presence of at least two kinds of cone photopigment, and normal color vision requires the presence of all three. Color vision testing is described in Chapter 2. In a broad sense, color vision defects are either congenital or acquired. While hereditary congenital color defects are almost always "red-green," affecting 8% of males and 0.5 % of females, acquired defects are more often of the "blue-yellow" variety and affect males and females equally. Congenital color vision defects affect both eyes equally, while acquired color defects frequently affect one eye more than the other. Most congenital color vision defects are X-linked recessive and are constant in type and severity throughout life. Acquired color vision defects generally vary in type and severity, depending upon the location and source of the usually ophthalmoscopically observable ocular pathology.

Dichromats are individuals whose cone photoreceptors contain only two of the three cone photopigments. Persons with a red-green color deficiency related to red-sensitive pigment loss were historically described first, and the condition is therefore referred to as **protanopia.** A second type of red-green deficiency involving green-sensitive pigment loss is known as **deuteranopia.** Blue-yellow color blindness is the third form and is referred to as **tritanopia.** While a color vision defect is present, there is no acuity loss in these patients.

Based on a color matching classification, the most common color vision deficit is that of **anomalous trichromats.** These individuals require three primaries for matching an unknown color but—unlike normal **trichromats**—use them in "anomalous" amounts. Each of the anomalous trichromats has a defect analogous to that of the dichromats described above.

There are two forms of monochromatism, and although both leave the affected individual completely without color discrimination, they are two quite separate entities. In **rod monochromatism,** the individual is born without functioning cones in the retina, and such a loss accounts for the associated symptoms of low visual acuity, absent color vision, photophobia, and nystagmus. The generalized loss of cones in this condition is shown unequivocally by the photopic electroretinogram. In **cone monochromatism,** affected individuals with this extremely rare condition have no hue discrimination but do have normal acuity and no photophobia or nystagmus. Cone monochromats do have cone photoreceptors, but all the cones contain the same visual pigment.

II. INTRAOCULAR TUMORS

J. Brooks Crawford, MD

PRIMARY BENIGN INTRAOCULAR TUMORS

Retinal Angioma*
Retinal hemangiomas occur as isolated tumors or associated with cerebellar hemangioblastomas, pancreatic cysts and carcinomas, renal cysts and carcinomas, and pheochromocytomas in von Hippel-Lindau syndrome (Figure 10–30). The retinal tumors are pink or red, endophytic, and usually supplied by a large feeder vessel. Juxtapapillary tumors are usually exophytic. Vision is affected by bleeding or exudation from the tumor vessels. Photocoagulation, diathermy, and cryotherapy are used to treat the retinal lesions.

Astrocytic (Glial) Hamartomas
Astrocytic hamartomas are translucent to whitish retinal and optic nerve head tumors most frequently associated with tuberous sclerosis (Bourneville's disease) (Figure 10–31). They may also be associated with neurofibromatosis (Recklinghausen's disease) or occur as isolated findings. These tumors are congenital, but they may enlarge; they do not tend to become calcified or acquire a mulberry configuration until after the age of 8 years.

---

* See also Retinocerebellar Angiomatosis in Chapter 14.

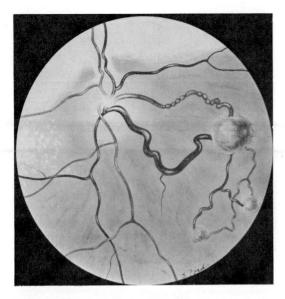

Figure 10–30. Angiomatosis retinae of Von Hippel-Lindau disease (drawing). (Courtesy of F Cordes.)

PRIMARY MALIGNANT TUMORS OF THE INTRAOCULAR STRUCTURES

Retinoblastoma
(Figure 10-32 to 10-34)

Retinoblastoma is a rare but life-endangering tumor of childhood. Two-thirds of cases appear before the end of the third year; rare cases have been reported at almost every age. The tumor is bilateral in about 30% of cases—these are the heritable cases. Retinoblastoma was formerly thought to result from mutation of an autosomal dominant gene, but it is now thought that an allele at a single locus within chromosomal band 13q14 controls both the heritable and nonheritable forms of

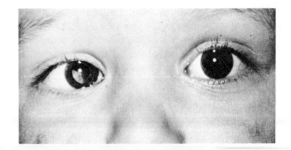

Figure 10–32. Retinoblastoma as viewed through the pupil.

the tumor. The normal retinoblastoma gene, present in every individual, is a suppressor gene or anti-oncogene. Individuals with the heritable form of the disease have one altered allele in every cell of the body; when the other allele in a developing retinal cell is affected by a spontaneous mutation, the tumor develops. In the nonheritable form of the disease, both alleles of the normal retinoblastoma gene in a developing retinal cell are inactivated by spontaneous mutation. Survivors of the heritable form of the disease (those 5% of new cases who had an affected parent or those who have had a germinal mutation) have almost a 50% chance of producing an affected child.

Retinoblastomas may grow outward (exophytic) or inward (endophytic). The latter then extend into the vitreous (Figure 10–33). Both types gradually fill the eye and extend through the optic nerve to the brain and along the emissary vessels and nerves in the sclera to the orbital tissues. Microscopically, most retinoblastomas are composed of small, closely packed, round or polygonal cells with large, darkly staining nuclei and scanty cytoplasm. They sometimes form characteristic Flexner-Wintersteiner rosettes, which are indicative of photoreceptor differentiation. Degenerative changes are frequent, accompanied by necrosis and calcification. A few spontaneous cures have been reported.

Retinoblastoma usually remains unnoticed until it has advanced far enough to produce a white pupil

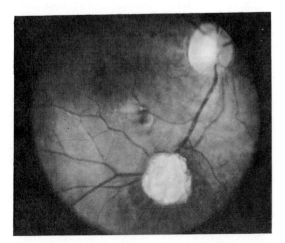

Figure 10–31. Retinal astrocytic hamartoma.

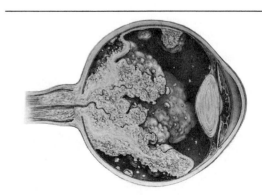

Figure 10–33. Endophytic retinoblastoma.

(leukocoria), strabismus, or inflammation. All children with strabismus or intraocular inflammation should be evaluated for the presence of retinoblastoma. The tumor is usually seen in the early stages only when sought for, as in children having a hereditary background or in cases where the other eye has been affected.

Retrolental fibroplasia, persistence of the primary vitreous, retinal dysplasia, Coats' disease, and nematode endophthalmitis may simulate retinoblastoma.

In general, the earlier the discovery and treatment of the tumor, the better the chance to prevent spread through the optic nerve and orbital tissues.

Enucleation is the treatment of choice for large retinoblastomas. Eyes with smaller tumors can be effectively treated with plaque or external beam radiotherapy (Figure 10–34), cryotherapy, or photocoagulation. Chemotherapy is occasionally necessary for recurrent disease, particularly to salvage the second eye of bilateral cases when the first eye has already been enucleated, and for metastatic disease.

Second primary malignant tumors, especially osteosarcomas, develop in a large number (estimates range

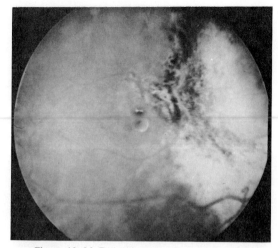

Figure 10–34. Retinoblastoma after radiotherapy.

from 20% to 90%) of survivors of bilateral retinoblastomas after a period of many years. These patients need to be carefully evaluated for the remainder of their lives.

REFERENCES

Retina & Retinal Disorders

Berson EL et al: A randomized trial of vitamin A and vitamin E supplementation for retinitis pigmentosa. Arch Ophthalmol 1993;111:761.

Byer NE: Long-term natural history of lattice degeneration of the retina. Ophthalmology 1989;96:1396.

Chan CK et al: The treatment of choroidal neovascular membranes by alpha interferon. Ophthalmology 1994; 101:289.

Cryotherapy for Retinopathy of Prematurity Cooperative Group: Multicenter trial of cryotherapy for retinopathy of prematurity. Arch Ophthalmol 1993;111:339.

Duane TD (editor): *Clinical Ophthalmology,* vol 3. Lippincott, 1987.

Early Treatment Diabetic Retinopathy Study Authors: Results from the Early Treatment Diabetic Retinopathy Study. Arch Ophthalmol 1991;85(Suppl 5):739.

Eye Disease Case-Control Study Group: Antioxidant status and neovascular age-related macular degeneration. Arch Ophthalmol 1993;111:104.

Flach AJ et al: Prophylaxis of aphakic cystoid macular edema without corticosteroids. Ophthalmology 1990;97:1253.

Flynn HW et al: Pars plana vitrectomy in the Early Treatment Diabetic Retinopathy Study. Ophthalmology 1992; 99:1351.

Freeman WR: Vitrectomy surgery for full-thickness macular holes. Am J Ophthalmol 1993;116:233.

Gass JDM: *Stereoscopic Atlas of Macular Diseases,* 3rd ed. 2 vols. Mosby, 1987.

Green WR, Enger C: Age-related macular degeneration histopathologic studies. Ophthalmology 1993;100: 1519.

Hayreh SS et al: Incidence of various types of retinal vein occlusion. Am J Ophthalmol 1994;117:429.

Hilton GF, McClean EB, Chuang EL: *Retinal Detachment,* 5th ed. American Academy of Ophthalmology, 1989.

Ho T et al: Vitrectomy in the management of diabetic eye disease. Surv Ophthalmol 1992;37:190.

Jiminez-Sierra J et al: *Inherited Retinal Diseases.* Mosby, 1989.

Klein R et al: The Wisconsin epidemiologic study of diabetic retinopathy. XIV: Ten-year incidence and progression of diabetic retinopathy. Arch Ophthalmol 1994;112:1217.

Macular Photocoagulation Study Group: Laser photocoagulation for juxtafoveal choroidal neovascularization. Arch Ophthalmol 1994;112:500.

Macular Photocoagulation Study Group: Visual outcome after laser photocoagulation for subfoveal choroidal neovascularization. Arch Ophthalmol 1994;112:480.

Moss SE, Klein R, Klein BEK: Ten-year incidence of visual loss in diabetic population. Ophthalmology 1994; 101:1061.

Moss SE et al: Ocular factors in the incidence and progression of diabetic retinopathy. Ophthalmology 1994;101:77.

Reichard P et al: The effect of long-term intensified insulin treatment on the development of microvascular complications of diabetes mellitus. N Engl J Med 1993;329:304.

Ryan SJ (editor): *Retina.* 3 vols. Mosby, 1989.

Ryan SJ: Traction retinal detachment. Am J Ophthalmol 1993;115:1.

Schaffer DB et al: Prognostic factors in the natural course of retinopathy of prematurity. Ophthalmology 1993; 100:230.

Smiddy WE et al: Results and complications in treated retinal breaks. Am J Ophthalmol 1991;112:623.

Smith R: Diabetes and retinal function. Br J Ophthalmol 1990;74:385.

Intraocular Tumors

Char DH: *Clinical Ocular Oncology.* Churchill Livingstone, 1989.

Gallie BL, Phillips RA: Retinoblastoma: A model of oncogenesis. Ophthalmology 1984;91:666.

Shields CL et al: Plaque radiotherapy in the management of retinoblastomas: Use as a primary and secondary treatment. Ophthalmology 1993;100:216.

Shields CL et al: Regression of retinoblastomas after plaque radiotherapy. Am J Ophthalmol 1993;115:181.

Singh AD et al: Relationship of regression pattern to recurrence in retinoblastoma. Br J Ophthalmol 1993; 77:12.

Spencer WH (editor): *Ophthalmic Pathology,* 3rd ed, 3 vols. Saunders, 1985.

11

Glaucoma

Daniel Vaughan, MD, & Paul Riordan-Eva, FRCS, FRCOphth

Glaucoma is characterized by elevated intraocular pressure associated with optic cupping and visual field loss. In the majority of cases, there is no associated ocular disease (primary glaucoma) (Table 11–1).

Almost 80,000 Americans are blind from glaucoma, making it the leading cause of preventable blindness in the United States. An estimated 2 million Americans have glaucoma. Primary open-angle glaucoma, the most common form, causes insidious asymptomatic progressive bilateral visual loss that is often not detected until extensive field loss has already occurred. Other forms of glaucoma are responsible for severe visual morbidity in individuals of all ages. Acute (angle-closure) glaucoma comprises 10–15% of cases in Caucasians. This percentage is higher in Asians, particularly among the Burmese and Vietnamese in southeast Asia.

The mechanism of raised intraocular pressure in glaucoma is impaired outflow of aqueous resulting from abnormalities within the drainage system of the anterior chamber angle (open-angle glaucoma) or impaired access of aqueous to the drainage system (closed-angle glaucoma) (Table 11–2). Treatment is directed toward reducing the intraocular pressure and, when possible, correcting the underlying pathogenesis.

Reducing aqueous production is a method of reducing intraocular pressure used in all forms of glaucoma. Several medications reduce aqueous production. Surgical procedures that reduce aqueous production are available but are generally used only after medical treatment has failed. Facilitating flow of aqueous through the trabecular meshwork is useful in open-angle glaucomas. Improving access of aqueous to the anterior chamber angle applies to closed-angle glaucoma when there is a reversible element of angle closure. This may be achieved by peripheral laser iridotomy if the cause is pupillary block, miosis if there is angle crowding, or cycloplegia if there is anterior lens displacement. Surgically bypassing the drainage system is useful in open-angle glaucoma and in angle closure that fails to respond to medical treatment. In the secondary glaucomas, consideration must always be given to treating the primary abnormality.

In all patients with glaucoma, the necessity for treatment and its effectiveness are assessed by regular determination of intraocular pressure (tonometry), inspection of optic disks, and measurement of visual fields.

The management of glaucoma is best left to the ophthalmologist, but the size of the problem and the importance of detecting asymptomatic cases call for the cooperation and assistance of all medical personnel. Ophthalmoscopy (noting optic nerve changes) and tonometry should be part of the routine physical examination of all patients old enough to cooperate and certainly all patients over 30 years of age. This is especially important in patients with a family history of glaucoma.

PHYSIOLOGY OF AQUEOUS HUMOR

The intraocular pressure is determined by the rate of aqueous production and the resistance to outflow of aqueous from the eye. Some knowledge of the physiology of aqueous humor is necessary for understanding glaucoma.

Composition of Aqueous

The aqueous is a clear liquid that fills the anterior and posterior chambers of the eye. Its volume is about 250 μL, and its rate of production, which is subject to diurnal variation, is 1.5–2 μL/min. The osmotic pressure is slightly higher than that of plasma. The composition of aqueous is similar to that of plasma except for much higher concentrations of ascorbate, pyruvate, and lactate and lower concentrations of protein, urea, and glucose.

Formation & Flow of Aqueous

Aqueous is produced by the ciliary body. An ultrafiltrate of plasma produced in the stroma of the ciliary processes is modified by the barrier function and secretory processes of the ciliary epithelium. Entering the posterior chamber, the aqueous passes through the pupil into the anterior chamber (Figure 11–1) and then to the trabecular meshwork in the anterior chamber

208

Table 11-1. Glaucoma classified according to etiology.

A. Primary glaucoma
1. Open-angle glaucoma
   a. Primary open-angle glaucoma (chronic open-angle glaucoma, chronic simple glaucoma)
   b. Normal-pressure glaucoma (low-pressure glaucoma)
2. Angle-closure glaucoma
   a. Acute
   b. Subacute
   c. Chronic
   d. Plateau iris

B. Congenital glaucoma
1. Primary congenital glaucoma
2. Glaucoma associated with other developmental ocular abnormalities
   a. Anterior chamber cleavage syndromes
      Axenfeld's syndrome
      Rieger's syndrome
      Peter's anomaly
   b. Aniridia
3. Glaucoma associated with extraocular developmental abnormalities
   a. Sturge-Weber syndrome
   b. Marfan's syndrome
   c. Neurofibromatosis
   d. Lowe's syndrome
   e. Congenital rubella

C. Secondary glaucoma
1. Pigmentary glaucoma
2. Exfoliation syndrome
3. Due to lens changes (phacogenic)
   a. Dislocation
   b. Intumescence
   c. Phacolytic
4. Due to uveal tract changes
   a. Uveitis
   b. Posterior synechiae (seclusio pupillae)
   c. Tumor
5. Iridocorneoendothelial (ICE) syndrome
6. Trauma
   a. Hyphema
   b. Angle contusion/recession
   c. Peripheral anterior synechiae
7. Postoperative
   a. Ciliary block glaucoma (malignant glaucoma)
   b. Peripheral anterior synechiae
   c. Epithelial downgrowth
   d. Following corneal graft surgery
   e. Following retinal detachment surgery
8. Neovascular glaucoma
   a. Diabetes mellitus
   b. Central retinal vein occlusion
   c. Intraocular tumor
9. Raised episcleral venous pressure
   a. Carotid-cavernous fistula
   b. Sturge-Weber syndrome
10. Steroid-induced

D. Absolute glaucoma: The end result of any uncontrolled glaucoma is a hard, sightless, and often painful eye.

Table 11-2. Glaucoma classified according to mechanism of intraocular pressure rise.

A. Open-angle glaucoma
1. Pretrabecular membranes: All of these may progress to angle-closure glaucoma due to contraction of the pretrabecular membranes.
   a. Neovascular glaucoma
   b. Epithelial downgrowth
   c. ICE syndrome
2. Trabecular abnormalities
   a. Primary open-angle glaucoma
   b. Congenital glaucoma
   c. Pigmentary glaucoma
   d. Exfoliation syndrome
   e. Steroid-induced glaucoma
   f. Hyphema
   g. Angle contusion or recession
   h. Iridocyclitis (uveitis)
   i. Phacolytic glaucoma
3. Posttrabecular abnormalities
   a. Raised episcleral venous pressure

B. Closed-angle glaucoma
1. Pupillary block (iris bombé)
   a. Primary angle-closure glaucoma
   b. Seclusio pupillae (posterior synechiae)
   c. Intumescent lens
   d. Anterior lens dislocation
   e. Hyphema
2. Anterior lens displacement
   a. Ciliary block glaucoma
   b. Central retinal vein occlusion
   c. Posterior scleritis
   d. Following retinal detachment surgery
3. Angle crowding
   a. Plateau iris
   b. Intumescent lens
   c. Mydriasis for fundal examination
4. Peripheral anterior synechiae
   a. Chronic angle closure
   b. Secondary to flat anterior chamber
   c. Secondary to iris bombé
   d. Contraction of pretrabecular membranes

Outflow of Aqueous

The trabecular meshwork is composed of beams of collagen and elastic tissue covered by trabecular cells that form a filter with a decreasing pore size as the canal of Schlemm is approached. Contraction of the ciliary muscle through its insertion into the trabecular meshwork increases pore size in the meshwork and hence the rate of aqueous drainage. Passage of aqueous into Schlemm's canal depends upon cyclic formation of transcellular channels in the endothelial lining. Efferent channels from Schlemm's canal (about 30 collector channels and 12 aqueous veins) conduct the fluid into the venous system. A small amount of aqueous leaves the eye between the bundles of the ciliary muscle and through the sclera (uveoscleral flow) (Figure 11-1).

The major resistance to aqueous outflow from the anterior chamber is the endothelial lining of Schlemm's canal and the adjacent portions of the trabecular meshwork—rather than the venous collector system. But the pressure in the episcleral venous net-

angle. During this period, there is some differential exchange of components with the blood in the iris.

Intraocular inflammation or trauma causes an increase in the protein concentration. This is called plasmoid aqueous and closely resembles blood serum.

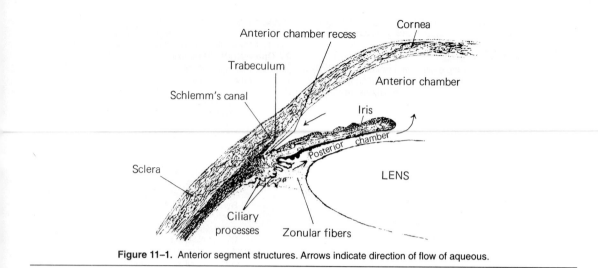

Figure 11–1. Anterior segment structures. Arrows indicate direction of flow of aqueous.

work determines the minimum level of intraocular pressure obtainable by medical therapy.

Pressure Dynamics*

Intraocular pressure is such an important feature of glaucoma that a review of pressure dynamics is desirable.

A. Pressure-Tension-Strain Relationships: The terms pressure, tension, and strain are frequently used interchangeably and are listed as synonyms in some dictionaries. However, the precise distinctions and interactions between these related but nonequivalent terms must be appreciated before pressure dynamics in glaucoma can be understood.

1. Pressure—Hydrostatic pressure is the force per unit area exerted by a fluid (gas or liquid) within a closed space. With the eye, as with other fluid-filled closed systems, the pressure force is exerted normal to the structural wall (the corneoscleral wall). Average pressure in the eye is about 14 mm Hg. For calculations, centimeters of water is a more convenient unit of pressure than millimeters of mercury. To convert millimeters of mercury to centimeters of water, multiply by 1.36. In more familiar terms, the average eye pressure is about 19 cm (7.5 inches) of water, or 0.25 psi (pounds per square inch). Glaucomatous damage usually begins at roughly double that value, and the eye ruptures at about 240 times average values.

Hydrostatic pressure per se causes no damage to the delicate neurons paralleling the scleral wall. A diver lying on the ocean bottom may be compared to a neuron lying on the uveoscleral bed. The diver will perceive no discomfort at a depth of 43 meters (141 feet) even through the pressure is about 3000 mm Hg, or approximately the pressure within an eye that results in rupture. The diver's body—though subjected to about 10

tons of hydrostatic pressure—will not be pushed against the ocean floor, and a neuron is not pushed against the sclera by hydrostatic pressure.

2. Tension (tensile stress)—A jack supporting a car is subjected to compressive stress. A towline pulling a car is subjected to tensile stress, or tension. Stresses are assigned a magnitude of force per unit area. Tensile stress, or the tension force vector, acts parallel to the scleral wall (attempting to pull the sclera apart). In the same way, the pressure of the abdomen at right angles to a belt is almost analogous to intraocular pressure, while the tension along the belt acting to pull the belt apart is analogous to scleral tension.

Trampolines and drumheads are examples of pure tension without pressure. The pressure is the same on either side of the tensed membrane. Tension levels in the sclera, cornea, and lamina cribrosa are not equal. The tension equation for thin-walled spheres can be used to obtain a close approximation of tensions in various parts of the corneoscleral wall. Tension in the sclera is directly proportionate to the intraocular pressure multiplied by the radius of curvature of the sclera and inversely proportionate to twice the thickness of the sclera:

$$\text{Tension} = \frac{\text{Pressure} \times \text{Radius}}{2 \times \text{Thickness}}$$

An inflated surgical glove or balloon (Figure 11–2) illustrates this relationship. The palm of the glove has relatively high tension and the thumb relatively low tension, though the pressure within the glove is equal at all locations. The thumb has low tension because the radius of curvature is small and the thickness large relative to the same factors at the palm. In the eye, tension is lower in the cornea or optic cup than in the sclera.

An eye under slowly increasing pressure usually ruptures beneath the lateral rectus where the sclera is thinner, as the tension equation would suggest. A pre-

*By Orson W. White, MD.

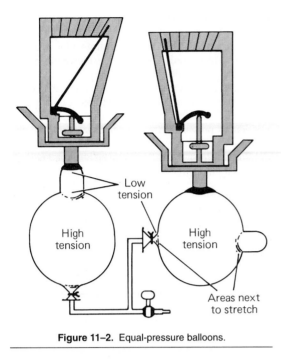

Figure 11–2. Equal-pressure balloons.

cipitous pressure rise due to trauma (eg, a blow from a club) frequently ruptures the eye at the limbus owing to the anvil effect of the more viscous vitreous.

3. Strain–Strain is stretch or displacement per unit length. A strain gauge measures displacement. Strain can result in damage and in the body can cause both pain and damage. Using the belt analogy, strain is the stretch per unit length of the belt resulting from the tension in the belt caused by the pressure of the abdomen.

To calculate the strain or stretch of a substance at a given pressure or tension, one of three moduli of elasticity is used. Each modulus is appropriate for a different type of structure. Thomas Young (1773–1829), an English physician, clarified these complex relationships as explained in the following paragraphs.

a. Young's modulus E–Young's modulus E is used for determining the elastic properties of structures such as cables, pressure vessels, submarines, biologic cells, unicellular organisms, *and eyes*. E is defined as the tension required to stretch a material of unit cross section to double its original length. This is represented by the following equation:

$$E = \frac{\text{Change in tension sclera}}{\text{Change in length of sclera per unit length}}$$

Thus, the stretch of the sclera per unit length (strain) is derived by dividing the change in tension of the sclera by Young's modulus of the sclera E.

b. Shear modulus G–Shear modulus G is used for determining the elastic properties of structures such

as drive shafts and bolts. G should not concern us in the discussion of elasticity of the eye. It is sometimes called the modulus of rigidity, and the unfortunate term "scleral rigidity" may have originated from inappropriate use of the shear modulus in ocular calculations.

c. Bulk modulus K–The bulk modulus K also should not concern us in our discussion of elasticity of the eye. But bulk modulus is the hydrostatic pressure (compressive stress) required to compress (strain) a solid material to half its original volume.

The empirical "scleral rigidity" equation found in some glaucoma literature resembles the bulk modulus equation. However, using the bulk modulus for the eye would be valid only if the eye were solid sclera and subjected to external hydrostatic pressure. However, the eye is a nearly spherical shell of elastic sclera filled with fluid under pressure and is therefore appropriately described only by Young's modulus, as are other thin-walled pressure vessels.

The belt analogy may now be used to illustrate the way in which neurons are damaged in glaucoma. Envision a very obese person wearing a large belt (sclera) with a delicate cloth liner (neurons). After fasting for several days, the obese subject feasts heavily, with the result that there is some ripping of the delicate cloth liner. The progression of the damage process is as follows: (1) The expanding abdomen (intraocular pressure) exerts gentle pressure at right angles to the belt, producing a summation tension parallel to the belt (sclera), tending to pull the belt apart. (2) The tension leads to stretching (strain) of the belt, following the rules of Young's modulus. (3) The stretching (strain) results in damage to the delicate cloth liner (neurons).

B. Devices for Measuring Ocular Tension and Pressure: The Goldmann applanation tonometer is designed to measure intraocular pressure, with results recorded in millimeters of mercury. The Schiotz device is a true tonometer, measuring primarily tension. Recordings should be in tension units or scale units, as originally proposed by Schiotz, but they are commonly converted to millimeters of mercury (which is a pressure unit, not a tension unit).

PATHOLOGY OF GLAUCOMA

The pathophysiology of intraocular pressure elevation—whether due to open-angle or to angle-closure mechanisms—will be discussed as each disease entity is considered (see below). The effects of raised intraocular pressure within the eye are common to all forms of glaucoma, their manifestations being influenced by the time course and magnitude of the rise in intraocular pressure.

The major mechanism of visual loss in glaucoma is diffuse ganglion cell atrophy, leading to thinning of the inner nuclear and nerve fiber layers of the retina and axonal loss in the optic nerve. The optic disk becomes atrophic, with enlargement of the optic cup (see below). The iris and ciliary body also become atrophic, and the ciliary processes show hyaline degeneration.

In acute angle-closure glaucoma, the intraocular pressure reaches 60–80 mm Hg, resulting in ischemic damage to the iris with associated corneal edema.

CLINICAL ASSESSMENT IN GLAUCOMA

Tonometry

Tonometry is the generic name for measurement of intraocular pressure. The most widely used instrument is the Goldmann applanation tonometer, which is attached to the slitlamp and measures the force required to flatten a fixed area of the cornea. Other applanation tonometers are the Perkins tonometer and the Tono-Pen, both of which are portable; the pneumatotonometer, which is useful when the cornea has an irregular surface and can be used with a soft contact lens in place. The Schiotz tonometer is portable and measures the corneal indentation produced by a known weight. (For further discussion of tonometry, see Chapter 2; for tonometer disinfection techniques, see Chapter 22).

The normal range of intraocular pressure is 10–24 mm Hg. A single normal reading does not rule out glaucoma. In primary open-angle glaucoma, many affected individuals will have a normal intraocular pressure when first measured. Conversely, isolated raised intraocular pressure does not necessarily mean that the patient has primary open-angle glaucoma, since other evidence in the form of a glaucomatous optic disk or visual field changes is necessary for diagnosis. If the intraocular pressure is consistently elevated in the presence of normal optic disks and visual fields (ocular hypertension), the patient may be observed periodically as a glaucoma suspect.

Gonioscopy
(See Chapter 2.)

The anterior chamber angle is formed by the junction of the peripheral cornea and the iris, between which lies the trabecular meshwork (Figure 11–3). The configuration of this angle—ie, whether it is wide (open), narrow, or closed—has an important bearing on the outflow of aqueous. The anterior chamber angle width can be estimated by oblique illumination of the anterior chamber with a penlight (Figure 11–4) or by slitlamp observation of the depth of the peripheral anterior chamber, but it is best determined by gonioscopy, which allows direct visualization of the angle structures (Figure 11–3). If it is possible to visualize the full extent of the trabecular meshwork, the scleral spur, and the iris processes, the angle is open. Being able to see only Schwalbe's line or a small portion of the trabecular meshwork means that the angle is narrow. Being unable to see Schwalbe's line means that the angle is closed.

Factors determining the configuration of the anterior chamber angle are the shape of the cornea—large myopic eyes have wide angles and small hyperme-

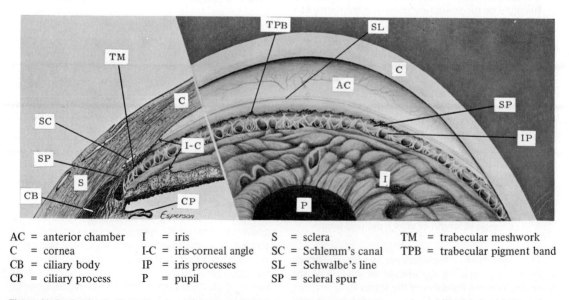

AC = anterior chamber	I = iris	S = sclera	TM = trabecular meshwork
C = cornea	I-C = iris-corneal angle	SC = Schlemm's canal	TPB = trabecular pigment band
CB = ciliary body	IP = iris processes	SL = Schwalbe's line	
CP = ciliary process	P = pupil	SP = scleral spur	

Figure 11–3. Composite illustration showing anatomic *(left)* and gonioscopic *(right)* view of normal anterior chamber angle. (Courtesy of R Shaffer.)

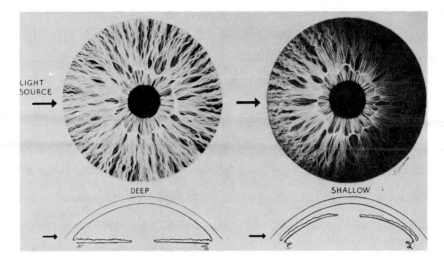

LIGHT
SOURCE

DEEP

SHALLOW

Figure 11–4. Estimation of depth of anterior chamber by oblique illumination (diagram). (Courtesy of R Shaffer.)

tropic eyes narrow ones. Enlargement of the lens with age tends to narrow the angle. Large myopic eyes have wide angles and small hyperopic eyes have narrow angles. Enlargement of the lens with age narrows the angle. This may account for the increased incidence of angle-closure glaucoma.

Myopic eyes have wide anterior chamber angles and hyperopic eyes have comparatively narrow ones. Enlargement of the lens with age tends to narrow the angle. Race is also a factor. The angles of Southeast Asians are much narrower than those of Caucasians.

Optic Disk Assessment

The normal optic disk has a central depression—the physiologic cup—whose size depends on the bulk of the fibers that form the optic nerve relative to the size of the scleral opening through which they must pass. In hypermetropic eyes, the scleral opening is small, and thus the optic cup is small; the reverse is true in myopic eyes. Glaucomatous optic atrophy produces specific disk changes characterized chiefly by loss of disk substance—detectable as enlargement of the optic disk cup—associated with disk pallor in the area of cupping. Other forms of optic atrophy cause widespread pallor without increased disk cupping.

Initially in glaucoma, there is concentric enlargement of the optic cup followed by preferential superior and inferior cupping with focal notching of the rim of the optic disk. The optic cup also increases in depth as the lamina cribrosa is displaced backward. As cupping develops, the retinal vessels on the disk are displaced nasally (Figure 11–5). The end result of glaucomatous cupping is the so-called "bean pot" cup in which no neural rim tissue is apparent (Figures 11–6 and 11–7).

The "cup-disk ratio" is a useful way of recording the size of the optic disk in glaucoma patients. It is the ratio of cup size to disk diameter, eg, a small cup is 0.1 and a large cup 0.9. In the presence of elevated intraocular pressure, a cup-disk ratio greater than 0.5 or significant asymmetry between the two eyes is highly suggestive of glaucomatous atrophy.

Clinical assessment of the optic disk can be performed by direct ophthalmoscopy or by examination with the 70-diopter lens, the Hruby lens, or special corneal contact lenses that give a three-dimensional view.

Other clinical evidence of neuronal damage in glaucoma is atrophy of the nerve fiber layer. This is detectable (Hoyt's sign) by ophthalmoscopy—particularly when red-free light is used—and precedes the development of optic disk changes.

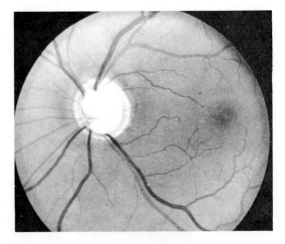

Figure 11–5. Typical glaucomatous cupping. Note the nasal displacement of the vessels and hollowed-out appearance of the optic disk except for a thin border. (Courtesy of S Mettier Jr.)

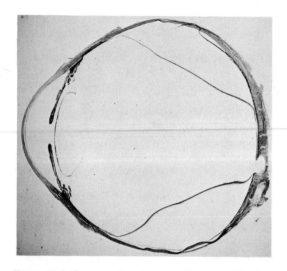

Figure 11–6. Cross-section of an eye with open-angle glaucoma. Note open anterior chamber angle (peripheral iris is not in contact with the posterior corneal surface). Deep glaucomatous cupping ("bean-pot" appearance) shows the process to be well advanced. (Courtesy of R Carriker.)

rum's area of the visual field—at 15 degrees from fixation—produces a Bjerrum scotoma and then an arcuate scotoma. Focal areas of more pronounced loss within Bjerrum's area are known as Seidel scotomas. Double arcuate scotomas—above and below the horizontal meridian—are often accompanied by a nasal step (of Roenne) because of differences in size of the two arcuate defects. Peripheral field loss tends to start in the nasal periphery as a constriction of the isopters. Subsequently, there may be connection to an arcuate defect, producing peripheral breakthrough. The temporal peripheral field and the central 5–10 degrees are affected late in the disease. Central visual acuity is not a reliable index of progress of the disease. In end-stage disease, there may be normal central acuity but only 5 degrees of visual field in each eye. In advanced glaucoma, the patient may have 20/20 visual acuity and be legally blind.

Various ways of testing the visual fields in glaucoma include the tangent screen, Goldmann perimeter, Friedmann field analyzer, and automated perimeter. (For technique and other details, see Chapter 2.)

Visual Field Examination

Regular visual field examination is essential to the diagnosis and follow-up of glaucoma. Glaucomatous field loss is not in itself specific, since it consists of nerve fiber bundle defects that may be seen in any form of optic nerve disease; but the pattern of field loss, the nature of its progression, and the correlation with changes in the optic disk are characteristic of the disease.

Glaucomatous field loss chiefly involves the central 30 degrees of field (Figure 11–8). The earliest change is baring of the blind spot. Contiguous extension into Bjer-

TREATMENT OF GLAUCOMA

MEDICAL TREATMENT

Suppression of Aqueous Production

Topical **beta-adrenergic blocking agents** are now the most widely used form of glaucoma therapy. They may be used alone or in combination with other drugs.

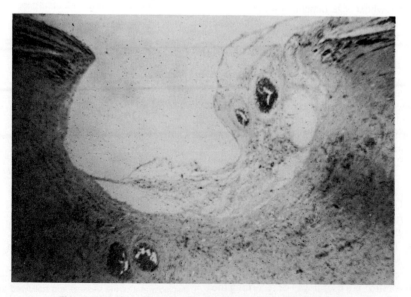

Figure 11–7. Glaucomatous ("bean-pot") cupping of the optic disk.

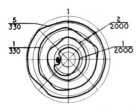

Baring of the blind spot. The earliest nerve fiber bundle defect.

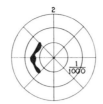

Incipient double nerve fiber bundle defect (Bjerrum scotoma).

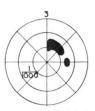

Bjerrum scotoma isolated from blind spot.

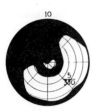

End stages in glaucoma field loss. Remnant of central field still shows nasal step.

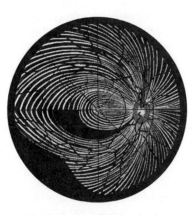

The basic visual field loss in glaucoma is the nerve fiber bundle defect with nasal step and peripheral nasal depression. It is here shown superimposed upon the nerve fiber layer of the retina and the retinal vascular tree. All perimetric changes in glaucoma are variations of these fundamental defects.

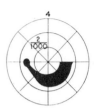

Fully developed nerve fiber bundle defect with nasal step (arcuate scotoma).

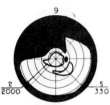

Peripheral depression with double nerve fiber bundle defect. Isolation of central field.

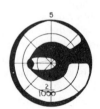

Double arcuate scotoma with peripheral breakthrough and nasal step.

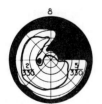

Nasal depression connected with arcuate scotoma. Nasal step of Rönne.

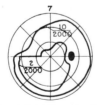

Peripheral breakthrough of large nerve fiber bundle defect with well developed nasal step.

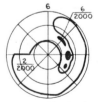

Seidel scotoma. Islands of greater visual loss within a nerve fiber bundle defect.

Figure 11–8. Visual field changes in glaucoma. (Reproduced, with permission, from Harrington DO: *The Visual Fields: A Textbook and Atlas of Clinical Perimetry,* 5th ed. Mosby, 1981.)

Timolol maleate 0.25% and 0.5%, betaxolol 0.25% and 0.5%, levobunolol 0.25% and 0.5%, and metipranolol 0.3% are the currently available preparations. The major contraindications to their use are chronic obstructive airways disease—particularly asthma—and cardiac conduction defects. In the case of betaxolol, the relative β_1-receptor selectivity—and the overall low affinity for all β receptors—account for a reduced but still significant risk of these systemic side-effects. Depression, confusion, and fatigue may occur with the topical beta-blocking agents.

Apraclonidine is a new α_2-adrenergic agonist that decreases aqueous humor formation without effect on outflow. **Epinephrine** and **dipivefrin** have some effect on aqueous production (see below).

Systemic **carbonic anhydrase inhibitors**—acetazolamide is the most widely used, but dichlorphenamide and methazolamide are alternatives—are used in chronic glaucoma when topical therapy is insufficient and in acute glaucoma when very high intraocular pressure needs to be controlled quickly. They are capable of suppressing aqueous production by 40–60%. Acetazolamide can be administered orally in a dosage of 125–250 mg up to four times daily or as Diamox Sequels 500 mg once or twice daily, or it can be given intravenously (500 mg). The carbonic anhydrase inhibitors are associated with major systemic side effects that limit their usefulness for long-term therapy.

Topical carbonic anhydrase inhibitors are being developed and show promise in having a beneficial effect with reduced systemic side effects.

Hyperosmotic agents influence aqueous production as well as dehydrating the vitreous body (see below).

Facilitation of Aqueous Outflow

Parasympathomimetic agents increase aqueous outflow by action on the trabecular meshwork through contraction of the ciliary muscle. The drug of choice is pilocarpine, 0.5–6% solution instilled several times a day, or 4% gel instilled at bedtime. Carbachol 0.75–3% is an alternative cholinergic agent. Irreversible anticholinesterase agents are the longest-acting parasympathomimetics available. These include demecarium bromide, 0.125% and 0.25%, and echothiophate iodide, 0.03–0.25%, which are generally restricted to aphakic or pseudophakic patients because of their cataractogenic potential. *Caution:* The irreversible anticholinesterase agents will potentiate succinylcholine administered during anesthesia, and anesthetists must be appropriately warned prior to surgery. These agents also produce extreme miosis that can lead to angle closure in patients with narrow angles. Patients must also be warned about the possibility of retinal detachment.

All parasympathomimetic agents produce miosis with dimness of vision, particularly in patients with cataract, and accommodative spasm that may be disabling to younger patients. Retinal detachment is a serious but uncommon occurrence.

Epinephrine, 0.25–2% instilled once or twice daily, increases aqueous outflow with some decrease in aqueous production. There are a number of external ocular side effects, including reflex conjunctival vasodilation, adrenochrome deposits, follicular conjunctivitis, and allergic reactions. Potential intraocular side effects are cystoid macular edema in aphakes and optic nerve head vasoconstriction. **Dipivefrin** is a prodrug of epinephrine that is metabolized intraocularly to its active state. Neither epinephrine nor dipivefrin should be used in eyes with narrow anterior chamber angles.

Reduction of Vitreous Volume

Hyperosmotic agents render the blood hypertonic, thus drawing water out of the vitreous and causing it to shrink. This is in addition to decreasing aqueous production. Reduction in vitreous volume is helpful in the treatment of acute angle-closure glaucoma and in malignant glaucoma when anterior displacement of the crystalline lens (caused by volume changes in the vitreous or choroid) produces angle closure (secondary angle-closure glaucoma).

Oral **glycerin (glycerol),** 1 mL/kg of body weight in a cold 50% solution mixed with lemon juice, is the most commonly used agent, but it should be used with care in diabetics. Alternatives are oral isosorbide and intravenous urea or mannitol (see Chapter 3 for dosages).

Miotics, Mydriatics, & Cycloplegics

Constriction of the pupil is fundamental to the management of primary angle-closure glaucoma and the angle crowding of plateau iris. Pupillary dilation is important in the treatment of angle closure secondary to iris bombé due to posterior synechiae.

When angle closure is secondary to anterior lens displacement, cycloplegics (cyclopentolate and atropine) are used to relax the ciliary muscle and thus tighten the zonular apparatus in an attempt to draw the lens backward.

SURGICAL & LASER TREATMENT

Peripheral Iridotomy & Iridectomy

Pupillary block is most satisfactorily overcome by forming a direct communication between the anterior and posterior chambers that removes the pressure difference between them. This can be achieved with the neodymium:YAG or argon laser (peripheral iridotomy) or by surgical peripheral iridectomy. Although more convenient to perform, laser treatment requires a relatively clear cornea and may produce a major rise in intraocular pressure, particularly if there is extensive synechial angle closure. Surgical peripheral iridotomy probably has a more guaranteed long-term success rate but has the potential for significant intraoperative and postoperative complications. YAG laser iridotomy is the essence of prevention when used in narrow angles prior to closure attacks.

Laser Trabeculoplasty

Application of laser (usually argon) burns via a goniolens to the trabecular meshwork facilitates aqueous outflow by virtue of its effects on the trabecular meshwork and Schlemm's canal or cellular events that enhance the function of the meshwork. The technique is applicable to many forms of open-angle glaucoma, and the results are variable depending upon the underlying cause. The pressure reduction usually allows decrease of medical therapy and postponement of glaucoma surgery. Treatments can be repeated (see Chapter 25). Recent studies suggest a role for laser trabeculoplasty in the initial treatment of primary open-angle glaucoma.

Glaucoma Drainage Surgery

Surgery to bypass the normal drainage mechanisms, allowing direct access of aqueous from the anterior chamber to the subconjunctival or orbital tissues, can be achieved by trabeculectomy or insertion of a drainage tube. Trabeculectomy has largely replaced full-thickness drainage procedures (eg, trephine, thermal sclerostomy, posterior lip sclerectomy). The major complication of trabeculectomy is bleb failure due to fibrosis in the episcleral tissues. This is more likely to occur in young patients, blacks, and patients who have previously undergone glaucoma drainage surgery or other surgery involving the episcleral tissues. Adjunctive treatment with antimetabolites such as fluorouracil and mitomycin is helpful in reducing the risk of bleb failure.

Implantation of a silicone tube to form a permanent conduit for aqueous flow out of the eye is an alternative procedure for eyes that have had unsuccessful trabeculectomy or are unlikely to respond to trabeculectomy. Patients in the latter group are chiefly those with secondary glaucomas, particularly neovascular glaucoma, glaucoma associated with uveitis, and glaucoma following corneal graft surgery.

Holmium laser sclerostomy is a new procedure that shows promise as an alternative to trabeculectomy.

Goniotomy is a useful technique in treating primary congenital glaucoma, in which there appears to be an obstruction to aqueous drainage in the internal portion of the trabecular meshwork.

Cyclodestructive Procedures

Failure of medical and surgical treatment may lead to consideration of laser or surgical destruction of the ciliary body to control intraocular pressure. Cryotherapy, diathermy, high-frequency ultrasound, and, most recently, thermal mode neodymium:YAG laser therapy can all be applied to the surface of the eye just posterior to the limbus to cause destruction of the underlying ciliary body. Transpupillary and transvitreal delivery of argon laser energy directly to the ciliary processes is also being developed. All cyclodestructive techniques may cause phthisis and should be reserved for the treatment of intractable glaucoma.

PRIMARY GLAUCOMA

PRIMARY OPEN-ANGLE GLAUCOMA

Primary open-angle glaucoma is the most common form of glaucoma. About 0.4–0.7% of persons over age 40 and 2–3% of persons over age 70 are estimated to have primary open-angle glaucoma. The disease is three times more common and generally more aggressive in blacks. There is a strong familial tendency in primary open-angle glaucoma, and close relatives of affected individuals should undergo regular screening.

The chief pathologic feature of primary open-angle glaucoma is a degenerative process in the trabecular meshwork, including deposition of extracellular material within the meshwork and beneath the endothelial lining of Schlemm's canal. This differs from the normal aging process. The consequence is a reduction in aqueous drainage leading to a rise in intraocular pressure.

Raised intraocular pressure precedes optic disk and visual field changes by many years. Although there is a clear association between the level of intraocular pressure and the severity of visual loss, there is great variability between individuals in the effect on the optic nerve of a particular level of pressure. Some people tolerate elevated intraocular pressure without developing disk or field changes (ocular hypertension; see below); others develop glaucomatous changes with consistently "normal" intraocular pressure (low-pressure glaucoma; see below).

The mechanism of neuronal damage in primary open-angle glaucoma and its relationship to the level of intraocular pressure is much debated. The major theories implicate intraocular pressure-dependent changes in the structural supportive elements in the optic nerve at the level of the lamina cribrosa or in the vascular supply to the optic nerve head.

Higher levels of intraocular pressure are associated with greater field loss at presentation. When there is glaucomatous field loss on first examination, the risk of further progression is much greater. Since intraocular pressure is the only treatable risk factor, it remains the focus of therapy. There is strong evidence that control of intraocular pressure slows disk damage and field loss.

In the patient with extensive disk changes or field loss, it is advisable to reduce the intraocular pressure as much as possible, whereas a patient with only a suspicion of disk or field changes may need less vigorous treatment. In all cases, the inconveniences and possible complications of treatment must be considered. Many glaucoma patients are old and frail and may not tolerate vigorous treatment. In order to gain a perspective on the need for treatment, an initial period of observation without treatment may be necessary to determine the rate of progression of disk and field changes. There is no justification for subjecting an elderly patient to extremes of treatment when the likelihood of their developing significant visual loss during their lifetime is small.

Diagnosis

The diagnosis of primary open-angle glaucoma is established when glaucomatous optic disk or field changes are associated with elevated intraocular pressures, a normal-appearing open anterior chamber angle, and no other reason for intraocular pressure elevation. Approximately 50% of patients with primary open-angle glaucoma have a normal intraocular pressure when first examined, so repeated tonometry is necessary prior to diagnosis.

Screening for Glaucoma

The major problem in detection of primary open-angle glaucoma is the absence of symptoms until relatively late in the disease. When patients first notice field loss, substantial glaucomatous cupping has already occurred. If treatment is to be successful, it must be started early in the disease, and this depends upon an active screening program. Unfortunately, specifically organized screening programs are plagued by the unreliability of a single intraocular pressure measurement in the detection of primary open-angle glaucoma and the complexities of relying on optic disk or visual field changes. Oculokinetic perimetry is a new technique that may offer a solution to this problem. At present it is necessary to rely for early diagnosis on regular ophthalmic assessment of relatives of affected individuals and on optic disk examination and tonometry becoming part of the routine physical of all adults over 30.

Treatment

Treatment is usually begun with topical beta-adrenergic blocking agents unless they are contraindicated. Epinephrine (or dipivefrin) and pilocarpine are the major alternatives. The usefulness of combining the various drug groups is debated. The combination of a beta-blocker and pilocarpine is certainly valuable. Laser trabeculoplasty has recently been reported as a possible initial treatment prior to starting any medical therapy.

If the intraocular pressure is not sufficiently controlled with topical therapy, laser trabeculoplasty may be helpful. Drainage surgery is held in reserve. Oral acetazolamide is usually employed only until these procedures have been undertaken or in the long-term management of patients unsuitable for surgery.

Cataract surgery will occasionally produce a significant improvement in intraocular pressure control and may be considered a therapeutic option if there is sufficient lens opacification or angle narrowing to justify it. But cataract surgery may also produce a transient rise in intraocular pressure that may be dangerous in the presence of poorly controlled intraocular pressure or extensive field loss. Combining trabeculectomy with cataract surgery may then be necessary.

Patients must be educated to understand that the treatment of primary open-angle glaucoma is a lifelong process and that regular reassessment by an ophthalmologist is essential.

Course & Prognosis

Without treatment, open-angle glaucoma may be insidiously progressive to complete blindness. If antiglaucoma drops control the intraocular pressure in an eye that has not suffered extensive glaucomatous damage, the prognosis is good (though visual field loss may progress in spite of normalized intraocular pressure). When the process is detected early, most glaucoma patients can be successfully managed medically.

NORMAL-PRESSURE GLAUCOMA (Low-Pressure Glaucoma)

A minority of patients with glaucomatous optic disk or visual field changes have an intraocular pressure consistently below 22 mm Hg. These patients have normal- or low-pressure glaucoma. The pathogenesis involves an abnormal sensitivity to intraocular pressure because of vascular or mechanical abnormalities at the optic nerve head. Disk hemorrhages are more frequently seen in normal-pressure than in primary open-angle glaucoma and often herald progression of field loss.

Before the diagnosis of low-pressure glaucoma can be established, a number of entities must be excluded:

(1) Prior episode of raised intraocular pressure, such as caused by iridocyclitis, trauma, or topical steroid therapy.

(2) Large diurnal variation in intraocular pressure with significant elevations, usually early in the morning.

(3) Postural changes in intraocular pressure with a marked elevation when lying flat.

(4) Intermittent elevations of intraocular pressure such as in subacute angle closure.

(5) Other causes of optic disk and field changes, including congenital disk abnormalities and acquired optic atrophy due to tumors or vascular disease.

OCULAR HYPERTENSION

Ocular hypertension is elevated intraocular pressure without disk or field abnormalities and is more common than primary open-angle glaucoma. The rate at which such individuals develop glaucoma is approximately 5–10 per 1000 per year. The risk increases with increasing intraocular pressure, increasing age, a positive family history for glaucoma, myopia, diabetes mellitus, and cardiovascular disease. It is also increased in blacks. The development of disk hemorrhages in a patient with ocular hypertension also indicates an increased risk for development of glaucoma.

Patients with ocular hypertension are considered glaucoma suspects and should undergo regular monitoring (one to three times a year) of the optic disk, intraocular pressure, and visual fields.

PRIMARY ACUTE ANGLE-CLOSURE GLAUCOMA

Primary acute angle-closure glaucoma occurs when sufficient iris bombé develops to cause occlusion of the anterior chamber angle by the peripheral iris. This blocks aqueous outflow and the intraocular pressure rises rapidly, causing severe pain, redness, and blurring of vision. Angle-closure glaucoma occurs in eyes with preexisting anatomic narrowing of the anterior chamber angle (found mainly in hypermetropes). The acute attack generally occurs in older patients when there has been enlargement of the crystalline lens associated with aging. In angle-closure glaucoma, the pupil is middilated, with associated pupillary block. This usually occurs in the evenings, when the level of illumination is reduced. It may also occur with pupillary dilation for ophthalmoscopy. If pupillary dilation is necessary in a patient with a shallow anterior chamber (easily detected by oblique illumination from a penlight [Figure 11–4] and then confirmed by gonioscopy), it is best to rely on the short-acting agent tropicamide and observe the patient carefully.

Clinical Findings

Acute angle-closure glaucoma is characterized by a sudden onset of severe blurring followed by excruciating pain, halos, and nausea and vomiting. Other findings include markedly increased intraocular pressure, a shallow anterior chamber, a steamy cornea, a fixed, moderately dilated pupil, and ciliary injection. It is important to perform gonioscopy on the fellow eye.

Differential Diagnosis

Acute iritis causes more photophobia than acute glaucoma. Intraocular pressure is usually not elevated; the pupil is constricted; and the cornea is usually not edematous. Marked flare and cells are present in the anterior chamber, and there is deep ciliary injection.

In acute conjunctivitis, there is little or no pain and no visual loss. There is discharge from the eye and an intensely inflamed conjunctiva but no ciliary injection. The pupillary responses and intraocular pressure are normal, and the cornea is clear.

Secondary acute angle-closure glaucoma may occur from anterior displacement of the lens-iris diaphragm associated with volume changes in the posterior segment of the eye. This may be seen in central retinal vein occlusion, in posterior scleritis, and after therapeutic procedures such as panretinal photocoagulation, retinal cryotherapy, and scleral buckling for retinal detachment. The clinical setting usually provides the diagnosis. Treatment is aimed at reducing the intraocular pressure with acetazolamide, topical beta-blockers, and hyperosmotic agents together with intensive cycloplegia (cyclopentolate and atropine) to encourage retrodisplacement of the lens through tightening of the zonular apparatus. This contrasts with the miotic therapy necessary in primary acute angle-closure glaucoma.

Complications & Sequelae

If treatment is delayed, the peripheral iris may adhere to the trabecular meshwork (anterior synechiae), producing irreversible occlusion of the anterior chamber angle requiring surgery. Optic nerve damage is common.

Treatment

Acute angle-closure glaucoma is an ophthalmic emergency!

Treatment is initially directed at reducing the intraocular pressure. Intravenous and oral acetazolamide—supplemented with hyperosmotic agents and topical beta-blockers—will usually reduce the intraocular pressure. Pilocarpine 4% can then be used intensively, eg, 1 drop every 15 minutes for 1–2 hours. Epinephrine must not be used because it will accentuate angle closure. Topical steroids in high doses are probably helpful to reduce the degree of damage to the iris and trabecular meshwork. A systemic analgesic may be necessary.

Once the intraocular pressure is under control, peripheral iridectomy should be undertaken to form a permanent connection between the anterior and posterior chambers, thus preventing recurrence of iris bombé. This is most often done with the neodymium:YAG laser, though the argon laser can also be used. Surgical peripheral iridectomy is indicated if laser treatment is unsuccessful.

If it is not possible to control the intraocular pressure medically, an emergency trabeculectomy or holmium laser sclerostomy is indicated. Preoperative intravenous mannitol is essential to lower the intraocular pressure as much as possible.

In all cases, the fellow eye should undergo prophylactic laser iridotomy.

SUBACUTE ANGLE-CLOSURE GLAUCOMA

The same etiologic factors operate in subacute as in acute angle-closure glaucoma except that episodes of elevated intraocular pressure are of short duration and are recurrent. The episodes of angle closure resolve spontaneously, but there is accumulated damage to the anterior chamber angle, with the formation of peripheral anterior synechiae. Occasionally, subacute angle closure will progress to acute closure.

The key to diagnosis is in the history. There will be recurrent short episodes of unilateral pain, redness, and blurring of vision associated with halos around lights. The attacks often occur in the evenings and resolve overnight. Examination between attacks may show only a narrow anterior chamber angle. The dark room provocative test can help identify which patients with narrow angles are at risk for the development of angle-closure glaucoma. In more advanced cases, there will be patchy peripheral anterior synechiae and chronically elevated intraocular pressure.

Treatment is similar to that of primary angle-closure glaucoma.

CHRONIC ANGLE-CLOSURE GLAUCOMA

A small number of patients with the predisposition to a anterior chamber angle closure never develop episodes of acute rise in intraocular pressure but form increasingly extensive peripheral anterior synechiae accompanied by a gradual rise in intraocular pressure. These patients present in the same way as those with primary open-angle glaucoma, often with extensive visual field loss in both eyes. Occasionally, they have attacks of subacute angle closure.

On examination, there is elevated intraocular pressure, narrow anterior chamber angles with variable amounts of peripheral anterior synechiae, and optic disk and visual field changes.

Once again, peripheral iridectomy is an important component of treatment. (Laser iridotomy in these patients is prone to produce a marked rise in intraocular pressure.) Intraocular pressure is then controlled medically if possible, but the extent of peripheral anterior synechia formation and sluggish outflow through the remaining trabecular meshwork make pressure control very difficult, so that drainage surgery is often required. Epinephrine and strong miotics must not be used unless there is a patent peripheral iridectomy because they will accentuate angle closure.

GLAUCOMA IN VIETNAMESE-AMERICANS

Glaucoma is different in most Asian than Caucasian populations because the anterior chamber angles of Asians are narrower. This is particularly true of Vietnamese people.

In a survey of 470 Vietnamese attending a health fair in San Jose, California, we found 94 (20%) with narrow angles. The mean age in this group was 55 years. Some of these individuals had closed angles when examined by gonioscopy but normal intraocular pressures, a condition seen much less commonly in Caucasians. In an associated study, 38 of 40 Vietnamese-American glaucoma patients (90%) had narrow angles.

Shiu Kwok in San Francisco studied 146 Chinese-American glaucoma patients and reported 74 open angles and 72 narrow angles—ie, 50% of the glaucoma patients had narrow anterior chamber angles.

Available information indicates that only 7–15% of Japanese and Filipino glaucoma patients have narrow anterior chamber angles—a rate similar to that of Caucasian patients.

The conclusion suggested by these scattered surveys is that with the growing significance of Asian societies in the world economy, persons of Asian ancestry will become the subjects of further large-scale studies and the objects of educational campaigns aimed at bringing more of them into the medical systems of their communities for early diagnosis and treatment of glaucoma before painful and sight-destroying attacks of angle-closure glaucoma occur.

PLATEAU IRIS

Plateau iris is an uncommon condition in which the central anterior chamber depth is normal but the anterior chamber angle is very narrow owing to a congenitally high level of insertion of the iris. Such an eye has little pupillary block, but dilation will cause bunching up of the peripheral iris, occluding the angle (angle crowding) even if a peripheral iridectomy has been performed. Affected individuals present with acute angle-closure glaucoma at a young age, with recurrences after peripheral iridectomy. Long-term miotic therapy or laser iridoplasty are required.

Pupillary dilation for fundus examination is apt to cause acute angle closure in patients with plateau iris and may precipitate a similar event in other eyes with deep anterior chambers—due to angle crowding rather than the pupillary block mechanism seen in eyes with shallow anterior chambers.

CONGENITAL GLAUCOMA

Congenital glaucoma (rare) can be subdivided into (1) primary congenital glaucoma, in which the developmental abnormalities are restricted to the anterior chamber angle; (2) the anterior segment developmental anomalies—Axenfeld's syndrome, Peter's anomaly, and Rieger's syndrome—in which iris and corneal development are also abnormal; and (3) a variety of other conditions—including aniridia, Sturge-Weber syndrome, neurofibromatosis, Lowe's syndrome, and congenital rubella—in which the developmental anomalies of the angle are associated with other ocular or extraocular abnormalities.

Clinical Findings

Congenital glaucoma is manifest at birth in 50%, diagnosed in the first 6 months in 70%, and diagnosed by the end of the first year in 80%. The earliest and most common symptom is epiphora. Photophobia and decreased corneal luster may be present. Increased intraocular pressure is the cardinal sign. Glaucomatous cupping of the optic disk is a relatively early—and the most important—change. Later findings include increased corneal diameter (above 11.5 mm is considered significant), epithelial edema, tears of Descemet's membrane, and increased depth of the anterior chamber (associated with general enlargement of the anterior segment of the eye) as well as edema and opacity of the corneal stroma (Figure 11–9).

Differential Diagnosis

Megalocornea, corneal clouding due to congenital dystrophy or mucopolysaccharidoses, and traumatic

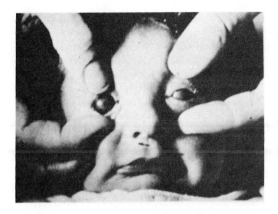

Figure 11–9. Congential glaucoma (buphthalmos).

rupture of Descemet's membrane should be ruled out. Measurement of intraocular pressure, gonioscopy, and evaluation of the optic disk are important in making the differential diagnosis. Assessment generally requires examination under general anesthesia.

Course & Prognosis

In untreated cases, blindness occurs early. The eye undergoes marked stretching and may even rupture with minor trauma. Typical glaucomatous cupping occurs relatively soon, emphasizing the need for early treatment.

1. PRIMARY CONGENITAL GLAUCOMA (Trabeculodysgenesis)

Primary congenital glaucoma is produced by an arrest of development of the anterior chamber angle structures at about the seventh month of fetal life. The iris is hypoplastic and inserts onto the trabecular surface in front of a poorly developed scleral spur, thus obscuring the trabecular meshwork and giving the appearance of a membrane (Barkan's membrane) across the angle.

Most patients present between 3 and 9 months of age. The treatment of choice is goniotomy. Single or repeated goniotomy produces permanent control of intraocular pressure in over 85% of cases. In patients presenting later, goniotomy is less successful and trabeculotomy or trabeculectomy becomes necessary. The long-term visual prognosis is then much less favorable.

2. ANTERIOR SEGMENT DEVELOPMENTAL ANOMALIES

These rare diseases represent a spectrum of improper development of the anterior segment, involving the angle, iris, cornea, and occasionally the lens. Usually there is some hypoplasia of the anterior stroma of the iris, with bridging filaments connecting the iris stroma to the cornea. If these bridging filaments occur peripherally and connect to a prominent, axially displaced Schwalbe's line (posterior embryotoxon), the disease is known as **Axenfeld's syndrome.** This resembles the trabeculodysgenesis of primary congenital glaucoma. If there are broader iridocorneal adhesions associated with the disruption of the iris, with polycoria and, in addition, skeletal and dental anomalies, the disorder is called **Rieger's syndrome** (an example of iridotrabecular dysgenesis). If adhesions are between the central iris and the central posterior surface of the cornea, the disease is known as **Peter's anomaly** (an example of iridocorneal trabeculodysgenesis).

These diseases are usually dominantly inherited, though sporadic cases have been reported. Glaucoma occurs in approximately 50% of such eyes and often does not present until late childhood or early adulthood. Goniotomy has a much lower success rate in these cases, and trabeculotomy or trabeculectomy may be recommended. Many such patients require long-term medical glaucoma therapy, and the prognosis is guarded for long-term retention of good visual function.

3. ANIRIDIA

The distinguishing feature of aniridia, as the name implies, is the vestigial iris. Often, little more than the root of the iris or a thin iris margin is present. Other deformities of the eye may be present, such as congenital cataracts, corneal dystrophy, and foveal hypoplasia. Vision is usually poor. Glaucoma frequently develops before adolescence and is usually refractory to medical or surgical management.

This rare syndrome is genetically determined. Examples of both autosomal dominant and recessive inheritance have been reported.

If medical therapy is ineffective, goniotomy or trabeculotomy may occasionally normalize the intraocular pressure. Filtering operations are often necessary, but the long-term visual prognosis is poor.

SECONDARY GLAUCOMA

Increased intraocular pressure occurring as one manifestation of some other eye disease is called secondary glaucoma. These diseases are difficult to classify satisfactorily. Treatment involves controlling intraocular pressure by medical and surgical means but also dealing with the underlying disease if possible.

PIGMENTARY GLAUCOMA

This syndrome seems to be primarily a degeneration of the pigmented epithelium of the iris and ciliary body. The pigment granules flake off from the iris as a result of friction against the underlying packets of zonular fibers, resulting in iris transillumination. The pigment is deposited on the posterior corneal surface (Krukenberg's spindle) and becomes lodged in the trabecular meshwork, impeding the normal outflow of aqueous. The syndrome occurs most often in myopic males between the ages of 25 and 40 who have a deep anterior chamber with a wide anterior chamber angle.

A number of pedigrees of autosomal dominant inheritance of pigmentary glaucoma have been reported. The pigmentary changes may be present without glaucoma (**pigment dispersion syndrome**), but such persons must be considered "glaucoma suspects."

The logical treatment in this condition is miotic therapy because it overcomes movement of the iris across the zonules. However, because the patients are usually young myopes, such therapy is poorly tolerated unless administered as pilocarpine once daily, preferably at bedtime. Beta-blockers and epinephrine are also effective.

The major problem, however, is the young age at which the disease develops, which increases the chance that drainage surgery will be necessary and enhances the advisability of combining such surgery with antimetabolite therapy. Laser trabeculoplasty is frequently used in this condition but is unlikely to obviate the need for drainage surgery.

EXFOLIATION SYNDROME (Pseudo-Exfoliation Syndrome)

In exfoliation syndrome, flake-like deposits of a fibrillary material are seen on the anterior lens surface (in contrast to the true exfoliation of the lens capsule caused by exposure to infrared radiation, ie, "glassblower's cataract"), ciliary processes, zonule, posterior iris surface, loose in the anterior chamber, and in the trabecular meshwork (along with increased pigmentation). These deposits can also be detected histologically in the conjunctiva, suggesting a more widespread abnormality. The disease is usually found in patients over the age of 65. Beta-blockers, miotics, and epinephrine are moderately effective. Laser trabeculoplasty or a filtering operation may be necessary.

GLAUCOMA SECONDARY TO CHANGES IN THE LENS

Lens Dislocation

The crystalline lens may be dislocated as a result of trauma or spontaneously, as in Marfan's syndrome. Anterior dislocation may cause obstruction of the pupillary aperture, leading to iris bombé and angle closure. Posterior dislocation into the vitreous is also associated with glaucoma, though the mechanism is obscure. It may be due to angle damage at the time of traumatic dislocation.

In anterior dislocation, the definitive treatment is lens extraction once the intraocular pressure has been controlled medically. In posterior dislocation, the lens is usually left alone and the glaucoma treated as primary open-angle glaucoma.

Intumescence of the Lens

The lens may take up considerable fluid during cataractous change, increasing markedly in size. It may then encroach upon the anterior chamber, producing both pupillary block and angle crowding and resulting in angle-closure glaucoma. Treatment consists of lens extraction once the intraocular pressure has been controlled medically.

Phacolytic Glaucoma

Some advanced cataracts may develop leakiness of the anterior lens capsule, which allows passage of liquefied lens proteins into the anterior chamber. The trabecular meshwork becomes edematous and obstructed with lens proteins, leading to an acute rise in intraocular pressure. Lens extraction is the definitive treatment once the intraocular pressure has been controlled medically, including intensive topical steroids.

GLAUCOMA SECONDARY TO CHANGES IN THE UVEAL TRACT

Uveitis

The intraocular pressure is usually below normal in uveitis because the inflamed ciliary body is functioning poorly. However, elevation of intraocular pressure may also occur through a number of different mechanisms. The trabecular meshwork may become blocked by inflammatory cells from the anterior chamber, with secondary edema, or may occasionally be involved in an inflammatory process specifically directed at the trabecular cells (trabeculitis). Chronic or recurrent uveitis produces permanent impairment of trabecular function, peripheral anterior synechiae, and occasionally angle neovascularization, all of which increase the chance of secondary glaucoma. Seclusio pupillae due to 360-degree posterior synechiae produces iris bombé and acute angle-closure glaucoma. The uveitis syndromes that tend to be associated with secondary glaucoma are Fuchs' heterochromic cyclitis, HLA-B27-associated acute anterior uveitis, and uveitis due to herpes zoster and herpes simplex.

Treatment is directed chiefly at controlling the uveitis with concomitant medical glaucoma therapy as necessary, avoiding miotics because of the increased chance of posterior synechia formation. Long-term therapy, including surgery, is often required because of irreversible damage to the trabecular meshwork.

Acute angle closure due to seclusion of the pupil may be reversed by intensive mydriasis but often requires laser peripheral iridotomy or surgical iridectomy. Any uveitis with a tendency to posterior synechia formation must be treated with mydriatics whenever the uveitis is active to reduce the risk of pupillary seclusion.

Tumor

Uveal tract melanomas may cause glaucoma by anterior displacement of the ciliary body, causing secondary angle closure, direct involvement of the anterior chamber angle, blockage of the filtration angle by pigment dispersion, and angle neovascularization. Enucleation is likely to be necessary.

IRIDOCORNEOENDOTHELIAL (ICE) SYNDROME (Essential Iris Atrophy, Chandler's Syndrome, Iris Nevus Syndrome)

This rare idiopathic condition of young adults is usually unilateral and manifested by corneal decompensation, glaucoma, and iris abnormalities.

GLAUCOMA SECONDARY TO TRAUMA

Contusion injuries of the globe may be associated with an early rise in intraocular pressure due to bleeding into the anterior chamber (hyphema). Free blood blocks the trabecular meshwork, which is also rendered edematous by the injury. Treatment is initially medical, but surgery may be required if the pressure remains elevated.

Late effects of contusion injuries on intraocular pressure are due to direct angle damage. The interval between the injury and the development of glaucoma may obscure the association. Clinically, the anterior chamber is seen to be deeper than in the fellow eye, and gonioscopy shows recession of the angle. Medical therapy is usually effective, but drainage surgery may be required.

Lacerations or contusional rupture of the anterior segment are associated with loss of the anterior chamber. If the chamber is not reformed soon after the injury—either spontaneously, by iris incarceration into the wound, or surgically—peripheral anterior synechiae will form and result in irreversible angle closure.

GLAUCOMA FOLLOWING OCULAR SURGERY

Ciliary Block Glaucoma (Malignant Glaucoma)

Surgery upon an eye with markedly increased intraocular pressure and a closed angle can lead to ciliary block glaucoma. Immediately after surgery, the in-

traocular pressure increases markedly, and the lens is pushed forward as a result of the collection of aqueous in and behind the vitreous body.

Treatment consists of cycloplegics, mydriatics, aqueous suppressants, and hyperosmotic agents. Hyperosmotic agents are used to shrink the vitreous body and let the lens fall more posteriorly.

Posterior sclerotomy, vitrectomy, and even lens extraction may be needed.

Peripheral Anterior Synechiae

Just as with trauma to the anterior segment (see above), surgery that results in a flat anterior chamber will lead to formation of peripheral anterior synechiae. Early surgical re-formation of the chamber is required if it does not occur spontaneously.

NEOVASCULAR GLAUCOMA

Neovascular of the iris (rubeosis iridis) and anterior chamber angle is most often secondary to widespread retinal ischemia such as occurs in advanced diabetic retinal vein occlusion. Glaucoma results initially form obstructin of the angle by the fibrovascular membrane, but subsequent contraction of the membrane leads to angle closure.

Treatment of established neovascular glaucoma is difficult and often unsatisfactory.

GLAUCOMA SECONDARY TO RAISED EPISCLERAL VENOUS PRESSURE

Raised episcleral venous pressure may contribute to glaucoma in Sturge-Weber syndrome, in which a developmental anomaly of the angle is also often present, and carotid-cavernous fistula, which may also cause angle neovascularization due to widespread ocular ischemia. Medical treatment cannot lower the intraocular pressure below the level of the abnormally elevated episcleral venous pressure, and surgery is associated with a high risk of complications.

STEROID-INDUCED GLAUCOMA

Topical and periocular corticosteroids may produce a type of glaucoma that simulates primary open-angle glaucoma, particularly in individuals with a family history of the disease, and will exaggerate the intraocular pressure elevation in those with established primary open-angle glaucoma. Withdrawal of the medication usually eliminates these effects, but permanent damage can occur if the situation goes unrecognized too long. If topical steroid therapy is absolutely necessary, medical glaucoma therapy will usually control the intraocular pressure. Systemic steroid therapy is less likely to cause a rise in intraocular pressure.

It is imperative that patients receiving topical or systemic steroid therapy undergo periodic tonometry and ophthalmoscopy, particularly if there is a family history of glaucoma.

REFERENCES

Adamis P et al: Fuchs' endothelial dystrophy of the cornea. Surv Ophthalmol 1993;38:149.

Anderson DR: Glaucoma: The damage caused by pressure. XLVI Edward Jackson Memorial Lecture. Am J Ophthalmol 1989;108:485.

Begg IS, Cottle RW: Epidemiologic approach to open-angle glaucoma: 2. Survival analysis of adverse drug reactions. Report of the Canadian Ocular Adverse Drug Reaction Registry Program. Can J Ophthalmol 1989;24:15.

Blasini M, Shields MB: Apraclonidine hydrochloride as an adjunct to timolol maleate therapy. J Glaucoma 1992;1:148.

Camras CB et al: Intraocular pressure reduction with PhXA34, a new prostaglandin analogue, in patients with ocular hypertension. Arch Ophthalmol 1992;110:1733.

Chisholm IA, Drance SM, To T: The glaucoma suspect: Differentiation of the future glaucoma eye from the non-glaucomatous suspect eye 2. visual field decay. Graefe's Arch Clin Exp Ophthalmol 1989;227:110.

Congdon N, Wang F, Tielsch JM: Issues in the epidemiology and population-based screening of primary angle-closure glaucoma. Surv Ophthalmol 1992;36:411.

David DR et al: Diurnal intraocular pressure variations: an analysis of 690 diurnal curves. Br J Ophthalmol 1992;76:280.

Farrar SM, Shields MB: Current concepts in pigmentary glaucoma. Surv Ophthalmol 1993;37:233.

Fechter RD, Weinreb RN: Mechanism of optic nerve damage in primary open angle glaucoma. Surv Ophthalmol 1994;39:23.

Fredrick DR et al: Narrow angle glaucoma in Vietnamese Americans. Tr Pac Coast Oto-Ophthalmol Soc 1993;73. [In press.]

Fristrom B, Nilsson SEG: Interaction of PhXA41, a new prostaglandin analogue, with pilocarpine. Arch Ophthalmol 1993;111:662.

Geyer O et al: Tono-Pen tonometry in normal and in post-keratoplasty eyes. Br J Ophthalmol 1992;76:538.

Glaucoma dialogue: (Editorial.) J Glaucoma 1992;1:143.

Gross FJ, Tingey D, Epstein DL: Increased prevalence of occludable angles and angle-closure glaucoma in patients with pseudoexfoliation. Am J Ophthalmol 1994; 117:333.

Harrington DO, Drake MV: *The Visual Fields: Test and Atlas of Clinical Perimetry,* 6th ed. Mosby, 1990.

Hitchings RA: Glaucoma screening. Br J Ophthalmol 1993;77:326.

Hoskins HD, Kass MA: *Becker-Shaffer's Diagnosis and Therapy of the Glaucomas,* 6th ed. Mosby, 1989.

Jampel HD, Jabs DA, Quigley HA: Trabeculectomy with 5-fluorouracil for adult inflammatory glaucoma. Am J Ophthalmol 1990;109:168.

Jay JL, Murdoch JR: The rate of visual field loss in untreated primary open angle glaucoma. Br J Ophthalmol 1993;77:176.

Jonas JB, Fernandez MC: Shape of the neuroretinal rim and position of the central retinal vessels in glaucoma. Br J Ophthalmol 1994;78:99.

Jonas JB, Xu L: Optic disk hemorrhages in glaucoma. Am J Ophthalmol 1994;117:1.

Kwok S et al: Glaucoma in Asian Americans: With special emphasis on Chinese and Vietnamese. Tr Pac Coast Oto-Ophthalmol Soc 1993;73. [In press.]

Lehto I: Longterm prognosis of pigmentary glaucoma. Acta Ophthalmologica 1991;69:437.

Leske MC et al: The Barbados Eye Study: Prevalence of open angle glaucoma. Arch Ophthalmol 1994;112:821.

Lippa EA et al: Multiple-dose, dose-response relationship for the topical carbonic anhydrase inhibitor MD-927. Arch Ophthalmol 1991;109:46.

Netland PA, Chaturvedi N, Dreyer EB: Calcium channel blockers in the management of low-tension and open-angle glaucoma. Am J Ophthalmol 1993;115:608.

O'Brien C et al: Intraocular pressure and the rate of visual field loss in chronic open-angle glaucoma. Am J Ophthalmol 1991;111:491.

O'Connor D, Zeyen T, Caprioli J: Comparisons of methods to detect glaucomatous optic nerve damage. Ophthalmol 1993;100:1498.

Optic nerve head analysis in the 1990s: (Editorial.) J Glaucoma 1993;2:77.

Psilas K et al: Comparative study of argon laser trabeculoplasty in primary open-angle and pseudoexfoliation glaucoma. Ophthalmologica 1989;198:57.

Quigley HA et al: Risk factors for the development of glaucomatous visual field loss in ocular hypertension. Arch Ophthalmol 1994;112:644.

Ritch R, Shields MB, Krupin T (editors): *The Glaucomas,* 2 vols. Mosby, 1989.

Ritch R et al: Argon laser trabeculoplasty in pigmentary glaucoma. Ophthalmology 1993;100:909.

Rossetti L et al: Randomized clinical trials on medical treatment of glaucoma. Arch Ophthalmol 1993;111:96.

Saunders DC: Acute closed-angle glaucoma and Nd-YAG laser iridotomy. Br J Ophthalmol 1990;74:523.

Schulzer M: Intraocular pressure reduction in normal-tension glaucoma patients. Ophthalmology 1992;99:1468.

Schumer R, Podos S: Medical treatment of newly diagnosed open-angle glaucoma. J Glaucoma 1993;2:211.

Shingleton BJ et al: Long-term efficacy of argon laser trabeculoplasty: A 10-year follow-up study. Ophthalmology 1993;100:1324.

Sommer A et al: Relationship between intraocular pressure and primary open angle glaucoma among white and black Americans: The Baltimore Eye Survey. Arch Ophthalmol 1991;109:1090.

Stewart WC, Shields MB: The peripheral visual field in glaucoma: Reevaluation in the age of automated perimetry. Surv Ophthalmol 1991;36:59.

Tielsch JM et al: Family history and risk of primary open angle glaucoma: The Baltimore Eye Survey. Arch Ophthalmol 1994;112:69.

Toris CB et al: Effects of PhXA41, a new prostaglandin F2 analog, on aqueous humor dynamics in human eyes. Ophthalmology 1993;100:1297.

Tsai CS et al: Visual field global indices in patients with reversal of glaucomatous cupping after intraocular pressure reduction. Ophthalmology 1991;98:1412.

Van Buskirk EM: *Clinical Atlas of Glaucoma.* Saunders, 1986.

Villumsen J, Alm A: PhXA34, a prostaglandin F2 analogue: Effect on intraocular pressure in patients with ocular hypertension. Br J Ophthalmol 1992;76:214.

Weinreb RN: Compliance with medical treatment of glaucoma. J Glaucoma 1992;1:134.

Whitacre MM, Emig M, Hassancien K: The effect of Perkins, Tono-Pen, and Schiotz tonometry on intraocular pressure. Am J Ophthalmol 1991;111:59.

Wilensky JT et al: Follow-up of angle-closure glaucoma suspects. Am J Ophthalmol 1993;115:338.

Wilkerson M et al: Four-week safety and efficacy study of dorzolamide, a novel, active topical carbonic anhydrase inhibitor. Arch Ophthalmol 1993;111:1343.

Zeyen TG, Caprioli J: Progression of disc and field damage in early glaucoma. Arch Ophthalmol 1993;111:62.

12

Strabismus

Taylor Asbury, MD, & Miles J. Burke, MD, MS

Under normal binocular viewing conditions, the image of the object of regard falls simultaneously on the fovea of each eye (bifoveal fixation) and the vertical retinal meridians are both upright. Either eye can be misaligned, so that only one eye at a time views the object of regard. Any deviation from perfect ocular alignment is called "strabismus." Misalignment may be in any direction—inward, outward, up, or down. The amount of deviation is the angle by which the deviating eye is misaligned. Strabismus present under binocular viewing conditions is **manifest strabismus, heterotropia, or tropia.** A deviation present only after binocular vision has been interrupted (ie, by occlusion of one eye) is called **latent strabismus, heterophoria, or phoria.**

Strabismus is present in about 4% of children. Treatment should be started as soon as a diagnosis is made in order to ensure the best possible visual acuity and binocular visual function. There is no such thing as "outgrowing" strabismus.

DEFINITIONS

Angle kappa: The angle between the visual axis and the central pupillary line. When the eye is fixing a light, if the corneal reflection is centered on the pupil, the visual axis and the central pupillary line coincide and the angle kappa is zero. Ordinarily, the light reflex is 2–4 degrees nasal to the pupillary center, giving the appearance of slight exotropia (positive angle kappa). A negative angle kappa gives the false impression of esotropia.

Conjugate movement: Movement of the eyes in the same direction at the same time.

Ductions: (Figure 12–1.) Monocular rotations with no consideration of the position of the other eye.

Adduction: Inward rotation.

Abduction: Outward rotation.

Supraduction (elevation): Upward rotation.

Infraduction (depression): Downward rotation.

Fusion: Formation of one image from the two images seen simultaneously by the two eyes. Fusion has two aspects:

Motor fusion: Adjustments made by the brain in innervation of extraocular muscles in order to bring both eyes into bifoveal and torsional alignment.

Sensory fusion: Integration in the visual sensory areas of the brain of images seen with the two eyes into one picture.

Heterophoria (phoria): Latent deviation of the eyes held straight by binocular vision.

Esophoria: Tendency for one eye to turn inward.

Exophoria: Tendency for one eye to turn outward.

Hyperphoria: Tendency for one eye to deviate upward.

Hypophoria: Tendency for one eye to deviate downward. (See Hypotropia.)

Heterotropia (tropia):

Strabismus: Manifest deviation of the eyes that cannot be controlled by binocular vision.

Esotropia: Convergent manifest deviation ("crossed eyes").

Exotropia: Divergent manifest deviation ("wall-eyes").

Hypertropia: Manifest deviation of one eye upward.

Hypotropia: Manifest deviation of one eye downward. By convention, in the absence of specific causation to account for the lower position of one eye, vertical deviations are designated by the higher eye (eg, right hypertropia, not left hypotropia, when the right eye is higher).

Incyclotropia: Inward rotation of one eye about the visual axis (ie, clockwise right eye, counterclockwise left eye).

Excyclotropia: Outward rotation of one eye about the visual axis (ie, counterclockwise right eye, clockwise left eye).

Orthophoria: The absence of any tendency of either eye to deviate when fusion is suspended. This state is rarely seen clinically. A small phoria is normal.

Primary deviation: The deviation measured with the normal eye fixing and the eye with the paretic muscle deviating (Figure 12–2).

Prism diopter (Δ): A unit of angular measurement used to characterize ocular deviations. A 1-diopter prism deflects a ray of light toward the base of the prism by 1 centimeter at 1 meter. One degree of arc equals approximately 1.7^{Δ}.

Secondary deviation: (Figure 12–2.) The deviation measured with the paretic eye fixing and the normal eye deviating.

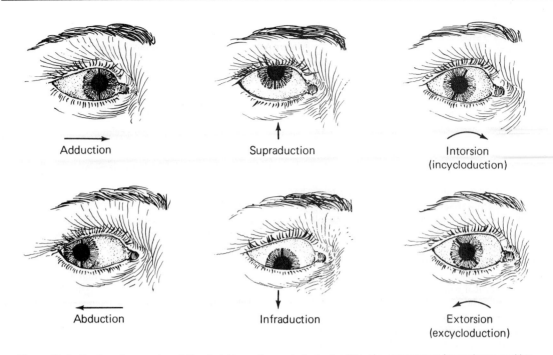

Figure 12–1. Ductions (monocular rotations), right eye. Arrows indicate direction of eye movement from primary position.

Torsion: Rotation of the eye about its anteroposterior axis (Figure 12–1).

Intorsion (incycloduction): Rotation of the 12 o'clock meridian of the eye toward the midline of the head.

Extorsion (excycloduction): Rotation of the 12 o'clock meridian of the eye away from the midline of the head.

Vergences (disjunctive movements): Movement of the two eyes in opposite directions.

Convergence: The eyes turn inward.

Divergence: The eyes turn outward.

Versions: Binocular rotations of the eyes in qualitatively the same direction.

PHYSIOLOGY

1. MOTOR ASPECTS

Individual Muscle Functions (Table 12–1)

Each of the six extraocular muscles plays a role in positioning the eye about three axes of rotation. The

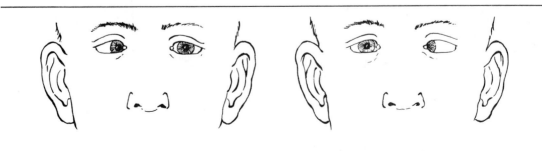

Primary deviation
(left eye fixing)

Secondary deviation (right eye fixing;
"overshoot" of sound left eye)

Figure 12–2. Paresis of horizontal muscle (right lateral rectus). Secondary deviation is greater than primary deviation because of Hering's law. With the left eye fixing, the right eye is deviated inward because of the paretic right lateral rectus. For the right eye to fix, the paretic right lateral rectus muscle must receive excessive stimulation. The yoke muscle, the left medial rectus, also receives the same excessive stimulation (Hering's law), which causes "overshoot" shown above (see p 210).

Table 12–1. Functions of the ocular muscles.

Muscle	Primary Action	Secondary Actions
Lateral rectus	Abduction	None
Medial rectus	Adduction	None
Superior rectus	Elevation	Adduction, intorsion
Inferior rectus	Depression	Adduction, extorsion
Superior oblique	Intorsion	Depression, abduction
Inferior oblique	Extorsion	Elevation, abduction

primary action of a muscle is the principal effect it has on eye rotation. Lesser effects are called secondary or tertiary actions. The exact action of any muscle depends on the direction of the eye in space.

The medial and lateral rectus muscles adduct and abduct the eye, respectively, with little effect on elevation or torsion. The vertical rectus and oblique muscles have vertical rotation and torsional functions. In general terms, the vertical rectus muscles are the main elevators and depressors of the eye, and the obliques are mostly involved with torsional positioning. The vertical effect of the superior and inferior rectus muscles is greater when the eye is abducted. The vertical effect of the obliques is greater when the eye is adducted.

Field of Action

The position of the eye is determined by the equilibrium achieved by the pull of all six extraocular muscles. The eyes are in the **primary position of gaze** when the head and the eyes are both aligned with the object of regard. To move the eye into another direction of gaze, the agonist muscle contracts to pull the eye in that direction and the antagonist muscle relaxes. The field of action of a muscle is the direction of gaze in which that muscle exerts its greatest contraction force as an agonist, eg, the lateral rectus muscle undergoes the greatest contraction in abducting the eye (Table 12–1). The fields of action of the vertical rectus and oblique muscles overlap to some extent.

Synergistic & Antagonistic Muscles (Sherrington's Law)

Synergistic muscles are those that have the same field of action. Thus, for vertical gaze, the superior rectus and inferior oblique muscles are synergists in moving the eye upward. Muscles synergistic for one function may be antagonistic for another. For example, the superior rectus and inferior oblique muscles are antagonists for torsion, the superior rectus causing intorsion and the inferior oblique extorsion. The extraocular muscles, like skeletal muscles, show reciprocal innervation of antagonistic muscles (Sherrington's law). Thus, in dextroversion (right gaze), the right medial and left lateral rectus muscles are inhibited while the right lateral and left medial rectus muscles are stimulated.

Yoke Muscles (Hering's Law)

For movements of both eyes in the same direction, the corresponding agonist muscles receive equal innervation (Hering's law). The pair of agonist muscles with the same primary action is called a yoke pair. The right lateral rectus and the left medial rectus muscles are a yoke pair for right gaze. The right inferior rectus and the left superior oblique muscles are a yoke pair for gaze downward and to the right. Table 12–2 lists the yoke muscle combinations.

Development of Binocular Movement

The neuromuscular system of an infant is immature, so that it is not uncommon in the first few months of life for ocular alignment to be unstable. Transient esodeviations are most common and may be associated with immaturity of the accommodation-convergence system. Gradually improving visual acuity together with maturation of the oculomotor system allows a more stable ocular alignment by age 4 months. Any ocular misalignment after this age should be investigated by an ophthalmologist.

Table 12–2. Yoke muscles in cardinal positions of gaze.

Eyes up and right	RSR and LIO
Eyes up and left	LSR and RIO
Eyes right	RLR and LMR
Eyes left	LLR and RMR
Eyes down and right	RIR and LSO
Eyes down and left	LIR and RSO

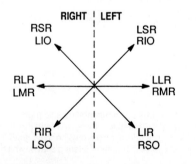

2. SENSORY ASPECTS

Binocular Vision

In each eye, whatever is imaged on the fovea is seen subjectively as being straight ahead. Thus, if two dissimilar objects were imaged on the two foveas, the two objects would be seen superimposed, but the dissimilarities would prevent fusion into a single impression. Because of the different vantage point in space of each eye, the image in each eye is actually slightly different from that in the other. Sensory fusion and stereopsis are the two different physiologic processes that are responsible for binocular vision.

Sensory Fusion & Stereopsis

Sensory fusion is the process whereby dissimilarities between the two images are not appreciated. On the peripheral retina of each eye, there are **corresponding points** that in the absence of fusion localize stimuli in the same direction in space. In the process of fusion, the direction values of these points can be modified. Thus, each point of the retina in each eye is capable of fusing stimuli that strike sufficiently close to the corresponding point in the other eye. This region of fusible points is called **Panum's area.**

Fusion is possible because subtle differences between the two images are ignored, and stereopsis, or binocular depth perception, occurs because of the cerebral integration of these two slightly dissimilar images.

Sensory Changes in Strabismus

Up to age 7 or 8, the brain usually develops responses to abnormal binocular vision that are unlikely to occur if the onset of strabismus is later. These changes include diplopia, suppression, anomalous retinal correspondence, and eccentric fixation.

A. Diplopia: If strabismus is present, each fovea receives a different image. The objects imaged on the two foveas are seen in the same direction in space. This process of localization of spatially separate objects to the same location is called **visual confusion.** The object viewed by one of the foveas is imaged on a peripheral retinal area in the other eye. The foveal image is localized straight ahead, while the peripheral image of the same object in the other eye is localized in some other direction. Thus, the same object is seen in two places (diplopia).

B. Suppression: Under binocular viewing conditions, the images seen by one eye become predominant and those seen by the other eye are not perceived (suppression). Suppression takes the form of a **scotoma** in the deviating eye only under binocular viewing conditions. (A scotoma is an area of reduced vision within the visual field, surrounded by an area of less depressed or normal vision.) Suppression scotomas in esotropia are usually approximately elliptical in shape, extending on the retina from just temporal to the fovea to the point in the peripheral retina where the object of regard for the other eye is imaged. In exotropia, the suppression area tends to be larger and extends from the fovea to usually the entire temporal half of the retina. When fixation shifts to the other eye, the suppression scotoma also switches to the newly deviating eye. In the absence of strabismus, a blurred image in one eye may also lead to suppression. The lack of simultaneous perception in the central retina prevents fine stereopsis, though crude stereopsis from the peripheral retina may still be present.

C. Amblyopia: Prolonged abnormal visual experience in a child under the age of 7 years may lead to amblyopia (reduced visual acuity in the absence of detectable organic disease in one eye). The two clinical contexts in which amblyopia occurs are strabismus and any disorder that causes a blurred retinal image in one or both eyes, eg, a significant refractive difference between the eyes **(anisometropia).**

In strabismus, the eye used habitually for fixation retains normal acuity and the nonpreferred eye often develops decreased vision (amblyopia). If spontaneous alternation of fixation is present, amblyopia does not develop. Suppression and amblyopia are different processes. Amblyopia is present when the affected eye is tested alone. Suppression occurs under binocular conditions and is a process in which the brain "ignores" a portion of the image received from the deviating eye so that the patient avoids diplopia. This visual field defect is termed a facultative scotoma, since no visual deficit can be demonstrated when the suppressing eye is tested alone.

D. Anomalous Retinal Correspondence: In strabismus under binocular viewing conditions, the peripheral retinal areas outside the suppression scotoma may take on new directional values in space shifted by the amount of the deviation. This results in an anomalous correspondence of directional values between the retinal points in the two eyes. The directional values in the deviating eye are changed just enough to avoid diplopia. Stereopsis is not possible under these conditions, and the new directional values may be labile, readjusting themselves from moment to moment as the deviation changes with direction of gaze. Should fixation shift to the opposite eye, the anomalous directional values also shift eyes. On monocular testing, the directional values are normal.

E. Eccentric Fixation: In eyes with sufficiently severe amblyopia, an extrafoveal retinal area may be used for fixation under monocular viewing conditions. It is always associated with severe amblyopia and unstable fixation. The eccentric fixation point is often not displaced in a direction appropriate to the direction of strabismus (eg, the nasal retina in esotropia). Gross eccentric fixation can be readily identified clinically by occluding the dominant eye and directing the patient's attention to a light source held directly in front. An eye with gross eccentric fixation will not point toward the light source but will appear to be looking in some other direction. More subtle degrees of eccentric fixation can be detected by an ophthalmoscope that projects a small fixation target onto the retina. If any area other than the macula is selected for fixation by the patient, the presence of eccentric fixation has been established.

EXAMINATION

History

A careful history is important in the diagnosis of strabismus.

A. Family History: Strabismus and amblyopia are frequently found to occur in families.

B. Age at Onset: This is an important factor in long-term prognosis. The earlier the onset of strabismus, the worse the prognosis for good binocular function.

C. Type of Onset: The onset may be gradual, sudden, or intermittent.

D. Type of Deviation: The misalignment may be in any direction. It may be greater in certain positions of gaze, including the primary position for distance or near.

E. Fixation: One eye may constantly deviate, or alternating fixation may be observed.

Visual Acuity

Visual acuity should be evaluated even if only a rough approximation or comparison of the two eyes is possible. Each eye is evaluated by itself, since binocular testing will not reveal poor vision in one eye. For the very young child, it may only be possible to establish that an eye is able to follow a moving target. The target should be as small as the child's age, interest, and level of alertness allow. Fixation is described as being normal if it is centrally (foveally) fixated and maintained while the eye follows a moving object. One technique for quantitatively measuring visual acuity in younger children is forced-choice preferential looking.

By the age of 2½–3 years, it is possible to perform recognition visual acuity testing using the Allen pictures. By age 4 years, many children will understand the Snellen tumbling "E" game and the HOTV recognition test. By age 5 or 6 years, most children can respond to Snellen alphabet visual acuity testing.

Determination of Refractive Error

It is important to determine the cycloplegic refractive error by retinoscopy (see Chapter 20). The standard drug for producing complete cycloplegia in children under age 2 years is atropine, which may be given as 0.5% or 1% eye drops or ointment instilled twice a day for 3 days. Atropine should not be used in older children, since prolonged cycloplegia lasting up to 2 weeks will interfere with near vision. After age 2, cyclopentolate 1% or 2% is the preferred cycloplegic.

Inspection

Inspection alone may show whether the strabismus is constant or intermittent, alternating or nonalternat-

ing, and variable or constant. Associated ptosis and abnormal position of the head may also be noted. The quality of fixation of each eye separately and of both eyes together should be noted. Nystagmoid movements indicate unstable fixation and often reduced visual acuity.

Prominent epicanthal folds that obscure all or part of the nasal sclera may give an appearance of esotropia (pseudoesotropia). Although this entity is confusing to lay persons as well as some physicians, these children have a normal corneal light reflection test. Prominent epicanthal folds gradually disappear by 4 or 5 years of age.

Determination of Angle of Strabismus (Angle of Deviation)

A. Prism and Cover Tests: (Figure 12–3.) Cover tests consist of four parts: (1) the cover test, (2) the uncover test, (3) the alternate cover test, and (4) the prism cover test. In all four tests, the patient looks intently at a target, which may be in any direction of gaze at distance or near.

1. Cover test–As the examiner observes one eye, a cover is placed in front of the other eye to block its view of the target. If the observed eye moves to take up fixation, it was not previously fixating the target, and a manifest deviation (strabismus) is present. The direction of movement reveals the direction of deviation (eg, the eye moves outwardly if there is esotropia).

2. Uncover test–As the cover is removed from the eye following the cover test, the eye emerging from under cover is observed. If the position of the eye changes, interruption of binocular vision has allowed it to deviate, and heterophoria is present. The direction of corrective movement shows the type of heterophoria.

3. Alternate cover test–The cover is placed alternately in front of first one eye and then the other. This test reveals the total deviation (heterotropia plus heterophoria if also present).

4. Prism plus cover testing–To quantitatively measure the deviation, an increasing strength of prism is placed in front of one or both eyes until there is neutralization of eye movement on alternate cover testing. For example, to measure full esodeviation, the cover is alternated while prisms of increasing base-out strength are placed in front of one or both eyes until the horizontal refixation movement of the deviated eye is neutralized.

B. Maddox Rod Test: (Figure 12–4.) This test is an accurate method of measuring a deviation if normal retinal correspondence is present. It is particularly useful for measurement of heterophoria but can also be used in heterotropia. A Maddox rod consists of a series of thin red cylinders placed side by side, mounted in a circular holder that can be held before the eye. When a target light is seen through the Maddox rod, its image is a red line perpendicular to the axes of the cylin-

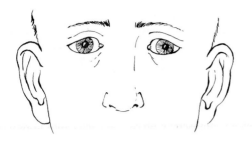

Eyes straight (maintained in position by fusion).

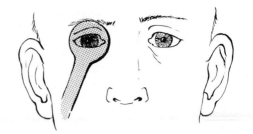

Position of eye under cover in orthophoria (fusion-free position). The right eye under cover has not moved.

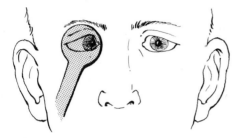

Position of eye under cover in esophoria (fusion-free position). Under cover, the right eye has deviated inward. Upon removal of cover, the right eye will immediately resume its straight-ahead position.

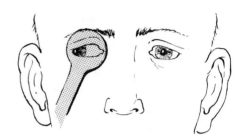

Position of eye under cover in exophoria (fusion-free position). Under cover, the right eye has deviated outward. Upon removal of the cover, the right eye will immediately resume its straight-ahead position.

Figure 12–3. Cover testing. The patient is directed to look at a target at eye level 6 m (20 feet) away. ***Note:*** In the presence of strabismus, the deviation will remain when the cover is removed.

ders. Thus, one eye sees the light directly while the other views its image through the Maddox rod. In orthophoria, the red line runs through the light. When the Maddox rod is held so that the cylinders are horizontal, a vertical red line is seen that is displaced to one side when a deviation is present. A prism can be held in front of one eye that allows the red line to run through the light. The strength of such a prism measures the angle of deviation. By rotating the Maddox

rod 90 degrees, a horizontal line is produced (cylinders of the rod are then vertical). Its vertical displacement can also be measured by prisms as described for horizontal deviations.

C. Objective Tests: Prism and cover measurements are objective in the sense that no report of sensory observations is required from the patient. However, cooperation and some degree of vision are required. The Maddox rod test is more subjective be-

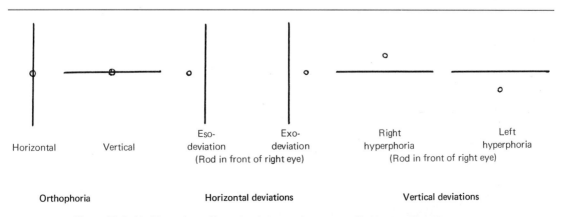

Horizontal	Vertical	Eso-deviation	Exo-deviation	Right hyperphoria	Left hyperphoria
		(Rod in front of right eye)		(Rod in front of right eye)	

Orthophoria   Horizontal deviations   Vertical deviations

Figure 12–4. Maddox rod test. Normal and abnormal responses. (Subjective view of the patient.)

cause the end point of the measurement is based on a report of sensory observations by the patient. Confused, uncooperative, or immature patients may be unable or unwilling to respond to this test. Clinical determinations of eye position that require no sensory observation by the patient (objective tests) are considerably less accurate, although still useful at times. Two methods commonly used depend on observing the position of the corneal reflection of a light. Results by both methods must be modified by allowing for the angle kappa.

1. Hirschberg method–The patient fixates a light at a distance of about 33 cm (13 inches). Decentering of the light reflection is noted in the deviating eye. By allowing 18^Δ for each millimeter of decentration, an estimate of the angle of deviation can be made.

2. Prism reflex method (Krimsky test)–The patient fixates a light. A prism is placed before the deviating eye, and the strength of the prism required to center the corneal reflection measures the angle of deviation.

Ductions
(Monocular Rotations)

With one eye covered, the other eye follows a moving light in all directions of gaze. Any decrease of rotation indicates weakness in the field of action of that muscle.

Versions
(Conjugate Ocular Movements)

Hering's law states that yoke muscles receive equal stimulation during any conjugate ocular movement. Versions are tested by having the eyes follow a light in the nine diagnostic positions: primary—straight ahead; secondary—right, left, up, and down; and tertiary—up and right, down and right, up and left, and down and left (Table 12–2). Apparent rotation of one eye relative to the other is noted as overaction or underaction. By convention, in the tertiary positions, the oblique muscles are said to be overacting or underacting with respect to the yoke rectus muscle. Fixation in the field of action of a paretic muscle results in overaction of the yoke muscle, since greater innervation is required for contraction of the underacting muscles (Figure 12–5). Conversely, fixation by the normal eye will lead to underaction of the paretic muscle.

Disjunctive Movements

A. Convergence: (Figure 12–6.) As the eyes follow an approaching object, they must turn inward in order to maintain alignment of the visual axes with the object of regard. The medial rectus muscles are contracting and the lateral rectus muscles are relaxing under the influence of neural stimulation and inhibition. (Neural pathways of supranuclear control are discussed in Chapter 14.)

Convergence is an active process with a strong voluntary as well as involuntary component. An important consideration in evaluating the extraocular muscles in strabismus is convergence.

To test convergence, a small object or light source is slowly brought toward the bridge of the nose. The patient's attention is directed to the object by saying, "Keep the light from going double as long as possible." Convergence can normally be maintained until the object is nearly to the bridge of the nose. An actual numerical value is placed on convergence by measuring the distance from the bridge of the nose (in centimeters) at which the eyes "break" (ie, when the nondominant eye swings laterally so that convergence is no longer maintained). This point is termed the **near point of convergence,** and a value of up to 5 cm (2 inches) is considered within normal limits.

The ratio of accommodative convergence to accommodation (AC/A ratio) is a way of quantitating the relationship of convergence to accommodation. Accommodative convergence is elicited by viewing an accommodative target, ie, one that has resolvable contours or letters that stimulate accommodation. The result is commonly expressed as prism diopters of convergence per diopter of accommodation. The AC/A ratio is useful as a research tool to further investigate and clarify this relationship and has contributed sig-

Figure 12–5. Testing versions. Example of paretic left superior oblique.

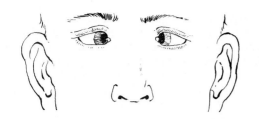

Figure 12–6. Convergence. The position of the eyes at the normal near point of convergence (NPC) is shown above. The break point is within 5 cm of the bridge of the nose.

nificantly to our understanding and therefore to the treatment of accommodative esotropia—particularly in using bifocals and miotics, as described later in this chapter.

B. Divergence: Electromyography has established that divergence is an active process, not merely a relaxation of convergence as previously believed by some authorities. Clinically, this function is seldom tested except in considering the amplitudes of fusion.

Sensory Examination

While many tests of the status of binocular vision have been devised, only a few need be mentioned here. The tests are for stereopsis, suppression, and fusion potential. All require the simultaneous presentation of two targets separately, one to each eye.

A. Stereopsis Testing: Many stereopsis tests are done with targets and Polaroid glasses to separate the stimuli. The monocularly observed targets have nearly imperceptible clues of depth. **Random dot stereograms** have no monocular depth clues. A field of random dots is seen by each eye, but the dot-to-corresponding-dot correlation between the two targets is such that if stereopsis is present, a form is seen in three dimensions.

B. Suppression Testing: The presence of suppression is readily demonstrated with the **Worth four-dot test.** Glasses containing a red lens over one eye and a green lens over the other are placed on the patient. A flashlight containing red, green, and white spots is viewed. The color spots are markers for perception through each eye, and the white dot, potentially visible to each eye, can indicate the presence of diplopia. The separation of the spots and the distance at which the light is held determine the size of the retinal area tested. Foveal and peripheral areas may be tested at distance and near.

C. Fusion Potential: In individuals with a manifest deviation, the status of binocular fusion potential can be determined by the red filter test. A red filter is placed over one eye. The patient is directed to look at a distance or near fixation light target. A red light and a white light are seen. Prisms are placed over one or both eyes in an attempt to bring the two images together. If fusion potential exists, the two images come together and are seen as a single pink light. If no fusion potential exists, the patient will continue to see one red and one white light.

OBJECTIVES & PRINCIPLES OF THERAPY OF STRABISMUS

The main objectives of strabismus treatment in children are (1) reversal of the deleterious sensory effects of strabismus (amblyopia, suppression, and loss of stereopsis) and (2) best possible alignment of the eyes by medical or surgical treatment. In all cases, the psychologic benefit of cosmetically straight eyes cannot be overestimated.

Timing of Treatment in Children

A child can be examined at any age, and treatment for amblyopia or strabismus should be instituted as soon as the diagnosis is made. Neurophysiologic studies in animals have shown that the infant brain is quite responsive to sensory experience, and the quality of function possible later in life is greatly influenced by early life experiences. It has been shown that overall results are favorably influenced by early alignment of the eyes, preferably by age 2. Good eye alignment can be achieved later, but normal sensory adaptation becomes more difficult as the child grows older. By age 8, the sensory status is generally so fixed that deficient stereopsis and amblyopia cannot be effectively treated.

Medical Treatment

Nonsurgical treatment of strabismus includes treatment of amblyopia, the use of optical devices (prisms and glasses), pharmacologic agents, and orthoptics.

A. Treatment of Amblyopia: The elimination of amblyopia is crucial in the treatment of strabismus and is always one of the first goals. The strabismic deviation may enlarge—rarely lessen—following the treatment of amblyopia. Surgical results are more predictable and stable if there is good visual acuity in each eye preoperatively.

1. Occlusion therapy–The mainstay of amblyopia treatment is occlusion. The sound eye is covered with a patch to simulate the amblyopic eye. Glasses are also used if there is a significant refractive error.

Two stages of successful amblyopia treatment are identified: initial improvement and maintenance of the improved visual acuity.

a. Initial stage–Full-time occlusion is the standard initial treatment. In some cases only part-time occlusion is used if the amblyopia is not too severe or the child is very young. As a guideline, full-time occlusion may be done for as many weeks as the child's age in years without risk of reduced vision in the sound eye.

Occlusion treatment is continued in some form as long as visual acuity improves (occasionally up to a year). It is not worthwhile continuing to patch for more than 4 months if there is no improvement.

Amblyopia is functional (ie, there is no identifiable organic lesion, although the adaptation must be cerebral). In most cases, if treatment is started soon enough, substantial improvement or complete normalization of visual acuity can be achieved. Occasionally, there is no improvement even under ideal conditions. Poor compliance with treatment (peeking around a patch or inadequate enforcement of patching by the parents) can always be a factor.

b. Maintenance stage–Maintenance treatment consists of part-time patching continued after the improvement phase to maintain the best possible vision beyond an age when amblyopia is likely to recur (about age 8).

2. Atropine therapy–A few children are intolerant to occlusion therapy. In such cases that have moderate or high hyperopia, atropine therapy may be effective. Atropine causes cycloplegia and therefore decreased accommodative ability. The sound eye is atropinized, and glasses are used to focus that eye for distance or near fixation only. This forces use of the amblyopic eye at all other times. Atropine 1%, 1 drop every few days, is usually sufficient for sustained cycloplegia.

B. Optical Devices:

1. Spectacles–The most important optical device in the treatment of strabismus is accurately prescribed spectacles. The clarification of the retinal image produced by glasses allows the natural fusion mechanisms to operate to the fullest extent. Small refractive errors need not be corrected. If there is significant hyperopia and esotropia, the esotropia probably is at least partially due to the hyperopia (accommodative esotropia). The prescription compensates for the full cycloplegic findings. If bifocals permit sufficient relaxation of accommodation to allow for near fusion, they should be used.

2. Prisms–Prisms produce optical redirection of the line of sight. Corresponding retinal elements are brought into line to eliminate diplopia. Correct sensory alignment of the eyes is also a form of antisuppression treatment. Used preoperatively, prisms can simulate the sensory effect that will follow successful surgery. In patients with horizontal deviation, prisms will show the patient's ability to fuse a simultaneous small vertical deviation, thus indicating whether surgery also needs to be done for the vertical component. In children with esotropia, prisms can be used preoperatively to predict a postoperative shift in position that might nullify the surgical result, and the planned surgery can be modified accordingly (prism adaptation test).

Prisms can be implemented in several ways. A particularly convenient form is the plastic Fresnel press-on prism. These plastic membranes can be placed on the glasses without the need for an optician and are very useful for diagnostic and temporary therapeutic purposes. For permanent wear, prisms are best ground into the spectacle prescription, but the amount is limited to about 5 prisms per lens since prismatic distortion becomes prominent at higher strengths.

C. Pharmacologic Agents:

1. Miotics–Echothiophate iodide and isoflurophate inactivate acetylcholinesterase at the neuromuscular junction and thus potentiate the effect of every nerve impulse. Accommodation becomes more effective relative to convergence than before treatment. Since accommodation controls the near reflex (the triad of accommodation, convergence, and miosis), less convergence will occur with reduced accommodation and the angle of deviation will be significantly reduced, often to zero.

Miotics have been used extensively for diagnosis and treatment of accommodative esotropia with or without an accompanying high accommodative convergence-to-accommodation (AC/A) ratio. In children who present with acquired esotropia and who have less than +3.00 spherical hyperopia, miotics can be used diagnostically. If after 4–6 weeks the esodeviation is eliminated, the diagnosis of accommodative esotropia is established. Miotic treatment can be continued, or fully corrected hyperopic glasses can be prescribed. Miotics may also be used in association with single vision glasses to avoid bifocals in many patients with a high AC/A ratio.

2. Botulinum toxin–The injection of botulinum toxin type A (Botox) into an extraocular muscle produces a dose-dependent duration of paralysis of that muscle. The injection is given under electromyographic positional control using a bipolar electrode needle. The toxin is tightly bound to the muscle tissue. The doses used are so small that systemic toxicity does not occur. The desired length of paralysis is dependent upon the angle of deviation. The larger the angle of deviation, the longer the duration of paralysis required. Paralysis of the muscle shifts the eye into the field of action of the antagonist muscle. During the time the eye is deviated, the paralyzed muscle is stretched, whereas the antagonist muscle is contracted. As the paralysis resolves, the eye will gradually return toward its original position but with a new balance of forces that permanently reduces or eliminates the deviation. Two or more injections are often necessary to obtain a lasting effect.

D. Orthoptics: An orthoptist is trained in methods of testing and treating patients with strabismus. Orthoptists offer significant help to the ophthalmologist, particularly in diagnosis and to a lessor extent in treatment. Evaluation of the sensory status may be very helpful in determining the fusion potential. An orthoptist may be able to aid in preoperative treatment, especially with patients who have amblyopia. At times, orthoptic training and instructions for "exercises" to be used at home can supplement and solidify surgical treatment.

Surgical Treatment
(Figures 12–7 and 12–8)

A. Surgical Procedures: A variety of changes in the rotational effect of an extraocular muscle can be achieved with surgery.

1. Resection and recession–Conceptually, the simplest procedures are strengthening and weakening. A muscle is strengthened by a procedure called **resection.** The muscle is detached from the eye, stretched out longer by a measured amount, and then resewn to the eye, usually at the original insertion site. The small amount of extra length is trimmed off. **Recession** is the standard weakening procedure. The muscle is detached from the eye, freed from fascial attachments, and allowed to retract. It is resewn to the eye a measured distance behind its original insertion.

The superior oblique is strengthened by tucking or advancing its tendon. This can be done by a graded amount. Superior oblique weakening is accomplished by a tenectomy (complete severing of the tendon) or one of several lengthening procedures. There is no effective strengthening procedure on the inferior oblique. The inferior oblique can be weakened by disinsertion, myectomy, or recession, with generally equivalent results.

2. Shifting of point of muscle attachment– In addition to simple strengthening or weakening, the point of attachment of the muscle can be shifted; this may give the muscle a rotational action it did not previously have. For example, a vertical shift of both horizontal rectus muscles on the same eye affects the vertical position of the eye. Vertical shifts of the horizontal rectus muscles in opposite directions affect the horizontal eye position in upgaze and downgaze. This is done for A or V patterns, in which the horizontal deviation is more of an esodeviation in upgaze or downgaze, respectively.

The torsional effect of a muscle can also be changed. Tightening of the anterior fibers of the superior oblique tendon, known as the Harada-Ito procedure, gives that muscle enhanced torsional action.

3. Faden procedure–A special operation for muscle weakening is called the posterior fixation (Faden) procedure (Figure 12–8). In this operation, a new insertion of the muscle is created well behind the original insertion. This causes mechanical weakening

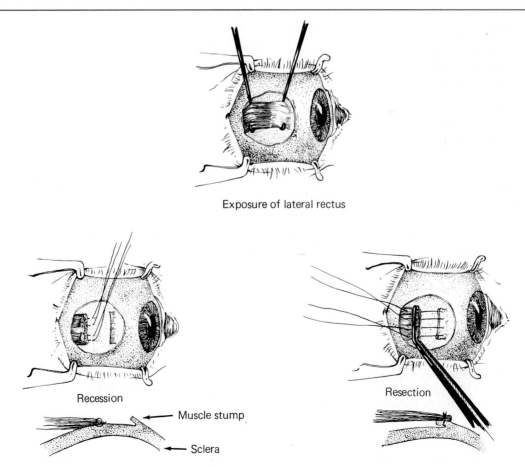

Exposure of lateral rectus

Recession

Muscle stump

Sclera

Resection

Figure 12–7. Surgical correction of strabismus (right eye).

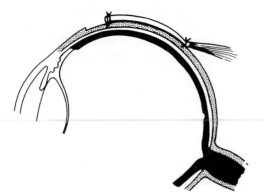

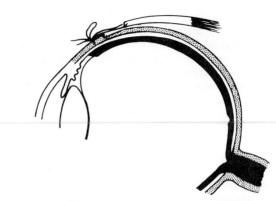

Figure 12–8. Posterior fixation (Faden) procedure. The rectus muscle is tacked to the sclera far posterior to its insertion. This prevents unwrapping of the muscle as the eye turns into the muscle's field of action. The muscle is progressively weakened in its field of action. If this procedure is combined with recession, the alignment in primary position is also affected.

Figure 12–9. Adjustable suture. The suture is placed on the sclera at any point that will be accessible to the surgeon. The bow is untied and the position of the muscle changed as desired.

of the muscle as the eye rotates into its field of action. When combined with recession of the same muscle, the Faden operation has a profound weakening effect on the muscle without significant alteration of the primary position of the eye. The procedure can be effective on vertical rectus muscles (dissociated vertical deviation) or horizontal muscles (high AC/A ratio, nystagmus, and other rare incomitant muscle imbalances).

B. Choice of Muscles for Surgery: The decision concerning which muscles to operate on is based on several factors. The first is the amount of misalignment measured in the primary position. Modifications are made for significant differences in distance and near measurements. The medial rectus muscles have more effect on the angle of deviation for near and the lateral rectus muscles more effect for distance. For esotropia greater at near, both medial rectus muscles should be weakened. For exotropia greater at distance, both lateral rectus muscles should be weakened. For deviations approximately the same at distance and near, bilateral weakening procedures or unilateral recession/resection procedures are equally effective.

Surgical realignment affects only the muscular or mechanical part of a neuromuscular imbalance. Although most individuals respond in a predictable manner, variable responses may be due to differing mechanical properties of the muscles and surrounding tissues as well as variable innervational input. For these reasons, more than one operation may be required to obtain a satisfactory result.

C. Adjustable Sutures: (Figure 12–9.) The development of adjustable sutures offers a great advantage in muscle surgery, particularly for reoperations and incomitant deviations. During the operation, the muscle is reattached to the sclera with a slip knot placed so that it is accessible to the surgeon. After the patient has recovered sufficiently from the anesthesia to cooperate in the adjustment process, a topical anes-

thetic drop is placed in the eye and the suture can be tightened or loosened to change the eye position as indicated by cover testing. Adjustable sutures can be used on any rectus muscle for either recession or resection and on the superior oblique muscle for correction of torsion. Although any patient willing to cooperate is suitable, the method is usually not applicable for children under age 12.

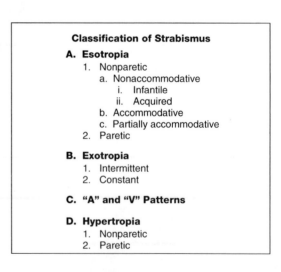

Classification of Strabismus

A. Esotropia
1. Nonparetic
   a. Nonaccommodative
      i. Infantile
      ii. Acquired
   b. Accommodative
   c. Partially accommodative
2. Paretic

B. Exotropia
1. Intermittent
2. Constant

C. "A" and "V" Patterns

D. Hypertropia
1. Nonparetic
2. Paretic

ESOTROPIA
(Convergent Strabismus, "Crossed Eyes")

Esotropia is by far the most common type of strabismus. It is divided into two types: **paretic** (due to paresis or paralysis of one or more extraocular muscles) and **nonparetic** (comitant). Nonparetic esotropia is the most common type in infants and children; it may be accommodative, nonaccommodative, or partially accommodative. Paretic strabismus is uncommon in childhood but accounts for most new cases of strabismus in adults. Most cases of childhood nonaccommodative esotropia are classified as **infantile esotropia,** with onset by age 6 months. The remainder occur after age 6 months and are classified as **acquired nonaccommodative esotropia.**

NONPARETIC ESOTROPIA

Nonaccommodative Esotropia

A. Infantile Esotropia: Nearly half of all cases of esotropia fall into this group. In most cases, the cause is obscure. The convergent deviation is manifest by age 6 months. The deviation is comitant, ie, the angle of deviation is approximately the same in all directions of gaze and is usually not affected by accommodation. The cause, therefore, is not related to the refractive error or dependent upon a paretic extraocular muscle. It is likely that the majority of cases are due to faulty innervational control, involving the supranucuelar pathways for convergence and divergence and their neural connections to the medial longitudinal fasciculus. A smaller number of cases are due to anatomic variations such as anomalous insertions of horizontally acting muscles, abnormal check ligaments, or various other fascial abnormalities.

There is also good evidence that strabismus does occur on a genetically determined basis. Esophoria and esotropia are frequently passed on as an autosomal dominant trait. Siblings may have similar ocular deviations. An accommodative element is often superimposed upon comitant esotropia, ie, correction of the hyperopic refractive error reduces but does not eliminate all of the deviation.

The deviation is often large ($\geq 40^\Delta$) and usually comitant. Abduction may be limited but can be demonstrated. Vertical deviations may be observed after 18 months of age, ie, overaction of the oblique muscles or dissociated vertical deviation. Nystagmus, manifest or latent, may be present. The most common refractive error is low to moderate hyperopia.

The eye that appears to be straight is the eye used for fixation. Almost without exception, it is the eye with better vision or lower refractive error (or both). If there is anisometropia, there will probably be some amblyopia as well. If at various times either eye is used for fixation, the patient is said to show spontaneous alternation of fixation; in this case, vision will be equal or nearly equal in both eyes. In some cases, the eye preference is determined by the direction of gaze. For example, with large-angle esotropia, there is a tendency for the right eye to be used in left gaze and the left eye in right gaze (cross fixation).

Infantile esotropia is treated surgically. Preliminary nonsurgical treatment may be indicated to ensure the best possible result. It is essential that amblyopia be fully treated prior to surgery. Glasses should be tried in hyperopic refractive errors of 3 D or more to determine if reducing accommodation has a favorable effect on the deviation. A miotic may be used successfully as an alternative to glasses.

Surgery is usually indicated after medical therapy and treatment of amblyopia have been completed. Once reproducible measurements are obtained, surgery should be performed since there is ample evidence that sensory results are better the sooner the eyes are aligned. Many procedures have been recommended, but the two most popular are (1) weakening of both medial rectus muscles, and (2) recession of the medial rectus and resection of the lateral rectus on the same eye.

B. Acquired Nonaccommodative Esotropia: This type of esotropia develops in childhood, usually after the age of 2 years. There is little or no accommodative factor. The angle of strabismus is often smaller than in infantile esotropia but may increase with time. Otherwise, clinical findings are the same as for congenital esotropia. Treatment is surgical and follows the same guidelines as for congenital esotropia.

Accommodative Esotropia

Accommodative esotropia occurs when there is a normal physiologic mechanism of accommodation with an associated overactive convergence response but insufficient relative fusional divergence to hold the eyes straight. There are two pathophysiologic mechanisms at work, singly or together: (1) sufficiently high hyperopia, requiring so much accommodation (and therefore convergence) to clarify the image that esotropia results; and (2) a high AC/A ratio, which is accompanied by mild to moderate hyperopia (1.5 D or more).

A. Accommodative Esotropia Due to Hyperopia: Accommodative esotropia due to hyperopia typically begins at age 2–3 but may occur earlier or later. Deviation is variable prior to treatment. Glasses with full cycloplegic refraction allow the eyes to become aligned.

B. Accommodative Esotropia Due to High AC/A Ratio: In accommodative esotropia due to a high ratio of accommodative convergence to accommodation (AC/A ratio), a deviation is greater at near than at distance. The refractive error is hyperopic. Treatment is with glasses with full cycloplegic refraction plus bifocals or miotics to relieve excess deviation at near.

Partially Accommodative Esotropia

A mixed mechanism—part muscular imbalance and part accommodative/convergence imbalance—may exist. Although antiaccommodative therapy decreases the angle of deviation, the esotropia is not eliminated. Surgery is performed for the nonaccommodative component of the deviation with the choice of surgical procedure as described for infantile esotropia.

PARETIC (INCOMITANT) ESOTROPIA
(Abducens Palsy)
(Figures 12–2 and 12–10)

In incomitant strabismus, there are always one or more paretic extraocular muscles. In the case of incomitant esotropia, the paresis is always one or both of the lateral rectus muscles, usually as a result of palsy of the abducens nerve. These cases are often seen in adults who have systemic hypertension or diabetes, but abducens palsy may occasionally be the first sign of a tumor or of inflammatory disease involving the central nervous system. Associated neurologic signs are then important clues. Head trauma is another frequent cause of abducens palsy.

Incomitant esotropia is also seen in infants and children, but much less commonly than comitant esotropia. These cases result from birth injuries affecting the muscle directly, from injury to the nerve, or, less commonly, from a congenital anomaly of the lateral rectus muscle or its fascial attachments.

If the lateral rectus muscle is totally paralyzed, the eye will not abduct past the midline. Esotropia is characteristically greater at distance than at near and greater to the affected side. Paresis of the right lateral rectus causes esotropia that becomes greater on right gaze and, if paresis is mild, little or no deviation on left gaze.

If, after 6–8 weeks following onset of the paresis there is no sign of improvement, botulinum toxin type A injections into the antagonist medial rectus muscle may be helpful or even curative in mild cases. In more severe cases, injections will decrease the likelihood of contracture of the antagonist muscle. If there is no improvement by 6 months, surgery is necessary. If there is little or no medial rectus contracture, its recession is indicated together with a large resection of the paretic lateral rectus muscle. For total abduction paralysis, the insertions of the superior and inferior rectus muscles may be transposed to the insertion of the lateral rectus muscle, and the medial rectus muscle may be recessed or temporarily paralyzed by botulinum toxin A. Adjustable sutures allow for fine gradations of surgery of the recessed muscle so that the largest possible area of single binocular vision is obtained. Abduction of the paretic muscle will always be limited.

Pseudoesotropia

Pseudoesotropia is the illusion of crossed eyes in an infant or toddler when no strabismus is present. This appearance is usually caused by a flat, broad nasal bridge and prominent epicanthal folds that cover a portion of the nasal sclera, giving the impression that the eyes are crossed. This very common condition may be differentiated from true misalignment by the corneal light reflection appearing in the center of the pupil of each eye when the child fixates a light. With normal fa-

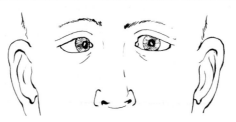

Primary position: right esotropia

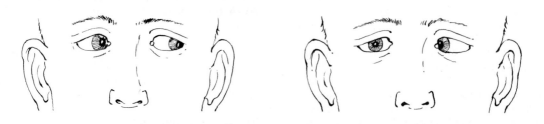

Left gaze: no deviation

Right gaze: left esotropia

Figure 12–10. Incomitant strabismus (paralytic). Paralysis of right lateral rectus muscle, with left eye fixing.

cial growth and increasing prominence of the nasal bridge, this pseudoestropic appearance gradually disappears. Of course, true esotropia may be present in association with this common infantile facial configuration.

EXOTROPIA
(Divergent Strabismus)

Exotropia is less common than esotropia, particularly in infancy and childhood. Its incidence increases gradually with age. Not infrequently, a tendency to divergent strabismus beginning as exophoria progresses to intermittent exotropia and finally to constant exotropia if no treatment is given. Other cases begin as constant or intermittent exotropia and remain stationary. As in esotropia, there may be a hereditary element in some cases. Exophoria and exotropia (considered as a single entity of divergent deviation) are frequently passed on as autosomal dominant traits, so that one or both parents of an exotropic child may demonstrate exotropia or a high degree of exophoria.

Alternative Classification of Exotropia

Constant or intermittent exotropia can also be classified on a descriptive basis as being an excess of divergence or an insufficiency of convergence. These descriptive terms do not imply that the cause of the deviation is understood.

A. Basic Exotropia: Distance and near deviations are approximately equal.

B. Divergence Excess: Distance deviation is significantly larger than near deviation.

C. Convergence Insufficiency: Near deviation is significantly larger than distance deviation.

D. Pseudodivergence Excess: Distance deviation is significantly larger than near deviation: however, use of a +3 diopter lens for near measurement will cause the near deviation to become approximately equal to the distance deviation.

INTERMITTENT EXOTROPIA

Clinical Findings

Intermittent exotropia accounts for well over half of all cases of exotropia. The onset of the deviation may be in the first year, and practically all have presented by age 5. The history often reveals that the condition has become progressively worse. A characteristic sign is closing one eye in bright light (Figure 12–11). The

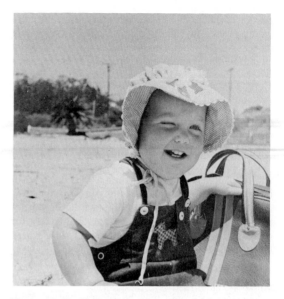

Figure 12–11. Child with intermittent exotropia squinting in sunlight.

manifest exotropia first becomes noticeable with distance fixation. The patient usually fuses at near, overcoming moderate to large angle exophoria. Convergence is frequently excellent. There is no correlation with a specific refractive error.

Since a child fuses at least part of the time, there is usually no gross sensory abnormality. For distance, with one eye deviated, there is suppression of that eye and normal retinal correspondence with little or no amblyopia.

Treatment

A. Medical Treatment: Nonsurgical treatment is largely confined to refractive correction and amblyopia therapy. If the AC/A ratio is high, the use of minus lenses may delay surgery for a while. Occasionally, antisuppression or convergence exercises may be of temporary benefit.

B. Surgical Treatment: Most patients with intermittent exotropia require surgery when their fusional control deteriorates. Deterioration of control is documented over time by an increasing percentage of time the manifest exotropia is observed, an enlarging angle of deviation, decreasing control for near fixation, and worsening in the patient's measured distance and near stereoscopic abilities. Surgery may also alleviate diplopia or other asthenopic symptoms.

The choice of procedure depends on the measurements of the deviation. Bilateral lateral rectus muscle recession is preferred when the deviation is greater at distance. If there is more deviation at near, it is best to undertake resection of a medial rectus muscle and recession of the ipsilateral lateral rectus muscle. Surgery on one or even two additional horizontal muscles may be necessary for very large deviations (>50$^\Delta$). It is desirable to obtain slight overcorrection in the immediate postoperative period for best long-term results.

CONSTANT EXOTROPIA (Figure 12–12)

Constant exotropia is less common than intermittent exotropia. It may be present at birth or may occur when intermittent exotropia progresses to constant exotropia. Some cases have their onset later in life, particularly following loss of vision in one eye. Except for cases due to loss of vision, the underlying cause is usually not known.

Clinical Findings

Constant exotropia may be of any degree. With chronicity or poor vision in one eye, the deviation can become quite large. Adduction may be limited, and hypertropia also may be present. There is suppression if the deviation was acquired by age 6–8; otherwise, diplopia may be present. If exotropia is due to very poor vision in one eye, there may be no diplopia. Amblyopia is uncommon in the absence of anisometropia, and spontaneous alternation of the fixating eye is frequently observed.

Treatment

Surgery is nearly always indicated. The choice and amount are as described for intermittent exotropia. Slight overcorrection in an adult may result in diplopia. Most patients adjust to this, especially if they have been forewarned of the possibility. If one eye has reduced vision, the prognosis for maintenance of a stable position is less favorable, with the strong possibility that the deviating eye will gradually become more exotropic. Botulinum toxin type A injections can be useful as primary treatment in small deviations or as supplementary treatment in significant surgical overcorrections or undercorrections.

A & V PATTERNS

A horizontal deviation may be vertically incomitant, ie, the deviation is different in upgaze versus downgaze (A or V pattern). An A pattern shows more esodeviation or less exodeviation in upgaze compared to downgaze. A V pattern shows less esodeviation or more exodeviation in upgaze compared to downgaze.

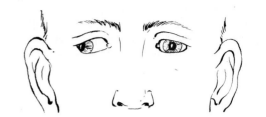

Figure 12–12. Right exotropia.

An A pattern is diagnostically significant when greater than 10$^\Delta$ and a V pattern when greater than 15$^\Delta$. These patterns are frequently associated with overaction of the oblique muscles, inferior obliques for V patterns and superior obliques for A patterns.

When surgically treating an A or V pattern, oblique muscle overaction must be treated if present. If little or no oblique overaction exists, vertical offsets of one-half tendon width of the horizontal muscles are utilized to collapse the pattern. The insertions of the medial rectus muscles are displaced toward the narrow end of the pattern (in V esotropia, recessed medial rectus muscles are moved down), and lateral rectus muscles are displaced toward the open end (in V exotropia, the insertions of the recessed lateral rectus muscles are moved up).

HYPERTROPIA (Figure 12–13)

Vertical deviations are customarily named according to the high eye, regardless of which eye has the better vision and is used for fixation. Hypertropias are less common than horizontal deviations and are usually acquired after childhood.

There are many causes of hypertropia. Congenital anatomic anomalies may result in muscle attachments in abnormal locations. Occasionally, there are anomalous fibrous bands that attach to the eye. Closed head trauma may produce paresis of the superior oblique

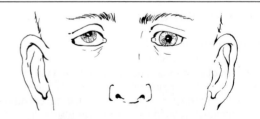

Figure 12–13. Right hypertropia.

muscle. Orbital tumors, brain stem lesions, and systemic diseases such as myasthenia gravis, multiple sclerosis, and Graves' disease can all produce hypertropias. Many of these specific entities are discussed in Chapter 14.

Clinical Findings

The clinical findings may vary, depending on the cause. The history is particularly important in diagnosis of hypertropias. Prism and cover measurements in primary and cardinal positions and head tilts are the mainstay of the clinical evaluation and may often be diagnostic. Observation of ocular rotations for limitations can also be of great value.

Diplopia is almost invariably present if strabismus develops past age 6–8. As in other forms of strabismus, sensory adaptation occurs if the onset is before this age range. Suppression and anomalous retinal correspondence may be present in gaze directions where there is strabismus. In gaze directions without strabismus, there may be no suppression and normal stereopsis.

There may be head tilt, turn, or abnormal posture of the head. The deviation may be of any magnitude and usually changes with the direction of gaze. Most hypertropias are incomitant. The deviation tends to be greatest in the field of action of one of the four vertically acting muscles. There may be an associated **cyclotropia,** especially with superior oblique dysfunction. To measure a cyclotropia, the **double Maddox rod test** is used. In a trial frame, a red and white Maddox rod are aligned vertically, one over each eye. With the patient's head held straight and fixing a light, one rod is gradually turned until the observed lines are parallel to each other and to normal horizontal orientation. The angle of tilt is then read from the angular scale on the trial frame (Figure 12–4).

The superior oblique is the most commonly paretic vertical muscle. The vertical rectus muscles are commonly involved in trauma, as with entrapment of the inferior rectus in an orbital floor fracture, and in thyroid eye disease, in which the inferior rectus becomes hypertrophied, inelastic, and fibrotic, which pulls the eye downward.

Paresis of the superior oblique may present in several patterns. It is not understood why different patients show different patterns. The simplest pattern is maximum deviation in the field of action of the muscle (ie, the lower field of gaze to the contralateral side). Another pattern is maximum deviation in the field of action of the ipsilateral antagonist, the inferior oblique. Deviation is then maximum in the upper field of gaze to the contralateral side. Deviation in the lower field need not be entirely lateralized and may have spread to the opposite side on downward gaze. Deviation may also be to one side only, without being much greater up or down; or it may be up and down the side and across the bottom as well. Most cases show some degree of excyclotropia.

The Bielschowsky head tilt test (Figure 12–14) is useful to confirm the diagnosis of superior oblique paresis. The test exploits the differing effects of each vertical muscle on torsion and elevation. Thus, with a paretic right superior oblique when the head is tilted to the right, the superior rectus and superior oblique contract to intort the eye and maintain the position of the retinal vertical meridian as much as possible. The superior rectus elevates the eye, and the superior oblique depresses the eye. Because of weakness of the superior oblique muscle, the vertical forces do not cancel out as they normally would, and right hypertropia increases. In head tilt to the left, the intorting muscles for the right eye relax and the inferior oblique and inferior rectus both contract to extort the eye. Both the paretic superior oblique and the superior rectus relax, and hypertropia is minimized. Hypertropia should be measured by prism plus cover with the head tilted to either side.

Treatment

A. Medical Treatment: For smaller and more comitant deviations, a prism may be all that is required. For constant diplopia, one eye may need to be occluded. Systemic disease must be treated if suspected to be the underlying cause.

B. Surgical Treatment: Surgery is often indicated if the deviation and diplopia persist. The choice of procedure depends on quantitative measurements. The use of adjustable sutures (Figure 12–9) is frequently a great help in fine-tuning the effect of vertical muscle surgery.

SPECIAL FORMS

DUANE'S RETRACTION SYNDROME

Duane's retraction syndrome is typically characterized by marked limitation of abduction, mild limitation of adduction, retraction of the globe and narrowing of the palpebral fissure on attempted adduction, and, frequently, upshoot or downshoot of the eye in adduction. Usually it is monocular, with the left eye more often affected. Most cases are sporadic, although some families with dominant inheritance have been described. A variety of other anomalies may be associated, such as dysplasia of the iris stroma, heterochromia, cataract, choroidal coloboma, microphthalmos, Goldenhar's syndrome, Klippel-Feil syndrome, cleft palate, and anomalies of the face, ear, or extremities. The causes of the motility defects are varied, and some anomalies of muscle structure have been found. Most cases can be explained by inappropriate innervation to the lateral rectus and sometimes to other muscles as well. Sher-

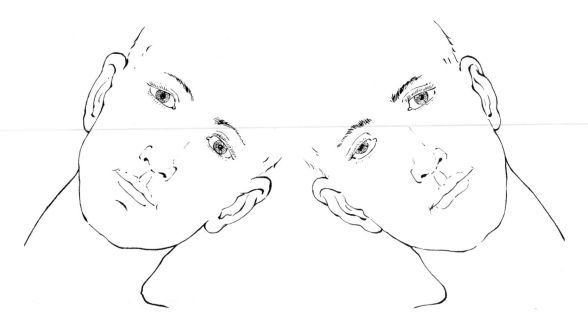

Figure 12–14. Head tilt test (Bielschowsky test). Paresis of right superior oblique. **Left:** Hypertropia is minimized on tilting the head to the sound side. The right eye may then extort and the intorting superior oblique and superior rectus relax. **Right:** When the head is tilted to the paretic side, the intorting muscles contract together, but their vertical actions do not cancel out as usual, because of superior oblique paresis. Hypertropia is worse with head tilt to the paretic side.

rington's law of reciprocal innervation is not obeyed, because nerve fibers to the medial rectus may also go to the lateral rectus. This accounts for simultaneous contraction of the medial and lateral rectus muscles (co-contraction), causing retraction of the globe. Cases with proved absence of the abducens nucleus and nerve have been documented.

Treatment

Only when a primary position misalignment or a significant compensatory head turn exists is surgical treatment indicated. The goal is to obtain straight eyes in the primary position and to horizontally expand the field of single vision. Recession of the medial rectus on the affected side is performed if any esotropia is present in the primary position. For more severe cases, temporal transposition of the vertical rectus muscles accompanied by weakening of the medial rectus muscle, either by adjustable recession or botulinum toxin A, is often indicated.

DISSOCIATED VERTICAL DEVIATION

Dissociated vertical deviation is frequently associated with congenital esotropia and rarely with an otherwise normal muscle balance. The exact cause is not known, though it is logical to assume it is from faulty supranuclear innervation of extraocular muscles.

Clinical Findings

Each eye drifts upward under cover, frequently with extorsion and a small exotropic shift, and then returns to its resting binocular position when the cover is removed. Occasionally, the upward drifting will occur spontaneously, causing a noticeable vertical misalignment. Most cases are bilateral, though asymmetry of involvement is common. There are usually no symptoms.

Treatment

Treatment is indicated if the frequency of the intermittent manifest vertical deviation is unacceptable. Nonsurgical treatment is limited to refractive correction to maximize the potential of motor fusion and therapy for amblyopia. Surgical results have been variable and can be disappointing. Currently, the most popular and successful procedures are very large recession of the superior rectus or recession of the superior rectus combined with the Faden procedure. A new procedure that involves transposing anteriorly the insertion of the inferior oblique muscle has also been effective.

BROWN'S SYNDROME (Superior Oblique Tendon Sheath Syndrome)

Brown's syndrome is due to fibrous adhesions in the superior nasal quadrant involving the superior oblique tendon and trochlea, which mechanically limit elevation of the eye. Limitation of elevation is most marked in the adducted position, and improvement in elevation occurs gradually as the eye is abducted. Differential diagnosis is concerned mainly with paresis of the inferior oblique muscle. Forced duction testing is diagnostic, since there is an upward restriction to elevation in adduction when Brown's syndrome is present. The condition is usually unilateral and idiopathic, though rarely it may be due to trauma or inflammation.

Surgical treatment is limited to those cases where there is an abnormal head position to compensate for hypotropia or cyclotropia of the involved eye. The objective is to free the mechanical adhesions and weaken the superior oblique muscle. Although controversial as to its timing, weakening of the ipsilateral inferior oblique may compensate for the induced fourth nerve palsy. Normalization of the head position may occur, but restoration of full motility is seldom achieved.

HETEROPHORIA

Heterophoria is deviation of the eyes that is held in check by binocular vision. Almost all individuals have some degree of heterophoria, and small amounts are considered normal. Larger amounts may cause symptoms depending on the level of effort required by the individual to control latent muscle imbalance.

Clinical Findings

The symptoms of heterophoria may be clear-cut (intermittent diplopia) or vague ("eyestrain" or asthenopia). Diplopia may come on only with fatigue or with poor lighting conditions, as in night driving. Usage requirements for the eyes and personality type are additional factors. Thus, there is no degree of heterophoria that is clearly abnormal, though larger amounts are more likely to be symptomatic. Except for hyperopia, high AC/A ratios, and mild cases of muscle paresis not resulting in frank heterotropia, the fundamental causes of heterophorias are unknown.

Asthenopia is sometimes caused by uncorrected refractive errors as well as by muscle imbalance. One possible mechanism is **aniseikonia,** in which an image seen by one eye is a different size and shape from that seen by the other eye. Spectacles with unequal lens powers in the two eyes can cause asthenopia by creating prismatic displacement of the image in one eye for gaze away from the optic axis that is too large to control (induced prism). Another mechanism that may produce symptoms is a change in spatial perception due to the curvature of the lenses or astigmatic corrections. (See Chapter 20.)

The symptoms encountered in asthenopia take a wide variety of forms. There may be a feeling of heaviness, tiredness, or discomfort of the eyes, varying from a dull ache to deep pain located in or behind the eyes. Headaches of all types occur. Easy fatigability, blurring of vision, and diplopia, especially after prolonged use of the eyes, also occur. Symptoms are more common for near visual work than for distance. Frequently, an aversion to reading develops. Symptoms can be brought on by fatigue or illness or following the ingestion of medications or alcohol.

Diagnosis

The diagnosis of heterophoria is based on prism and cover measurements. Relative fusional vergence amplitudes are measured. While the patient views an accommodative target at distance or near, prisms of increasing strength are placed in front of one eye. The fusional vergence amplitude is the amount of prism the patient is able to overcome and still maintain single vision. Measurements are done with base-out, base-in, base-up, and base-down prisms. The important feature is the size of the amplitudes in comparison to the angle of heterophoria. While one cannot give exact norms for normal relative fusion vergence, guidelines for typical normal findings are as follows: at distance, convergence is 14^Δ, divergence is 6^Δ, and vertical is 2.5^Δ; at near, convergence is 35^Δ, divergence is 15^Δ, and vertical is 2.5^Δ.

Treatment

Heterophoria requires treatment only if symptomatic. Untreated heterophoria or asthenopia does not cause any permanent damage to the eyes or vision. Treatment methods are designed to facilitate fusion either by medical or surgical means.

A. Medical Treatment:

1. Accurate refractive correction–Occasionally, poor visual acuity is found in the presence of symptomatic heterophoria. Spectacles providing clear vision are sometimes all that is needed to alleviate symptoms. The clearer image allows the patient's fusional capacity to function to its fullest.

2. Manipulation of accommodation–In general, esophorias are treated with antiaccommodative therapy and exophorias by stimulating accommodation. Plus lenses often work well for esophoria, especially if hyperopia is present, by reducing accommodative convergence. A high AC/A ratio may be effectively treated with plus lenses, sometimes combined with bifocals or miotics.

3. Prisms–The use of prisms requires the wearing of glasses; for some patients, this is unacceptable. A trial of plastic Fresnel press-on prisms should be made before ground-in prisms are ordered. For optical reasons, larger amounts of prismatic correction produce visual distortions limiting the use of prisms in higher strengths. Furthermore, very thick lenses can result. The usual practice is to prescribe about one-third to one-half of the measured deviation, which often allows fusion to occur. Prisms can be useful for esophoria, exophoria, and vertical phorias as well.

4. Botulinum toxin type A (Botox) injection—This treatment is well suited to producing small to moderate shifts in ocular alignment and has been used as a substitute for surgical weakening of one muscle. The main disadvantage is that the resulting effect may be variable or wear off completely months later.

B. Surgical Treatment: Surgery should be done only after medical methods have failed. As in strabismus, muscles are chosen for correction according to the measured deviation at distance and near in various directions of gaze. Sometimes only one muscle needs

REFERENCES

Burke MJ: *Intermittent Exotropia.* In: *Strabismus Surgery International Ophthalmology Clinics.* Vol 25, No 4. Nelson LB, Wagner RS (editors). Little, Brown, 1985.

Collins C, O'Mear DM, Scott AB: Muscle tension during unrestrained human eye movement. J Physiol 1975;245:363.

Duke-Elder S, Wybar K: *Ocular Motility and Strabismus.* Vol 6 of: *System of Ophthalmology.* Duke-Elder S (editor). Mosby, 1973.

Eggers HM: Functional anatomy of the extraocular muscles. In: *Biomedical Foundations of Ophthalmology.* Tasman W (editor). Lippincott, 1993.

Helveston EM: 19th Annual Frank Costenbader Lecture: The origins of congenital esotropia. J Pediatr Ophthalmol Strabismus (July–Aug) 1993;30:215.

Helveston EM: *Surgical Management of Strabismus: An Atlas of Strabismus Surgery,* 4th ed. Mosby, 1993.

Huber AL, Electrophysiology of the retraction syndrome. Br J. Ophthalmol 1974;58:293.

Ing MR: Early surgical alignment for congenital esotropia. Trans Am Ophthalmol Soc 1981;79:625.

Jampolsky A: Current techniques of adjustable strabismus surgery. Am J Ophthalmol 1979;88:406.

Knapp P: Diagnosis and surgical treatment of hypertropia. Am Orthop J 1971;21:29.

Kratz RE et al: Anterior tendon displacement of the inferior oblique for DVD. J Pediatr Ophthalmol Strabismus (Sept–Oct) 1989;26:212.

Kushner J: Binocular field expansion in adults after surgery for esotropia. Arch Ophthalmol 1994;112:636.

Parks MM: The monofixation syndrome. Trans Am Ophthalmol Soc 1969;67:609.

Prism Adaptation Study Research Group: Efficacy of prism adaptation in the surgical management of acquired esotropia. Arch Ophthalmol 1990;108:1248.

Rogers GL et al: Strabismus surgery and its effects upon infant development in congenital esotropia. Ophthalmology 1982;89:479.

Romano PE, Robinson JA: General anesthesia morbidity and mortality in eye surgery at a children's hospital. J Pediatr Ophthalmol Strabismus 1981;18:17.

Rosenbaum AL, Kushner BJ, Kirschen D: Vertical rectus muscle transposition and botulism toxin (Oculinum) to medial rectus for abducens palsy. Arch Ophthalmol 1989;107:820.

Scott AB: *Botulism Toxin: Treatment of Strabismus.* Vol 7, Module 12, in: *Focal Points: Clinical Modules for Ophthalmologists.* American Academy of Ophthalmology, 1989.

Shauly Y, Prager TC, Mazow ML: Clinical characteristics and long-term postoperative results of infantile esotropia. Am J Ophthalmol 1994;117:183.

Tasman W, Jaeger EA (editors): *Duane's Clinical Ophthalmology,* rev ed, vol 1. Lippincott, 1993.

von Noorden GK: *Burian–von Noorden's Binocular Vision and Ocular Motility,* 4th ed. Mosby, 1990.

von Noorden GK: *von Noorden-Maumenee's Atlas of Strabismus,* 4th ed. Mosby, 1983.

Wiesel TN, Hubel DM: Extent of recovery from the effects of visual deprivation in kittens. J Neurophysiol 1965; 28:1060.

Wright KW: *Color Atlas of Ophthalmic Surgery: Strabismus.* Lippincott, 1991.

Wright KW et al: High-grade stereo acuity after early surgery for congenital esotropia. Arch Ophthalmol 1994;112:913.

Orbit

13

John H. Sullivan, MD

PHYSIOLOGY OF SYMPTOMS

Owing to the rigid bony structure of the orbit, with only an anterior opening for expansion (Chapter 1), any increase in the orbital contents taking place to the side of or behind the eyeball will displace that organ forward (**proptosis**). Protrusion of the eyeball is the hallmark of orbital disease. Expansive lesions may be benign or malignant and may arise from bone, muscle, nerve, blood vessels, or connective tissue. A mass may be inflammatory, neoplastic, cystic, or vascular. Protrusion is not in itself injurious unless the lids are unable to cover the cornea. The underlying cause, however, is usually serious and sometimes life-threatening. **Pseudoproptosis** is apparent proptosis in the absence of orbital disease. Such confusion may arise with high myopia, buphthalmos, and lid retraction.

History and examination provide many clues to the cause of proptosis. The position of the eye is determined by the location of the mass. Expansion within the muscle cone displaces the eye straight ahead (**axial proptosis**), whereas a mass arising outside the muscle cone will also cause sideways or vertical displacement of the globe directly away from the mass (**nonaxial proptosis**). Bilateral involvement generally indicates systemic disease, such as Graves' disease. The term "exophthalmos" is often used when describing proptosis associated with Graves' disease. **Pulsating proptosis** reflects the pulse of an orbital vascular malformation or transmission of cerebral pulsations in the absence of the superior orbital roof, as in neurofibromatosis. **Positional proptosis**—which changes with Valsalva's maneuver—is a sign of orbital varices or meningocele. **Intermittent proptosis** may be the result of a sinus mucocele. The Hertel exophthalmometer (see Chapter 2) is the standard method of quantifying the magnitude of proptosis. Serial measurements are most accurate if performed by the same individual with the same instrument.

With the change in position of the eyeball, especially if it takes place rapidly, there may be enough mechanical interference with the movement of the eye to cause dissociation of ocular movements and diplopia (double vision). Pain may occur as a result of rapid expansion, inflammation, or infiltration of sensory nerves. Vision is not usually affected early unless the lesion arises from the optic nerve. Pupillary signs and color vision testing may identify subtle optic nerve compression or involvement before acuity is reduced significantly. Involvement of the superior orbital fissure by trauma or tumor produces a characteristic combination of diplopia resulting from disturbance of function of the oculomotor, trochlear, and abducens nerves and corneal and facial anesthesia (ophthalmic division of trigeminal nerve), known as the **orbital fissure syndrome.** Expanding lesions at the orbital apex result in the **orbital apex syndrome,** characterized by proptosis; and optic nerve compression, variably accompanied by the diplopia and corneal and facial anesthesia seen in the orbital fissure syndrome.

DIAGNOSTIC STUDIES

1. IMAGING

CT & MRI

Imaging by **computed tomography (CT scan)** (Figures 13–1 and 13–2) was a major advance in orbital diagnosis. Continued improvement in resolution quality—as well as three-dimensional reconstructions— have made CT the single most important diagnostic study in the investigation of orbital disease. Contrast enhancement with CT during study of vascular lesions sometimes provides additional information. **Magnetic resonance imaging (MRI)** is capable of displaying subtle changes within soft tissue that cannot be imaged with CT, but it is less useful for bony changes. A surface coil applied directly to the orbit enhances image resolution. MRI is contraindicated in the presence of a ferrous intraorbital or intracranial foreign body.

Ultrasonography

The use of ultrasonography in the diagnosis of orbital disease has largely been supplanted by CT and MRI. Although it is a noninvasive and inexpensive form of imaging, its usefulness in both A and B mode is limited to the anterior portion of the orbit. It is of greatest value in the hands of the clinician-ultrasonographer capable of interpreting "real time" images.

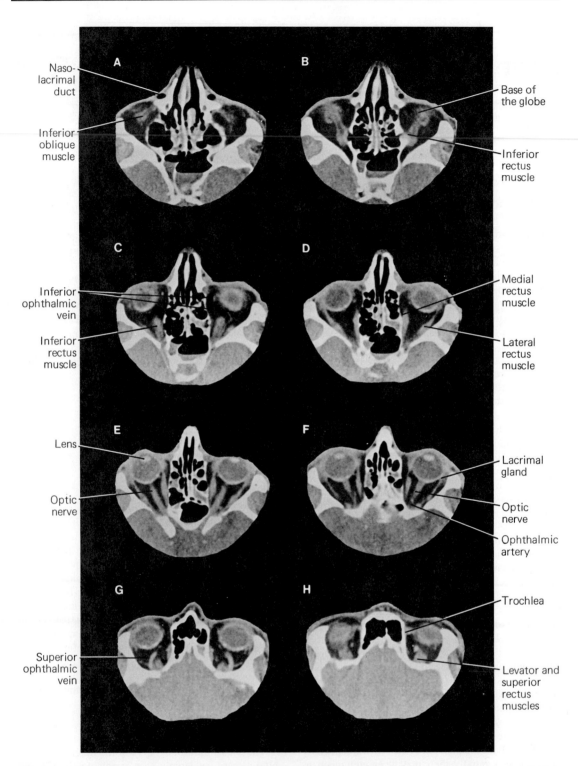

Figure 13–1. Normal CT scan showing the anatomy of the orbit. Axial CT sections, thickness 1.5 mm. **A:** Lowest section. **B:** Highest section. Note clear delineation of individual muscles, optic nerve, and major veins within the orbital fat.

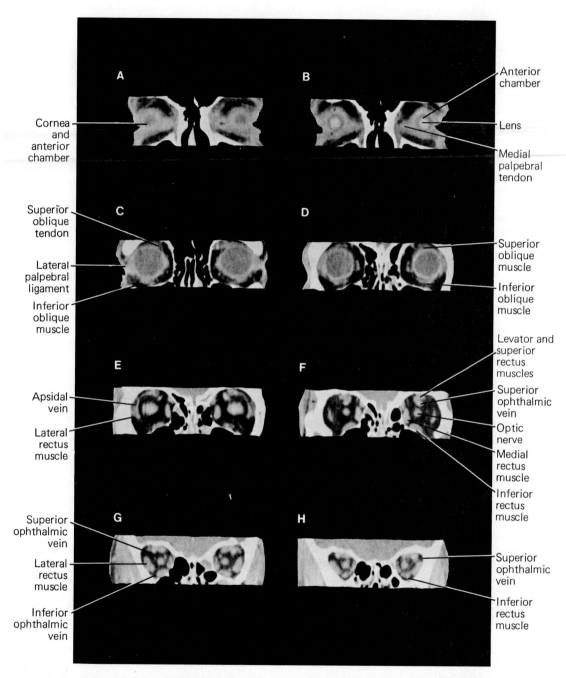

Figure 13–2. Coronal computer reconstructions from axial CT sections. *A:* Most anterior section. *H:* Most posterior section. Note detailed demonstration of ocular and orbital structures.

Venography

Venography is occasionally useful in defining the extent of orbital venous disease. Although the diagnosis can usually be made by MRI, contrast injection into the orbital veins via a scalp vein can sometimes reveal the presence of varices that have escaped detection by CT.

Angiography

Selective carotid angiography with bone subtraction is sometimes necessary to make the diagnosis of certain orbital vascular disorders. In spontaneous, low-flow dural carotid artery-cavernous sinus fistula, angiography is required for delineation of the extent of involvement and for treatment by embolization.

Radiography

Plain x-rays are sufficient for diagnosis of many orbital disorders such as fractures. However, the thin walls of the orbit are difficult to visualize even with tomography, and CT or MRI imaging is used to determine the extent of injury. Dacryocystography and radionuclide scanning can sometimes be helpful in localizing the site of lacrimal obstructions, but these procedures are seldom used. The results are difficult to interpret, and treatment is seldom altered by the findings. Positive contrast radiography and pneumoorbitography are no longer used. Orbital thermography is a research procedure.

Fine-Needle Aspiration

Fine-needle aspiration is an invasive procedure that has proved very useful in orbital diagnosis. Cytology specimens can be aspirated from a lesion the exact location of which is determined by CT imaging. Cytopathology can be inconclusive but is often invaluable.

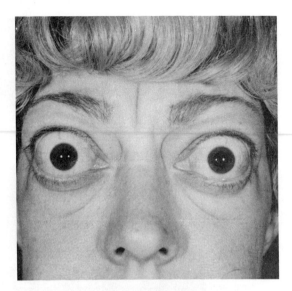

Figure 13–3. Graves' ophthalmopathy.

DISEASES & DISORDERS OF THE ORBIT

INFLAMMATORY DISORDERS

1. GRAVES' OPHTHALMOPATHY

The most common cause of unilateral or bilateral proptosis in adults or children is Graves' disease.

The terminology used to describe ocular involvement in thyroid disease is often confusing. Some degree of ophthalmopathy—usually mild—occurs in a high percentage of hyperthyroid patients. Severe infiltrative orbital myopathy with significant proptosis and restricted motility occurs in about 5% of cases of Graves' disease (Figure 13–3). This severe form, however, can also occur with hypothyroidism or with no detectable thyroid abnormality.

Thyroid ophthalmopathy is thought to be an autoimmune disease. It is often seen in autoimmune (Hashimoto's) thyroiditis. Antithyroglobulin, antimicrosomal, and other antibodies can usually be demonstrated, but their role in pathogenesis is in question.

Clinical Findings

Proptosis associated with thyroid disease is characterized by lid retraction, which serves to distinguish it from other causes of proptosis. Lagophthalmos results from proptosis and lid retraction, and corneal exposure is a factor even in mild cases. Ocular myopathy usually begins with lymphocytic infiltration and edema of the rectus muscles. In time, the inflamed muscles may become fibrotic and permanently restricted. The eye

may be tethered so as to raise the intraocular pressure when it is measured in upgaze.

Diplopia usually begins in the upper field of gaze because of infiltrative myopathy involving the inferior rectus muscle. All extraocular muscles may eventually be involved, and there may be no position of gaze free of diplopia. The extraocular muscles may become massively enlarged and—in addition to restricting eye movement—may compress the optic nerve. Compressive optic neuropathy is most common with enlargement of the posterior aspect of the muscles that occurs without severe proptosis. Early signs include an afferent pupillary defect, impairment of color vision, and slight loss of visual acuity. Blindness is liable to occur if compression is unrelieved.

Treatment

The goal of treatment of Graves' ophthalmopathy is initially to maintain corneal hydration. As the disease progresses it becomes necessary to address the problems of diplopia, proptosis, and compressive optic neuropathy. Management of severe cases is difficult and multidisciplinary. An endocrinologist should monitor the metabolic activity, administer ^{131}I for ablation, or provide supplemental hormone therapy as indicated. Oral corticosteroids (prednisone, 60–100 mg/d) may be helpful in controlling the acute phase of infiltrative myopathy. Complications and side effects limit the use of corticosteroids in long-term maintenance. Orbital radiation is effective during the active phase of the disease. Soft tissue signs of swelling and chemosis are usually relieved. Diplopia and proptosis may be improved.

Early compression neuropathy may also be relieved by radiation therapy, but neuropathy unresponsive to medical management is an indication for surgical decompression of the orbit. Several approaches have been devised to expand the orbital volume by fracture of the bony walls. The method of choice is fracture of the orbital floor into the maxillary sinus and the media wall into the ethmoid sinus. Proptosis can be reduced by surgery, but there is a significant risk of intractable diplopia and a lesser risk of orbital infection. For these reasons, decompression for cosmetic reasons alone is controversial.

Eyelid retraction is often more disturbing than proptosis—both functionally, because of exposure keratitis, and cosmetically. Decompression does not usually relieve lid retraction, but correction of the retraction camouflages proptosis to some extent. Lid retraction is corrected by surgery. The upper and lower lid retractors (aponeurosis and sympathetic muscles) can be lengthened by inserting a spacer such as eye bank sclera. Small amounts (2 mm) of lid retraction can be corrected by simply disinserting the retractors from the upper tarsal border.

Strabismus surgery should not be undertaken until the myopathy has stabilized. The adjustable suture technique is useful. Most patients can achieve at least a small area of single-image binocular vision in a useful position of gaze. Torsional diplopia, the result of oblique muscle involvement, complicates management.

Some patients have intractable diplopia despite all attempts at correction.

2. PSEUDOTUMOR

A frequent cause of proptosis in adults and children is inflammatory pseudotumor. The term "pseudotumor" was coined to indicate a nonneoplastic process that produces the sentinel sign of an orbital neoplasm, ie, proptosis. This entity consists of a heterogeneous group of inflammatory diseases of unknown cause. The site of inflammation is usually diffuse and not amenable to excision. The process can involve any orbital structure (eg, myositis, dacryoadenitis, lymphogranuloma) or cell type (eg, lymphocytes, fibroblasts, histiocytes, plasma cells). Onset is usually rapid, and pain is often present.

Pseudotumor is usually unilateral; when both orbits are involved, it is more often a manifestation of systemic disease. In addition to lymphoma, the condition may be confused with Graves' ophthalmopathy, Wegener's granulomatosis, and systemic vasculitis.

Treatment with systemic corticosteroids or with radiation is usually effective. Surgery often exacerbates the inflammatory reaction.

ORBITAL INFECTIONS

1. ORBITAL CELLULITIS
(Figure 13–4)

Orbital cellulitis is the most common cause of proptosis in children. Immediate treatment is essential. For

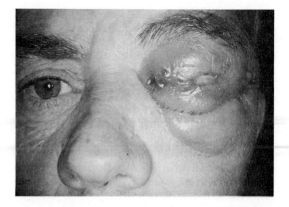

Figure 13–4. Orbital cellulitis. Abscess draining through upper eyelid.

tunately, the diagnosis usually is not difficult, because the clinical findings are characteristic. Although most cases occur in children, aged and immunocompromised individuals may also be affected.

Trauma may be responsible for introduction of contaminated material into the orbit through the skin or paranasal sinuses. In the preantibiotic era, orbital cellulitis frequently led to blindness or death resulting from septic cavernous sinus thrombosis.

The orbit is surrounded by the paranasal sinuses, and part of their venous drainage is through the orbit. Most cases of orbital cellulitis arise from extension of sinusitis through the thin ethmoid bones. The organisms usually responsible are those most frequently found in sinuses: *Haemophilus influenzae, Streptococcus pneumoniae,* other streptococci, and staphylococci.

Clinical Findings

Preseptal cellulitis is the most common presentation. CT scan or MRI is helpful in distinguishing between pre- and postseptal involvement as well as identifying and localizing an orbital abscess or foreign body. Plain x-rays alone can only identify the presence of sinusitis.

It is important to distinguish between preseptal and orbital infections. Both present with edema, erythema, hyperemia, pain, and leukocytosis. Chemosis, proptosis, limitation of eye movement, and reduction of vision indicate deep orbital involvement. Extension to the cavernous sinus may cause bilateral involvement of cranial nerves II–VI, with severe edema and septic fever. Erosion of the orbital bones may cause brain abscess and meningitis.

In children, few orbital diseases develop as rapidly as cellulitis. Confusion may exist with rhabdomyosarcoma, pseudotumor, and Graves' ophthalmopathy.

Treatment

Treatment should be initiated before the causative organism is identified. As soon as nasal, conjunctival, and blood cultures are obtained, intravenous antibiotics should be administered. A β-lactamase-resistant antibiotic should be given for staphylococcal infection and amoxicillin with clavulanic acid (Augmentin) or chloramphenicol for *H influenzae.* Posttraumatic cellulitis—especially following animal bites—must be covered for gram-negative and gram-positive bacilli. Hot compresses help localize the inflammatory reaction. Nasal decongestants and vasoconstrictors help drain the paranasal sinuses. Early surgical drainage is indicated in suppurative preseptal cellulitis. MRI is useful in deciding when and where to drain an orbital abscess. Most cases respond promptly to antibiotics. Those that do not may require drainage of the paranasal sinuses. Early consultation with an otolaryngologist may be helpful.

2. MUCORMYCOSIS

Diabetics and immunocompromised patients have a propensity to develop severe and often fatal fungal infections of the orbit. The organisms are of the Zygomycetes group, which have a tendency to invade vessels and create ischemic necrosis. Infection usually begins in the sinuses and erodes into the orbital cavity. A necrotizing reaction destroys muscle, bone, and soft tissue, frequently without causing signs of orbital cellulitis.

The patient is usually quite ill and presents with pain and proptosis. Examination of the nose often reveals a necrotic area of mucosa, a smear of which shows broad branching hyphae.

Without treatment, the infection gradually erodes into the cranial cavity, resulting in meningitis, brain abscess, and death usually within days to weeks. Treatment is difficult and often inadequate. It consists of correction of the underlying disease combined with surgical debridement and administration of amphotericin B intravenously. Recurrences are common.

CYSTIC LESIONS INVOLVING THE ORBIT

1. DERMOID

Dermoids are not true neoplasms but benign choristomas arising from embryonic tissue not usually found in the orbit. Orbital dermoids arise from surface ectoderm and often contain epithelial structures such as keratin, hair, and even teeth. Most are cystic and filled with an oily fluid that can incite a severe inflammatory reaction if liberated into the orbit. Most dermoids occur in the superior temporal quadrant of the orbit, but they can occur at any bony suture line.

X-rays show a sharp, round bony defect from the pressure of a slowly growing mass affixed to the periosteum.

Epidermoid cyst is a superficial keratin-filled mass, usually near the superior orbital rim. It may be congenital or posttraumatic. Excision is usually not difficult.

A **lipodermoid** is a solid mass of fatty material that occurs below the conjunctival surface. Hair growth on the overlying conjunctiva is not uncommon. Lipodermoids are often much larger than they appear to be, and excision may cause considerable damage to vital structures. If treatment is necessary, limited excision is usually advised.

2. SINUS MUCOCELE

The proximity of the orbit to the paranasal sinuses may lead to invasion of the bony walls and extension of an obstructed sinus into the orbit. Plain x-ray will usually make the diagnosis, but CT or MRI may be required to differentiate sinus mucocele from dermoid cyst and to define the extent of the lesion (Figure 13–5). Otolaryngologic and neurosurgical assistance may be necessary for surgical removal.

3. MENINGOCELE

Erosion of the meninges into the orbital cavity through a congenital dehiscence in the bony sutures creates a cystic mass filled with cerebrospinal fluid known as a **meningocele**. Both brain and meninges are frequently included in a **meningoencephalocele.** The resultant fluctuant mass in the superior medial orbit typically enlarges with Valsalva's maneuver. Most cases are present at birth, but those arising from the sphenoid bone may not become apparent until adolescence.

VASCULAR ABNORMALITIES INVOLVING THE ORBIT

1. ARTERIOVENOUS MALFORMATION

Arteriovenous malformations are an uncommon cause of proptosis. Varices produce intermittent prop-

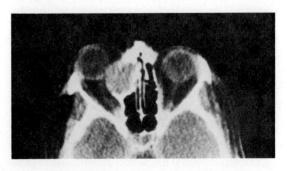

Figure 13–5. CT scan of orbital mucocele.

tosis, sometimes associated with pain and transient reduction of vision. Some degree of proptosis can be induced with Valsalva's maneuver or by placing the head in a dependent position. MRI scan is usually diagnostic, and venography is seldom indicated.

Surgery is the only method of treatment available and is fraught with hazard. Morbidity following eradication of the varix may jeopardize visual function. Most varices are best left untreated unless vision is at risk.

2. CAROTID ARTERY–CAVERNOUS SINUS FISTULA

Carotid artery-cavernous sinus fistulas with high-flow shunts are easily diagnosed. Although sometimes occurring spontaneously, they usually follow trauma. Physical signs include severe congestion and chemosis, with pulsating proptosis and a loud bruit.

Low-flow shunts (dural carotid cavernous sinus fistula) are usually spontaneous and often misdiagnosed. Mild congestion, venous engorgement and arterialization, elevated intraocular pressure, mild proptosis, and a faint bruit are the usual features. Diagnosis is by subtraction angiography, and treatment is by selective intra-arterial embolization.

PRIMARY ORBITAL TUMORS

CAPILLARY HEMANGIOMA

Capillary hemangiomas are common benign tumors that sometimes involve the eyelids and orbit (Figure 13–6). Superficial lesions are reddish (strawberry ne-

vus), and deeper lesions are more bluish. Over 90% become apparent before the age of 6 months. They tend to enlarge rapidly in the first year of life and regress slowly over 6–7 years. Lesions within the orbit may cause strabismus or proptosis. Involvement of the eyelids may induce astigmatism or occlude vision, resulting in amblyopia.

Small superficial lesions require no treatment and are best allowed to spontaneously regress. Deep orbital lesions are often associated with significant morbidity with or without treatment. The most common dilemma, however, is the rapidly growing lid lesion in a preverbal infant. Parents are often unwilling to wait for spontaneous regression and plead for treatment even if amblyopia is not a threat. The use of intralesional sustained-release corticosteroids has been found to be effective in many instances and has evolved as the preferred method of treatment in most cases. Corticosteroids are thought to have an antiangiogenic effect that inhibits capillary proliferation and induces vascular constriction.

Other forms of treatment are less effective but sometimes necessary. These include prolonged compression, systemic corticosteroids, sclerosing agents, cryotherapy, laser surgery, radiation, and surgical resection.

CAVERNOUS HEMANGIOMA (Figure 13–7)

Cavernous hemangiomas are benign, grow slowly, and usually become symptomatic in middle life. Most occur in women. They most often lie within the muscle cone, producing axial proptosis, hyperopia, and, in many cases, choroidal folds. Unlike capillary hemangiomas, they do not tend to regress spontaneously. Surgical excision is usually successful and is indicated if the patient is symptomatic.

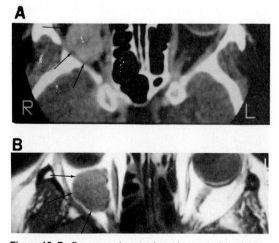

Figure 13–7. Cavernous hemangioma (arrows) of the right orbit as demonstrated by both CT scan **(A)** and MRI **(B).** The left side demonstrates the appearance of a normal orbit and globe. (Courtesy of D Char.)

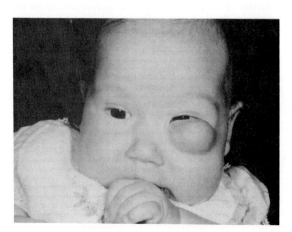

Figure 13–6. Capillary hemangioma.

LYMPHANGIOMA

In its early stages, lymphangioma may be very similar to hemangioma—even histologically. Both usually begin in infancy, though lymphangioma may present later in life. Lymphangioma does not regress and is characterized by intermittent hemorrhage and gradual worsening. Large blood cysts may cause proptosis and diplopia and require evacuation.

The tumor is often multifocal and frequently occurs in the soft palate and other areas of the face as well as the orbit. On histologic examination, it consists of large serum-filled channels and lymphoid follicles. Treatment can be for the purpose of either acute decompression of a hemorrhagic blood cyst or eradication of the tumor. Needle aspiration of blood or extirpation of a specific cyst may be temporarily effective. Excision of tumor by any method is seldom satisfactory. The risk of amblyopia is similar to that associated with capillary hemangioma.

RHABDOMYOSARCOMA
(Figure 13–8)

Rhabdomyosarcoma is the most common primary malignant tumor of the orbit in childhood. Presentation is before age 10, and rapid growth is characteristic. The tumor may destroy adjacent orbital bone and spread into the brain. The combination of external megavoltage radiation and chemotherapy has improved the survival rate of these patients from less than 50%, when orbital exenteration was used, to over 90% today.

NEUROFIBROMA

Neurofibromatosis 1 (Recklinghausen's disease) is inherited as an autosomal dominant trait. The responsible gene is on chromosome 17. Plexiform neurofibromas are characteristic and can distort the eyelids

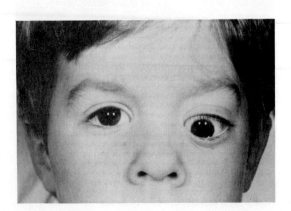

Figure 13–8. Rhabdomyosarcoma.

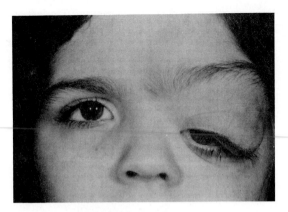

Figure 13–9. Neurofibromatosis.

(Figure 13–9) and orbit. The presence of café au lait spots helps confirm the diagnosis. The sphenoid bone is often defective; the associated orbital defect may lead to pulsating exophthalmos or enophthalmos. Optic nerve gliomas produce signs (proptosis) and symptoms (visual loss) in 5% of affected individuals; imaging has shown that many more patients harbor asymptomatic optic nerve gliomas. Some of these patients also develop meningiomas and, rarely, malignant peripheral nerve sheath tumors.

OPTIC NERVE GLIOMA

Approximately 75% of symptomatic optic nerve gliomas become apparent before age 10. Twenty-five to 50 percent are associated with neurofibromatosis 1. Most are low-grade astrocytomas and astrocytic hamartomas. Those anterior to the chiasm behave in a benign fashion; those in and posterior to the chiasm may be more aggressive. Visual loss and optic atrophy are the most common signs. Proptosis occurs if the tumor is in the orbit.

Treatment is controversial. There are no compelling statistics to indicate that either surgery or radiation is effective. Some believe these tumors to be benign hamartomas that do not require treatment. Others believe that they require surgical excision or radiotherapy. If progressive growth and visual loss are documented, radiotherapy is often effective in stabilizing or even improving vision. In blind eyes with marked proptosis, the patient's cosmetic appearance can often be improved by excising the tumor through a lateral orbitotomy.

LACRIMAL GLAND TUMORS

Fifty percent of masses presenting in the lacrimal gland are epithelial tumors; one-half of these are malignant. Inflammatory masses and lymphoproliferative tumors comprise the other 50%. The most common epithelial tumor is the pleomorphic adenoma (benign mixed tumor). These tumors should be excised—not biopsied—because of their propensity for recurrence and malignant transformation.

A malignant tumor of the lacrimal gland is suspected when the patient presents with pain and destructive bony changes are evident on x-ray. Biopsy should be performed through the eyelid to avoid tumor seeding in the orbit. Orbital exenteration with ostectomy is required if there is to be any chance of survival. Even with radical treatment, the prognosis is poor.

LYMPHOMA

Lymphomatous tumors of the orbit are divided into malignant lymphomas and reactive lymphoid hyperplasia, or pseudolymphoma. Immunologic and DNA hybridization techniques can help the pathologist determine whether a given lesion is a monoclonal proliferation (and presumably malignant) or a benign polyclonal proliferation. However, malignant lymphomas can have associated benign reactive lesions; benign polyclonal lesions can have small clones of B lymphocytes; and monoclonal tumors often remain localized and behave in a benign fashion.

The differential diagnosis includes orbital infection and systemic diseases such as collagen disease, histiocytosis, Wegener's granulomatosis, sinusitis, and sarcoidosis. Pain is more common with benign inflammatory processes than with malignant lymphomas.

The prognosis for both polyclonal lymphoid proliferations and well-differentiated B cell monoclonal lesions is excellent. If disease is confined to the orbit, treatment for both monoclonal and polyclonal lesions is with radiation. In one study, only 13% of these patients who were free of systemic disease after 6 months developed nonocular lymphomatous lesions.

HISTIOCYTOSIS

Proliferation of Langerhans cells with characteristic cytoplasmic granules comprises a spectrum of disease that includes what were formerly classified as unifocal and multifocal eosinophilic granuloma, Hand Schüller

Christian disease (multifocal lytic skull lesion, proptosis, and diabetes insipidus), and Letterer Siwe disease (cutaneous, visceral, and lymph node involvement). The younger the child at the time of diagnosis, the greater the chance of multifocal disease.

The orbital lesions can be treated with surgical curettement, corticosteroid injections, or low-dose radiation.

METASTATIC TUMORS

Metastatic tumors reach the orbit by hematogenous spread, since the orbit is devoid of Lymphatics. Metastasis is usually from the breast in women and from the lung in men. In children, the most common metastatic tumor is neuroblastoma, which is often associated with spontaneous periocular hemorrhage as the rapidly growing tumor becomes necrotic. Metastatic tumors are much more common in the choroid than in the orbit, probably because of the nature of the blood supply.

Many metastatic orbital tumors respond to radiation, some to chemotherapy. Small localized tumors that are symptomatic can sometimes be completely or partially excised. Neuroblastomas in children under 11 months have a relatively good prognosis. Adults with metastatic tumors in the orbit have a very limited life expectancy.

SECONDARY TUMORS

Basal cell, squamous cell, and sebaceous gland carcinomas may spread locally into the anterior orbit. Nasopharyngeal carcinomas—most commonly from the maxillary sinus—and meningiomas invade the posterior orbit.

REFERENCES

Avery G, Tang RA, Close LG: Ophthalmic manifestations of mucoceles. Ann Ophthalmol 1983;15:734.

Beard C, Quickert MH: *Anatomy of the Orbit.* Aesculapius, 1969.

Char DH: *Clinical Ocular Oncology.* Churchill Livingstone, 1989.

Char DH: *Thyroid Eye Disease.* Williams & Wilkins, 1985.

Dorfman RE, Spickler EM: Current status of magnetic reso-

nance imaging of the orbit. Top Magn Reson Imaging 1990;2:17.

Dutton J, Slamovits T (editors): Viewpoints: Management of blow˜2Dout fractures of the orbital floor. Surv Ophthalmol 1991;35:1.

Fells P et al: Extraocular muscle problems in thyroid eye disease. Eye 1994;8:497.

Ferry AP, Abedi S: Diagnosis and management of rhino-

Dorbitocerebral mucormycosis (phycomycosis): A report of 16 personally observed cases. Ophthalmology 1983; 90:1096.

Grove AS: Evaluation of exophthalmos. N Engl J Med 1975;292:1005.

Haik BG et al: Capillary hemangioma of the lids and orbit: An analysis of the clinical features and therapeutic results in 101 cases. Ophthalmology 1979;86:760.

Henderson JW: *Orbital Tumors,* 2nd ed. Decker, 1980.

Holds JB: The spectrum of orbital disease. Int Ophthalmol Clin 1992;32:59.

Hoyt WF, Baghdassarian SA: Optic glioma of childhood: Natural history and rationale for conservative management. Br J Ophthalmol 1969;53:793.

Jacobson DM et al: Maternal orbital hematoma associated with labor. Am J Ophthalmol 1988;105:547.

Jakobiec FA, Bonanno PA, Sigelman J: Conjunctival adnexal cysts and dermoids. Arch Ophthalmol 1978;96:1404.

Jakobiec FA, Knowles DM: An overview of ocular adnexal lymphoid tumors. Tr Am Ophthalmol Soc 1989;97:420.

Jones IS, Jakobiec FA: *Diseases of the Orbit.* Harper & Row, 1979.

Keltner JL et al: Dural and carotid cavernous sinus fistulas: Diagnosis, management, and complications. Ophthalmology 1987;94:1585.

Kennerdell JS, Maroon JC, Rootman J: Orbital decompression for dysthyroid orbitopathy. J Neurosurg 1989;70:816.

Kodsi SR et al: A review of 340 orbital tumors in children during a 60-year period. Am J Ophthalmol 1994;117:177.

Leone CR Jr, Wissinger JP: Surgical approaches to diseases of the orbital apex. Ophthalmology 1988;95:391.

Lyons CJ, Rootman J: Orbital decompression for disfiguring exophthalmos in thyroid orbitopathy. Ophthalmology 1994;101:223.

Macy JI, Mandelbaum SH, Minckler DS: Ocular pathology for clinicians. 8. Orbital cellulitis. Ophthalmology 1980; 87:1309.

Osguthorpe JD, Hochman M: Inflammatory sinus diseases affecting the orbit. Otolaryngol Clin North Am 1993; 26:657.

Prummel MF et al: Randomised double blind trial of prednisone versus radiotherapy in Graves' ophthalmopathy. Lancet 1993;342:949.

Rootman J, Nugent R: The classification and management of acute orbital pseudotumors. Ophthalmology 1982;89: 1040.

Rootman J et al: Orbital adnexal lymphangiomas: A spectrum of hemodynamically isolated vascular hamartomas. Ophthalmology 1986;93:1558.

Sergott RC, Glaser JS: Graves' ophthalmopathy: A clinical and immunologic review. Surv Ophthalmol 1981;26:1.

Shields CL et al: Orbital metastasis from a carcinoid tumor: Computed tomography, magnetic resonance imaging, and electron microscopic findings. Arch Ophthalmol 1987; 105:968.

Shields JA, Shields CL, Eagle RC: Cavernous hemangioma of the orbit. Arch Ophthalmol 1987;105:853.

Spencer WH (editor): *Ophthalmic Pathology,* 3rd ed. 3 vols. Saunders, 1985.

Volpe NJ, Jakobiec FA: Pediatric orbital tumors. Int Ophthalmol Clin 1992;32:201.

Warwick R: *Eugene Wolff's Anatomy of the Eye and Orbit,* 7th ed. Saunders, 1977.

Wharam M et al: Localized orbital rhabdomyosarcoma. Ophthalmology 1987;94:251.

Wilson WB, Manke WF: Orbital decompression in Graves' disease: The predictability of reduction of proptosis. Arch Ophthalmol 1991;109:343.

Neuro-Opthalmology

14

Pamela S. Chavis, MD, & William F. Hoyt, MD

The eyes are intimately related to the brain and frequently give important diagnostic clues to central nervous system disorders. Indeed, the optic nerve is a part of the central nervous system. Intracranial disease frequently causes visual disturbances because of destruction of or pressure upon some portion of the optic pathways. Cranial nerves III, IV, and VI, which control ocular movements, may be involved, and nerves V and VII are also intimately associated with ocular function.

Figure 14–1 shows the normal brain as portrayed by the technique of magnetic resonance imaging (MRI).

THE SENSORY VISUAL PATHWAY

Topographic Overview (Figure 14–2)

Cranial nerve II subserves the special sense of vision. Light is detected by the rods and cones of the

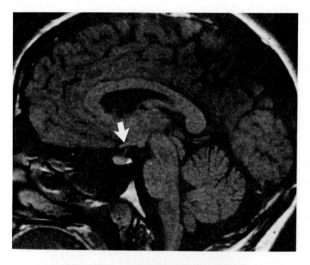

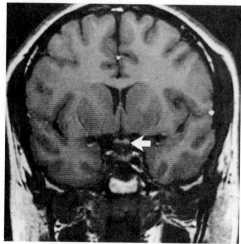

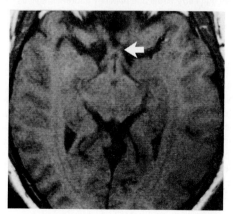

Figure 14–1. Magnetic resonance imaging (MRI) of normal brain in sagittal section *(upper left),* coronal section *(upper right),* and axial section *(lower left).* The white arrows indicate the chiasm. The future impact of this technique on localization of lesions affecting the intracranial visual and ocular motor pathways will be profound.

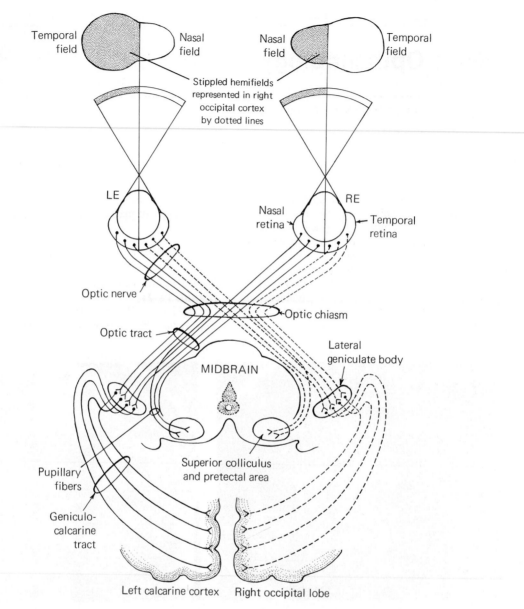

Figure 14–2. The optic pathway. The dotted lines represent nerve fibers that carry visual and pupillary afferent impulses from the left half of the visual field.

retina, which may be considered the special sensory end organ for vision. The cell bodies of these receptors extend processes that synapse with the bipolar cell, the second neuron in the visual pathway. The bipolar cells synapse, in turn, with the retinal ganglion cells. Ganglion cell axons comprise the nerve fiber layer of the retina and converge to form the optic nerve. The nerve emerges from the back of the globe and travels posteriorly within the muscle cone to enter the cranial cavity via the optic canal.

Intracranially, the two optic nerves join to form the optic chiasm. At the chiasm, more than half of the fibers (those from the nasal half of the retina) decussate and join the uncrossed temporal fibers of the opposite nerve to form the optic tracts. Each optic tract sweeps around the cerebral peduncle toward the lateral geniculate nucleus, where it will synapse. All of the fibers receiving impulses from the right hemifields of each eye thus make up the left optic tract and project to the left cerebral hemisphere. Similarly, the left hemifields project to the right cerebral hemisphere. Twenty percent of the fibers in the tract subserve pupillary function. These fibers leave the tract just anterior to the nucleus and pass via the brachium of the superior colliculus to the midbrain pretectal nucleus. The remaining fibers synapse in the lateral geniculate nucleus. The cell bodies of this structure give rise to the geniculocalcarine tract. This tract passes through the posterior limb of the internal capsule and then fans into the optic radiations that traverse parts of the temporal and parietal lobes en route to the occipital cortex (calcarine cortex).

Analysis of Visual Fields in Localizing Lesions in the Visual Pathways

In clinical practice, lesions in the visual pathways are localized by means of central and peripheral visual field examination. The technique (perimetry) is discussed in Chapter 2. Figure 14–3 shows the types of field defects caused by lesions in various locations of the pathway. Lesions anterior to the chiasm (of the retina or optic nerve) cause unilateral field defects; lesions anywhere in the visual pathway posterior to the chiasm cause contralateral homonymous defects. These may be congruous (ie, identical in size, shape, and location) or incongruous. Chiasmal lesions usually cause bitemporal defects.

Multiple isopters (test objects of different sizes) should be used in order to evaluate the defects thoroughly. A field defect shows evidence of edema or compression when there are areas of "relative scotoma" (ie, a larger field defect for a smaller test object). Such visual field defects are said to be "sloping." This is in contrast to ischemic or vascular lesions with steep borders (ie, the defect is the same size no matter what size test object is used). Such visual field defects are said to be "absolute."

Another important generalization is that the more congruous the homonymous field defects (ie, the more similar the two hemifields), the farther posterior the lesion is in the visual pathway. A lesion in the occipital region causes identical defects in each field, whereas optic tract lesions cause incongruous (dissimilar) homonymous field defects. In addition, the more posterior the lesion, the more likely there is to be macular sparing and, therefore, maintenance of good visual acuity in both hemifields. A complete homonymous hemianopia should still have intact visual acuity in the spared visual field (intact retrochiasmatic pathway), since that part of the visual system contains both macular and peripheral functions. Occipital lesions may cause a discrepancy between static and kinetic testing (Riddoch phenomenon) with fuller fields to a kinetic or "moving" object.

THE OPTIC NERVE

OPTIC NEURITIS & MULTIPLE SCLEROSIS (Figures 14–4 and 14–5)

"Optic neuritis" and "papillitis" are broad terms denoting inflammation, or demyelinization of the optic nerve due to a wide variety of diseases (Table 14–1). Loss of vision is the cardinal symptom and serves to differentiate papillitis from papilledema, which it may resemble on ophthalmoscopic examination.

Retrobulbar neuritis is an optic neuritis that occurs far enough behind the optic disk so that early changes at the optic disk are not visible by means of the ophthalmoscope; however, visual acuity is markedly reduced. ("The patient sees nothing, and the doctor sees nothing.") Papillitis is disk swelling caused by local inflammation at the nerve head (intraocular optic nerve) (Figure 14–4).

The Optic Neuritis Treatment Trial (ONTT) confirmed some of the known demographics of acute optic neuritis and papillitis. More than 77% of the patients were women; 85% were white; and the mean age was 32 years.

Retrobulbar neuritis is associated with multiple sclerosis in 13–85% of patients in different population groups in the world. The percentage of progression to multiple sclerosis after an episode of optic neuritis tends to be higher everywhere with increased length of patient follow-up.

Clinical Findings

According to the ONTT, approximately one-third of patients have vision better than 20/40 initially with their first attack, and slightly more than one-third have vision worse than 20/200. There may be pain in the region of the eye (92.2%) which worsens with specific eye movement (51.3%). Vision characteristically improves dramatically within 2–6 weeks.

Central scotomas are the most common visual field defect. They are usually circular, varying widely in size and density, and may break out to an altitudinal defect. A central scotoma that has broken out to the periphery, however, should make the clinician suspect a compressive lesion. Almost any unilateral field change is possible. The pupillary light reflex is sluggish, and if the optic nerves are asymmetrically involved an afferent pupillary defect will be present.

The optic disk was initially normal in 65% and compatible with retrobulbar neuritis, while papillitis occurred in 35% patients in the ONTT.

Ophthalmoscopically, hyperemia of the optic disk and distention of large veins are early signs in papilli-

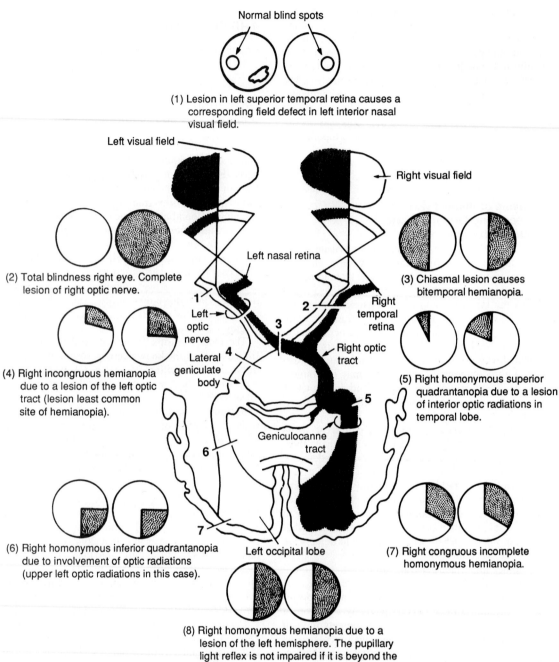

Normal blind spots

(1) Lesion in left superior temporal retina causes a corresponding field defect in left interior nasal visual field.

Left visual field

Right visual field

(2) Total blindness right eye. Complete lesion of right optic nerve.

Left nasal retina

(3) Chiasmal lesion causes bitemporal hemianopia.

1

Left optic nerve

Right temporal retina

2

3

Right optic tract

(4) Right incongruous hemianopia due to a lesion of the left optic tract (lesion least common site of hemianopia).

Lateral geniculate body

4

(5) Right homonymous superior quadrantanopia due to a lesion of interior optic radiations in temporal lobe.

5

Geniculocanne tract

6

(6) Right homonymous inferior quadrantanopia due to involvement of optic radiations (upper left optic radiations in this case).

7

Left occipital lobe

(7) Right congruous incomplete homonymous hemianopia.

(8) Right homonymous hemianopia due to a lesion of the left hemisphere. The pupillary light reflex is not impaired if it is beyond the tract.

Figure 14–3. Visual field defects due to various lesions of the optic pathways.

Table 14–1. Etiologic classification of diseases of the optic nerve.

A. Idiopathic optic neuritis

B. Demyelinating diseases
1. Multiple sclerosis
2. Other rare demyelinating syndromes, eg, neuromyelitis optica (Devic's disease)

C. Viral infections
1. Postviral optic neuritis (measles, mumps, chickenpox, influenza)
2. Postinfectious encephalomyelitis
3. Polyradiculoneuronitis (Guillain-Barré syndrome)
4. Infectious mononucleosis
5. Herpes zoster

D. Local extension of inflammatory disease
1. Sinusitis
2. Intracranial disease: meningitis, encephalitis
3. Orbital disease: cellulitis, vasculitis
4. Intraocular disease: chorioretinitis, endophthalmitis, iridocyclitis

E. Systemic infections and inflammation
1. Syphilis
2. Tuberculosis
3. Cryptococcosis
4. Coccidioidomycosis
5. Infective endocarditis
6. Sarcoidosis

F. Nutritional and metabolic
1. Diabetes mellitus
2. Vitamin deficiencies: vitamin B_{12} deficiency, beriberi, pellagra

G. Toxic
1. Tobacco-alcohol amblyopia
2. Heavy metal: arsenic, lead, thallium
3. Drugs: ethambutol, isoniazid, streptomycin, disulfiram, digitalis, chloramphenicol, chloroquine, chlorpropamide, halogenated hydroxyquinones (eg, iodochlorhydroxyquin)
4. Methanol

H. Hereditary optic atrophy
1. Leber's disease
2. Dominant (juvenile) optic atrophy
3. Recessive (infantile) optic atrophy
4. Heredodegenerative diseases
5. Optic nerve anomalies

I. Vascular disease
1. Temporal arteritis
2. Arteriosclerosis (anterior ischemic optic neuropathy): diabetes mellitus, hypertension
3. Polyarteritis nodosa
4. Takayasu's disease

J. Neoplastic disease
1. Direct infiltration of optic nerve, leukemic or malignant
2. Compressive neuropathy: tumors, thyroid eye disease
3. Paraneoplastic syndrome

K. Trauma

L. Radiation neuropathy

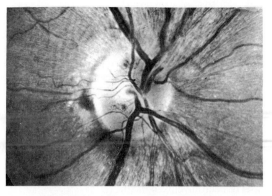

Figure 14–4. Mild disk swelling in papillitis.

tis. Blurred disk margins and filling of the physiologic cup are common and may advance to marked edema of the nerve head, but elevations of more than 3 diopters (1 mm) are unusual. Retinal exudates and edema in the papillomacular bundle may rarely occur and may be associated with a lower rate of progression to multiple sclerosis. Flame-shaped hemorrhages may occur in the nerve fiber layer near the optic disk (6%), and vitreous cells can be localized to the prepapillary area in papillitis (3%).

Differential Diagnosis

Papilledema is the most common differential diagnostic problem (Figure 14–5). In papilledema, there is often greater elevation of the optic nerve head, nearly normal visual acuity, normal pupillary response to

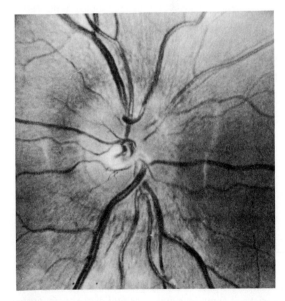

Figure 14–5. Early papilledema. The disk margins are blurred superiorly and inferiorly by the thickened layer of nerve fibers entering the disk.

light, associated increased intracranial pressure, and an intact visual field except for an enlarged blind spot. If there has been acute papilledema with vascular decompensation (ie, hemorrhages and cotton wool spots) or chronic papilledema with secondary ischemia to the optic nerve, then visual field defects can include nasal nerve fiber bundle defects and nasal quadrantanopias. Papilledema is usually bilateral, whereas papillitis is usually unilateral. Despite these obvious differences, differential diagnosis can be difficult because of the similarity of the ophthalmoscopic findings and because papilledema can be quite asymmetric and papillitis bilateral in some postviral events (eg, Devic's disease, or neuromyelitis optica).

NEUROMYELITIS OPTICA
(Devic's Disease)

This rare demyelinating disease of the central nervous system—considered by many to be a severe and acute form of multiple sclerosis—is characterized by bilateral optic neuritis and Brown-Séquard's syndrome. At 2–3 weeks post-viral infection or postimmunization, it presents with a subacute onset of loss of vision in one eye, followed soon by involvement of the other eye and paraplegia. Approximately 50% of patients progress to death within the first decade due to the paraplegia, but the remainder may have a prolonged remission and, ultimately, a better prognosis than patients with chronic demyelinating disease or multiple sclerosis.

Treatment may begin with a loading dose of intravenous methylprednisolone followed by a 2-month tapering course of oral steroids with monitoring of oligoclonal bands in the cerebrospinal fluid. With early institution of this treatment, visual recovery can be excellent.

MULTIPLE SCLEROSIS

Multiple sclerosis is a chronic, relapsing demyelinating disorder of the central nervous system of unknown cause. Characteristically, the lesions occur at different times and in noncontiguous locations in the nervous system—ie, "lesions are disseminated in time and space." Onset is usually in young adult life; this disease rarely begins before 15 years or after 55 years of age. There is a tendency to involve the optic nerves and chiasm, brainstem, cerebellar peduncles, and spinal cord, though no part of the central nervous systems is protected. The peripheral nervous system is seldom involved.

Clinical Findings

A. Symptoms and Signs: Clinically, there are a variety of symptoms and signs that may vary in number and character from time to time. In addition to ocular disturbances, there may be motor weakness with pyramidal signs, ataxia, urinary disturbances, paresthesias, dysarthria, and intention tremors. Sensory hyperesthesias and urinary incontinence are common early signs. Other problems can evolve over months to years.

Patients may first complain of blurring of vision, as if a mist or film covers the eye. This is due to optic neuritis (especially retrobulbar neuritis). Because of the transient nature of the visual defect and the absence of physical findings, the complaint is sometimes misdiagnosed as hysteria. The other eye is involved eventually. The overall incidence of optic neuritis in multiple sclerosis is 90%.

Diplopia is a common early symptom, due most frequently to internuclear ophthalmoplegia. This condition, caused by a lesion of the medial longitudinal fasciculus, is characterized by saccadic paresis of the ipsilateral medial rectus muscle on conjugate lateral gaze to the opposite side and nystagmus in the opposite (abducting) eye; thus, diplopia can occur on lateral gaze. In multiple sclerosis, the medial longitudinal fasciculus lesions are commonly bilateral. Medial rectus function can be normal for convergence if its nucleus is not involved by the demyelinating lesion. Ptosis may also occur; less commonly, weakness of the lateral rectus or other muscles, singly or together, occurs.

Nystagmus is a common early sign, and—unlike most manifestations of the disease (which tend toward remission)—it is often permanent (70%).

Peripheral retinal vasculitis and low-grade uveitis are occasionally associated with multiple sclerosis. This can be either a granulomatous or lymphocytic retinal periphlebitis with venous sheathing and gray-white perivascular dots. Focal retinitis is less common.

B. Laboratory Findings: The cerebrospinal fluid gamma globulin concentration is frequently high, and oligoclonal bands can be elevated, representing local production of IgG and IgA; these may indicate a response to viral infection or an aberrant immune response to a viral antigen. CD8 levels in the cerebrospinal fluid may also be abnormal. Some patients with multiple sclerosis have no spinal fluid abnormalities, especially if their disease process is in a less acute or milder phase. Oligoclonal bands can be followed in the cerebrospinal fluid as a marker of disease activity in patients being treated with steroids or immunosuppressives.

Pathologically, multiple areas of demyelination are present in the white matter. Early, there is degeneration of myelin sheaths and relative sparing of the axons. Glial tissue overgrowth and complete nerve fiber destruction with some round cell infiltration are seen later. The disease affects the optic nerve and chiasm more than the rest of the visual sensory system.

C. Special Examinations: Retinal nerve fiber layer defects consistent with a subclinical optic neuritis can be detected in 68% of multiple sclerosis patients. The visual evoked response (VER) may help confirm involvement of the visual pathway. The VER has been reported to be abnormal in 80% of definite, 43% of probable, and 22% of suspected cases of multiple sclerosis. A normal VER in cases with suspected multiple sclerosis makes the diagnosis questionable, but with positive oligoclonal bands or abnormal contrast sensitivity the diagnosis can be made with more certainty. CT scan and especially MRI can detect subclinical white matter demyelinating lesions even in the optic nerve and can confirm that there are disseminated lesions compatible with the diagnosis of multiple sclerosis. While over 25% of patients with retrobulbar neuritis had two or more T2-weighted MRI lesions, a visual acuity worse than 20/200 in the ONTT was associated with more demyelinating lesions in the brain on MRI.

Course, Treatment, & Prognosis

A. Optic Neuritis: Loss of vision occurs within the first few hours after onset and is maximal within several days. Without treatment, visual acuity usually begins to improve 2–3 weeks after onset and sometimes returns to normal in a few days. Improvement may continue slowly over a period of 6 weeks. Other autoimmune disease such as lupus erythematosus should be considered, especially in those patients with poor recovery from the initial attack of retrobulbar neuritis. Other causes of optic neuropathy include toxic amblyopias, other demyelinating diseases, Leber's optic atrophy, diabetes mellitus, and vitamin B_{12} deficiency. If the process is sufficiently destructive, retrograde optic atrophy results, and nerve fiber bundle defects appear in the retinal nerve fiber layer (Figure 14–6). The disk loses its normal pink color and becomes pale. In very severe recurrent cases, a chalky-white disk with sharp outlines and moderately decreased vision results. Disk pallor does not necessarily correlate with visual acuity. Optic neuritis in demyelinating disease has a favorable prognosis without treatment for an individual attack, but over a period of years significant visual loss is the rule since permanent damage results from recurrent attacks. Complete recovery of vision occurs in 65%, but despite normal visual acuity, contrast sensitivity (92%) and visual evoked responses (36%) can be abnormal. Longer optic nerve demyelinating lesions, especially in the optic canal, can be associated with poor visual outcome.

B. Multiple Sclerosis: The course of this disease is unpredictable; risk factors that can predispose to the evolution of optic neuritis to multiple sclerosis include female sex, HLA-DR2 and -DR3, retinal perivenous sheathing, cerebral MRI abnormalities, and cerebrospinal fluid oligoclonal banding. Remissions and exacerbations may occur and are sometimes preceded by general malaise corresponding to T cell changes in the peripheral blood or are initiated by elevations in body temperature (Uhthoff's phenomenon). Pregnancy or the number of pregnancies has no effect on disability. Onset during pregnancy has a more favorable outcome than onset unrelated to pregnancy. Lactation, however, is associated with recurrent optic neuritis.

C. Treatment of Optic Neuritis and Multiple Sclerosis: The Optic Neuritis Treatment Trial (ONTT) was specifically designed to compare 3 days of intravenous methylprednisolone (1 g/d) followed by 11 days of oral prednisone (1 mg/kg/d), oral prednisone (1 mg/kg/d) for 14 days, and placebo in the treatment of optic neuritis. The recovery of vision was faster with the steroid treatments, but the ultimate visual outcome was no different from that of the placebo group. Oral prednisone appeared to increase the risk of recurrent optic neuritis. In comparison with the placebo group at the 2-year follow-up point, the intravenous methylprednisolone group had experienced a greater than 50% reduction in the incidence of neurologic episodes consistent with the development of multiple sclerosis. This apparent benefit from intravenous methylprednisolone was greater for patients with multiple white matter lesions on brain MRI at presentation. It remains to be seen whether this protective effect from intravenous methylprednisolone combined with oral prednisone persists with longer follow-up.

Steroid treatment, particularly intravenous methylprednisolone, is useful in hastening recovery from acute relapses in multiple sclerosis but does not influence the final disability or the rate of further relapses. Systemic interferon may provide long-term benefit in patients with remitting and relapsing disease. For patients with chronic progressive disease, intensive immunosuppression with either azathioprine or pulsed cyclophosphamide may be beneficial.

ISCHEMIC OPTIC NEUROPATHY

Ischemic optic neuropathy is characterized by acute, pallid disk swelling, associated with loss of vision; often there are one or two peripapillary splinter hemorrhages (Figure 14–7). The disorder is due to occlusion of the posterior ciliary arteries in the retrolaminar cribrosa area (a few millimeters behind the optic nerve head) where the optic nerve capillaries are relatively less abundant; hence, acute visual loss due to ischemic optic neuropathy should be associated with ophthalmoscopic evidence of disk edema within 24 hours after the onset of visual symptoms.

Ischemic optic neuropathy occurs generally in the sixth or seventh decade and is associated with arteriosclerosis, diabetes, hypertension, and hyperlipidemia, but any thrombotic condition capable of producing intracranial stroke can affect the posterior ciliary arteries as well. In younger patients, vasculitis, migraine, inherited prothrombotic states (deficiencies of protein C, protein S, or antithrombin III), and possible cardiac disease should be explored. A significantly reduced cup:disk ratio with crowding of axons in a relatively small scleral canal, drusen, and increased intraocular pressure may be predisposing factors. Embolic disease uncommonly produces ischemic optic

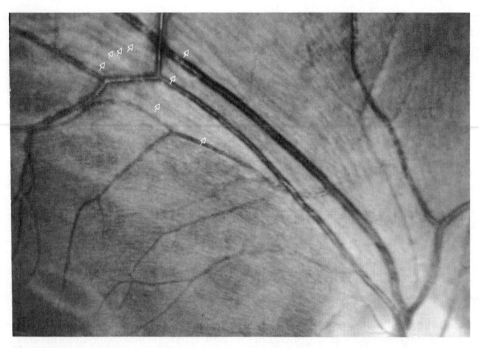

Figure 14–6. Retinal nerve fiber layer in demyelinating optic neuropathy of multiple sclerosis. The upper temporal nerve fiber bundles show multiple slit-like areas of thinning (arrows) representing retrograde axonal atrophy from subclinical disease in the optic nerve. Vision in the eye was 20/20.

neuropathy. Most important to the ophthalmologist is giant cell arteritis, which can present with bilateral visual loss; this occurs generally in elderly people and is associated with a high sedimentation rate, painful and tender temporal arteries, pain on mastication, general malaise, anorexia, weight loss, fever of unknown origin, anemia, and muscular aches and pains. It may represent an autoimmune response to internal elastic lamina that is bared to the systemic circulation by ulcerated arteriosclerotic plaques.

Impairment of visual acuity in ischemic optic neuropathy may vary from slight—with a corresponding decrease in color vision—to no light perception; visual field defects are commonly altitudinal (inferior defects more commonly than superior), and quadrantanopias and nerve fiber bundle defects may be evident. Central scotomas occasionally occur. The initial visual loss tends to be more severe in arteritic than nonarteritic ischemic optic neuropathy, and the subsequent visual recovery parallels this as well. While the visual loss is generally precipitous, it can uncommonly be progressive over hours to days—rarely over weeks. Progression may occur due to a cycle of ischemia, edema, and compression and may be halted by optic nerve sheath fenestration—especially if the optic nerve sheath is enlarged on ultrasound. As the acute process resolves, a pale disk with or without "glaucomatous" cupping results (Figure 14–8). Recurrences in the same eye are rare, presumably related to decompression in the scleral canal due to infarction of some axons.

PAPILLEDEMA
(Figures 14–5 and 14–9 to 14–11)

Papilledema (choked disk) is a noninflammatory congestion of the optic disk associated with increased intracranial pressure (Figure 14–5). Papilledema will occur in any condition causing persistent increased intracranial pressure; the most common causes are cerebral tumors, abscesses, subdural hematoma, acquired hydrocephalus, arteriovenous malformations, and malignant hypertension. It can also occur in spinal tumors, uremia, and the mucopolysaccharidoses. In an ophthalmology practice where patients walk in and are usually healthy except for visual complaints, it is often due to idiopathic intracranial hypertension, a disorder characterized by papilledema and a normal neurologic examination except for perhaps a sixth nerve paresis and, rarely, Bell's palsy, with normal CT, MRI, and cerebrospinal fluid studies (except for increased intracranial pressure).

For papilledema to occur, the subarachnoid spaces around the optic nerve must be patent and connect the retrolaminar optic nerve through the bony optic canal to the intracranial subarachnoid space, thus allowing increased intracranial pressure to be transmitted to the retrolaminar optic nerve. There slow and fast axonal transport is blocked, and axonal distention occurs as the first sign of papilledema. Hyperemia of the disk, dilated surface capillary telangiectases, blurring of the peripapillary disk margin, and loss of spontaneous ve-

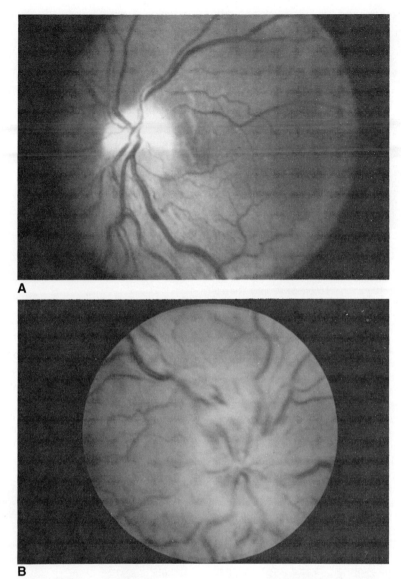

A

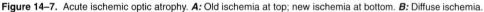

B

Figure 14–7. Acute ischemic optic atrophy. **A:** Old ischemia at top; new ischemia at bottom. **B:** Diffuse ischemia.

nous pulsations occur later. Edema around the disk can cause a decreased sensitivity to small isopters on visual field testing, but circumferential retinal folds with changes in the internal limiting membrane reflexes (Paton's lines) will eventually become evident as the retina is pushed away from the choked disk; when the retina is pushed away, the blind spot will be enlarged to large isopters on visual field testing as well. Fully developed papilledema is associated with peripapillary edema (which can extend to the macula), choroidal folds, hemorrhages, and cotton-wool spots (Figures 14–9 and 14–10). Hemorrhages and cotton-wool spots herald vascular and axonal decompensation and then nerve fiber layer infarcts, and nasal quadrantanopia will occur.

Papilledema can occur if ocular hypotony is present and intracranial pressure is normal; for in this situation, intracranial pressure would appear falsely high relative to low pressure within the globe. Uveitis has also been associated with papilledema, either due to hypotony or to posterior vitreous permeability at the optic nerve head.

It takes 24–48 hours for early papilledema to occur and 1 week to develop fully. It takes 6–8 weeks for fully developed papilledema to resolve during adequate treatment. Papilledema can be associated with sudden visual loss after sudden intracranial decompression (ventriculography) or decreased systolic perfusion pressure. Visual loss can occur as a result of macular lesions, progressive optic nerve decompensation or

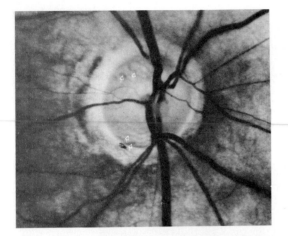

Figure 14–8. Chronic ischemic optic atrophy with loss of neuroglial tissue and exposure of the lamina cribrosa. The pale disk has a shallow cup without nasal displacement of the central retinal vessels. Multiple dark holes are present in the disk surface. The disk is ringed by a zone of choroidal atrophy. The retinal arterioles are narrowed irregularly.

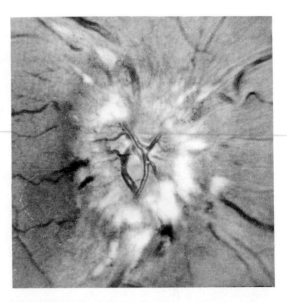

Figure 14–10. Papilledema with cotton wool spots and hemorrhages.

sudden decompensation due to secondary ischemia, or central retinal artery occlusion. In chronic papilledema (Figure 14–11), the hyperemic, elevated disk becomes gray-white as a result of astrocytic gliosis and neural atrophy with secondary constriction of retinal blood vessels. There can be opticociliary collateral vessels and fine exudates or drusen (Figure 14–12). Opticociliary collateral vessels link the central retinal vein and the peripapillary choroidal veins when the retinal venous circulation is obstructed in the prelaminar region of the optic nerve. Central retinal vein obstruction, optic disk drusen, myopia, congenital anomaly, glaucoma, optic nerve gliomas, and meningiomas are common causes; the latter three causes also have optic

atrophy associated with the opticociliary collateral vessel. In chronic papilledema, there is loss of peripheral visual field, and transient visual obscurations occur.

Papilledema is often asymmetric and will be greater on the side of a supratentorial lesion. It can be strictly unilateral if there is an orbital lesion. Papilledema will

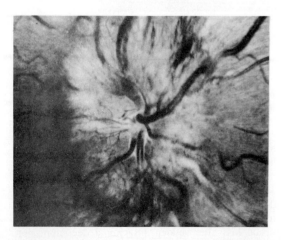

Figure 14–9. Fully developed papilledema. The disk tissue is swollen, elevated, and congested, and the retinal veins are markedly dilated.

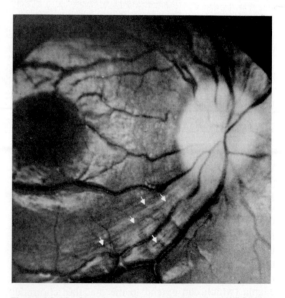

Figure 14–11. Chronic atrophic papilledema in a child with a cerebellar medulloblastoma. The disk is pale and slightly elevated and has blurred margins. The white areas surrounding the macula are reflected light from the vitreoretinal interface. The inferior temporal nerve fiber bundles are partially atrophic (arrows).

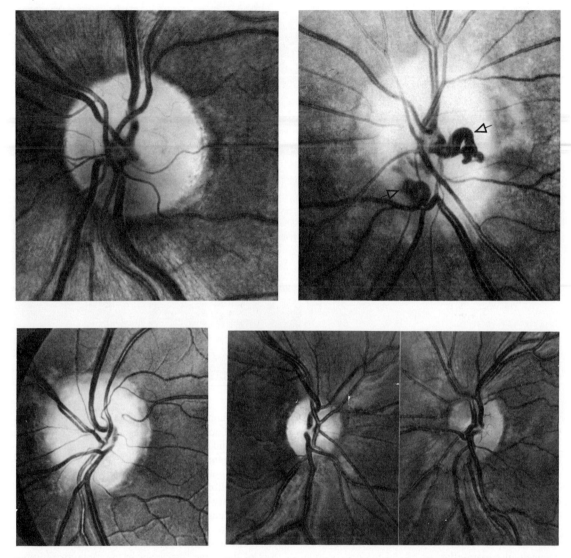

Figure 14–12. Examples of optic atrophy. ***Upper left:*** Primary optic atrophy due to nutritional amblyopia. ***Upper right:*** Secondary optic atrophy with opticociliary shunts (arrows) due to optic nerve sheath meningioma. ***Lower left:*** Optic atrophy with optic disk drusen. ***Lower right:*** Pallor (atrophy) of right optic disk due to nerve compression by sphenoid meningioma. The left disk is normal.

occur late in glaucoma, but it will not occur at all if there is optic atrophy or if the optic nerve sheath on that side is not patent. Foster Kennedy's syndrome is papilledema on one side with optic atrophy on the other (optic nerve and sheath compressed by neoplasm) (Figure 14–12). This is commonly due to meningiomas of the sphenoid wing and classically to meningiomas of the olfactory groove. However, this clinical presentation can be mimicked (pseudo-Foster Kennedy syndrome) by ischemic optic neuropathy when an old ischemic optic neuropathy with atrophy is associated with a new hyperemic ischemic optic neuropathy.

Papilledema can be mimicked by buried drusen of the optic nerve, small hyperopic disks, and myelinated nerve fibers (Figure 14–13). The treatment of pa-

pilledema must be directed to the underlying cause. In benign intracranial hypertension, it can include lumbar puncture, diuretics, corticosteroids, lumboperitoneal shunt, and fenestration of the optic nerve sheath.

OPTIC NERVE ATROPHY
(Figure 14–12)

Etiologic Classification

A. Vascular: Occlusion of the central retinal vein or artery; arteriosclerotic changes within the optic nerve itself, disturbing its vascular supply; or posthemorrhagic, due to sudden massive blood loss (eg, bleeding peptic ulcer).

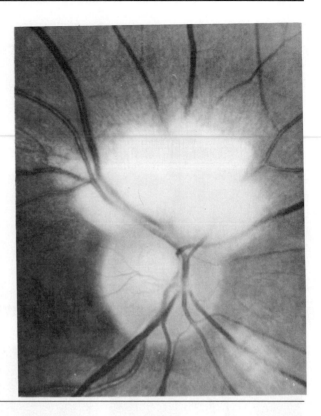

Figure 14–13. Large patch of myelinated nerve fibers originating from superior edge of disk. Another smaller patch is present near the inferior nasal border of the disk. (Right eye.)

B. Degenerative: Consecutive atrophy secondary to retinal disease, with destruction of ganglion cells (eg, retinitis); or as part of a systemic degenerative disease (eg, cerebromacular degeneration).

C. Secondary to Papilledema.

D. Secondary to Optic Neuritis: (including retrobulbar neuritis).

E. Pressure Against the Optic Nerve: Aneurysm of the anterior circle of Willis; bony pressure at the optic foramen (eg, osteitis deformans); intracanalicular, parasellar, or orbital tumors, or even thyroid eye disease.

F. Toxic: End result of toxic amblyopia (see below).

G. Metabolic: Diabetes, ganglioside disease, etc.

H. Traumatic: Direct injury to a nerve (severing, avulsion, or contusion).

I. Glaucomatous: See Chapter 11.

Clinical Findings

Loss of visual acuity, visual field, and color vision are the only symptoms; pallor of the optic disk and loss of pupillary reaction are usually proportionate to visual loss except in compressive lesions. Compressive lesions can produce extensive central visual acuity changes and peripheral visual field changes long before there are fundus changes of relative severity (axons can be dysfunctional long before they become atrophic).

Changes in visual function occur very slowly over weeks or months. It is difficult to assess prognosis on the basis of ophthalmoscopic findings alone. Even with experimental chiasmal section, it can take 2 months for axonal degeneration to extend from the chiasm to the retinal ganglion cell. Treatment and outcome are variable depending on the cause.

Hereditary optic neuropathies produce bilateral temporal segmental disk pallor with preferential loss of papillomacular axons. Central retinal artery occlusion produces segmental retinal arteriolar narrowing and loss of the nerve fiber layer in the same distribution. Attenuated retinal blood vessels plus segmental or diffuse disk pallor, with or without "glaucomatous" optic nerve cupping, can signify prior ischemic optic neuropathy. Peripapillary exudates are the hallmark of papillitis and occasionally papilledema. Peripapillary gliosis and atrophy, chorioretinal folds, and internal limiting membrane wrinkling can also be helpful signs of prior disk edema.

TOXIC-NUTRITIONAL OPTIC NEUROPATHIES

1. TOBACCO-ALCOHOL AMBLYOPIA

Nutritional amblyopia is another term for this entity. It occurs more commonly in males with poor dietary habits, particularly if the diet is deficient in thiamine.

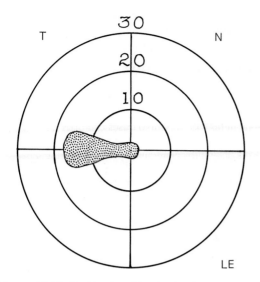

Figure 14–14. Nutritional amblyopia showing centrocecal scotoma. VA = 20/200.

Heavy drinking with or without heavy smoking is most often associated with a poor nutritional state. Bilateral loss of central vision is present in over 50% of patients, reducing visual acuity to less than 20/200, but can be asymmetric. Central visual fields reveal scotomas that nearly always include both fixation and the blind spot (centrocecal scotoma) (Figure 14–14). Centrocecal scotomas are usually of constant density, but when density of the scotoma varies, the most dense portion usually lies between fixation and the blind spot in the papillomacular bundle.

Much consideration has been given in the literature to other toxic causes such as cyanide from tobacco, producing low vitamin stores and low levels of sulfur-containing amino acids, but experimental studies with cyanide in primates have not confirmed this theory. Rarely, pernicious anemia, methanol poisoning, retrobulbar neuritis, or macular degeneration may cause diagnostic confusion.

Adequate diet plus thiamine, folic acid, and vitamin B_{12} is nearly always effective in completely curing the disease if it is recognized early. Withdrawal of tobacco and alcohol is advisable and may hasten the cure, but innumerable cases are known in which adequate nutrition or vitamin B_{12} supplements effected the cure despite continued excessive intake of alcohol or tobacco. Improvement usually begins within 1–2 months, though in occasional cases significant improvement may not occur for a year. Visual function can but may not return to normal; permanent optic atrophy or at least temporal disk pallor can occur depending upon the stage of disease at the time treatment was started (Figure 14–13). Loss of the ganglion cells of the mac-

ula and destruction of myelinated fibers of the optic nerve—and sometimes of the chiasm as well—are the main histologic changes.

2. DRUG TOXICITY

Ethambutol, isoniazid (INH), rifampin, and disulfiram can all produce a retrobulbar neuritis picture, or a swollen disk which will improve with prompt cessation of the drug with or without nutritional supplements. Serial color vision screening is the most sensitive clinical test and must be done prophylactically.

Either chronic lead exposure or thallium (present in depilatory creams) can produce a toxic effect on the optic nerve.

Quinine is toxic to ganglion cells and will cause optic neuropathy with severely narrowed retinal arteries. Chloramphenicol in high doses causes optic neuropathy. Chloroquine and ethchlorvynol can cause bitemporal hemianopia. Amiodarone toxicity can produce bilateral disk edema, but it characteristically also induces a verticillate keratopathy as well as other central nervous system signs.

3. METHANOL POISONING

Methanol is used widely in the chemical industry as antifreeze, solvent varnish, or paint remover; it is also present in fumes of some industrial solvents such as those used in old photocopier machines. Significant systemic absorption can occur from fumes inhaled in a room with inadequate ventilation and (rarely) can be absorbed through the skin.

Clinical Findings

The principal manifestations of methanol poisoning are visual disturbances and acidosis. The metabolites of methanol are formic acid and formaldehyde, which produce an acidosis and cause gastroenteritis, pulmonary edema, and retinal ganglion cell and diffuse retinal damage.

Visual impairment can be the first sign and begins with mild blurring of vision and then progresses to contraction of visual fields and sometimes to complete blindness. Visual disturbances range from "spots before the eyes" to complete blindness. The field defects are quite extensive and nearly always include the centrocecal area (Figure 14–15).

Hyperemia of the disk is the first ophthalmoscopic finding. Within the first 2 days, a whitish, striated edema of the disk margins and nearby retina appears. Disk edema can last up to 2 months and is followed by optic atrophy of mild to severe degree (Figure 14–16).

Decreased pupillary response to light occurs in proportion to the amount of visual loss. In severe cases,

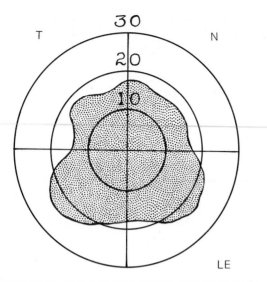

Figure 14–15. Methyl alcohol amblyopia showing very large centrocecal scotoma. VA = hand movements only.

the pupils become dilated and fixed. Extraocular muscle palsies and ptosis may also occur.

Treatment

Treatment consists of correction of the acidosis with intravenous sodium bicarbonate and oral or intravenous administration of ethanol to compete with and thus prevent the slower metabolism of methanol into its by-products. Hemodialysis is indicated for blood methanol levels over 50 mg/dL.

OPTIC NERVE TRAUMA

Visual loss due to indirect optic nerve trauma can occur in 1% of all skull injuries. Intravenous dexamethasone in high or very high doses can offer good results to patients with subperiosteal hemorrhage, orbital hemorrhage, or intracanalicular edema. Transethmoidal optic canal decompression of the optic nerve appears safe and effective in combination with corticosteroids.

GENETICALLY DETERMINED OPTIC ATROPHY

1. LEBER'S OPTIC NEUROPATHY

Leber's hereditary optic neuropathy is a rare disease characterized by sequential and progressive acute or subacute optic neuropathy; it occurs in young men aged 20–30 years (occasionally in women). The pattern of transmission is nonmendelian, being an example of maternal inheritance (with a female carrier rate of 95–100%; see Chapter 18) due to a mutation in mitochondrial DNA (mtDNA) which is exclusively derived from the mother. Worldwide there is greater than 90% prevalence of a point mutation of mtDNA at position 11778, 14484, or 3460. Blurred vision and a central scotoma appear first in one eye and later—within days, weeks, or months—in the other eye. The diagnosis of this familial disorder can only be confirmed

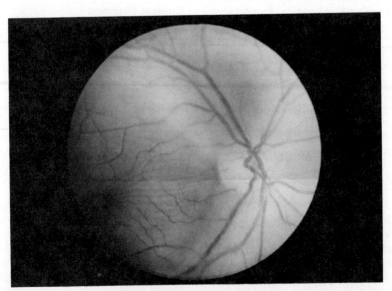

Figure 14–16. Methanol poisoning.

during the acute episode by documenting a hyperemic, edematous disk that does not leak during fluorescein angiography despite dilated capillary telangiectases on the disk surface and the immediate peripapillary retina. The nerve fiber layer around the disk can appear gray owing to the pseudoedema of axonal congestion. Eventually, both optic nerves may become atrophic; vision may then be about 20/200 or worse. Some specific point mutations (eg, at position 14484) may be associated with a better visual outcome. Total loss of vision or recurrences of visual loss usually do not occur. MRI of the optic nerves shows a lesion over 10 mm and is mostly posterior within the orbit and optic canal.

This disorder may be associated with a multiple sclerosis-like illness, heredofamilial ataxias, and Charcot-Marie-Tooth disease as well as cardiac anomalies. Other mitochondrial diseases include myoclonic epilepsy and ragged red fibers, mitochondrial myopathy, lactic acidosis and stroke-like episodes, and chronic progressive external ophthalmoplegia.

2. CONGENITAL OR INFANTILE HEREDITARY OPTIC ATROPHY

This disorder occurs in a severe autosomal recessive form and a milder autosomal dominant form. The recessive form is present at birth or within 2 years and is accompanied by nystagmus. The more common dominant form has an insidious onset in childhood, with little progression thereafter. There is characteristically a centrocecal scotoma with variable loss of central visual acuity.

The dominant form can be associated with congenital or progressive deafness and ataxia. The recessive form can be associated with progressive hearing loss, spastic quadriplegia, and dementia, though an inborn error of metabolism must be first considered. There is another recessive form consisting of juvenile diabetes insipidus, diabetes mellitus, optic atrophy, and deafness (DIDMOAD syndrome).

3. OPTIC ATROPHY WITH NEURODEGENERATIVE DISEASES

Various neurodegenerative diseases with onset in the years from childhood to early adult life are manifested by steadily progressive neurologic and visual signs. Examples are hereditary ataxias and Charcot-Marie-Tooth disease. Most of the sphingolipidoses late in their course are associated with optic atrophy. The leukodystrophies (Krabbe's, metachromatic leukodystrophy, adrenoleukodystrophy, globoid dystrophy, Pelizaeus-Merzbacher disease, Schilder's disease) are associated with optic atrophy earlier. Canavan's spongy degeneration and glioneuronal dystrophy (Alper's disease) are associated with optic atrophy as well. Peroxisome disorders (Zellweger's disease, Ref-

sum's disease, etc) can have optic atrophy with cataract, glaucoma, and a pigmentary retinopathy. Optic atrophy can occur in the mucopolysaccharidoses due to hydrocephalus from mucopolysaccharides in the meninges or due to mucopolysaccharides in glial cells of the optic nerve.

Optic atrophy secondary to retinal ganglion cell atrophy can also occur in Alzheimer's disease. Large retinal ganglion cells project to the superior colliculus, and eye movement abnormalities occur as well.

OPTIC NERVE ANOMALIES

Tilted disks, optic nerve hypoplasia, dysplasia, and coloboma are all congenital optic nerve anomalies. Closure of the fetal fissure, ocular melanogenesis, and disk development occur at the same time as development of the skull, face, and limbs. Accordingly, tilted disks, which occur in 3% of normals, may also be seen with hypertelorism or the craniofacial dysostoses (Crouzon's disease, Apert's disease). They are oval disks with usually an inferior crescent and an associated area of fundus hypopigmentation (Figure 14–17).

Optic nerve hypoplasia, dysplasia, and coloboma have all been associated with basal encephaloceles as well and with varying intracranial anomalies, from Duane's retraction syndrome to agenesis of the corpus callosum (de Morsier's syndrome) and pituitary-hypothalamic dysfunction (especially growth hormone deficiency). Hypoplastic optic nerves are small, with normal-sized retinal blood vessels (Figure 14–18). They are associated with a wide range of visual acuities, astigmatism, a peripapillary halo that may have a pigmented rim also (double-ring sign), and various visual field defects. Dysplastic optic disks usually are associated with poor vision and show abnormal vasculature, retinal pigment epithelium, and glial tissue. They are often surrounded by a chorioretinal pigmentary disturbance. Dysplastic disks have been reported with trisomy 4q. The papillorenal syndrome has been reported with dysplastic disks and colobomas. Colobomas of the optic nerve have been called "pseudoglaucoma" because of their resemblance to glaucomatous cupping. Disk colobomas or hypoplasia when associated with chorioretinal lacunae, absence of the corpus callosum, and focal seizures constitute Aicardi's syndrome. This can also include retrobulbar cysts.

Optic nerve drusen can be deeply buried in the optic nerve head in children and mimic papilledema, even causing enlarged blind spots. They can be seen by retroillumination as "lumpy-bumpy," yellow, crystalline excrescences, becoming more apparent with increasing age and the loss of overlying axons; fluorescein angiography can help in the diagnosis by showing local dye pooling, and the calcium in drusen can be seen on ultrasound and CT scan. They can rarely cause visual loss by choroidal neovascularization and vitreous hemorrhage.

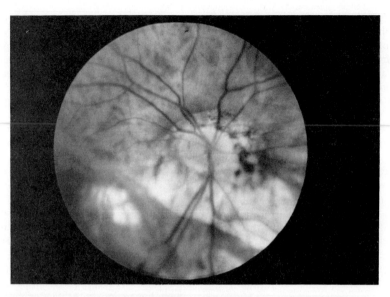

Figure 14–17. Tilted disk.

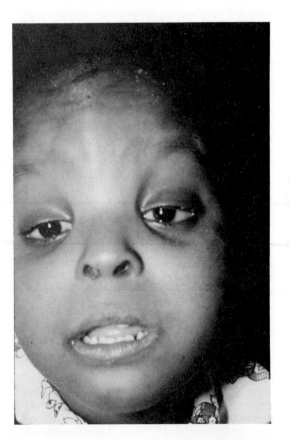

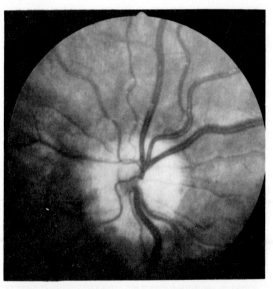

Figure 14–18. *At left:* Hypertelorism. *Above:* Optic nerve hypoplasia.

THE OPTIC CHIASM

In general, lesions of the chiasm cause bitemporal hemianopic defects. Early, these defects are typically incomplete and are often asymmetric. However, as compression progresses, the temporal hemianopia becomes complete, the inferior and superior nasal fields will then be involved, and central visual acuity will decrease. Most diseases that affect the chiasm are neoplastic, with vascular or inflammatory processes only occasionally producing chiasmatic visual field loss.

PITUITARY TUMORS

The anterior lobe of the pituitary gland is the site of origin of pituitary tumors (Figure 14–19). Symptoms and signs include loss of vision, field changes, pituitary dysfunction, extraocular nerve palsies, and evidence on CT scan or MRI of sellar and suprasellar tumor.

Combination therapy with radiation and surgery has been challenged by medical treatment with bromocriptine, which has been effective not only in tumors associated with galactorrhea but also in some null cell (or endocrinologically inactive) tumors. Visual loss or endocrine dysfunction is an indication for treatment. Visual acuity and visual fields may improve dramatically after pressure has been removed from the chiasm. The initial appearance of the optic nerve head does not predict the ultimate visual outcome.

CRANIOPHARYNGIOMA

Craniopharyngiomas are an uncommon group of tumors arising from epithelial remnants of Rathke's pouch (80% of the population normally have such remnants) and characteristically become symptomatic between the ages of 10 and 25 years but occasionally not until the 60s and 70s. They are usually suprasellar, occasionally intrasellar. The signs and symptoms vary tremendously with the age of the patient and the exact location of the tumor as well as its rate of growth. When a suprasellar tumor occurs, asymmetric chiasmatic or tract field defects are prominent. Papilledema is more common than in pituitary tumors. Optic nerve hypoplasia can be seen in those tumors presenting in infancy. Pituitary deficiency may result, and involvement of the hypothalamus may cause stunted growth. Calcification of parts of the tumor contributes to a characteristic radiologic appearance, especially in children.

Treatment consists of surgical removal—as complete as possible at the first procedure, since reoperation tends to involve the hypothalamus, and patients then do poorly. Adjunctive radiotherapy is often used, particularly if there has been incomplete surgical removal.

SUPRASELLAR MENINGIOMAS

Suprasellar meningiomas arise from the meninges covering the tuberculum sellae and the planum sphenoidale, with a high proportion of patients being female. The tumor is usually anterior and superior to the chiasm. Visual field changes due to involvement of the optic nerves and chiasm often occur early (but asymmetrically) followed by slowly progressive damage to the visual pathway. CT scans with contrast enhancement easily demonstrate these tumors (Figure 14–20). Hyperostoses associated with bony erosion and a dense calcified tumor are the radiologic hallmarks of meningioma. Treatment consists of surgical removal.

CHIASMATIC & OPTIC NERVE GLIOMAS

Optic nerve and chiasm gliomas are rare, usually indolent disorders of children that sometimes occur as part of the clinical picture of neurofibromatosis. Onset may be sudden, with rapid loss of vision. Optic atrophy occurs, and visual field defects reveal an optic

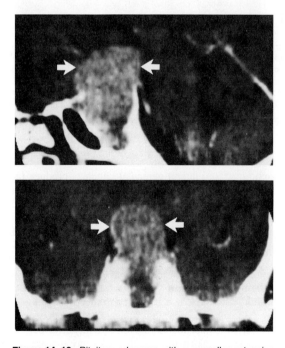

Figure 14–19. Pituitary adenoma with suprasellar extension (arrows) causing bitemporal hemianopia. CT scans with contrast enhancement. Sagittal re-formation *(top)*. Coronal re-formation *(bottom)*.

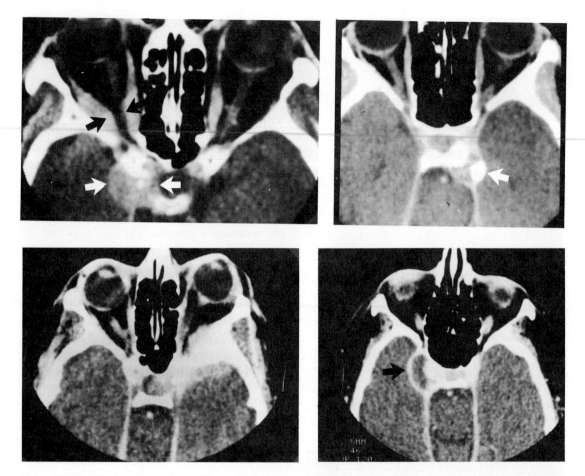

Figure 14–20. CT scans of four patients with eye signs of basal cranial tumors. ***Upper left:*** Optic nerve compression due to thyroid myopathy (black arrows) and meningioma (white arrows). ***Upper right:*** Sixth nerve palsy due to chordoma of petrous tip (arrow). ***Lower left:*** Proptosis due to sphenoid ridge meningioma. ***Lower right:*** Third nerve palsy due to intracavernous aneurysm (black arrow).

nerve or chiasmatic syndrome. CT scans may reveal enlarged optic nerves and a mass in the region of the chiasm and hypothalamus. Treatment depends on the location of the tumor and its clinical course. Irradiation can be given during a tumor growth spurt, and optic nerve resection is sometimes done when an optic nerve tumor aggressively starts to extend intracranially toward the chiasm.

THE RETROCHIASMATIC VISUAL PATHWAYS

Cerebrovascular disease and tumors are responsible for most lesions of the retrochiasmatic visual path-

ways, though almost any intracranial disease process can involve these structures. Retrochiasmatic visual field defects are homonymous. Partial lesions in the optic tract and lateral geniculate nucleus produce incongruous (or dissimilar) visual field defects due to a 90-degree medial rotation of axons in each tract and the decussation of half of the axons through the chiasm. Thus, there may be more involvement of a nasal hemifield than of its corresponding temporal hemifield. Once the lesion becomes complete, however, incongruity cannot be assessed, and this sign loses its localizing ability. Retrochiasmatic visual field defects should spare visual acuity since the visual pathway from the other hemibrain is intact. The optic tracts and lateral geniculate nucleus are infrequently affected. After several weeks to months, the disks may appear pale, and the retinal nerve fiber layer is deficient. The optic tract and lateral geniculate nucleus have at least a dual blood supply, so that primary vascular lesions are uncommon. Most cases are due to trauma, tumors, arteriovenous malformations, abscesses, and demyelinating diseases.

Lesions involving the geniculocalcarine pathway to the occipital cortex produce homonymous field defects but do not result in optic atrophy (due to the synapse at the geniculate nucleus). Generally, the more posterior a lesion is located, the more congruous the homonymous visual field defect. The inferior geniculocalcarine pathway passes through the temporal lobe and the superior pathway through the parietal lobe, with macular function between them. Lesions of the inferior pathway result in superior visual field defects. Processes affecting the anterior and midtemporal lobes are commonly neoplastic; posterior temporal lobe and parietal processes can be either vascular or neoplastic. An insidious onset with mild and multiple neurologic deficits would be more typically neoplastic, whereas an acute cataclysmic neurologic event would be more typically vascular. Vascular lesions of the occipital lobe, on the other hand, are common and account for over 80% of cases of isolated homonymous visual field loss in patients over age 50 years. The most posterior tip of each occipital lobe projects to homonymous macular fields. Anterior to the macular representation lies the peripheral field; thus, vascular occlusions can selectively involve the posterior occipital cortex and produce homonymous defects with congruous macular scotomas or spare the posterior cortex, and homonymous defects with macular sparing will result. The cortical centers involved in the generation of optokinetic nystagmus lie in the area between the occipital and temporal lobes and in the posterior parietal area, which are within the vascular territory of the middle cerebral artery. Optokinetic nystagmus asymmetry characteristically occurs in parietal lesions but not in occipital lesions. An asymmetric optokinetic nystagmus combined with an occipital visual field defect indicates a process not respecting vascular territories and thus suggests a tumor (Cogan's sign). CT scans demonstrate vascular and neoplastic disease of the occipital lobe with remarkable clarity (Figures 14–21 and 14–22).

THE PUPIL

The size of the normal pupil varies at different ages, from person to person, and with different emotional states, levels of alertness, degrees of accommodation, and ambient room light. The normal pupillary diameter is about 3–4 mm, smaller in infancy, and tending to be larger in childhood and again progressively smaller with advancing age. Pupillary size relates to varying interactions between the parasympathetically innervated iris

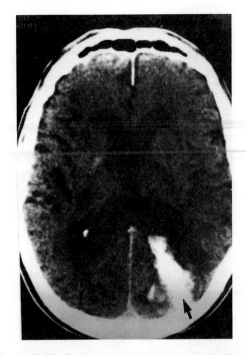

Figure 14–21. Occipital hematoma (arrow) resulting from a bleeding arteriovenous malformation. This lesion produced homonymous hemianopia and headache.

dilator, with supranuclear control from the frontal (alertness) and occipital lobes (accommodation). The pupil also normally responds to respirations (ie, hippus). Twenty to 40 percent of normal patients have a slight difference in pupil size (physiologic anisocoria), usually of about 0.5 mm. Mydriatic and cycloplegic drugs work more effectively on blue eyes than on brown eyes.

Neuroanatomy of the Pupillary Pathways

Evaluation of the pupillary reactions is important in localizing lesions involving the optic pathways. The examiner should be familiar with the neuroanatomy of the pathway for reaction of the pupil to light and the miosis associated with accommodation (Figure 14–23).

A. Light Reflex: (Figure 14–24.) The pathway for the light reflex is entirely subcortical. The afferent pupillary fibers are included within the optic nerve and visual pathways until they exit the optic tract just prior to the lateral geniculate nucleus. They enter the midbrain through the brachium of the superior colliculus and synapse in the pretectal nucleus. Each pretectal nucleus decussates neurons dorsal to the cerebral aqueduct to the ipsilateral and contralateral Edinger-Westphal nucleus via the posterior commissure and the periaqueductal gray matter. A synapse then occurs in the Edinger-Westphal nucleus of the oculomotor nerve. The efferent pathway is via the third nerve to the

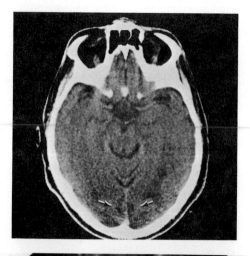

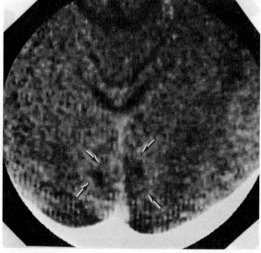

Figure 14–22. CT scans showing bilateral small infarctions of the visual cortex causing a ring-like scotoma in the middle field of vision. **Top:** Axial section. **Bottom:** Magnified view of the occipital cortex. The infarcted areas appear as zones of low density between the splenium and the occipital pole.

ciliary ganglion in the lateral orbit. The postganglionic fibers go via the short ciliary nerves to innervate the sphincter muscle of the iris.

B. The Near Reflex: When the eyes look at a near object, three reactions occur—accommodation, convergence, and constriction of the pupil—bringing a sharp image into focus on corresponding retinal points. There is convincing evidence that the final common pathway is mediated through the oculomotor nerve with a synapse in the ciliary ganglion. The afferent pathway enters the midbrain ventral to the Edinger-Westphal nucleus and sends fibers to both sides of the cortex. Although the three components are closely associated, the near reflex cannot be considered a pure reflex, since each component can be neutralized while leaving the other two intact—ie, by prism (neutraliz-

ing convergence), by lenses (neutralizing accommodation), and by weak mydriatic drugs (neutralizing miosis). It can occur even in a blind person who is instructed to look at his nose. Bilateral overaction of the near reflex is accommodative spasm. Bilateral accommodative paresis occurs in botulism poisoning and in the Fisher variant of Guillain-Barré syndrome.

ARGYLL ROBERTSON PUPIL

A typical Argyll Robertson pupil is strongly suggestive of central nervous system syphilis associated with tabes dorsalis or general paresis. The pupil is less than 3 mm in diameter (miotic) and does not respond to light stimulation but does accommodate; this finding is nearly always bilateral. The pupils are commonly irregular, eccentric, and dilate poorly with mydriatics as a consequence of concomitant iris atrophy. Less commonly, the sign is incomplete (slow response to light) or unilateral or associated with tonic pupils (mimicking Adie's syndrome). Some degree of Argyll Robertson pupil is present in over 50% of patients with central nervous system syphilis. A wide variety of other central nervous system diseases infrequently cause incomplete Argyll Robertson pupil. These include diabetes, chronic alcoholism, encephalitis, multiple sclerosis, central nervous system degenerative disease, and tumors of the midbrain. The periaqueductal gray matter of the midbrain is the usual site of the lesion and thus affects the light reflex. The near reflex pathway is more ventral and thus is spared.

TONIC PUPIL

Tonic pupil occurs because of an abnormal pupillary constrictor mechanism in which all or a segment of the sphincter muscle contracts slowly (tonically) to near stimulation and relaxes even slower, but either response is better than the light response. It is usually associated with loss of deep tendon reflexes (Adie's syndrome). It results from damage to the ciliary ganglion, which carries 30 nerves destined for the ciliary body to one destined for the iris sphincter. Thus, accommodation is more apt to be preserved by a ciliary body lesion and is also—as a consequence of preferential innervation—more likely to reinnervate after an injury. This can produce segmental pupillary innervation. A weak (0.1%) solution of pilocarpine instilled into the conjunctival sac causes a tonic pupil to constrict as a result of denervation hypersensitivity; normal pupils are not affected. Some preganglionic oculomotor nerve lesions have, however, been shown to have denervation hypersensitivity probably related to a direct iris pathway that does not synapse at the ciliary ganglion. Bilateral tonic pupils should raise a question of autonomic neuropathy.

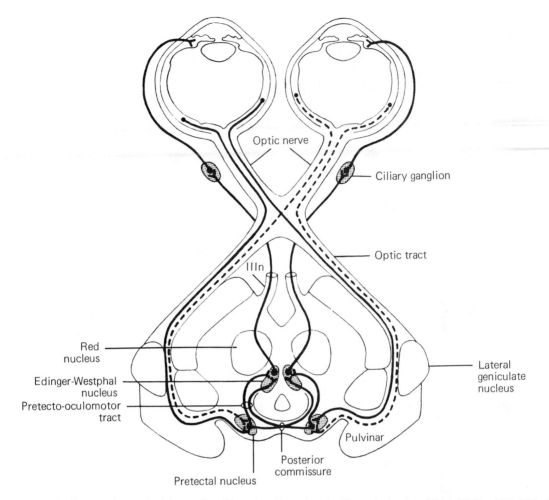

Figure 14–23. Diagram of the path of the pupillary light reflex. (Reproduced, with permission, from Walsh FB, Hoyt WF: *Clinical Neuro-ophthalmology,* 3rd ed. Vol 1. Williams & Wilkins, 1969.)

HORNER'S SYNDROME

Horner's syndrome is caused by a lesion of the sympathetic pathway, either (1) in its **central portion,** which extends from the posterior hypothalamus through the brainstem to the upper spinal cord (C8–T2); or (2) in its **preganglionic portion,** which exits the spinal cord and synapses in the superior cervical (stellate) ganglion; or (3) in its **postganglionic portion,** from the superior cervical ganglion via the carotid plexus and the ophthalmic division of the trigeminal nerve, by which it enters the orbit. The sympathetic fibers then follow the nasociliary branch of the ophthalmic division of the trigeminal nerve and the long ciliary nerves to the iris and innervate Müller's muscle and the iris dilator. Iris dilator muscle paresis causes miosis, which is more evident in dim light. Melanocyte maturation in the iris of a neonate depends upon sympathetic innervation; thus, less pigmented (bluer) irides occur if a con-

genital sympathetic lesion is present. Unilateral miosis, ptosis, and absence of sweating on the ipsilateral face and neck make up the complete syndrome. Postganglionic fibers to the face for sweating and vasoconstriction follow the external carotid. Causes of Horner's syndrome include cervical vertebral fractures, tabes dorsalis, syringomyelia, cervical cord tumor, cervical rib, Lyme disease, apical bronchogenic carcinoma, aneurysm of the carotid or subclavian artery, brachial plexus injuries, and injuries to or dissection of the carotid artery high in the neck. Pharmacologic testing with topical cocaine in the conjunctival sac can differentiate Horner's syndrome from central anisocoria, and hydroxyamphetamine can further localize the process to the postganglionic neuron, thus assisting in defining the cause of the syndrome.

Raeder's paratrigeminal syndrome is Horner's syndrome associated with unilateral headache or facial pain in the distribution of the trigeminal nerve. If as-

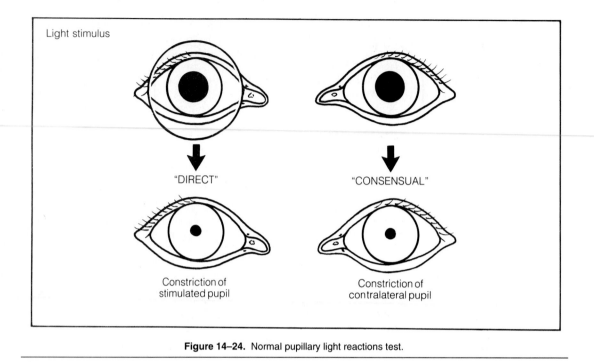

Figure 14–24. Normal pupillary light reactions test.

sociated with a sixth, third, fourth, or second cranial nerve palsy, complete neurologic evaluation for basilar skull tumor is required. Without these additional cranial nerves, Raeder's syndrome is a benign condition perhaps related to cluster headache.

AFFERENT PUPILLARY DEFECT

Optic nerve fibers from the right eye decussate at the chiasm to enter the left tract as well as continuing into the right tract, and the same is true on the left side. The pupillary light pathways enter the midbrain through the brachium of the superior colliculus to synapse in the pretectal nucleus; here, they decussate also, as each pretectal nucleus connects to the ipsilateral and contralateral Edinger-Westphal nucleus. For this reason, light shone into the right eye produces an immediate direct response in the right and an immediate indirect consensual response in the left eye (Figure 14–24). The intensity of this response in each eye is proportionate to the light-carrying ability of the directly stimulated optic nerve.

One of the most important assessments to make for the patient complaining of decreased vision is whether it is due to a local ocular problem, eg, cataract, or to a more serious optic nerve problem. Even dense cataracts do not change the light afferent pathways to the brain; hence, a comparison is possible. If an optic nerve lesion is present, the direct light response in the involved eye is less intense than the consensual response (in the involved eye) evoked when the normal

eye is stimulated. This phenomenon is called a relative afferent pupillary defect (RAPD) (Figure 14–25). It will be positive also if there is a large retinal lesion. Causes of unilateral decreased vision without an afferent pupillary defect include refractive error, cloudy media (cataract), amblyopia, hysteria or malingering, a macular lesion, and chiasmatic problems. It is anatomically possible for a relative afferent defect with normal visual function to occur if the brachium of the superior colliculus is damaged by a thalamic hemorrhage.

Amaurotic pupillary defect is the term applied to an eye that does not even see light owing to severe unilateral retinal or optic nerve disease. Obviously, a blind eye would not have a direct light response, nor could it induce a consensual response in the normal eye. However, a light shown directly into the normal eye would induce a direct response there and a consensual response in the blind eye (Figure 14–26).

EXTRAOCULAR MOVEMENTS

This section deals with the neural apparatus that controls eye movements and causes them to move simultaneously, up or down and side to side, as well as in convergence or divergence.

The neural control of eye movements is ultimately

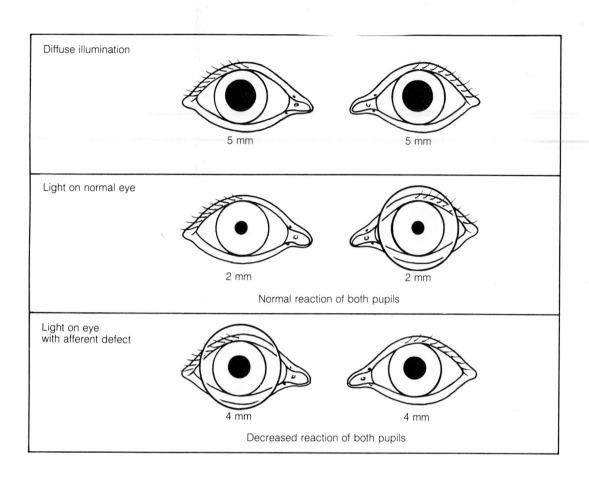

Figure 14–25. Afferent pupillary defect (Marcus Gunn pupil).

effected by alterations in activity in the nuclei and nerve fibers of the oculomotor, trochlear and abducens nerves. These are referred to as the nuclear and infranuclear pathways. Coordination of eye movements requires connections between these ocular motor nuclei; the internuclear pathways. The supranuclear pathways are responsible for generation of the commands necessary for the execution of the appropriate movement, whether it be voluntary or involuntary.

Classification & Examination of Eye Movements

Eye movements are either fast or slow. Fast eye movements include voluntary or involuntary refixation movements (saccades) and the fast phases of vestibular and optokinetic nystagmus (see below). The fast eye movement system is tested by command refixation movements and by the fast phase of vestibular and optokinetic nystagmus.

Slow eye movements include pursuit movements,

which track a slowly moving target once the saccadic system has placed the target on the fovea, and which are tested by asking a patient to follow a slow, smoothly moving target, the slow phase movements generated by vestibular stimuli, the slow phase of optokinetic nystagmus, and vergence movements which—unlike all the other forms of eye movements—involve dysconjugate movements of the two eyes.

Under physiologic conditions, vestibular stimulation occurs from head movements. The resulting slow eye movements, known as the **vestibulo-ocular responses (VOR),** compensate for the head motion such that the position of the eyes in space remains static and steady visual fixation can be maintained. The **doll's head maneuver** is a clinical method of testing the vestibulo-ocular response. The patient is asked to fixate on a target while the examiner moves the head in a horizontal or vertical plane. If the vestibulo-ocular response is deficient, the compensatory eye movements are insufficient and must be supplemented by saccadic movements to maintain fixation. The head motion

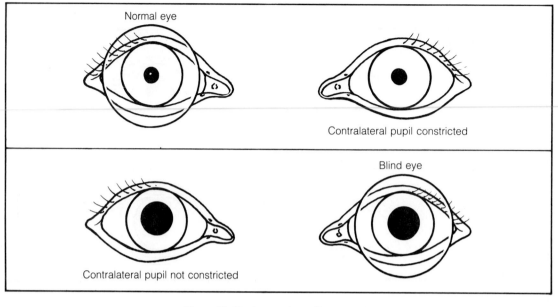

Normal eye

Contralateral pupil constricted

Blind eye

Contralateral pupil not constricted

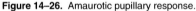

Figure 14–26. Amaurotic pupillary response.

must be rapid—otherwise, pursuit mechanisms dominate the ocular motor response. In the unconscious patient, the doll's head maneuver is used to assess brainstem function. Since the pursuit and saccadic systems are not operative, the head movements can be slow. Absence of the vestibulo-ocular response leads to failure of the eyes to move within the orbit. Other methods of vestibular stimulation are whole body rotation and caloric testing (see below).

Generation of Eye Movements
A. Physiology:
1. Fast eye movements–Understanding of the control of eye movements is most complete in the case of saccadic movements. Similar mechanisms are thought to apply to the fast phases of nystagmus. The generation of a saccade involves a **pulse** of increased innervation to move the eye in the required direction and a **step** increase in tonic innervation to maintain the new position in the orbit by counteracting the visco-elastic forces working to return the eye to the primary position. The pulse is produced by the **burst cells of the saccadic generator.** The step change in tonic innervation is produced by the **tonic cells of the neural integrator,** so-called because it effectively integrates the pulse to produce the step. Saccades are effectively ballistic movements—ie, once initiated, their trajectory can not be altered—and there is a close relationship between the amplitude of movement and its peak velocity, larger movements having greater peak velocities. Loss of the saccadic generator function leads to slowing of saccades. Loss of the neural integrator function leads to a failure of maintenance of the desired final position, ie, a failure of gaze holding. Clinically,

this usually manifests as a gaze-evoked nystagmus, with a drift of the eyes toward the primary position followed by a corrective saccade back to the desired position of gaze.

2. Slow eye movements–The slow phase movements generated by vestibular stimuli are a direct response to the detection of movement by the semicircular canals. The canals are acceleration detectors, but their output is integrated to produce a velocity signal which is then conveyed to the ocular motor nuclei. The generation of pursuit movements is less well understood. The slow phase of optokinetic nystagmus is in part a pursuit movement, but there is also an additional specific optokinetic movement generated by the perception of movement of the background of the visual scene. This optokinetic movement appears to be generated by the pathways involved in generating slow phase vestibular movements but with an input from the retina, either via cortical centers or directly via a subcortical pathway. Vergence eye movements are generated in response to retinal disparity, ie, stimulation of noncorresponding retinal loci by the object of regard. Electromyography has established divergence as an active process, not a relaxation of convergence.

B. Anatomy:
1. Brainstem centers for fast eye movements–The saccadic generator for horizontal eye movements lies in the paramedian pontine reticular formation. The output from this structure is channeled through the abducens nucleus, which contains both the motor neurons for the abducens nerve and the cell bodies of interneurons which pass via the medial longitudinal fasciculus to innervate the motor neurons in the contralateral medial rectus subnucleus of the oculo-

motor nerve. The neural integrator for horizontal eye movements appears to be located close to the paramedian pontine reticular formation in the nucleus prepositus hypoglossi.

The saccadic generator for vertical movements is in the rostral interstitial nucleus of the medial longitudinal fasciculus in the rostral midbrain. The pathway to the ocular motor nuclei for upward movements involves the posterior commissure, dorsal to the cerebral aqueduct, and its nucleus. The corresponding pathway for downward eye movements is less well defined. Neural integration for vertical eye movements seems to take place in both the interstitial nucleus of Cajal, close to the rostral interstitial nucleus of the medial longitudinal fasciculus in the midbrain and in the vestibular nuclei in the medulla.

2. Cortical centers for fast eye movements—Voluntary saccades are initiated in the frontal lobe (frontal eye field area 8). The pathway descends through the basal ganglia and the anterior limb of the internal capsule into the brainstem, terminating in the midbrain pretectal area for vertical movements and crossing to the paramedian pontine reticular formation in the opposite side of the pons for horizontal movements. The generation of involuntary (reflexive) saccades, in response to a target appearing in the peripheral field of vision, depends upon activity within the superior colliculus, which receives information from the occipital cortex and also directly from the retina in a purely subcortical pathway.

3. Brainstem centers for slow eye movements—The processing of information from the semicircular canals occurs in the vestibular nuclei, which then connect directly to the ocular motor nuclei. These pathways from the vestibular nuclei in the medulla to the pons and midbrain pass in a number of fiber tracts, including the medial longitudinal fasciculus.

4. Cortical centers for slow eye movements—Pursuit movements originate in the occipital cortex. The pathway descends through the posterior limb of the internal capsule to the midbrain and ipsilateral paramedian pontine reticular formation. The slow phase of optokinetic nystagmus is likely to be generated at least in part in area V5 (or MT) at the junction of the occipital and temporal lobes, which is involved in motion detection. The descending pathway probably accompanies the pathway for pursuit movements. Vergence eye movements are generated in the occipital cortex, and the pathway also probably descends via the posterior limb of the internal capsule, together with the pathway for pursuit movements, to terminate in the rostral midbrain near or in the oculomotor nucleus. Impulses then pass directly to each medial rectus subnucleus and via the medial longitudinal fasciculus to the abducens nuclei. It is not clear whether convergence and divergence are controlled by the same or separate brainstem centers.

ABNORMALITIES OF EYE MOVEMENTS

Owing to the multiplicity of pathways involved in the supranuclear control of eye movements, with origins in different areas of the brain and an anatomic separation in the brainstem of the horizontal and vertical eye movement systems, disorders of the supranuclear pathways characteristically produce a dissociation of effect upon the various types of eye movements. Thus, the clinical clues to a supranuclear lesion are a differential effect on horizontal and vertical eye movements or upon saccadic, pursuit, and vestibular eye movements. In diffuse brainstem disease, such features may not be apparent, and differentiation from disease at the neuromuscular junction or within the extraocular muscles on clinical grounds can be difficult.

Disease of the internuclear pathways results in a disruption of the conjugacy of eye movements. In infranuclear disease, the pattern of eye movement disturbance usually complies with that expected of a lesion involving one or more cranial nerves or their nuclei.

1. LESIONS OF THE SUPRANUCLEAR PATHWAYS

Frontal Lobe

A seizure focus in the frontal lobe may cause involuntary turning of the eyes to the opposite side. Destructive lesions cause transient deviation to the same side, and the eyes cannot be turned quickly and voluntarily (saccadic movement) to the opposite side. This is called frontal gaze palsy, and recovery occurs when the opposite frontal eye field substitutes. Ocular pursuit to the opposite side is retained. There is no diplopia. Phenytoin can significantly affect saccades.

Occipital Lobe

Smooth ocular pursuit may be lost with posterior lesions of the hemispheres. The patient is unable to follow a slowly moving object in the direction of the gaze palsy. The command (fast) eye movement is not lost, so pursuit is "saccadic." Sedative agents and carbamazepine can alter smooth pursuit eye movements.

Midbrain

Lesions of the posterior commissure cause impairment of conjugate upgaze. Lesions dorsal and medial to the red nuclei produce a downgaze paresis (trauma, infarcts).

Parinaud's syndrome (pretectal syndrome) is characterized by loss of voluntary upward gaze and convergence-retraction nystagmus and (usually) loss of the pupillary light response with retention of miosis in response to the near reflex. Convergence-retraction movements of the globe on attempted upward gaze is due to simultaneous firing of the rectus muscles due to loss of supranuclear control. There may also be an apparent accommodative spasm, a loss of conjugate voluntary downward gaze associated with loss of convergence and accommodation, ptosis or lid retraction, papilledema, or third nerve palsy. Surrounding structures may also be involved depending on the size and location of the lesion. Conjugate horizontal ocular movements are usually not affected. The syndrome results from tectal or pretectal lesions affecting the periaqueductal area. Pinealomas, infiltrating gliomas, vascular lesions (arteriovenous malformations), demyelinating disease, and trauma may produce this picture.

Pons

Lesions of the paramedian pontine reticular formation produce an ipsilateral horizontal gaze palsy affecting saccadic and pursuit movements. Vestibular slow phase movements are preserved owing to the direct pathway from the vestibular nuclei to the abducens and oculomotor nuclei.

Lesions of the brain stem that cause gaze palsies include vascular accidents, arteriovenous malformations, multiple sclerosis, tumors (pontine gliomas, cerebellopontine angle tumors), and encephalitis.

2. SUPRANUCLEAR SYNDROMES INVOLVING DISJUNCTIVE OCULAR MOVEMENTS

Spasm of the Near Reflex

The near reflex consists of three components: convergence, accommodation, and constriction of the pupil. Spasm of the near reflex is usually caused by hysteria, though encephalitis, tabes dorsalis, and meningitis may cause spasm by irritation of the supranuclear pathway. It is characterized by convergent strabismus with diplopia, miotic pupils, and spasm of accommodation (induced myopia).

If hysteria is the cause, atropine 1%, 2 drops in each eye twice daily, or minus (concave) lenses may give temporary relief. Psychiatric consultation is indicated for treatment of an underlying mental cause.

Convergence Paralysis

Convergence paralysis is characterized by a sudden onset of diplopia for near vision, with absence of any individual extraocular muscle palsy. It is caused by hysteria or destructive lesions of the supranuclear pathway for convergence. The combination of motor convergence failure and pupillary miosis confirms patient effort and an organic lesion. Multiple sclerosis, myasthenia gravis, head trauma, encephalitis, tabes dorsalis, tumors, aneurysms, minor cerebrovascular accidents, and Parkinson's disease are the most common organic causes.

INTERNUCLEAR OPHTHALMOPLEGIA

The medial longitudinal fasciculus is an important fiber tract extending from the rostral midbrain to the spinal cord. It contains many pathways connecting nuclei within the brainstem, particularly those concerned with extraocular movements. The most common manifestation of damage to the medial longitudinal fasciculus is an internuclear ophthalmoplegia, in which conjugate horizontal eye movements are disrupted owing to failure of coordination between the abducens nerve nucleus in the pons and the oculomotor nerve nucleus in the midbrain. The lesion in the brainstem is ipsilateral to the eye with the adduction failure or opposite to the direction of horizontal gaze that is abnormal. In the mildest form of internuclear ophthalmoplegia, the clinical abnormality is restricted to a slowing of saccades in the adducting eye. In the most severe form, there is a complete loss of adduction on horizontal gaze. Convergence is characteristically preserved in internuclear ophthalmoplegia except when the lesion is in the midbrain, when the convergence mechanisms may also be affected. Another feature of internuclear ophthalmoplegia is nystagmus in the abducting eye on attempted horizontal gaze, which is at least in part a result of compensation for the failure of adduction in the other eye. In bilateral internuclear ophthalmoplegia, there may also be an upbeating nystagmus on upgaze due to failure of control of gaze holding in the upward direction, and the eyes may be divergent; this is known as the WEBINO (wall-eyed bilateral internuclear ophthalmoplegia) syndrome.

Internuclear ophthalmoplegia may be due to multiple sclerosis (particularly in young adults), brainstem infarction (particularly in older patients), tumors, arteriovenous malformations, Wernicke's encephalopathy, and encephalitis. Bilateral internuclear ophthalmoplegia is most commonly due to multiple sclerosis.

A horizontal gaze palsy combined with an internuclear ophthalmoplegia, due to a lesion of the abducens nucleus or paramedian pontine reticular formation extending into the ipsilateral medial longitudinal fasciculus, affects all horizontal eye movements in the ipsilateral eye and adduction in the contralateral eye. This is known as a "one-and-a-half syndrome," or paralytic pontine exotropia.

NUCLEAR & INFRANUCLEAR CONNECTIONS

Oculomotor Nerve (III)

The motor fibers arise from a group of nuclei in the central gray matter ventral to the cerebral aqueduct at the level of the superior colliculus. The midline central caudal nucleus innervates both levator palpebrae superioris muscles. The paired superior rectus subnuclei innervate the contralateral superior rectus. The efferent fibers decussate immediately and pass through the opposite superior rectus subnucleus. The subnuclei for the medial rectus, inferior rectus, and inferior oblique muscles are also paired structures but innervate the ipsilateral muscles. The fascicle of the oculomotor nerve courses through the red nucleus and the inner side of the substantia nigra to emerge on the medial side of the cerebral peduncles. The nerve runs alongside the sella turcica, in the outer wall of the cavernous sinus, and through the superior orbital fissure to enter the orbit.

The parasympathetics arise from the Edinger-Westphal nucleus just rostral to the motor nucleus of the third nerve and pass via the inferior division of the third nerve to the ciliary ganglion. From there the short ciliary nerves are distributed to the sphincter muscle of the iris and to the ciliary muscle.

A. Oculomotor Paralysis: Lesions of the third nerve nucleus affect the ipsilateral medial and inferior rectus and inferior oblique muscles, both levator muscles, and both superior rectus muscles. There will be bilateral ptosis and bilateral limitation of elevation as well as limitation of adduction and depression ipsilaterally. From the fascicle of the nerve in the midbrain to its eventual termination in the orbit, all other lesions produce purely ipsilateral results. Just before entering the orbit, the nerve divides into a superior and inferior branch; the former innervates the levator palpebrae and superior rectus muscles and the latter all other muscles and the sphincter.

If the lesion involves the third nerve anywhere from the nucleus (midbrain) to the peripheral branches in the orbit, the eye is turned out by the intact lateral rectus muscle and slightly depressed by the intact superior oblique muscle. (Incyclotorsion from the action of the intact superior oblique muscle can be observed by watching a small blood vessel on the medial conjunctiva as depression of the eye is attempted.) There can be a dilated fixed pupil, absent accommodation, and ptosis of the upper lid, often severe enough to cover the pupil. The eye may only be moved laterally. Trauma, aneurysm, viral infections, and vascular disease are the most common causes. Aneurysm usually arises from the junction of the internal carotid and posterior communicating arteries. Vascular disease includes diabetes mellitus, migraine, hypertension, and the collagenoses. The common location for vascular palsies is in the cavernous sinus region, where the pupillary fibers are peripheral and nourished better by the vasa vasorum. Compressive lesions such as aneurysms involve the external pupillary fibers early and produce pupillary dilation. Thus, aneurysm and vascular disease can be differentiated clinically, since in vascular lesions the pupillary responses are usually spared, whereas aneurysmal compression causes a completely fixed and dilated pupil. Less than 5% of vascular third nerve palsies are associated with complete pupillary palsy, and in only 15% is there partial pupillary palsy.

Some apparently vascular oculomotor palsies with or without pupillary sparing can be seen on MRI to have focal mesencephalic infarcts without the usual rubral tremor or other local signs. In compressive lesions, the pupil may become constricted because of aberrant regeneration (see below), or a concomitant Horner's syndrome (sympathetic paresis) can produce a "frozen" pupil of 3–4 mm.

Bilateral nuclear third nerve palsies can also be associated with sparing of the lids. Bilateral peripheral third nerve palsies can occur secondary to interpeduncular lesions such as basilar artery aneurysm or a herniated hippocampus of the temporal lobe.

Monocular elevator paralysis or inability to elevate in both abduction (superior rectus) and adduction (inferior oblique) can occur as a congenital defect or as a complication of thyroid ophthalmopathy, orbital myositis, orbital floor fracture, myasthenia gravis, paresis of the superior division of the third nerve (tumor, sinusitis, postviral), or midbrain stroke.

Third nerve palsies in children may be congenital or may be due to ophthalmoplegic migraine, meningitis, or postviral.

B. Oculomotor Synkinesis (Aberrant Regeneration of the Third Nerve): This phenomenon is characterized by (1) lid dyskinesias on horizontal gaze (ie, the levator palpebrae superioris fires when the medial rectus fires); (2) adduction on attempted upgaze (ie, the medial rectus fires when the superior rectus fires); (3) retraction on attempted upgaze (ie, cofiring of recti, which are retractors); (4) pseudo-Argyll Robertson pupil (ie, no light response, no near response in the primary position but a "near" response on adduction or adduction-depression—pupillary innervation from medial or inferior rectus); (5) pseudo-Graefe's sign (ie, no lid lag on downgaze but lid retraction due to lid innervation from the inferior rectus); and (6) a monocular vertical optokinetic nystagmus response (due to co-firing muscles fixing the involved eye, allowing only the normal eye to respond to the moving target). This oculomotor synkinesis probably occurs not only as a combination of misdirection of sprouting axons into the wrong sheaths and subsequent muscle co-firing but also as a consequence of ephaptic transmission or cross-talk between axons without covering myelin sheaths.

Oculomotor synkinesis can occur secondary to severe trauma or compression of the third nerve by a posterior communicator artery aneurysm, or primarily due to an internal carotid aneurysm or meningioma in the cavernous sinus. If compression lasts several weeks, strabismus surgery is often required to achieve binocular single vision.

C. Cyclic Oculomotor Palsy: Cyclic oculomotor palsy can complicate a congenital third nerve palsy; it is a rare predominantly unilateral event with a typical third nerve paresis showing cyclic spasms every 10–30 seconds. During these intervals, ptosis improves and accommodation increases. This phenomenon continues unchanged throughout life but decreases with sleep and increases with greater arousal. It is probably a periodic discharge by damaged neurons of the oculomotor nucleus which summate subthreshold stimuli until a discharge occurs.

D. Marcus Gunn Phenomenon (Jaw-Winking Syndrome): This rare congenital condition consists of elevation of a ptotic eyelid upon movement of the jaw. Acquired cases occur after damage to the oculomotor nerve with subsequent innervation of the lid (levator palpebrae superioris) by a branch of the fifth cranial nerve. Muscular palsies may be present.

Trochlear Nerve (IV)

Motor (entirely crossed) fibers arise from the trochlear nucleus just caudal to the third nerve at the level of the inferior colliculus; they then run posteriorly, decussate in the anterior medullary velum, and wind around the cerebral peduncles. The fourth nerve travels near the third nerve along the wall of the cavernous sinus to the orbit, where it supplies the superior oblique muscle. The fourth nerve is unique among the cranial nerves in arising from the dorsal brainstem.

A. Trochlear Paralysis: Lesions of the fourth nerve are commonly vascular, traumatic, or idiopathic (congenital or developmental with later decompensation). However, cerebellar tumors can also present with a fourth nerve lesion as an early sign. The nerve is vulnerable to injury at the site of exit from the dorsal aspect of the brainstem. Both nerves may be damaged by severe trauma as they decussate in the anterior medullary velum, resulting in bilateral superior oblique palsies.

Superior oblique palsy results in upward deviation (hypertropia) of the eye. The hypertropia increases when the patient looks down and with adduction. In addition, there is excyclotropia; therefore, one of the diplopic images will be tilted with respect to the other. Torsional symptoms suggest an acquired late-onset superior oblique palsy: correspondingly, the lack of torsional symptoms suggest an early onset of the deviation. Tilting the head toward the involved side increases the deviation. Tilting the head away from the side of the involved eye may relieve the diplopia, and patients frequently present with a head tilt. Miscellaneous causes include multiple sclerosis, a brainstem arteriovenous malformation, orbital pseudotumor, and myasthenia gravis. Strabismus surgery is effective in patients who fail to improve with time.

B. Superior Oblique Myokymia: A monocular microtremor of the superior oblique muscle can rarely occur. It is an acquired, haphazard, and episodic overaction of the superior oblique muscle characterized by rapid torsional movements of one eye. Patients notice oscillopsia when this occurs, and the symptoms can be improved by carbamazepine. The cause may be compression of the trochlear nerve by an aberrant artery.

Abducens Nerve (VI)

Motor (entirely uncrossed) fibers arise from the nucleus in the floor of the fourth ventricle in the lower portion of the pons near the internal genu of the facial nerve. Piercing the pons, the fibers emerge anteriorly, the nerve running a long course over the tip of the petrous portion of the temporal bone into the cavernous sinus. It enters the orbit with the third and fourth nerves to supply the lateral rectus muscle.

A. Abducens Nucleus Lesion: The abducens nucleus contains the motor neurons to the ipsilateral lateral rectus and the cell bodies of interneurons innervating the motor neurons to the contralateral medial rectus. It is the final common relay point for all horizontal conjugate eye movements, and a lesion within the nucleus will produce an ipsilateral horizontal gaze palsy affecting all types of eye movement including vestibular movements. This contrasts with a lesion of the paramedian pontine reticular formation, in which vestibular movements are preserved.

B. Abducens Nerve Paralysis: (See also Chapter 12.) This is the most common single muscle palsy. Abduction of the eye is absent; esotropia is present in the primary position and increases upon gaze to the affected side. Movement of the eye to the opposite side is normal. Möbius' syndrome (congenital facial diplegia) can be associated with a sixth nerve or conjugate gaze palsy. Vascular disorders (arteriosclerosis, diabetes, migraine, and hypertension) are common causes. However, dural arteriovenous fistula, basilar artery disease, increased intracranial pressure, lumbar puncture, tumors at the base of the skull, meningitis, and trauma are other frequent causes. Arnold-Chiari malformation (congenital downward displacement of the cerebellar tonsils) can also produce brainstem traction and sixth nerve palsies. Lyme disease can produce an isolated sixth nerve palsy as well as those that occur secondary to meningeal involvement. A child with a sixth nerve palsy should be evaluated for a brainstem tumor (glioma) or inflammation if trauma was not present or if trauma was minimal. Pseudo-sixth nerve palsies can occur in Duane's retraction syndrome, spasm of the near reflex, thyroid eye disease, myasthenia, dorsal midbrain compression (Parinaud's syndrome), or long-standing strabismus and in medial rectus entrapment by an ethmoid fracture.

C. Duane's Syndrome: Duane's syndrome is uncommon (< 1% of cases of strabismus) and in almost all cases congenital. It is a stationary, nearly always unilateral condition consisting of deficient horizontal ocular motility characterized by complete or partial deficiency of abduction. Evidence based on pathologic studies has determined that Duane's syndrome can be due to congenital absence of the sixth nerve with coinnervation of the lateral rectus by a branch of the third nerve. Therefore, attempted adduction movements result in retraction of the globe and narrowing of the lid fissure. The visual handicap is seldom severe. Visual acuity can be normal, and the eye is otherwise normal. Unless the deviation is very large, strabismus surgery is best avoided.

Cochlear nucleus lesions producing sensorineural hearing loss occur in 6.8% of cases of Duane's syndrome. Congenital malformations may also include the facial and skeletal bones, the ribs, and the external ear. Ocular anomalies can include epibulbar dermoids. Acquired Duane's syndrome is a rare event occurring after a peripheral nerve palsy.

D. Gradenigo's Syndrome: Gradenigo's syndrome is characterized by pain in the face (from irritation of the trigeminal nerve) and abducens palsy. The syndrome is produced by meningeal inflammation at the tip of the petrous bone and most often occurs as a rare complication of otitis media with mastoiditis or petrous bone tumors.

Symptoms and Signs of Extraocular Muscle Palsies

Diplopia occurs when the visual axes are not aligned. This is especially true when the onset of strabismus is after age 6 (suppression and abnormal retinal correspondence do not develop). Dizziness or dysequilibrium may be associated but disappears with monocular patching. Head tilt occurs, especially in paresis of the superior oblique muscle, when the tilt is to the opposite side to avoid diplopia by moving the eye out of the field of action of the paralyzed muscle. Vertical saccadic velocity can differentiate a superior oblique palsy from inferior rectus palsy. Horizontal saccadic velocity can differentiate a restricted globe with pseudo-sixth nerve from sixth nerve paresis. Forced duction tests should also be done, since a paresis could be simulated by a restricted yoke muscle.

Ptosis is caused by weakness or paralysis of the levator muscle. Any extraocular muscle palsy that occurs with minor head trauma (subconcussive injuries) should be investigated for a basal tumor. The minimally positive edrophonium test is unreliable because it can be nonspecific. Fascicular lesions involving the portion of a cranial nerve within the brainstem resemble peripheral nerve lesions but can be differentiated on the basis of other brainstem signs and their subsequent poor recovery. For vascular causes of cranial nerve palsies, recovery by 4 months is the rule. Palsies that persist longer than 6 months—especially those involving the sixth nerve—should be evaluated for an underlying structural compressive lesion (tumor, arteriovenous fistula, aneurysm).

Syndromes Affecting Cranial Nerves III, IV, & VI

A. Superior Orbital Fissure Syndrome: All extraocular peripheral nerves pass through the superior orbital fissure and can be involved by trauma or by tumor encroaching on the fissure.

B. Orbital Apex Syndrome: This syndrome is similar to the superior orbital fissure syndrome with the addition of optic nerve signs and usually greater proptosis and less pain. It is caused by an orbital tumor, inflammation, or trauma that damages the optic and extraocular nerves.

C. Complete Ophthalmoplegia (Sudden): Complete ophthalmoplegia of sudden onset can be due to brainstem vascular disease, Wernicke's encephalopathy, pituitary apoplexy, Fisher's syndrome, myasthenia crisis, bulbar poliomyelitis, diphtheria, botulism, meningitis, and syphilitic or arteriosclerotic basilar aneurysm.

THE CEREBELLUM

The cerebellum has an important modulating influence on the function of the neural integrators. Thus, it is involved in gaze holding and the control of saccades, particularly the relationship between the pulse and the step of saccade generation. Cerebellar dysfunction produces gaze-evoked nystagmus, by its influence on gaze holding, and abnormalities of saccades, including saccadic dysmetria, in which the saccadic amplitude is inaccurate, and postsaccadic drift due to a mismatch between the pulse and step of the saccade.

The cerebellum is also important in the control of pursuit eye movements, and cerebellar dysfunction may thus result in broken (saccadic) pursuit.

MYASTHENIA GRAVIS

Myasthenia gravis is characterized by abnormal fatigability of striated muscles after repetitive contraction which improves after rest and often is first manifested by weakness of the extraocular muscles. Unilateral fatiguing ptosis is a frequent first sign, with subsequent bilateral involvement of extraocular muscles, so that diplopia is often an early symptom. Unusual ocular presentations may simulate gaze palsies, internuclear ophthalmoplegias, vertical nystagmus, and progressive external ophthalmoplegia. Generalized weakness of the arms and legs, difficulty in swallowing, weakness of jaw muscles, and difficulty in breathing may follow rapidly in untreated cases. This weakness shows diurnal variations and often worsens as the day progresses but can be improved by a nap. There are no sensory changes.

The incidence of the disease is in the range of 1:30,000 to 1:20,000. Myasthenia gravis usually affects young adults aged 20–40 (70% are under 40 years of age), though it may occur at any age and is often misdiagnosed as hysteria, especially because the weakness can be greater in exciting or embarrassing situations. Older patients are more commonly male and are more likely to have a thymoma.

The onset may follow an upper respiratory infection, stress, pregnancy, or any injury, and the disease has been noted as a transitory condition in newborn infants of myasthenic mothers. Myasthenia gravis has been associated with hyperthyroidism (5%), thyroid abnormalities (15%), autoimmune diseases (5%), and diffuse metastatic carcinoma (7%).

In about one-third of cases, the disease is confined to the extraocular muscles at onset. In about two-thirds of these cases, the disease will become generalized with time, usually within the first year.

The differential diagnosis includes progressive external ophthalmoplegia, brainstem lesions, epidemic encephalitis, bulbar and pseudobulbar palsy, postdiphtheritic paralysis, botulism, multiple sclerosis, and toxic reactions to the beta-blockers (eg propranolol) or penicillamine. Many other drugs may unmask or exacerbate myasthenia gravis; they include lithium, aminoglycoside antibiotics, chloroquine, and phenytoin.

Substantial neurophysiologic evidence indicates that the disease has its origin at the neuromuscular junction, especially at the postsynaptic site, probably due to antibodies against it and the presynaptic site. A commercial test of anti-acetylcholine receptor antibodies can diagnose the disease in 80–90% of patients with systemic myasthenia and 40–60% of patients with pure ocular myasthenia; the titers do not correlate with severity of disease, however.

Most patients have merely histologic thymic hyperplasia, often apparent on lateral oblique chest x-rays or CT scans of the mediastinum or noted at surgical removal of the thymus. Thymomas occur in 15% of patients.

Cholinesterase destroys acetylcholine at the myoneural junction, and cholinesterase-inhibiting drugs improve the condition by increasing the amount of acetylcholine available to the damaged postsynaptic site. The edrophonium chloride test is used in addition to the neostigmine diagnostic test. Edrophonium, 2 mg (0.2 mL), is given intravenously over 15 seconds. Relief of ptosis constitutes a positive response and confirms the diagnosis of myasthenia gravis. If no response occurs in 30 seconds, an additional 5–7 mg (0.5–0.7 mL) is given. The test is most helpful when marked ptosis is present, but myasthenia can affect any muscle or combination of muscles, and significant improvement in function is also helpful. Slightly positive edrophonium tests can occur in neurogenic palsies, however, and there may be false-negative results when myasthenia is complicated by muscle wasting.

A regional curare test can diagnose systemic involvement in patients with only ocular involvement clinically. Myasthenic patients are sensitive to one-tenth the usual curarizing dose. Repetitive nerve stimulation, especially of the facial or proximal muscles, can also demonstrate abnormal muscle fatigability (a more than 10% decrease in the response is diagnostic of myasthenia).

Myasthenia can be treated with pyridostigmine, systemic steroids, azathioprine, cyclosporine, immunoglobulins, and plasmapharesis according to the severity of disease. During severe exacerbations, artificial ventilation may be necessary. Thymectomy may be indicated in patients with thymoma (though it may not influence the severity of the myasthenia) and in patients with early-onset generalized disease without evidence of thymoma—in one third of whom it may produce complete remission without the need for immunosuppressants. Ocular myasthenia tends to respond less well to anticholinesterase agents than generalized disease, but the response to systemic steroids is usually good. Extraocular muscle surgery can be undertaken but should be delayed until the ocular motility deficit has been stable for a long time.

Myasthenia is generally a chronic disease with a tendency to pursue a relapsing and remitting course. The prognosis depends upon the extent of the disease, the response to medication and thymectomy, and the careful management of severe exacerbations.

CHRONIC PROGRESSIVE EXTERNAL OPHTHALMOPLEGIA

This rather rare disease is characterized by a slowly progressive inability to move the eyes and very often is associated with severe early ptosis yet normal pupillary reactions and accommodation. It may begin at any age and progresses over a period of 5–15 years to complete external ophthalmoplegia. It is a form of mitochondrial myopathy and may be associated with other manifestations of mitochondrial disease such as pigmentary degeneration of the retina, deafness, cerebellar-vestibular abnormalities, seizures, cardiac conduction defects, and peripheral sensorimotor neuropathy, in which case the term "ophthalmoplegia-plus" may be applied. The combination of chronic progressive external ophthalmoplegia, heart block, and retinitis pigmentosa is known as the Kearns-Sayre syndrome. Chronic progressive external ophthalmoplegia is associated with deletions of mitochondrial DNA, which are more frequent and more extensive in the cases with nonocular manifestations.

The differential diagnosis includes ophthalmoplegia with motor neuron disease, progressive supranuclear palsy, Möbius' syndrome, spinocerebellar degeneration, Bassen-Kornzweig syndrome, Refsum's disease, and juvenile sphingolipidosis.

NYSTAGMUS

Nystagmus (Figure 14–27) is defined as repetitive, rhythmic oscillations of one or both eyes in any or all fields of gaze. The waveform may be pendular, in which the movements in each direction have equal speed, amplitude, and duration; or jerk, in which the slow movement in one direction is followed by a rapid corrective return to the original position (fast component).

Jerk nystagmus is classified as grade I, present only with the eyes directed toward the fast component; grade II, present also with the eyes in primary position; or grade III, present even with the eyes directed toward the slow component. The movements may be horizontal, vertical, torsional, oblique, circular, or a combination of these. The direction may change depending upon the direction of gaze.

The **amplitude** of nystagmus is the extent of the movement; the **rate** of nystagmus is the frequency of oscillation. Generally speaking, the faster the rate, the smaller the amplitude and vice versa. Nystagmus is usually conjugate but is occasionally dysconjugate, as in physiologic end-gaze nystagmus, convergence-retraction nystagmus, and seesaw nystagmus.

Nystagmus is also occasionally dissociated (more marked in one eye than the other), as in internuclear ophthalmoplegia, spasmus nutans, seesaw nystagmus, monocular visual loss, and acquired pendular nystagmus and with asymmetric muscle weakness in myasthenia gravis.

Physiology of Symptoms

Reduced visual acuity is caused by inability to maintain steady fixation. False projection is evident in vestibular nystagmus, where past-pointing is present. Head tilting is usually involuntary, to decrease the nystagmus. The head is turned toward the fast components in jerk nystagmus or set so that the eyes are in a posi-

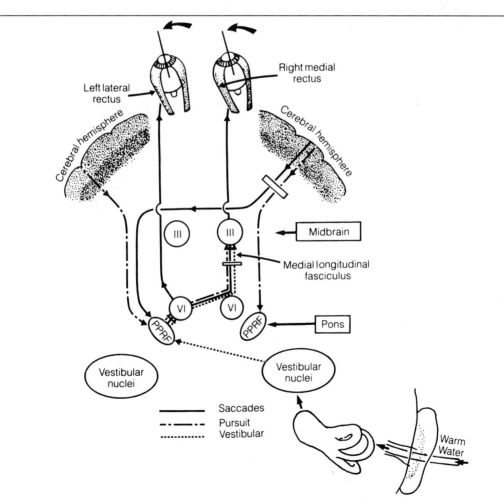

Figure 14–27. Nystagmus.

tion that minimizes ocular movement in pendular nystagmus. The patient sometimes complains of illusory movements of objects (oscillopsia). This is more apt to be present in nystagmus due to lesions of lower centers, such as the labyrinth, or associated with the sudden onset of nystagmus in an adult. The apparent movement of the environment occurs during the slow component and causes an extremely distressing vertigo, so that the patient is unable to stand. Head nodding is most apt to accompany congenital nystagmus, spasmus nutans, and miner's nystagmus. Nystagmus is noticeable and cosmetically disturbing except when excursions of the eye are very small.

Classification of Nystagmus
  A. Physiologic nystagmus
    1. End-point nystagmus
    2. Optokinetic nystagmus
    3. Stimulation of semicircular canals
  B. Pathologic nystagmus
    1. Congenital
      a. Poor vision
      b. Congenital nystagmus
      c. Latent nystagmus
    2. Spasmus nutans
    3. Down-beat nystagmus
    4. Upbeat nystagmus
    5. Convergence retraction nystagmus
    6. Seesaw nystagmus
    7. Horizontal nystagmus
      a. Voluntary nystagmus
      b. Acquired pendular nystagmus
      c. Periodic alternating nystagmus
      d. Gaze-evoked nystagmus
    8. Vestibular nystagmus
  C. Mimics of nystagmus

PHYSIOLOGIC NYSTAGMUS

Three types of nystagmus can be elicited in the normal person.

End Point (End-Gaze) Nystagmus
Normal individuals have a wide null or quiet zone but can have horizontal nystagmus on end-horizontal gaze (ie, pupillary light reflex just on both corneas); physiologic end-gaze nystagmus disappears as the eyes move in a few degrees. It is primarily horizontal but may have a slight torsional component and greater amplitude in the abducting eye; it is a normal form of gaze-evoked nystagmus.

Optokinetic Nystagmus
This type of nystagmus may be elicited in all normal individuals, most easily by means of a rotating drum with alternating black and white lines but in fact by any repetitive targets in the visual field such as repetitive telephone poles as seen from a window of a fast-moving vehicle. The slow component follows the object and the fast component moves rapidly in the opposite direction to fixate on each succeeding object. A unilateral or asymmetric horizontal response usually indicates a deep parietal lobe lesion, especially a tumor. It occurs as a result of a deficit in the slow (pursuit) phase. Anterior cerebral (ie, frontal lobe) lesions may inhibit this response only temporarily when an acute saccadic gaze palsy is present, which suggests the presence of a compensatory mechanism that is much greater than for lesions situated farther posteriorly. Asymmetry of response in the vertical plane suggests a brainstem lesion. Since it is an involuntary response, this test is especially useful in detecting hysteria or malingering. A large mirror filling the patient's central field at near can be rotated from side to side and will induce an optokinetic nystagmus if vision is present.

Stimulation of Semicircular Canals
Endolymph flow in the semicircular canals inputs into the vestibular nuclei; they then maintain resting vestibular tonus on the oculomotor nuclei via the paramedian pontine reticular formation and the medial longitudinal fasciculus, also to the cerebellum and to the cortex.

  A. Bárány Rotating Chair: The horizontal canals are parallel to the floor when the head is tilted 30 degrees forward. Rotation of the subject causes a jerk nystagmus in the direction of the turning. The slow component is in the opposite direction, the same as the flow of endolymph in the semicircular canals.

  B. Caloric Stimulation: With the subject supine and the head flexed on the chest, cold water ear irrigation produces nystagmus with the fast component away from the side of irrigation while warm water produces nystagmus with the fast component toward the side of irrigation. (The mnemonic device is "COWS": cold–opposite, warm–same.) This is named for the obvious or fast phase, but the true component is the slow or vestibular component; the fast or saccadic movement is a corrective movement that occurs in the alert patient with an intact reticular activating system. Hence, a comatose patient with an intact pons will show only the true vestibular component.

PATHOLOGIC NYSTAGMUS

Nystagmus can be thought of as a disorder of the mechanisms that hold the eyes or fixation steady—thus, the neural systems involved in nystagmus include cerebellovestibular, optokinetic, and pursuit systems.

Congenital Nystagmus
Congenital impairment of vision or visual deprivation due to lesions in any part of the eye or optic nerve can result in pendular nystagmus. Causes include

corneal opacity, cataract, albinism, Chédiak-Higashi syndrome, corectopia, achromatopsia, posterior polar chorioretinitis, aniridia, and optic atrophy. At least in part, it occurs because of poor fixation.

Pendular nystagmus, which occurs in children with poor vision, has been called "sensory nystagmus," while jerk nystagmus, which occurs in children with good vision, has been called "motor nystagmus." However, eye movement recordings delineate jerk and pendular waveforms that are irrespective of visual acuity. Jerk nystagmus will be associated with a "foveating or breaking saccade" to achieve good vision; however, in pendular nystagmus, the eyes oscillate across the target, whereas on eye movement recording, a jerk component can often be seen.

Congenital nystagmus is present at birth or shortly thereafter. It is usually horizontal and conjugate, but occasionally there may be a vertical vector in the waveform. However, whatever movement is observed on horizontal gaze is also present on vertical gaze. Horizontal optokinetic nystagmus is absent or an "inverted pursuit" can be seen on optokinetic drum testing with the fast phase to the drum; vertical optokinetic nystagmus is still present. This latter point differentiates it from poor vision, in which optokinetic nystagmus is absent or deficient whether horizontal or vertical repetitive targets are viewed. Most patients with congenital nystagmus have a relatively quiet or null zone that can be eccentric to the primary position, and they will adjust a head turn to keep this eccentric position straight ahead. Since this nystagmus is decreased by convergence, some patients will adopt an esotropia, but it is increased by anxiety or increased "effort to see." Mechanical esotropia by prisms or ocular surgery can decrease this effort and improve vision.

Latent Nystagmus

Latent nystagmus is a common nonprogressive variant of congenital nystagmus that only appears when one eye is covered, when both eyes develop nystagmus with the slow phase toward the cover and the fast phase away.

Spasmus Nutans

Spasmus nutans is a bilateral, generally horizontal (occasionally vertical) nystagmus in which each eye has a very different amplitude or is dissociated; it is associated with head nodding as a compensatory vestibular mechanism. It is benign, but central nervous system visual disorders must be eliminated, especially if there is a vertical component to the waveform. It may appear at about 4 months of age and should resolve by 3 years of age or rarely later.

Downbeat Nystagmus

Downbeat nystagmus is associated with cervicomedullary junction abnormalities. It is often evident in the primary position as a slow upward drift with a rapid corrective saccade down. Occasionally it is evident only on oblique downgaze. The mechanism for the eyes "drifting up" may be loss of inhibition of the central vestibular connections from the anterior semicircular canals, a vertical pursuit imbalance, or vestibulocerebellar disease affecting the vertical neural integrators. Disorders known to produce it include, notably, Arnold-Chiari malformation and basilar invagination but also demyelinating disease, cerebellar atrophy, hydrocephalus, and side effects of anticonvulsants.

Upbeat Nystagmus

Upbeat nystagmus occurs in the primary position of gaze and is increased on upgaze or downgaze.

A. Upgaze Nystagmus: Increase of upbeat nystagmus on upgaze is due to disorders of the anterior superior cerebellar vermis or the medulla. It can also occur in meningitis and as a toxic side effect of barbiturates, alcohol, and anticonvulsants. It is characterized by a tendency of the eyes to drift down, with corrective saccades upward that increase in amplitude with increasing upgaze. It may be due to loss of influence of the anterior semicircular canals, which mediate upward vestibular tone.

B. Downgaze Nystagmus: A fine upbeat nystagmus on downgaze has been associated with medullary abnormalities. This phenomenon is rarely seen.

Convergence-Retraction Nystagmus

Convergence-retraction nystagmus occurs on attempted upgaze in patients with Parinaud's syndrome from dorsal midbrain lesions, and occasionally with upper midbrain gliomas and demyelinating disease. Here the fast phases of nystagmus are convergent and horizontal, and there is a defective or absent upward saccade. The globes appear to converge and retract during each fast phase of the nystagmus, which is best elicited as the patient watches down-moving stripes on an optokinetic nystagmus tape or drum. Electromyographic studies show cocontraction of extraocular muscles and loss of normal agonist-antagonist reciprocal innervation.

Seesaw Nystagmus

Seesaw nystagmus is characterized by rising intorsion of one eye and falling extorsion of the other—and then the reverse. Although it is uncommon, it occurs with chiasmatic tumors, head trauma, and midbrain infarction and is often associated with a bitemporal hemianopia. A congenital form can occur without bitemporal hemianopia. The generator of this nystagmus may be the interstitial nucleus of Cajal.

Horizontal Nystagmus

A. Voluntary Nystagmus: Voluntary nystagmus is a high-frequency burst of horizontal oscillations that are saccadic in each direction. This is self-induced by convergence in normals and is an ill-sustained shuddering or shivering movement.

B. Acquired Pendular Nystagmus: This uncommon disorder occurs in multiple sclerosis and other white matter or brainstem abnormalities and may be associated with palatal myoclonus. It can be congenital or acquired and may be horizontal, vertical, or both. Both vectors—whatever their direction—have the same amplitude. Lesions in the dentato-rubro-olivary connections may be responsible. Treatment with valproic acid, trihexyphenidyl, clonazepam, isoniazid, and base-out prisms may be helpful.

C. Periodic Alternating Nystagmus: This is a direction-reversing nystagmus in which each direction can take 1–2 minutes before reversing. It occurs in pontomedullary junction abnormalities (Arnold-Chiari malformation), multiple sclerosis, heredodegenerative ataxias, and congenitally; it has been reported—especially in acquired cases—to be abolished by baclofen.

D. Gaze-Evoked Nystagmus: This type of nystagmus is induced by directing gaze out of the primary position either horizontally or vertically. Such a movement depends on a neural integrator to correlate pursuit, saccadic, and vestibular input, but if this integrator is defective, the eyes cannot be maintained in eccentric gaze out of the primary position and will drift back. Smooth pursuit or ocular stabilization can also be faulty. Cerebellar diseases, sedatives, and anticonvulsant medications can be associated with gaze-evoked nystagmus and faulty smooth pursuit. Cerebellopontine angle neoplasms can produce a unilateral gaze paresis with coarse gaze-evoked nystagmus and rapid vestibular nystagmus to the opposite side (due to asymmetric vestibular input).

Vestibular Nystagmus

Vestibular nystagmus is always of the jerk type but can originate as a consequence of peripheral (semicircular canal) or central imbalance (inputs from semicircular canals or vestibulocerebellar connection). The slow component is considered to be a response to impulses originating in the semicircular canals; the fast component is a corrective movement originating in the reticular activating system. Vestibular nystagmus is not dependent upon visual stimuli, ie, it is present with the lids closed as well as open and can be elicited in blind individuals also. Peripheral nystagmus is inhibited or dampened by visual fixation and can be deconditioned by training, which is why ballet dancers stare fixedly after several spinning turns and another reason why they train. Torsional movements are especially characteristic of vestibular nystagmus, but horizontal or vertical vestibular nystagmus also occurs. In peripheral vestibular (occasionally central) nystagmus, the movement can be enhanced or elicited by a specific head position that stimulates the impaired semicircular canal. Smooth pursuit and saccades are abnormal in central vestibular lesions.

The characteristics of vestibular nystagmus due to labyrinthine or vestibular nerve disease are as follows: (1) vertigo, tinnitus, and deafness are apt to be associated; (2) nystagmus is maximal early in the disease and tends to improve or disappear in 2–3 weeks (unless the vestibular nuclei are affected directly, in which case nystagmus may be permanent); and (3) the lesion is usually destructive, and its direction (fast component) is away from the side the lesion is on.

Vestibular nystagmus may be due to labyrinthitis, Meniere's disease, trauma (including surgical destruction of one labyrinth); vascular, inflammatory, or neoplastic lesions of the vestibular nerves; lesions of the vestibular nuclei (encephalitis, multiple sclerosis, syringobulbia, poliomyelitis, thrombosis of the posteroinferior cerebellar artery); or cerebellar tumors and abscesses (probably as a result of pressure on the vestibular pathways).

Mimics of Nystagmus

Several cerebellar abnormalities can simulate nystagmus. These include macrosquare wave jerks around a visual fixation point, ocular dysmetria, ocular flutter, and opsoclonus (constant conjugate chaotic saccades).

CEREBROVASCULAR DISORDERS OF OPHTHALMOLOGIC IMPORTANCE

Vascular Insufficiency & Occlusion of the Internal Carotid Artery

Amaurosis fugax is a fleeting or transient loss of vision that is usually associated clinically with carotid occlusive disease, though it can occur with any microembolic or thrombotic disorder, including cardiac valvular disease, cardiac arrhythmia, temporal arteritis, migraine, severe hypotension or shock, papilledema, orbital tumors, and hyperviscosity states. Antiphospholipid antibodies have been associated with transient and permanent cerebral and retinal vascular occlusions in patients younger than the usual stroke population. These antibodies may be the key determinant in patients with existing structural lesions of the carotid artery, mitral valve, etc. In embolization, vision can be suddenly lost or slowly disappear like a curtain rising or falling. In hypotension, the visual field constricts from the periphery to the center.

Perhaps 95% of episodes of amaurosis fugax occur as a result of atherosclerotic lesions of the ipsilateral internal carotid artery. Cerebral and retinal disturbances occur as a result of small emboli breaking loose from the sclerotic plaque and lodging in cerebral or retinal arterioles (occlusion of the central retinal artery or a major branch can occur). Cholesterol emboli (Hollenhorst plaques) may be visible with the ophthalmoscope as small, glistening, yellow-red crystals situated at bifurcations of the retinal arteries. A finding of reduced ophthalmic artery pressure (as determined by ophthalmodynamometry), bruits over the internal carotid artery, and angiography helps to confirm the diagnosis. Removal of a high-grade stenotic plaque by carotid endarterectomy may improve the quality of life for the patient and decrease the likelihood of embolic stroke to the cerebral hemisphere.

Retinovascular occlusions can occur from calcific and platelet emboli. Duller, white-gray embolic fragments in the retinal blood vessels are the hallmark of calcific emboli from cardiac valvular disease, whereas gummy, white, nonreflective plugs neatly filling a blood vessel are platelet fibrin material and can be from carotid occlusive disease. Most embolic fragments can be readily seen with the ophthalmoscope in the posterior pole but—most especially Hollenhorst plaques–will also eventually pass through the retinal microvasculature, and only 10% remain in place. To induce more rapid passage and better visual results, they are treated acutely with a varying combination of aspirin, dipyridamole, CO_2-O_2 mixture, paracentesis, ocular massage, and intravenous acetazolamide. After 24 hours, the clinical picture is usually irreversible, though many exceptions to this rule have been reported. Visual acuity better than counting fingers on presentation has a better prognosis with vigorous treatment. Central retinal or branch artery occlusion, especially when due to Hollenhorst plaques, has a poorer 5-year survival rate due to attendant cardiac disease or stroke than does occlusion due to thrombotic disease.

Venous stasis retinopathy is a sign of internal carotid artery occlusion. It is characterized by venous dilation and tortuosity, retinal hemorrhages, macular edema, and eventual neovascular proliferation. It resembles diabetic retinopathy, but the changes occur more in the retinal midperiphery than the posterior pole. The treatment is endarterectomy and, if necessary, panretinal laser photocoagulation. Untreated ischemic signs can become chronic with vasodilation of the conjunctiva, iris neovascularization, neovascular glaucoma, cloudy cornea, anterior chamber cells, and a rapidly developing cataract.

Occlusion of the Middle Cerebral Artery

This disorder may produce severe contralateral hemiplegia, hemianesthesia, and homonymous hemianopia. The lower quadrants of the visual fields (upper radiations) are most apt to be involved. Aphasia may be present if the dominant hemisphere is involved.

Vascular Insufficiency of the Vertebrobasilar Arterial System

Brief episodes of transient bilateral blurring of vision commonly precede a basilar artery stroke. An at-

tack seldom leaves any residual visual impairment, and the episode may be so minimal that the patient or doctor does not heed the warning. The blurring is described as a graying of vision just as if the house lights were being dimmed at a theater. Episodes seldom last more than 5 minutes (often only a few seconds) and may be associated with other transient symptoms of vertebrobasilar insufficiency. Antiplatelet drugs can decrease the frequency and severity of vertebrobasilar symptoms.

Occlusion of the Basilar Artery

Complete or extensive thrombosis of the basilar artery nearly always causes death. With partial occlusion or basilar "insufficiency" due to arteriosclerosis, a wide variety of brainstem and cerebellar signs may be present. These include nystagmus, supranuclear oculomotor signs, and involvement of cranial nerves III, IV, VI, and VII.

Prolonged anticoagulant therapy has become the accepted treatment of partial basilar artery thrombotic occlusion.

Occlusion of the Posterior Cerebral Artery

Occlusion of the posterior cerebral artery seldom causes death. Occlusion of the cortical branches (most common) causes homonymous hemianopia, usually superior quadrantic (the artery supplies primarily the inferior visual cortex). Lesions on the left in right-handed persons can cause aphasia, agraphia, and alexia if extensive with parietal and occipital involvement. Involvement of the occipital lobe and splenium of the corpus callosum can cause alexia (inability to read) without agraphia (inability to write); such a patient would not be able to read his or her own writing. Occlusion of the proximal branches may produce the thalamic syndrome (thalamic pain, hemiparesis, hemianesthesia, choreoathetoid movements) and cerebellar ataxia.

Subdural Hemorrhage

Subdural hemorrhage results from tearing or shearing of the veins bridging the subdural space from the pia mater to the dural sinus. It leads to an encapsulated accumulation of blood in the subdural space, usually over one cerebral hemisphere. It is nearly always caused by head trauma. The trauma may be minimal and may precede the onset of neurologic signs by weeks or even months.

In infants, subdural hemorrhage produces progressive enlargement of the head with bulging fontanelles. The diagnosis is established by the finding of bloody spinal fluid on tapping the subdural space and by enlarged head measurements. Ocular signs include strabismus, pupillary changes, papilledema, and retinal hemorrhages.

In adults, the symptoms of chronic subdural hematoma are severe headache, drowsiness, and mental confusion, usually appearing hours to weeks (even months) after trauma. Symptomatology is similar to that of cerebral tumors. Papilledema is present in 30–50% of cases. Retinal hemorrhages occur in association with papilledema. Ipsilateral dilation of the pupil is the most common and most serious pupillary sign and is an urgent indication for immediate surgical evacuation of blood. Unequal, miotic, or mydriatic pupils can occur, or there may be no pupillary signs. Other signs, including vestibular nystagmus and cranial nerve palsies, also occur. Many of these signs result from herniation and compression of the brainstem and therefore often appear late with stupor and coma.

Skull films may show a shift of a calcified pineal gland. CT scan or MRI frequently confirms the diagnosis.

Treatment of acute large subdural hematoma consists of surgical evacuation of the blood; small hematomas may be treated with steroids or simply followed with careful observation. Without treatment, the course of large hematomas is progressively downhill to coma and death. With early and adequate treatment, the prognosis is good.

Subarachnoid Hemorrhage

Subarachnoid hemorrhage (Figure 14–28) most commonly results from ruptured congenital berry aneurysms of the circle of Willis in the subarachnoid space. It may also result from trauma, birth injuries, intracranial hemorrhage, hemorrhage associated with tumors, arteriovenous malformations, or systemic bleeding disorders.

The most prominent symptom of subarachnoid hemorrhage is sudden, severe headache, usually occiptal and often associated with signs of meningeal irritation (eg, stiff neck). Drowsiness, loss of consciousness, coma, and death may occur rapidly once an aneurysm ruptures and produces a subarachnoid hemorrhage. Ocular symptoms are not always present. A posterior communicating artery aneurysm may produce a third nerve palsy with pupillary involvement by distention of an aneurysmal sac before the aneurysm ruptures and produces a subarachnoid hemorrhage. Oculomotor palsy with associated numbness and pain in the distribution of the ipsilateral trigeminal nerve is pathognomonic of a supraclinoid, internal carotid, or posterior communicating artery aneurysm. Papilledema usually appears late when it does occur and after there has been a subarachnoid hemorrhage. Various types of retinal hemorrhage occur infrequently (preretinal hemorrhages are the most common—Terson's syndrome) and carry a poor prognoses for life when they are both early and extensive, since they reflect rapid severe elevation of intracranial pressure.

Exophthalmos may occur as a result of extravasation of blood into orbital tissues. Pressure of an aneurysm on the optic nerve may cause blindness in one eye.

Arteriography following injection of radiopaque substances may help to demonstrate and localize the aneurysms. Blood is present in the cerebrospinal fluid.

Ligation of aneurysmal vessels or of parent arterial trunks may be advisable. Supportive treatment, including control of blood pressure, is all that can be offered during the acute phase of subarachnoid hemorrhage. Thus, it is important to diagnose the posterior communicating artery aneurysm when it first produces a third nerve palsy with pupillary involvement.

Migraine

Migraine is a common episodic illness of unknown cause and varied symptomatology characterized by severe unilateral headache (which alternates sides), visual disturbances, nausea, and vomiting. The neurologic symptoms that usually precede the headache occur in the vasoconstrictive phase; the headache follows in the vasodilative phase. There is usually a family history of a similar disorder. The disease usually becomes manifest between ages 15 and 30 years. It is more common and more severe in women. Many factors, particularly emotional ones, may predispose or contribute to the attacks. Prodromal symptoms are common and include drowsiness, paresthesias, "scintillating" scotomas, blurred vision, and other symptoms. In some patients, homonymous hemianopia can be accurately recorded on the tangent screen during attacks. There are no other objective findings. Visual symptoms usually last only 15–30 minutes. Antiphospholipid antibodies have been associated with migrainous headaches and severe atypical migraine.

Ergotamine tartrate, when given early in an attack,

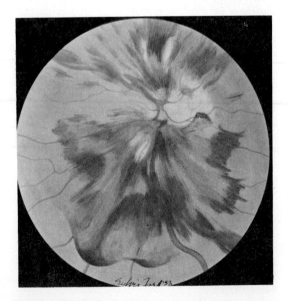

Figure 14–28. Subhyaloid hemorrhage around optic disk associated with subarachnoid hemorrhage. (Drawing.)

is often effective. Once the attack is well under way, treatment is of little value. Sumatriptan is effective in the acute and well-established migraine attack. The headaches last several hours to several days. Bed rest is often helpful and sometimes essential for relief of discomfort.

PHAKOMATOSES

The phakomatoses (Gr *phakos* "birthmark" + *-oma* "swelling") are a group of diseases characterized by multiple hamartomas occurring in various organ systems and at variable times.

NEUROFIBROMATOSIS

Neurofibromatosis is a generalized hereditary disease characterized by multiple tumors of the skin, central nervous system, peripheral nerves, and nerve sheaths. Other developmental anomalies, particularly of the bones, may be associated. There are two distinct dominant conditions. Neurofibromatosis 1 (peripheral) (Recklinghausen's disease) consists of multiple café au lait spots (99%), peripheral neurofibromas, and Lisch nodules (iris hamartomas) (93%), and its gene lies on the pericentromeric region of chromosome 17. The frequency is 1:3000 live births, with 100% penetrance. In neurofibromatosis 2 (central), there may be few or no café au lait spots or peripheral neurofibromas, but bilateral acoustic neuromas are present, and its gene lies on chromosome 22. The frequency is 1:35,000. Neurofibromatosis 1 is associated with tumors primarily of astrocytes and neurons, whereas neurofibromatosis 2 is associated with tumors of the meninges and Schwann cells. There is no racial predominance. Signs may be present at birth but are activated during pregnancy, during puberty, and at menopause.

Clinical Findings

Tumors may occur anywhere in the body, including the eye. Café au lait spots (small pigmented areas of skin) tend to enlarge and darken with age. A few may occur in 5–10% of the normal population, but in neurofibromatosis 1 there are five or six such spots greater than 1.5–2 cm in diameter; axillary freckles are especially significant. Cutaneous neurofibromatosis occurs especially on the trunk and spares the palms and soles. Tumors of the lids can be isolated cutaneous neurofibromas or plexiform (rubbery "bag of worms") neurofibromas. The latter may be associated with glaucoma.

Tumors of the optic nerve, meninges (menin-

gioma), and glial cells (astrocytomas) also occur. Bilaterally thickened optic nerves are pathognomonic of neurofibromatosis 1, and many are asymptomatic (30–80%), raising the question of hamartomas or optic nerve hyperplasia. A subgroup with nerves having a thickened nerve core and a low-density perineural proliferation are often symptomatic, with proptosis and decreased visual acuity. This latter group may represent a low-grade astrocytoma or optic nerve glioma. About 70% of optic nerve gliomas present before the age of 7 years. MRI shows lengthening and kinking of the optic nerve, and bright spots in brain parenchyma can be seen on T2-weighted images. Optic nerve glioma can cause papilledema or optic atrophy. There may be Lisch nodules and enlarged corneal nerves. About 75% of patients with neurofibromatosis 2 have early posterior subcapsular lens opacities. Pigment epithelial and retinal hamartomas with optic disk gliomas also occur with increased frequency in neurofibromatosis 2.

Spinal cord neurofibromas occur frequently. The acoustic nerve is the cranial nerve most commonly involved by bilateral acoustic neuromas, resulting in the cerebellopontine angle syndrome.

Bone development is affected when the tumor involves periosteum. Pulsating exophthalmos occasionally occurs when an osseous developmental defect of the sphenoid wing of the posterior orbit is present.

Treatment & Prognosis

Visual function in optic nerve gliomas does not change much after diagnosis. Chiasmal gliomas are less aggressive in neurofibromatosis than when they occur in its absence. The risk is greatest during the early follow-up period, and survival relates to the surrounding brain involvement.

When lesions are confined to the skin, the prognosis is good. Intracranial and intraspinal lesions are usually multiple and have a poor prognosis. The disease tends to be fairly stationary, with only slow progression over long periods of time. Neurofibromas of the peripheral nerves occur also and may undergo sarcomatous degeneration (5%).

RETINOCEREBELLAR ANGIOMATOSIS (Von Hippel–Lindau Disease)

This rare disease occurs most commonly in men in the third decade but can appear at any time up to age 60. Its incidence is 1:10,000, and there is neither gender nor racial predilection. About 25% of patients show autosomal dominant inheritance. The earliest signs are dilation and tortuosity of the retinal vessels, which later develop into an angiomatous formation with hemorrhages and exudates (retinal capillary angioblastomas) (Figure 10–30). A stage of massive exudation, retinal detachment, and secondary glaucoma occurs later and will cause blindness if untreated. The disease is unilateral in 65% of cases. Patients must be followed expectantly with periodic, presymptomatic screening because in up to 25% of cases the retinal angiomatosis is associated with a similar generalized process, most often affecting the cerebellum (hemangioblastoma) and less commonly the pancreas, kidney (renal cell carcinoma), adrenal gland, and other organs. The evidence at present suggests that this is all one genetically determined disease showing autosomal dominant inheritance with variable expression.

Treatment & Prognosis

Early treatment of retinal lesions with photocoagulation, diathermy, or cryotherapy has been effective in some cases. Cerebral and cerebellar tumors have been successfully removed, but recurrences are common. MRI scanning revolutionizes follow-up of these patients, since it can be done without radiation hazard and detects presymptomatic lesions.

STURGE-WEBER SYNDROME

This uncommon nonfamilial disease with unknown inheritance is recognizable at birth by a characteristic nevus flammeus (port wine stain, or venous angioma) on one side of the face following the distribution of one or more branches of the fifth cranial nerve. There is corresponding angiomatous involvement (leptomeningeal angiodysplasia) of the meninges and brain, which causes jacksonian seizures (85%), mental retardation (60%), and cerebrocortical atrophy. Since these cortical lesions calcify, they can be seen on plain skull x-rays after infancy. Unilateral infantile glaucoma on the affected side frequently develops if there is extensive involvement of the conjunctiva with hemangioma of the episclera and anterior chamber anomalies. Lid or conjunctival involvement nearly always implies ultimate intraocular involvement and glaucoma. Forty percent of patients with a port wine stain on the face develop choroidal hemangioma on the same side. There is at least one cytogenic study reporting trisomy 22.

Treatment & Prognosis

There is no effective treatment for Sturge-Weber syndrome, though the glaucoma can be controlled in rare cases by surgery.

WYBURN-MASON SYNDROME

Wyburn-Mason syndrome is a rare disorder of multiple arteriovenous malformations, variably involving the retina, other portions of the anterior visual pathway,

the midbrain, the maxilla, and the mandible, all on the same side of the head.

Headaches and seizures are common central nervous system presenting signs. Large, tortuous, dilated vessels covering extensive areas of the retina are an important diagnostic clue and can cause cystic retinal degeneration with decreased vision. Optic atrophy without retinal lesions can also occur.

ATAXIA-TELANGIECTASIA

Ataxia-telangiectasia is an autosomal recessive disorder characterized by skin and conjunctival telangiectases, cerebellar ataxia, and recurrent sinopulmonary infections. All signs and symptoms are progressive with time, but the ataxia appears first as the child begins to walk, and the telangiectases appear between 4 and 7 years of age. Mental retardation also occurs. The recurrent infections relate to thymic deficiencies and corresponding T cell abnormalities as well as to decreased or absent immunoglobulins. Saccadic and eventual pursuit abnormalities produce a supranuclear ophthalmoplegia.

TUBEROUS SCLEROSIS
(Bourneville's Disease)

Tuberous sclerosis is characterized by the triad of adenoma sebaceum, epilepsy, and mental retardation, though 30–50% of affected individuals have normal intelligence. Adenoma sebaceum (angiofibromas) occur in 90% of patients over the age of 4 years, and the number of lesions increases with puberty. These flesh-colored papules are 1–2 mm in diameter and have a butterfly distribution on the nose and malar area; they can also occur in the subungual and periungual areas. Ashleaf-shaped hypopigmented ovals can be present on the skin even of neonates but are best seen under Wood's (ultraviolet) light.

Retinal hamartomas appear as oval or circular white areas in the peripheral fundus and characteristically have a mulberry-like appearance (Figure 10–31). Renal hamartomas occur in 80% of patients. Subependymal nodules in the periventricular areas of the brain can calcify and appear as candle wax gutterings or drippings on radiologic studies (25–30% of skull x-rays and 90% of CT scans) in patients with clinical tuberous sclerosis. MRI can show actively growing subependymal nodules. These can become astrocytomas. Seizures occur in 90% of patients, usually within the first 3 years of life.

The disease is inherited sporadically (80%) or as an autosomal dominant with low penetrance. The prevalence may be 1:9400 if patients with the incomplete form of the disease are included. Vision is generally normal, and progression of retinal hamartomas is rare. The prognosis for life relates to the degree of central nervous system involvement. In severe cases, death can occur in the second or third decade; if there is minimal central nervous system involvement, life expectancy should be normal.

CEREBROMACULAR DEGENERATION

Genetically determined (autosomal recessive) neuronal lipid storage disease of the brain may affect the neural elements of the retina as well. The clinical forms are classified by the age at onset and the enzyme deficiency. The pathologic changes are present prenatally. Clinical manifestations occur as a critical level of intraneuronal lipidosis is reached, resulting in a progressive disease with dementia, visual disturbances, and neuromotor signs. A definitive diagnosis can be established readily by conjunctival biopsy, rectal biopsy, or appendectomy showing ganglioside accumulation even before clinical signs are present.

The striking ocular finding of a cherry-red spot in the macula is seen in congenital and infantile cases. A halo occurs from loss of transparency of the ganglion cell ring of the macula, which accentuates the central red or the normal choroidal vasculature. A cherry-red spot will occur in central retinal artery occlusion, sphingolipidosis, mucolipidosis, commotio retinae, and methanol toxicity. The sphingolipidoses include

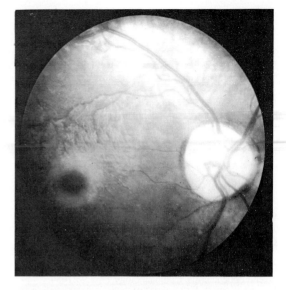

Figure 14–29. Cherry-red spot of Tay-Sachs disease in an 18-month-old child.

Niemann-Pick disease type A and type B, Tay Sachs disease, Sandhoff's disease, neuronal ceroid lipofuscinosis, and generalized gangliosidosis. Optic atrophy will occur early in Tay-Sachs disease, and the cherry-red spot can be pigmented in dark retinas (Figure 14–29).

Extraocular muscle involvement can occur in juvenile sphingolipidoses, Refsum's disease, and beta-lipoproteinemia, the latter two disorders being associated with retinitis pigmentosa.

REFERENCES

Ashworth B, Aspinall PA, Mitchell JD: Visual function in multiple sclerosis. Doc Ophthalmol 1990;73:209.

Baker RS, Epstein AD: Ocular motor abnormalities from head trauma. Surv Ophthalmol 1991;35:245.

Barondes M et al: Bilaterality of drusen. Br J Ophthalmol 1990;74:180.

Beck RW et al: A randomized, controlled trial of corticosteroids in the treatment of acute optic neuritis. N Engl J Med 1992;326:581.

Beck RW et al: Brain magnetic resonance imaging in acute optic neuritis. Arch Neurol 1993;50:841.

Beck RW et al: The effect of corticosteroids for acute optic neuritis on the subsequent development of multiple sclerosis. N Engl J Med 1993;329:1764.

Beck RW for the Optic Neuritis Study Group: Corticosteroid treatment of optic neuritis: A need to change treatment practices. Neurology 1992;42:1133.

Bever CT Jr et al: Prognosis of ocular myasthenia. Ann Neurol 1983;14:516.

Bogousslavsky J et al: Correlates of brain-stem oculomotor disorders in multiple sclerosis: Magnetic resonance imaging. Arch Neurol 1986;43:460.

Brey RL et al: Antiphospholipid antibodies and cerebral ischemia in young people. Neurology 1990;40:1190.

Brodsky MV: Congenital optic disk anomalies. Surv Ophthalmol 1994;39:89.

Brown GC, Shields JA: Tumors of the optic nerve head. Surv Ophthalmol 1985;29:239.

Burde RM: Optic disk risk factors for nonarteritic anterior ischemic optic neuropathy. Am J Ophthalmol 1993;116:759.

Celesia GG et al: Optic neuritis: A prospective study. Neurology 1990;40:919.

David NJ: Optokinetic nystagmus: A clinical review. J Clin Neurol Ophthalmol 1989;9(4):258.

De Palma P et al: The incidence of optic neuropathy in 84 patients treated with ethambutol. Metab Pediatr Syst Ophthalmol 1989;12:80.

De Potter P, Zografos L: Survival prognosis of patients with retinal artery occlusion and associated carotid artery disease. Graefes Arch Clin Exp Ophthalmol 1993;231:212.

deGroot J, Chusid JG: *Correlative Neuroanatomy,* 20th ed. Appleton & Lange, 1988.

Durelli L et al: High-dose intravenous methylprednisolone in the treatment of multiple sclerosis: Clinical-immunologic correlations. Neurology 1986;336:238.

Dutton JJ, Burde RM, Klingele TG: Autoimmune retrobulbar optic neuritis. Am J Ophthalmol 1982;94:11.

Dutton JJ: Glioma of the anterior visual pathway. Surv Ophthalmol 1994;38:427.

Elbol P, Work K: Retinal nerve fiber layer in multiple sclerosis. Acta Ophthalmol 1990;68(4):481.

Farris BK, Pickard DR: Bilateral postinfectious optic neuritis and intravenous steroid therapy in children. Ophthalmology 1990;97:339.

Garrett SN, Kearney JJ, Schiffman JS: Amiodarone optic neuropathy. J Clin Neuroophthalmol 1988;8(2):105.

Gross-Jendroska M et al: Kearns-Sayre syndrome: A case report and review. Eur J Ophthalmol 1992;2(1):15.

Guy JR et al: T-lymphocyte subpopulations in acute unilateral optic neuritis. Ophthalmology 1989;96:1054.

Guy M et al: Gadolinium-DTPA-enhanced magnetic resonance imaging in optic neuropathies. Ophthalmology 1990;97:592.

Halliday AM, McDonald WI: Visual evoked potentials. In *Clinical Neurophysiology.* Stalberg E, Young RR (editors). Butterworths, 1981.

Hardwig P, Robertson DM: Von Hippel-Lindau disease: A familial, often lethal, multisystem phakomatosis. Ophthalmology 1984;91:263.

Harrington DO, Drake MV: *The Visual Fields: Text and Atlas of Clinical Perimetry,* 6th ed. Mosby, 1990.

Hoffman HJ: How is pseudotumor cerebri diagnosed? Arch Neurol 1986;43:167.

Hopf HC, Gutmann L: Diabetic 3rd nerve palsy: Evidence for a mesencephalic lesion. Neurology 1990;40:1041.

Hoyt WF: Ophthalmoscopy of the retinal nerve fiber layer in neuro-ophthalmologic diagnosis. Aust NZ J Ophthalmol 1976;4:14.

Huber A: *Eye Signs and Symptoms in Brain Tumors,* 3rd ed. Mosby, 1976.

Imes RK, Hoyt WF: Childhood chiasmal gliomas: Update on the fate of patients in the 1969 San Francisco Study. Br J Ophthalmol 1986;70:179.

Ishibashi Y, Hori Y (editors): Tuberous sclerosis and neurofibromatosis: Epidemiology, pathophysiology, biology and management. Proceedings of the International Symposium on Neurocutaneous Syndrome. Excerpta Medica, 1990.

Jacobson D: Pupillary responses to dilute pilocarpine in preganglionic 3rd nerve disorders. Neurology 1990;40:804.

Joseph MP et al: Extracranial optic nerve decompression for traumatic optic neuropathy. Arch Ophthalmol 1990; 108:1091.

Kelman SE: The ischemic optic neuropathy decompression trial. Arch Ophthalmol 1993;111:1616.

Keltner JL et al: Visual field profile of optic neuritis: One-year follow-up in the Optic Neuritis Treatment Trial. Arch Ophthalmol 1994;112:946.

Lam BL, Weingeist TA: Corticosteroid-responsive traumatic optic neuropathy. Am J Ophthalmol 1990;109:99.

Landau K, Yasargil GM: Ocular fundus in neurofibromatosis type 2. Br J Ophthalmol 1993;77:646.

Leigh JR, Zee DS: *The Neurology of Eye Movement.* Vol 23 of *Contemporary Neurology Series.* Davis, 1983.

Lesser RL et al: Neuro-ophthalmologic manifestations of Lyme disease. Ophthalmology 1990;97:699.

Levine SR et al: Cerebrovascular and neurologic disease associated with antiphospholipid antibodies: 48 cases. Neurology 1990;40:1181.

Lindenberg R, Walsh FB, Sacks JG: *Neuropathology of Vision: An Atlas.* Lea & Febiger, 1973.

Lorenz B et al: Retrobulbar cysts in Aicardi's syndrome. Ophthalmic Paediatr Genet 1991;12(2):105.

Mackey D: Three subgroups of patients from the United Kingdom with Leber hereditary optic neuropathy. Eye 1994;8:431.

Maimone D, Reder AT: Soluble CD8 levels in the CSF and serum of patients with multiple sclerosis. Neurology 1991;41:851.

Martin N et al: Gadolinium-DTPA enhanced MR imaging in tuberous sclerosis. Neuroradiology 1990;31:492.

Masuyama Y et al: Clinical studies on the occurrence and the pathogenesis of opticociliary veins. J Clin Neuroophthalmol 1990;10:1.

McDonald WI: Optic neuritis and its significance. Clin Exp Neurol 1989;26:1.

McHenry JC, Spoor TC: Optic nerve sheath fenestration for treatment of progressive ischemic optic neuropathy. Arch Ophthalmol 1993;111:1601.

McHenry JC, Spoor TC: Spontaneous improvement of progressive anterior ischemic optic neuropathy. Arch Ophthalmol 1993;111:1602.

Newman NJ: Mitochondrial disease and the eye. Ophthalmol Clin N Am 1992;5(3):405.

Nikoskelainen E et al: Recent advances in Leber's hereditary optic neuroretinopathy. Eye 1991;5:291.

North American Symptomatic Carotid Endarterectomy Trial Collaborators: Beneficial effect of carotid endarterectomy in symptomatic patients with high-grade carotid stenosis. N Engl J Med 1991;325:445.

Nucci P, Mets MB, Gabianelli EB: Trisomy 4q with morning glory disc anomaly. Ophthalmic Paediatr Genet 1990; 2:143.

Optic Neuritis Study Group: The clinical profile of optic neuritis: Experience of the Optic Neuritis Treatment Trial. Arch Ophthalmol 1991;109:1673.

Patel U, Gupta SC: Wyburn-Mason syndrome: A case report and review of the literature. Neuroradiology 1990;31:544.

Ragge NK: Clinical and genetic patterns of neurofibromatosis 1 and 2. Br J Ophthalmol 1993;77:662.

Robb R: Idiopathic superior oblique palsies in children. J Pediatr Ophthalmol Strabismus 1990;27:66.

Rush JA et al: Optic glioma: Long-term follow-up of 85 histopathologically verified cases. Ophthalmology 1982; 89:1213.

Sadun AA: The efficacy of optic nerve sheath decompression for anterior ischemic optic neuropathy and other optic neuropathies. Am J Ophthalmol 1993;115:384.

Sadun AA: The optic neuropathy of Alzheimer's disease. Metab Pediatr Syst Ophthalmol 1989;12:64.

Sanders EA et al: Estimation of visual function after optic neuritis: A comparison of clinical tests. Br J Ophthalmol 1986;79:918.

Sebag J et al: Optic disc cupping in arteritic anterior ischemic optic neuropathy resembles glaucomatous cupping. Ophthalmology 1986;93(3):357.

Spoor TC et al: Progressive and static nonarteritic ischemic optic neuropathy treated by optic nerve sheath decompression. Ophthalmology 1993;100:306.

Spoor TC et al: Treatment of pseudotumor cerebri by primary and secondary optic nerve sheath decompression. Am J Ophthalmol 1991;112:177.

Thompson DS et al: The effects of pregnancy in multiple sclerosis: A retrospective study. Neurology 1986;36:1097.

Traccis S et al: Successful treatment of acquired pendular elliptical nystagmus in multiple sclerosis with isoniazid and base-out prisms. Neurology 1990;40:492.

Trobe JD: High-dose corticosteroid regimen retards development of multiple sclerosis in optic neuritis treatment trial. Arch Ophthalmol 1994;112:35.

Van Dorp DB, Kwee ML: Tuberous sclerosis. Ophthalmic Paediatr Genet 1990;2:95.

Vargas ME et al: Endovascular treatment of giant aneurysms which cause visual loss. Ophthalmology 1994;101:1091.

15

Ocular Disorders Associated With Systemic Diseases

M.D. Sanders, FRCP, FRCS, & Elizabeth M. Graham, FRCP, FRCOphth

Examination of the eye provides the ophthalmologist an opportunity to make a unique contribution to the diagnosis of systemic disease. Nowhere else in the body can a microcirculatory system be investigated with such precision, and nowhere else are the results of minute focal lesions so devastating. Many systemic diseases involve the eyes, and therapy demands some knowledge of the vascular, rheologic, and immunologic nature of these diseases.

VASCULAR DISEASE

NORMAL ANATOMY & PHYSIOLOGY

The blood supply to the eye is from the ophthalmic artery, which is the first branch of the internal carotid artery (see Chapter 1). The first branches of the ophthalmic artery are the central retinal artery and the long posterior ciliary arteries. The retina is perfused by retinal and choroidal vessels that provide contrasting anatomic and physiologic circulations. The retinal arteries correspond to arterioles in the systemic circulation. They function as end arteries and feed a capillary bed consisting of small capillaries (7 μm) with tight endothelial junctions. Dependent on this anatomic arrangement is the maintenance of the blood-retina barrier, and this system is autoregulated, since there are no autonomic nerve fibers. Most of the blood within the eye, however, is in the choroidal circulation, which is characterized by a high flow rate, autonomic regulation, and an anatomic arrangement with collateral branching and large capillaries (30 μm), all of which have fenestrations in juxtaposition to Bruch's membrane. Examination of the retinal vessels is facilitated by the use of red-free light and fluorescein angiography, whereas indocyanine green angiography gives further information about the choroidal vessels.

PATHOLOGIC APPEARANCES IN RETINAL VASCULAR DISEASE

Hemorrhages

Retinal hemorrhages result from diapedeses from veins or capillaries, and the morphologic appearances depend upon the size, site, and extent of damage to the vessel (Figure 15–1). Hemorrhages may be caused by any condition that alters the integrity of the endothelial cells. They usually indicate some abnormality of the retinal vascular system, and systemic factors should be considered in relation to (1) vessel wall disease (eg, hypertension, diabetes), (2) blood disorders (eg, leukemia, polycythemia), and (3) reduced perfusion (eg, carotid cavernous fistula, acute blood loss).

A. Preretinal Hemorrhages: These result from damage to the superficial disk or retinal vessels and are usually large, producing a gravity-dependent fluid level.

B. Linear Hemorrhages: These usually small

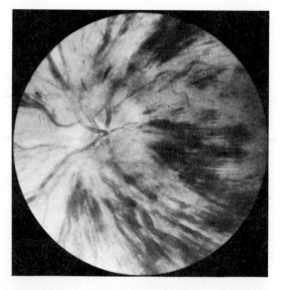

Figure 15–1. Flame-shaped retinal hemorrhages in the nerve fiber layer radiate out from the optic disk. Three days before the photograph was taken, the patient experienced sudden loss of vision, which left him with light perception only.

hemorrhages lie in the superficial nerve fiber layers and hence have a characteristic linear appearance, conforming to the alignment of nerve fibers in any particular area of the fundus.

C. Punctate Hemorrhages: Hemorrhages situated deeper in the substance of the retina are punctate and derived from capillaries and smaller venules. The circular appearance is related to the anatomic arrangement of structures in the retina.

D. Subretinal Hemorrhages: These hemorrhages are less common because normally there are no blood vessels between the retina and the choroid. Such hemorrhages are large and red, with a well-defined margin and no fluid level. They are seen in relation to the disk and in any condition where abnormal vessels pass from the choroidal circulation into the retina.

E. Hemorrhages Under the Pigment Epithelium: Hemorrhages situated under the pigment epithelium are usually dark and large, so that they must be differentiated from choroidal melanomas and hemangiomas.

F. White Central Hemorrhages (Roth's Spots): Superficial retinal hemorrhages with pale or white centers are not pathognomonic of any disease process but may arise in a variety of circumstances: (1) retinal infarction (cotton wool spot) with surrounding hemorrhage; (2) retinal hemorrhage in combination with extravasation of white corpuscles (eg, leukemia); and (3) retinal hemorrhage with central resolution.

Acute Ocular Ischemia

A. Optic Disk Infarction (Ischemic Optic Neuropathy): Impairment of the blood supply to the optic disk produces sudden visual loss, usually with an altitudinal field defect and pallid swelling of the optic disk (see p 269). The primary abnormality is complete or partial interruption of the choroidal blood supply to the disk, while the retinal capillaries on the surface of the disk appear dilated. Fluorescein angiography confirms the circulatory alterations (Figure 15–2). Pathologic studies show infarction of the retrolaminar region of the optic nerve. The explanation for the vulnerability of the short posterior ciliary vessels supplying this region is unknown. Optic disk infarction is often caused by giant cell arteritis in old age and by hypertension and arteriosclerotic disease in middle age. Small optic disks are particularly prone to infarction.

Investigations should include serum lipids, blood glucose, serologic tests for syphilis, and assessment of blood viscosity by hemoglobin, hematocrit, and fibrinogen determinations. Giant cell arteritis merits measurement of the erythrocyte sedimentation rate and temporal artery biopsy on an urgent basis. Corticosteroids are essential in the management of giant cell arteritis, but the results of use of these drugs are equivocal in nonarteritic disorders. Surgical decompression of the optic nerve sheath has been advocated in the uncommon progressive form of nonarteritic ischemic optic neuropathy. The results, however, have failed to show any significant benefit.

B. Choroidal Infarction: This is extremely rare, though certain clinical appearances have been attributed to ciliary vessel occlusion. These include small pale areas in the equatorial region that resolve to leave mottled pigmentary areas (Elschnig's spots) due to necrosis of the pigment epithelium. Larger infarcts may occur and may be triangular or linear.

C. Retinal Infarction: The funduscopic appearance of arteriolar occlusion depends on the size of the vessel occluded, the duration of occlusion, and the time course. Occlusion of major arterioles produces a total, hemispheric, or segmental pallid swelling of the retina. Occlusion of a precapillary retinal arteriole produces the pathognomonic appearance of a cotton wool spot (Figure 15–3). This consists of a pale, slightly elevated swelling usually one-fourth to one-half the size of the optic disk. Pathologic examination shows distention of neurons, with cytoid bodies (Figure 15–4); electron microscopy shows the accumulation of axoplasm and organelles. Occlusion of arterioles, whether due to intrinsic vessel wall disease or to intramural factors, may produce these pathognomonic signs.

D. Transient Retinal Ischemia (Amaurosis Fugax): Transient episodes of monocular visual loss lasting 5–10 minutes are characteristic of amaurosis fugax. Patients often describe a curtain coming down from above or across their vision, usually with complete return of vision within seconds or minutes. Paresthesias in the contralateral limbs localize the disorder to the carotid artery and suggest involvement of the ophthalmic artery and middle cerebral artery. It is important for the ophthalmologist to auscultate the carotid for a systolic bruit and to search the fundus for emboli. Amaurosis fugax is most commonly due to retinal emboli, of which there are three main types.

1. Cholesterol emboli–These so-called Hollenhorst plaques usually arise from an atheromatous plaque in the carotid artery and consist of cholesterol and fibrin. They lodge at the bifurcation of retinal arterioles, are refractile, and may appear larger than the vessel that contains them (Figure 15–5).

2. Calcific emboli–Originating from damaged cardiac valves, these emboli lodge within the arteriole, producing complete occlusion and infarction of the distal retina. Calcific emboli are solid and calcified and occur in younger patients with a variety of cardiac lesions.

3. Platelet-fibrin emboli–Most cases of amaurosis fugax are probably due to the transit of platelet aggregates through the retinal and choroidal circulations. The emboli are usually broken up as they traverse the retinal circulation and hence are rarely seen, though occasionally they produce retinal infarction. Arising from abnormalities of the heart or great vessels, they may be reduced by drugs that reduce platelet coagulability (eg, aspirin).

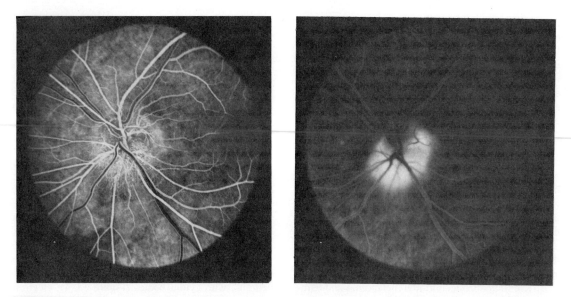

Figure 15–2. Ischemic optic neuropathy. Sudden visual loss in a 48-year-old man produced a complete inferior altitudinal field loss. *Left:* Fluorescein angiography shows impaired filling of the upper part of the disk with dilation of retinal capillaries at the lower part of the disk. *Right:* Photograph 10 minutes after injection shows leakage of dye mainly at the lower part of the disk.

Patients with retinal emboli who are under 40 years of age should undergo cardiac studies (24-hour electrocardiographic recording, echocardiography) to exclude atrial fibrillation, mitral valve prolapse, or subacute infective endocarditis. In older patients, carotid disease should be suspected.

There are several other causes of amaurosis fugax, including factors that induce temporary reduction in ocular perfusion, eg, arterial disease, cardiac disorders, hematologic disorders, and, rarely, elevation of intraocular pressure (Table 15–1).

Central Retinal Vein Occlusion (Figure 15–6)

Central retinal vein occlusion is an important cause of visual morbidity in elderly people, particularly those with hypertension or glaucoma.

Fundus examination shows dilated tortuous veins

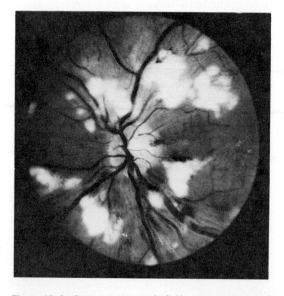
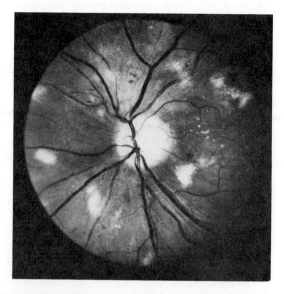

Figure 15–3. Cotton wool spots. *Left:* Numerous cotton wool spots are seen in the posterior pole in a patient with accelerated hypertension. *Right:* One month after hypotensive treatment. Note resolution of the infarcts.

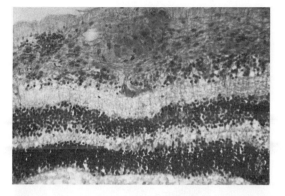

Figure 15–4. Cotton wool spot. Histologic examination shows cytoid bodies and distended neurons in the superficial retinal layers. Deeper retinal layers are normal. (Courtesy of Professor N Ashton.)

Table 15–1. Causes of amaurosis fugax.

Retinal emboli	Cholesterol emboli Calcific emboli Platelet-fibrin emboli

Arterial disease	Carotid artery stenosis
	Carotid artery ulceration
	  Bifurcation
	  Carotid siphon

Cardiac disease	Dysrhythmias (eg, atrial fibrillation)
	Valvular disease (eg, mitral leaflet
	  prolapse)
	Left ventricular aneurysm or mural
	  thrombus secondary to myocardial
	  infarction

Hematologic disease	Anemia Polycythemia Macroglobulinemia Sickle cell disease

Other	Mechanical compression of vertebral
	  or carotid arteries
	Hypertensive episode
	Hypotensive episode
	  Drugs
	  Spontaneous (eg, diabetes mellitus,
	    Addison's disease)
	Arteritis
	Raised intraocular pressure

with retinal and macular edema, hemorrhages all over the posterior pole, and cotton wool spots. The arterioles are usually attenuated, indicating generalized microvascular disease.

The prognosis for vision is poor. Fluorescein angiography demonstrates two types of response: a nonischemic type, with dilation of retinal vessels and edema; and an ischemic type, with large areas of capillary nonperfusion or evidence of retinal or anterior segment neovascularization. In 93% of ischemic and 50% of nonischemic central retinal vein occlusions, the ultimate visual acuity is less than 20/200.

Central retinal vein occlusion has an increased incidence in certain systemic conditions such as diabetes mellitus, hypertension, collagen vascular diseases, and hyperviscosity syndromes (eg, Waldenström's macroglobulinemia, angioimmunoblastic lymphadenopathy). However, the prevalence of cerebrovascular or cardiovascular disease is not increased

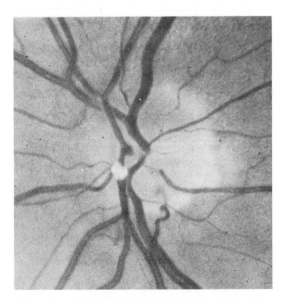

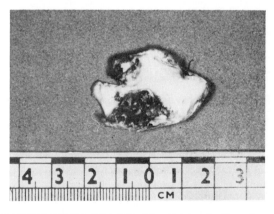

Figure 15–5. Cholesterol embolus (Hollenhorst plaque). *Left:* A cholesterol embolus at the optic disk, which is refractile and appears larger than the vessel that contains it. A collateral vessel is seen at the lower border of the disk. *Right:* Surgical specimen from a patient with a similar embolus shows an atheromatous ulcer at the bifurcation of the common carotid artery.

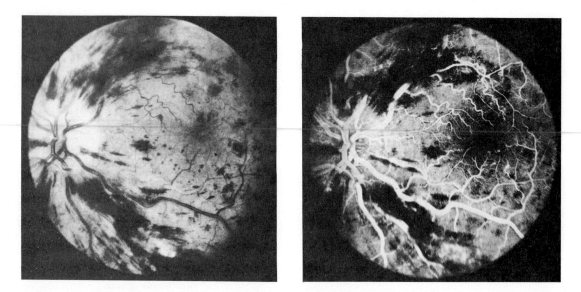

Figure 15–6. Central retinal vein occlusion. **Left:** Photograph shows linear hemorrhages in the nerve fiber layer and punctate hemorrhages in the deeper retinal layers. **Right:** Fluorescein angiogram shows dilation of the veins.

compared to the general population. Investigations include measurement of serum lipids, plasma proteins, plasma glucose, and assessment of blood viscosity by hemoglobin, hematocrit, and fibrinogen estimations. In young patients, protein C, protein S, and antithrombin III levels should be measured to exclude abnormalities of the thrombolytic system. If hypertension is present, simple renal function tests, including urea and electrolytes, estimation of creatinine clearance, microscopic examination of the urine, and renal ultrasound are indicated.

Treatment of retinal vein occlusion is unsatisfactory. Trials with anticoagulants and fibrinolytic agents have not been successful. In ischemic central retinal vein occlusion, panretinal laser photocoagulation is effective in preventing and treating secondary neovascular glaucoma.

Occasionally, central retinal vein occlusion occurs in young people and may be associated with cells in the vitreous. Rheologic investigations are usually negative, and the prognosis for vision is good.

Retinal Branch Vein Occlusion (Figure 15–7)

Occlusion of a branch vein should be viewed as part of the spectrum of central retinal vein occlusion. Investigations are similar in the two conditions, but arterial disease—particularly hypertension—is common. Branch retinal vein occlusion occurs more frequently in the superotemporal and inferotemporal regions and particularly at sites where arteries cross over veins, and only rarely where veins cross over arteries.

The value of laser treatment in the management of

the complications of branch retinal vein occlusion is discussed in Chapters 10 and 24.

ATHEROSCLEROSIS & ARTERIOSCLEROSIS

The process of atherosclerosis occurs in larger arteries and is due to fatty infiltration of a patchy nature occurring in the intima and associated with fibrosis. Involvement of smaller vessels (ie, < 300 μm) by diffuse fibrosis and hyalinization is termed arteriosclerosis. The retinal vessels beyond the disk are less than 30 μm; therefore, involvement of the retinal arterioles should be termed arteriosclerosis, whereas involvement of the central retinal artery is properly termed atherosclerosis.

Atherosclerosis is a progressive change developing in the second decade, with lipid streaks in larger vessels, progressing to a fibrous plaque in the third decade. In the fourth and fifth decades, ulceration, hemorrhages, and thrombosis occur, and the lesion may be calcified. Destruction of the elastic and muscular elements of the media produces ectasia and rupture of the large vessels, though in smaller vessels obstruction is usually seen. The clinical results of atherosclerosis are seen several decades after the onset of the process. Factors contributing to atheroma include hyperlipidemia, hypertension, and obesity.

Arteriosclerosis is characterized by an enhanced light reflection, focal attenuation, and irregularity of caliber. These signs may also be seen in the arterioles of normotensive individuals in middle age. In elderly individuals with arteriosclerosis and associated mild

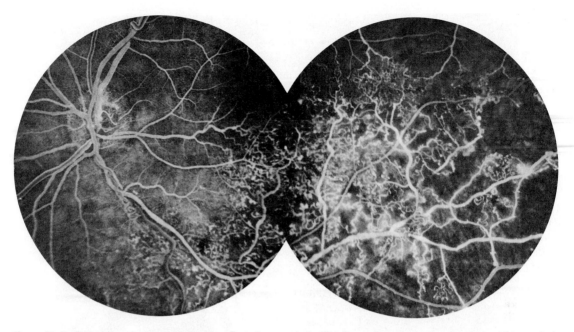

Figure 15–7. Retinal branch vein occlusion. The affected segment of retina shows changes of reduced perfusion. This results in irregularity of the arterioles and veins, areas of capillary closure, and dilated capillaries with microaneurysms.

hypertension, it is difficult to differentiate the changes of arteriosclerosis from those due to hypertension.

Appearance of Retinal Vessels

A normal arteriolar wall is transparent, so that what is actually seen is the column of blood within the vessel. A thin, central light reflection in the center of the blood column appears as a yellow refractile line about one-fifth the width of the column. As the walls of the arterioles become infiltrated with lipids and cholesterol, the vessels become sclerotic. As this process continues, the vessel wall gradually loses its transparency and becomes visible; the blood column appears wider than normal, and the thin light reflection becomes broader. The grayish yellow fat products in the vessel wall blend with the red of the blood column to produce a typical "copper wire" appearance. This indicates moderate arteriosclerosis. As sclerosis proceeds, the blood column-vessel wall light reflection resembles "silver wire," which indicates severe arteriosclerosis; at times, even occlusion of an arteriolar branch may occur.

Red-free light (a white light with a green filter) allows details of hemorrhages, focal irregularity of blood vessels, and nerve fibers to be seen more clearly (Figure 15–8).

HYPERTENSIVE RETINOPATHY

Wagener and Keith in 1939 classified patients with hypertensive retinopathy into four groups (Figures 15–9 to 15–12). Stages I and II were restricted to arteriolar changes with attenuation and an increased light reflection ("copper" or "silver" wiring). More emphasis has been placed on stages III and IV, which include cotton wool spots, hard exudates, hemorrhages, and extensive microvascular changes. Stage IV is differentiated by the additional feature of edema of the optic disk.

The appearance of the fundus in hypertensive retinopathy is determined by the degree of elevation of the blood pressure and the state of the retinal arterioles. Thus, in young patients with accelerated hypertension, an extensive retinopathy is seen, with hemorrhages, retinal infarcts (cotton wool spots), choroidal infarcts (Elschnig's spots), and occasionally serous detachment of the retina (Figure 15–13). Severe disk edema is a prominent feature. Vision may be impaired but is restored if blood pressure is reduced with caution.

In contrast, elderly patients with arteriosclerotic vessels are unable to respond in this manner, and their vessels are thus protected by the arteriosclerosis. It is for this reason that elderly patients seldom exhibit florid hypertensive retinopathy (Figure 15–14).

Fluorescein angiography has made possible accurate documentation of these microcirculatory changes. In young patients with hypertension, arteriolar attenuation and occlusion are seen, and capillary nonperfusion can be verified in relation to a cotton wool spot, which is surrounded by abnormal dilated capillaries and microaneurysms with increased permeability on fluorescein angiography.

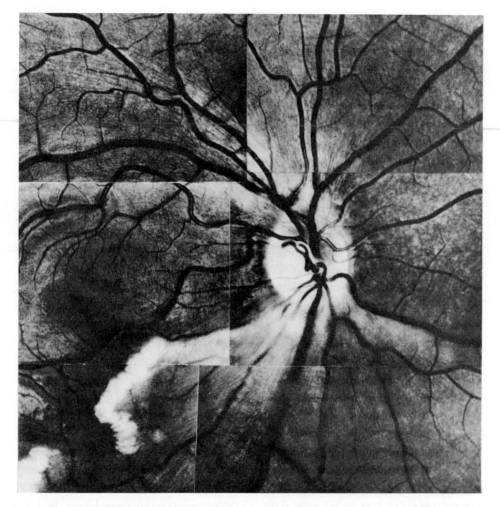

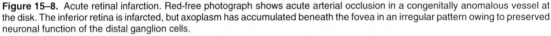

Figure 15–8. Acute retinal infarction. Red-free photograph shows acute arterial occlusion in a congenitally anomalous vessel at the disk. The inferior retina is infarcted, but axoplasm has accumulated beneath the fovea in an irregular pattern owing to preserved neuronal function of the distal ganglion cells.

Resolution of the cotton wool spots and the arteriolar changes occurs with successful hypotensive therapy. In elderly patients, the underlying arteriosclerotic changes are irreversible.

Other Forms of Hypertensive Retinopathy

A severe retinopathy may be seen in advanced renal disease, in patients with pheochromocytoma, and in preeclampsia-eclampsia. All such patients should receive a complete medical workup to establish the nature of the hypertension.

CHRONIC OCULAR ISCHEMIA

Reduction in the retinal arteriovenous pressure gradient may produce acute signs of ocular ischemia (see preceding pages) or the less frequently recognized chronic changes.

Carotid Occlusive Disease

Carotid occlusive disease usually presents in middle-aged and elderly patients and is due to involvement of both the carotid artery and its smaller branches. Contributory factors include hypertension, smoking, and hyperlipidemia.

In anterior segment ischemia, patients develop iritis, intraocular pressure changes, and pupillary abnormalities. In retinal ischemia (Figure 15–15A), patients show evidence of capillary dilation and hemorrhages, capillary occlusion, new vessels at the optic disk, and cotton wool patches.

Carotid Cavernous Fistula

Carotid cavernous fistula results from a communication between the carotid artery or its branches and

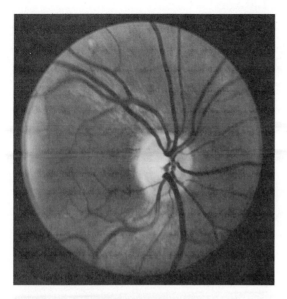

Figure 15–9. Keith-Wagener retinopathy stage I. Minimal vascular changes; a nearly normal fundus.

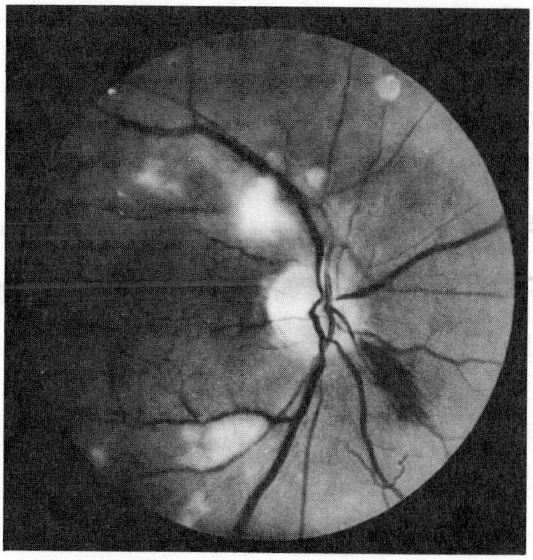

Figure 15–11. Keith-Wagener retinopathy stage III. Marked attenuation of retinal arterioles is apparent, with numerous microinfarcts and a large retinal hemorrhage.

the cavernous sinus, producing characteristic vascular signs. Direct carotid fistulas are usually acute, florid, and posttraumatic, whereas fistulas from dural vessels are usually chronic, mild, and not associated with trauma. Clinical features include elevated intraocular pressure, dilated conjunctival vessels, dilated retinal vessels with hemorrhages and fluorescein leakage

(Figure 15–15B), ophthalmoplegia (usually lateral rectus), and bruit. CT and MRI show thickened ocular muscles and a dilated superior ophthalmic vein. The condition must be differentiated from thyroid eye disease, and interventional radiology is the ultimate diagnostic and therapeutic resource.

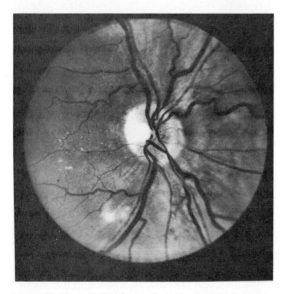

Figure 15–10. Keith-Wagener retinopathy stage II. There is irregularity of caliber of the arterioles and focal attenuation. Signs of retinal vascular disease include hard exudates at the macula, a cotton wool patch below the macula, and grooves in the nerve fiber layer beneath the disk, suggesting previous microinfarcts.

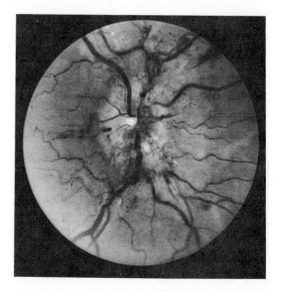

Figure 15–12. Keith-Wagener retinopathy stage IV. This may include the same retinal changes as stage III, but in addition there is disk swelling.

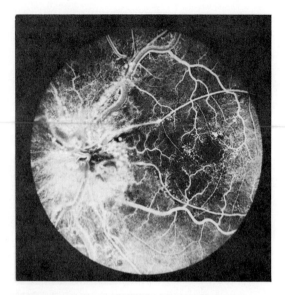

Figure 15–13. Accelerated hypertension. Fluorescein angiogram in a young man showing arteriolar constriction, dilation of capillaries with microaneurysms, and areas of closure. Marked disk edema is present.

BENIGN INTRACRANIAL HYPERTENSION (Pseudotumor Cerebri)

Benign intracranial hypertension is raised intracranial pressure without other cerebrospinal fluid abnormalities and with normal radiologic studies. Patients

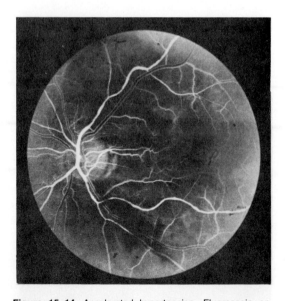

Figure 15–14. Accelerated hypertension. Fluorescein angiogram in an elderly woman showing marked arteriolar constriction and irregularity but few signs of florid retinopathy.

A

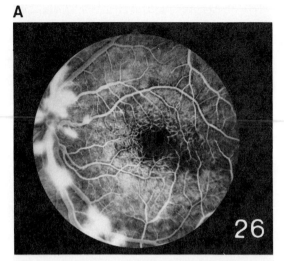

B

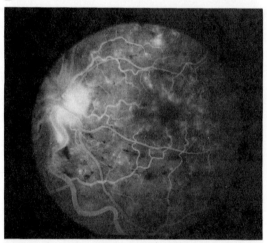

Figure 15–15. **A:** Fluorescein angiography of left fundus in a patient with chronic ocular ischemia secondary to Takayasu's disease. Note capillary dilation, leakage of dye, retinal hemorrhages, cotton-wool spots, and neovascularization of the optic nerve head. **B:** Fluorescein angiography, showing leakage at optic disk and macula in a patient with chronic ocular ischemia secondary to dural arteriovenous fistula.

present with headache, tinnitus, and dizziness; blurred vision, and diplopia are the ophthalmologic features. Etiologic factors include (1) drug therapy, particularly oral contraceptives, nalidixic acid, tetracyclines, sulfonamides, vitamin A, and prolonged steroid therapy or steroid withdrawal in children; (2) endocrine abnormalities; and (3) blood dyscrasias. In many cases there is no obvious cause; in this (idiopathic) group, the patients are usually young overweight women with irregular menstrual cycles. Benign intracranial hypertension is very rare in men.

The cause of the increased intracranial pressure is unknown, though diminished absorption of cerebrospinal fluid due to impaired venous sinus drainage is suspected.

On examination, visual fields are initially normal apart from enlarged blind spots due to gross papilledema. Generalized field constriction and inferonasal and arcuate defects occur in advanced cases. Cerebrospinal fluid pressure is raised. MRI shows distended nerve sheaths, an empty sella, and absence of a mass lesion. MR angiography complements the examination and detects any venous sinus occlusion. The aims of treatment are to reduce spinal fluid pressure and prevent permanent visual loss associated with optic atrophy, which occurs in up to 50% of patients. Treatment includes strict diet, oral acetazolamide, optic nerve sheath decompression, and lumboperitoneal shunt procedures. Optic nerve sheath decompression functions either as a fistula or by producing subarachnoid fibrous tissue in the nerve sheath and thus protects the disk from the raised sheath pressure. This procedure is relatively free of side effects and complications.

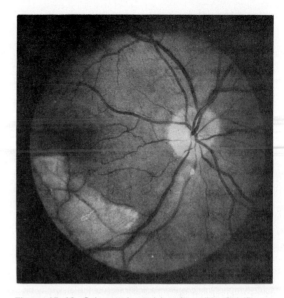

Figure 15–16. Subacute bacterial endocarditis. Calcific embolus impacted in arteriole below the disk, producing a distal area of retinal infarction.

SUBACUTE INFECTIVE ENDOCARDITIS

Inflammatory changes on the cardiac valves may produce multiple embolization with frequent ocular manifestations that range from retinal and choroidal infarction to a mild infective vitritis. The emboli may arise from vegetations on the cardiac valves and may be composed of platelet and fibrinogen aggregates or calcified endocardial vegetations (Figure 15–16).

HEMATOLOGIC & LYMPHATIC DISORDERS

LEUKEMIA

The ocular changes of leukemia occur primarily in those structures with a good blood supply, including the retina, the choroid, and the optic disk (Figure 15–17). Changes are most common in the acute leukemias, where hemorrhages are seen in the nerve fiber and preretinal layers.

HYPERVISCOSITY SYNDROMES

Increased viscosity results in a reduced flow of blood through the eye. This produces a characteristic dilation of the retinal arteries and veins, hemorrhages, microaneurysms, and areas of capillary closure (Fig-

ure 15–18). Polycythemia, either primary or secondary, may produce a hyperviscosity syndrome; the other main causes are macroglobulinemia and multiple myeloma. Reduction of the abnormalities producing hyperviscosity can reverse the retinal changes.

SICKLE CELL DISEASE

Sickle cell hemoglobinopathies are heritable disorders in which the normal adult hemoglobin is replaced by sickle hemoglobin in the red cell. This causes "sickle-shaped" deformity of the red cell on deoxygenation.

Ocular abnormalities include conjunctival changes, with "comma-shaped capillaries," and retinal changes, including arterial occlusions and peripheral capillary closure which leads to new vessel formation, particularly a sea fan pattern. Retinal detachment may develop. Laser therapy is rarely needed, since the complexes fibrose and reperfusion can occur.

NEOPLASTIC DISEASE
(Figure 15–19)

Neoplastic disease may involve the eye and optic pathways by direct spread, by metastases, or by immunologic mechanisms.

The consequences of metastatic spread depend upon the size and site of the metastatic tumor and the site of the primary lesion. The most frequent primary tumor metastasizing to the eye is carcinoma of the breast in

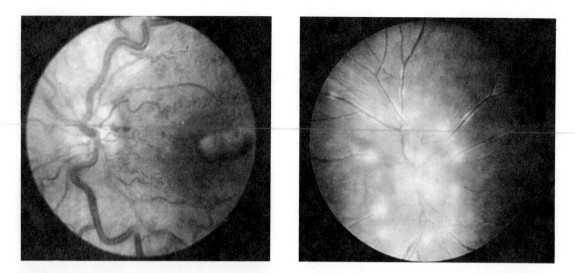

Figure 15–17. *Left:* Retinal changes in chronic myeloid leukemia, where dilated veins and hemorrhages may be seen. *Right:* In acute lymphoblastic leukemia, infiltration of the disk may be seen.

women and bronchial carcinoma in men. Choroidal metastases probably represent the commonest choroidal neoplasm. Visual loss may occur from non-metastatic disease with consequent retinal degeneration. The syndromes are called cancer-associated retinopathy, melanoma-associated retinopathy, both associated with specific retinal autoantibody, and diffuse uveal melanocytic proliferation.

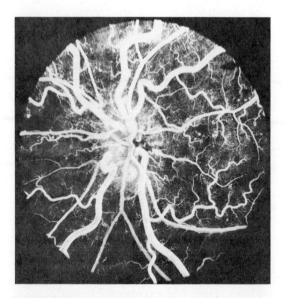

Figure 15–18. Hyperviscosity syndrome. Dilated arteries and veins, with hemorrhages and microaneurysms in a patient with hyperviscosity due to elevated IgM levels.

METABOLIC DISORDERS

DIABETES MELLITUS

Diabetes mellitus is a complex metabolic disorder that also involves the small blood vessels, often causing widespread damage to tissues, including the eyes.

The ocular complications occur approximately 20 years after onset despite apparently adequate diabetic control. Improved treatment measures (eg, improved insulins, antibiotics) that have lengthened the life span of diabetics have actually resulted in a marked increase in the incidence of retinopathy and other ocular complications. The visual outlook for adult (maturity-onset) diabetics is considerably better than for juvenile diabetics.

The possibility of diabetes should be considered in all patients with unexplained retinopathy, cataract, extraocular muscle palsy, optic neuropathy, or sudden changes in refractive error. Absence of glycosuria or a normal fasting blood glucose level does not exclude a diagnosis of diabetes.

Diabetic Retinopathy
(Figures 15–20 to 15–23)

Diabetic retinopathy is a common cause of blindness and now accounts for almost one-fourth of blind registrations in the western world.

The presence and degree of retinopathy seem to be more closely related to the duration of the disease than

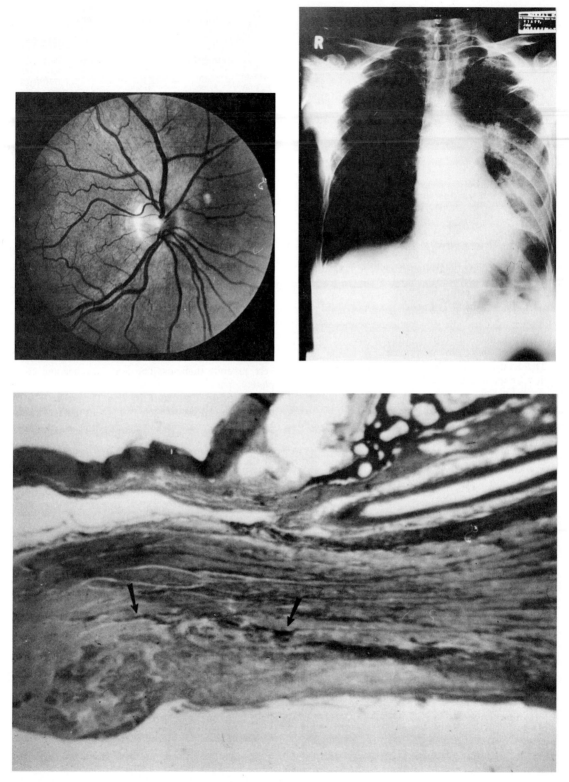

Figure 15–19. Neoplastic disease. ***Top left:*** Normal fundus of a patient with rapid visual loss in his only eye. ***Top right:*** Chest x-ray showed left lower lobe consolidation and a hilar mass. ***Bottom:*** Carcinoma of the bronchus was confirmed at autopsy, and metastasis was found in the optic nerve in the region of the canal (arrows).

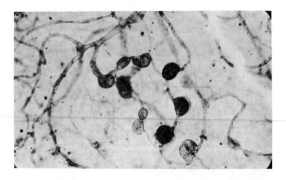

Figure 15–20. Diabetic retinopathy stage I. Trypsin-digested whole mount showing microaneurysms of the retinal capillaries.

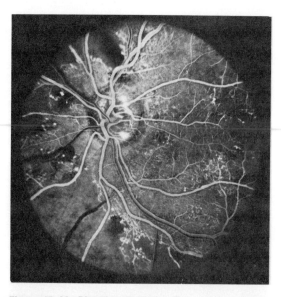

Figure 15–22. Diabetic retinopathy. Fluorescein angiogram shows florid retinopathy of diabetes with extensive areas of capillary closure, dilated capillaries with microaneurysms, and early new vessel formation at the optic disk.

to its severity. Good diabetes control retards the development of retinopathy and other diabetic complications.

The juvenile diabetic develops a severe form of retinopathy within 20 years in 60–75% of cases even if under good control. The retinopathy is usually proliferative. In older diabetic patients, retinopathy is more often nonproliferative, with the risk of severe central visual loss from maculopathy.

The details of characteristics and treatment of diabetic retinopathy are presented in Chapter 10.

Lens Changes

A. True Diabetic Cataract (Rare): Bilateral cataracts occasionally occur with a rapid onset in severe juvenile diabetes. The lens may become completely opaque in several weeks.

B. Senile Cataract in the Diabetic (Common): Typical senile nuclear sclerosis, posterior subcapsular changes, and cortical opacities occur earlier and more frequently in diabetics.

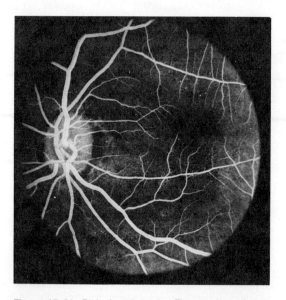

Figure 15–21. Diabetic retinopathy. Fluorescein angiogram shows earliest stage with microaneurysm in the macular region.

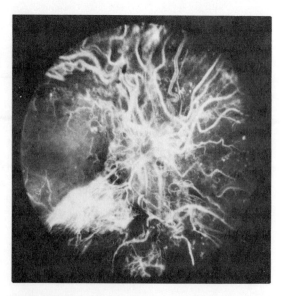

Figure 15–23. Proliferative diabetic retinopathy. Fluorescein angiogram shows extensive growth of vessels into the vitreous with marked fluorescein leakage.

C. Sudden Changes in the Refraction of the Lens: Especially when diabetes is not well controlled, changes in blood glucose levels cause changes in refractive power by as much as 3 or 4 diopters of hyperopia or myopia. This results in blurred vision. Such changes do not occur when the disease is well controlled.

Iris Changes

Glycogen infiltration of the pigment epithelium and sphincter and dilator muscles of the iris may cause diminished pupillary responses. The reflexes may also be altered by the autonomic neuropathy of diabetes.

Rubeosis iridis is a serious complication of the retinal ischemia that is also the stimulus to retinal neovascularization in severe diabetic retinopathy. Numerous small intertwining blood vessels develop on the anterior surface of the iris. Spontaneous hyphema may occur. The formation of peripheral anterior synechiae is aided by the vascularization of anterior chamber structures, eventually blocking aqueous outflow sufficiently to cause secondary glaucoma.

Extraocular Muscle Palsy
(Figure 15–24)

This common occurrence in diabetes is manifested by a sudden onset of diplopia caused by paresis of an extraocular muscle. This may be the presenting sign and is due to infarction of the nerve. When the third nerve is involved, pain may be a prominent symptom. Differentiation from a posterior communicating aneurysm is important; in diabetic third nerve palsy, the pupil is usually spared. Recovery of ocular motor function usually occurs within a year. The fourth and sixth nerves may be similarly involved.

Optic Neuropathy

Visual loss is usually due to infarction of the optic disk or nerve. A characteristic telangiectatic pattern is visible at the optic disk in some younger diabetics with sudden visual loss.

ENDOCRINE DISEASES

Disturbances of the endocrine glands have a number of important ocular manifestations. By far the most important of these are due to disturbances of the thyroid gland, though parathyroid and pituitary abnormalities also produce significant ocular changes.

THYROID GLAND DISORDERS

1. GRAVES' DISEASE

The general term Graves' disease has been used to denote hyperthyroidism due to an autoimmune process. Patients with the eye signs of Graves' disease but without clinical evidence of hyperthyroidism are referred to as having ophthalmic Graves' disease. Apart from signs of hyperthyroidism, patients may have pretibial myxedema and clubbing of the fingers, and when these signs occur in combination with the ocular signs, the condition is termed thyroid acropachy.

Various laboratory tests are used in the diagnosis of thyroid disease (Table 15–2).

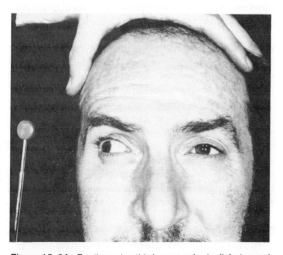

Figure 15–24. Pupil-sparing third nerve palsy in diabetes mellitus. Sudden painful ophthalmoplegia, left ptosis, failure of adduction, and normal pupillary responses.

Table 15–2. Thyroid function tests.

	Hyper-thyroid	Hypo-thyroid	Comments
Plasma T_4	+	−	
T_3 resin uptake	−	+	Thyopac technique. Other tests may vary.
Free thyroxine index	+	−	
Plasma TSH levels	−	+	In pituitary hypothyroidism, TSH is reduced.
Autoantibodies	May be present	May be present (Hashimoto's)	

Clinical Findings

Patients may present with nonspecific complaints such as dryness of the eyes, discomfort, or prominence of the eyes. The American Thyroid Association has graded the ocular signs in order of increasing severity from 0 (no signs or symptoms) to 6 (sight loss due to optic nerve involvement).

Class	Signs
0	No signs or symptoms
1	Only signs, which include upper lid retraction, with or without lid lag, or proptosis to 22 mm. No symptoms.
2	Soft tissue involvement
3	Proptosis > 22 mm
4	Extraocular muscle involvement
5	Corneal involvement
6	Sight loss due to optic nerve involvement

Lid retraction is almost pathognomonic of thyroid disease, particularly when associated with exophthalmos. Lid retraction may be unilateral or bilateral and involve the upper and lower lids. It is often accompanied by restrictive myopathy, initially involving the inferior rectus and resulting in impaired elevation of the eyes. The pathogenesis of lid retraction is diverse. Hyperstimulation of the sympathetic nervous system has long been considered a prime element. Reversal of retraction by topical guanethidine eye drops* supports this concept. Direct inflammatory infiltration of the levator muscle is also believed to be a factor in some instances of lid retraction. Restrictive myopathy of the inferior rectus muscle can cause lid retraction from the increased stimulation of the levator on attempted upgaze.

A. Exophthalmos: (Figure 15–25.) The degree of exophthalmos may be extremely variable. Measurements using the Hertel or Krahn exophthalmometer range from minimal (20 mm) to excessive (28 mm or more). The condition is usually asymmetric and may be unilateral, and it is important clinically to assess the resistance to manual retropulsion of the globe. The increase in orbital contents that produces the exophthalmos is largely due to an increase in the bulk of the ocular muscles. Visualization of the ocular muscles by CT scan (Figure 15–25) can differentiate exophthalmos from an orbital tumor. In some cases, thickening of the ocular muscles may be restricted to certain muscles only (eg, medial or inferior rectus muscles).

B. Ophthalmoplegia: This is seen more commonly in ophthalmic Graves' disease, which usually affects older people and may be grossly asymmetric. Limitation of elevation is the most frequent finding,

and this is mainly due to adhesions between the inferior rectus and inferior oblique muscles. Confirmation may be gained by measuring the intraocular pressure on elevation, when a substantial increase in the intraocular pressure suggests tethering. Often there is mild limitation of ocular movements in all positions of gaze. Patients complain of diplopia, which may be relieved by corticosteroid treatment, may spontaneously return to normal, or, if it remains static for 6–12 months, can frequently be relieved by operation on one or more extraocular muscles.

C. Retinal and Optic Nerve Changes: Compression of the globe by the orbital contents may produce elevation of the intraocular pressure and retinal or choroidal striae. The optic disk may become swollen and progress to visual loss from optic atrophy. Optic neuropathy associated with Graves' disease occasionally occurs as a result of compression and ischemia of the optic nerve as it traverses the tense orbit, particularly at the orbital apex.

D. Corneal Changes: In some patients, a superior limbic keratoconjunctivitis may be seen, though this is not specific for thyroid disease. In severe exophthalmos, corneal exposure and ulceration may occur.

Pathogenesis of the Ocular Signs

The main feature is gross distention of the ocular muscles due to the deposition of mucopolysaccharides. The mucopolysaccharides are strongly hygroscopic, which accounts for the increased water content of the orbits.

The pathogenesis of Graves' disease remains unknown, though an immunologic disorder involving both cellular and humoral elements has been implicated. Long-acting thyroid stimulator (LATS) is unlikely to be of significance in humans, because it is not always found in patients with ocular signs. There has, however, been good correlation between hyperthyroidism and human-specific thyroid stimulator, previously known as LATS protector, although this correlation is not seen in patients with Graves' disease. Thyroid autoantibodies against thyroglobulin and the microsome fraction of thyroid cells are frequently found in Hashimoto's disease and less often in Graves' disease. There are now thought to be two pathogenetic components to Graves' disease: (1) immune complexes of thyroglobulin-antithyroglobulin bind to extraocular muscles and produce a myositis; and (2) exophthalmos-producing substance acts with ophthalmic immunoglobulins to displace thyroid-stimulating hormones from the retro-orbital membranes, which results in the increase of retro-orbital fat.

Treatment

A. Medical Treatment: Medical treatment includes adequate control of the hyperthyroidism as a primary measure. However, thyroid ophthalmopathy

---

*Not commercially available in the USA. Available under protocol in Canada as Ismelin (guanethidine monosulfate 5%) Eye Drops (Ciba).

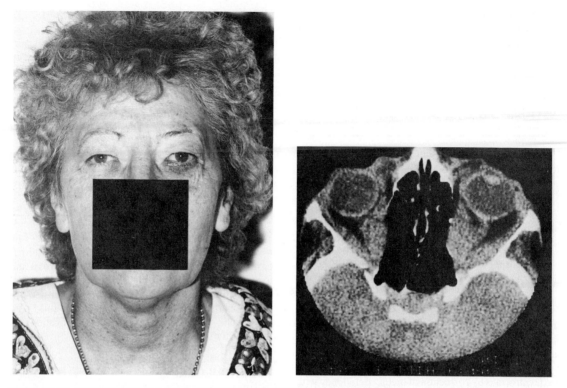

Figure 15–25. Thyroid ophthalmopathy. *Left:* Proptosis, visual loss, and ophthalmoplegia occurred in this elderly woman with a history of thyroid disease. *Right:* CT scans showed gross thickening of the ocular muscles, particularly in relation to the orbital apex. The increased intraorbital pressure is producing convexity of the medial orbital wall.

may occur in the euthyroid or hypothyroid states. Severe cases with visual loss, disk edema, or corneal ulceration merit urgent medical treatment with corticosteroids in high doses (eg, prednisolone, 100 mg); low doses are ineffective. Plasmapheresis is occasionally used with good results in the treatment of refractory cases, but full immunosuppression must follow plasmapheresis to prevent rebound increase of immunoglobulins and recurrence of disease. Immunosuppressive agents (eg, azathioprine) may play a supportive role and allow a lower maintenance dose of corticosteroids. In most cases, medical treatment produces adequate control, and surgical decompression is now performed less frequently. Orbital radiotherapy may be useful to avoid operation or as a sequel to surgical decompression. Guanethidine eye drops, 5% (see above and footnote), may produce temporary resolution of the lid retraction, which may be useful for cosmetic reasons.

B. Surgical Treatment: Decompression of the orbit is usually performed by removing the medial and inferior walls via an ethmoidal approach. Decompression of the orbital apex is essential for a successful outcome.

2. HYPOTHYROIDISM (Myxedema)

Significant ocular signs are not common in myxedema, though the signs of thyroid ophthalmopathy may be seen. Hyperthyroid patients who subsequently become hypothyroid are at greater risk of ophthalmic involvement.

HYPOPARATHYROIDISM

Occasionally at thyroidectomy, the parathyroid glands are removed inadvertently, causing hypoparathyroidism. Spontaneous cases of hypoparathyroidism, though rare, should be suspected in young patients with cataracts. The blood calcium decreases, and serum phosphates are increased. Tetany may ensue and can be severe enough to cause generalized convulsions. The ocular manifestations consist of blepharospasm and twitching eyelids. Small, discrete, punctate opacities of the lens cortex develop that may eventually require lens extraction.

Treatment with calcium salts, calciferol, and dihydrotachysterol usually prevents further development of lens opacities, but any that have occurred prior to treatment remain.

VITAMINS & EYE DISEASE

VITAMIN A

Vitamin A is essential for the maintenance of epithelium throughout the body. Ocular changes resulting from vitamin A deficiency (see Figure 15–26) are described in Chapter 6.

VITAMIN B

Vitamin B_1 (thiamine) deficiency produces **beriberi,** and 70% of patients with beriberi have ocular abnormalities. Epithelial changes in the conjunctiva and cornea produce dry eyes. Visual loss may occur as a result of optic atrophy.

Treatment is by correction of dietary deficiency with liver, whole wheat bread, cereals, eggs, and yeast, or with parenteral injection of thiamine.

Nicotinic acid deficiency (pellagra) is quite common in alcoholics and is characterized by dermatitis, diarrhea, and dementia. Ocular involvement is rare, but optic neuritis or retinitis may develop.

Riboflavin deficiency has been said to cause a number of ocular changes. Rosacea keratitis, vascularization of the limbal cornea, seborrheic blepharitis, and secondary conjunctivitis have all been attributed to riboflavin deficiency.

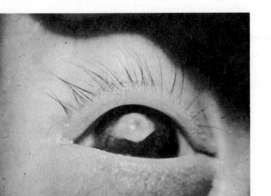

Figure 15–26. Keratomalacia. Case of xerophthalmia in a 5-month-old child.

VITAMIN C

In vitamin C deficiency (scurvy), hemorrhages may develop in a variety of sites, eg, skin, mucous membranes, body cavities, the orbits, and subperiosteally in the joints. Hemorrhages may also occur into the lids, subconjunctival space, anterior chamber, vitreous cavity, and retina.

Treatment of vitamin C deficiency is with proper diet, particularly adequate amounts of citrus juice.

GRANULOMATOUS DISEASES

Many of the so-called granulomatous infectious diseases, including tuberculosis, brucellosis, leprosy, and toxoplasmosis, undergo a chronic course with frequent exacerbations and remissions. The eye is often involved, particularly by anterior uveitis. The following paragraphs deal with other ocular complications of these systemic diseases.

TUBERCULOSIS

Ocular tuberculosis results from endogenous spread from systemic foci. The incidence of eye involvement is less than 1% in known cases of pulmonary tuberculosis; granulomatous panuveitis and retinal "cold" abscesses may occur.

Tuberculosis of the Uveal Tract

A. Iritis (Anterior Uveitis): (See Chapter 7.) Local treatment of iritis with mydriatics and corticosteroids is indicated. Systemic tuberculosis therapy is useful in the treatment of established cases of tuberculous uveitis.

B. Miliary Tuberculosis: In this usually fatal form of tuberculosis, many small discrete yellowish nodules are visible ophthalmoscopically in the choroid at the posterior pole of the eye.

SARCOIDOSIS
(Figure 15–27)

Sarcoidosis is a multisystem disease with pulmonary, ocular (uveitis), cutaneous, and reticuloendothelial system manifestations. A granulomatous uveitis may be accompanied by cells in the vitreous periphlebitis, disk swelling, retinal neovascularization, and choroidal disease. New vessels may require photocoagulation. The systemic disease is controlled by the administration of oral corticosteroids and occasionally immunosuppressants. Infiltrative optic neuropathy is a rare cause of progressive severe visual loss.

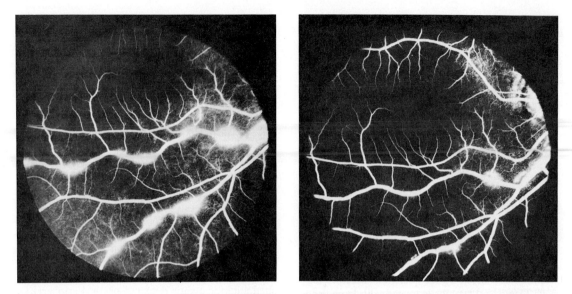

Figure 15–27. Sarcoidosis. Focal periphlebitis is a feature of ocular sarcoid and responds dramatically to corticosteroids. *Left:* Before treatment. *Right:* After treatment.

EALES' DISEASE

This disease was originally reported to occur in young men in poor general health who experienced recurrent vitreous hemorrhages from areas of retinal neovascularization. However, such symptoms are also known to occur in tuberculosis, sarcoidosis, systemic lupus erythematosus, sickle cell disease, and diabetes. Extensive investigations are therefore indicated to exclude these conditions in patients with consistent clinical features. If test results are negative, Eales's disease is then appropriate as a diagnosis arrived at by exclusion. Photocoagulation of the new vessels can reduce the chance of further vitreous hemorrhage.

LEPROSY
(Hansen's Disease)

Leprosy is a chronic granulomatous disorder caused by *Mycobacterium leprae,* an acid-fast bacillus. It is estimated that 12–15 million people in the world have leprosy and that of this number, 20–50% (2.4 million to 6 or 7 million) have ocular involvement. In tropical countries, the infection is endemic.

Three major types of leprosy are recognized: lepromatous, tuberculoid, and dimorphous. The eye may be affected in any type of leprosy, but ocular involvement is more common in the lepromatous type. Ocular lesions are due to direct invasion by *M leprae* of the ocular tissues or of the nerves supplying the eye and adnexa. Since the organism appears to grow better at lower temperatures, infection is more apt to involve the anterior segment of the eye than the posterior segment.

Clinical Findings

The early clinical signs of ocular leprosy are lagophthalmos, loss of the lateral portions of the eyebrows and eyelashes (madarosis), conjunctival hyperemia, and superficial keratitis (Figure 15–28), with interstitial keratitis—beginning typically in the superior temporal quadrant of the cornea—often supervening.

Scarring of the cornea from interstitial or exposure keratitis (or both) causes blurred vision and often blindness. Granulomatous iritis with lepromas (iris pearls) is common, and a low-grade iritis associated with iris atrophy and a pinpoint pupil may also occur. Hypertrophy of the eyebrows with deformities of the lids and trichiasis late in the course of the disease, and exposure keratitis, typically in the inferior and central

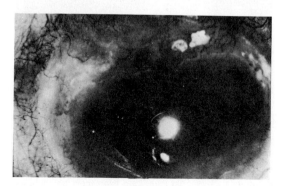

Figure 15–28. Leprosy keratitis, left eye. (Courtesy of W Richards.)

cornea, can result from facial motor nerve palsy and absence of corneal sensation.

Ocular leprosy can be diagnosed on the basis of characteristic signs combined with a characteristic skin biopsy.

Treatment

Leprosy is now treated with multidrug therapy, which includes dapsone, rifampin, and clofazimine, and the results in patients with early disease have been encouraging.

SYPHILIS

Congenital Syphilis

The most common eye lesion in congenital syphilis is interstitial keratitis (discussed in Chapter 6). Chorioretinitis unassociated with interstitial keratitis may occur. Congenital syphilis is treated with large doses of penicillin.

Acquired Syphilis

Ocular chancre (primary lesion) occurs rarely on the lid margins and follows the same course as a genital chancre.

Iritis and iridocyclitis occur in the secondary stage of syphilis along with the rash in about 5% of cases. The inflammation may involve the posterior segment, including the pigment epithelium and the retinal capillaries (Figure 15–29).

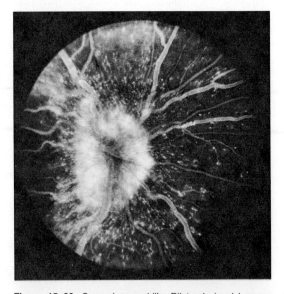

Figure 15–29. Secondary syphilis. Bilateral visual loss occurred in a 24-year-old man. Late fluorescein photographs showed disk leakage with dilation and leakage of peripapillary capillaries.

TOXOPLASMOSIS

This disease is of great ocular importance. The etiologic organism is a protozoal parasite that infects a great number of animals and birds and has worldwide distribution. Felids are the definitive host.

Congenital Toxoplasmosis (Figure 15–30)

Infection occurs in utero, and one-third of infants born to mothers who acquired toxoplasmosis during pregnancy—particularly during the third trimester—will be affected.

A focal choroiditis is seen, usually in the posterior pole, and an active lesion is often related to an old healed lesion. Episodes of posterior uveitis and chorioretinitis usually represent reactivation of a congenital infection. Rarely, panuveitis may occur, or optic neuritis progressing to optic atrophy. Isolated anterior uveitis does not occur. Peripheral vision is usually preserved, but because of macular involvement in at least 50% of cases, central vision is reduced.

Treatment with systemic corticosteroids and antibiotics reduces inflammation but does not prevent scar formation. Subconjunctival or retrobulbar injection of corticosteroids is contraindicated, because it may cause severe exacerbation of disease. Other forms of treatment are discussed in Chapter 7.

Acquired Toxoplasmosis

Acquired toxoplasmosis affects young adults and is characterized by general malaise, lymphadenopathy, sore throat, and hepatosplenomegaly similar to that

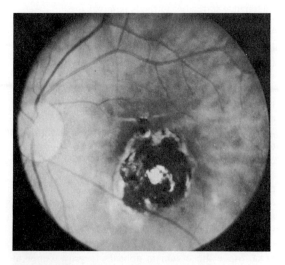

Figure 15–30. Healed toxoplasmic chorioretinitis. Note scaring in left macular area.

seen in infectious mononucleosis. It is endemic in South America. Toxoplasmic retinochoroiditis may rarely follow acquired systemic toxoplasmosis. The diagnosis is confirmed by the finding of both IgG and IgM antibodies.

VIRAL DISEASES

HERPES SIMPLEX

The most common manifestation of herpes simplex is fever blisters on the lips. The most common and serious eye lesion is keratitis (see Chapter 6). Vesicular skin lesions can also appear on the skin of the lids and the lid margins. Herpes simplex may cause iridocyclitis and may rarely cause severe encephalitis.

There are two morphologic strains of the virus: type 1 and type 2. Ocular infections are usually produced by type 1, whereas genital infections are caused by type 2. Retinitis due to herpes simplex virus type 1 occurs in adults suffering from herpes encephalitis or in immunosuppressed patients. Severe occlusive retinal vasculitis develops, followed by retinal necrosis and detachment. Type 1 antigens have been found in all layers of the retina, pigment epithelium, and choroid. Intravenous acyclovir prevents spread of the disease, and prophylactic retinal buckling may be useful.

Herpes simplex virus type 1, varicella-zoster virus, and cytomegalovirus have all been implicated in **acute retinal necrosis syndrome,** which produces a similar clinical picture but affects healthy young individuals. A 3-month course of oral acyclovir reduces the chances of involvement of the second eye.

VARICELLA-ZOSTER
(Chickenpox & Herpes Zoster)

First infection with varicella-zoster virus causes chickenpox (varicella). Swollen lids, conjunctivitis, vesicular conjunctival lesions, and (rarely) uveitis and optic neuritis may occur.

Herpes zoster is the response to the same virus in a partially immune person, ie, someone who has previously had chickenpox. It is usually confined to a single dermatome on one side and presents with malaise, headache, and fever followed by burning, itching, and pain in the affected area. The commonest ophthalmic manifestation is herpes zoster ophthalmicus, and the ocular complications are caused by ischemia, viral spread, or a granulomatous reaction. The acute stage is characterized by a virulent rash, conjunctivitis, kerati-

tis, episcleritis, and uveitis when the nasociliary nerve is involved.

Treatment in the acute stages with high doses of oral acyclovir; 800 mg five times a day for 10 days, started within 72 hours after eruption of the rash, reduces ocular complications including postherpetic neuralgia. Anterior uveitis requires topical steroids and cycloplegics.

The acute retinal necrosis syndrome has been described following chickenpox and herpes zoster (see above). In immunocompromised individuals, both herpes zoster, which may become disseminated, and varicella are likely to be severe and may be fatal.

CYTOMEGALIC INCLUSION DISEASE

Infection with cytomegalovirus, also a member of the herpesvirus group, may range from a subclinical infection to classic manifestations of cytomegalic inclusion disease. The virus most frequently affects newborn infants and compromised hosts, and the disease can be acquired or congenital. The ocular findings in the newborn include focal necrotizing retinitis and choroiditis with perivascular infiltrates and retinal hemorrhages. Other reported ocular findings include microphthalmia, cataract, optic atrophy, and optic disk malformation.

Histopathologic examination of the retinal and choroidal lesion shows large inclusion-bearing cells characteristic of cytomegalovirus infections. There is disruption of the normal architecture of the retina and choroid, with evidence of necrosis and mononuclear and perivascular infiltration. Calcifications in the retina may be observed.

The differential diagnosis in the congenital disease should include toxoplasmosis, rubella, herpes simplex infection, and syphilis.

Ganciclovir is the drug of choice for cytomegalic inclusion retinitis. It halts the progression of the disease without eradicating the virus. (See section on AIDS, below.)

POLIOMYELITIS

Bulbar poliomyelitis severe enough to cause lesions of the third, fourth, or sixth cranial nerve is usually fatal. In survivors, any type of internal or external ophthalmoplegia may result. Supranuclear abnormalities ("gaze" palsies, paralysis of convergence or divergence) are rare residual defects. Optic neuritis is uncommon. Treatment is purely symptomatic, though occasionally a residual extraocular muscle imbalance can be greatly improved by strabismus surgery.

GERMAN MEASLES
(Rubella)

Maternal rubella during the first trimester of pregnancy causes serious congenital anomalies. The most common eye complication is cataract, which is bilateral in 75% of cases. Other congenital ocular anomalies are frequently associated with the cataracts, eg, uveal colobomas, nystagmus, microphthalmos, strabismus, retinopathy, and infantile glaucoma. Congenital cataract, especially if bilateral, may require surgical removal, but the prognosis is always guarded.

Cataract surgery should be delayed until at least age 2, since the live virus is present in ocular tissues for many months after birth.

MEASLES
(Rubeola)

Acute conjunctivitis is common early in the course of measles. Koplik's spots may be seen on the conjunctiva, and epithelial keratitis occurs frequently.

The treatment of the eye complications of measles is symptomatic unless there is secondary infection, in which case local antibiotic ointment is used.

MUMPS

The most common ocular complication of mumps is dacryoadenitis. A diffuse keratitis with corneal edema resembling the disciform keratitis of herpes simplex occurs rarely.

INFECTIOUS MONONUCLEOSIS

The disease process can affect the eye directly, causing nongranulomatous uveitis, scleritis, conjunctivitis, retinitis, choroiditis, or optic neuritis. Complete recovery is usual, but residual visual loss can result.

FUNGAL DISEASE

CANDIDIASIS

Ocular involvement accompanies systemic *Candida* infection and candidemia in approximately two-thirds of cases. The initial *Candida* lesion is a focal necrotizing granulomatous retinitis with or without choroiditis, characterized by fluffy white exudative lesions associated with cells in the vitreous overlying the lesion. Such lesions may spread to involve the optic nerve and macula. Endophthalmitis, Roth's spots, and exudative retinal detachment may occur. Spread into the vitreous cavity may result in the formation of a vitreous abscess. Anterior uveitis occurs, and a hypopyon may form.

Treatment consists of systemic administration of amphotericin B, flucytosine, and ketoconazole. Early vitrectomy may prevent macular damage.

MUCORMYCOSIS

Mucormycosis is a rare, often fatal infection occurring in debilitated patients, particularly poorly controlled diabetics. The fungi (*Rhizopus, Mucor,* and *Absidia*) attack through the upper respiratory tract and invade the arterioles, producing necrotic tissue. Clinical features are the pathognomonic black hemipalate, proptosis, and an ischemic globe with blindness due to central retinal artery occlusion. Death occurs from cerebral abscess.

Treatment includes removal of the affected tissue, intravenous amphotericin B (preferably liposomal), and management of the underlying medical condition.

ACQUIRED IMMUNODEFICIENCY SYNDROME
(AIDS)

AIDS is caused by a retrovirus called human immunodeficiency virus (HIV). The virus infects mature T helper cells and leads to immunosuppression, the severity of which depends on the balance between the rates of destruction and replacement of T cells. The persistent immunodeficiency gives rise to opportunistic infections. The virus has been recovered from various body fluids, including blood, semen, saliva, tears, and cerebrospinal fluid.

Transmission & Prevention of AIDS

Transmission of HIV is primarily by exchange of bodily fluids during sexual contact or through the use of contaminated needles by intravenous drug abuse. Transmission may also occur when contaminated blood products are transfused. The virus is not transmitted by casual contact, but because it is found in tears, conjunctival cells, and blood, health care workers must take reasonable precautions when handling infectious waste or when at risk of contact with body fluids.

Clinical Findings

The spectrum of clinical disease is wide, presumably due to the degree of immunologic damage and the frequency and nature of opportunistic infections. Typically, an acute flu-like illness occurs a few weeks after infection, followed months later by weight loss, fever, diarrhea, lymphadenopathy, and encephalopathy. The com-

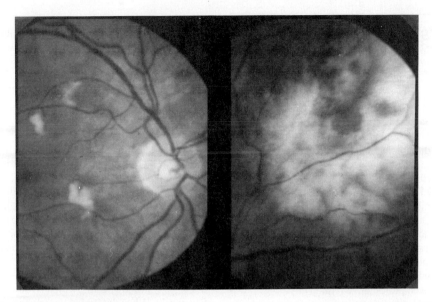

Figure 15–31. Retinal changes in AIDS. Multiple cotton wool spots *(left)* and retinal necrosis with hemorrhage *(right)* due to opportunistic infection. (Courtesy of R Marsh.)

monest ocular findings are retinal microvasculopathy with cotton wool spots (Figure 15–31) and hemorrhages and conjunctival vasculopathy characterized by comma vessels, sludging of the blood, and linear hemorrhages. The cause of these findings is unknown, but they are sometimes associated with increased plasma viscosity and may represent immune complex deposition.

The hallmark of AIDS is the high incidence of infections, which are frequently multiple, opportunistic, and severe. The eye is involved in 30% of cases, and both the anterior segment and the retina may be affected. Viral opportunistic infections of the retina are most common, particularly cytomegalovirus retinitis, which is a grave prognostic sign when found at the initial examination. Typically there is as a hemorrhagic necrotic retinopathy spreading from vascular arcades and associated with arteriolar occlusions (Figure 15–3). The vitreous is quiet; retinal detachment may occur. Involvement of the optic nerve results in gross optic disk edema and severe sudden and irreversible visual loss. Diagnosis is usually based on circumstantial evidence of positive antibody titers in blood, urine, or cerebrospinal fluid. Ocular fluids and retinal specimens are rarely examined. Treatment is with either ganciclovir or foscarnet. Both are virostatic drugs that stop progression of disease but do not eradicate the virus from the eye. Maintenance therapy is thus required, with attendant problems of long-term intravenous therapy. Neutropenia is the most important side effect of ganciclovir, and renal damage of foscarnet. Local administration of both drugs is effective in controlling ocular infection but not systemic spread.

Herpes simplex retinitis begins in the peripheral retina, advances to involve the entire fundus, and is associated with arteriolar occlusion. The retinitis almost always occurs concurrently with herpes simplex encephalitis, and this serves to distinguish herpes simplex from cytomegalovirus retinitis, which is rarely complicated by encephalitis. Treatment is with acyclovir, but maintenance therapy is required. A virulent form of retinitis, progressive outer retinal necrosis, is attributed to herpes zoster.

Toxoplasma chorioretinitis is usually bilateral, acquired (congenital infections are rarely reactivated in AIDS), and associated with substantial vitreous reaction; candidal endophthalmitis is rarely seen except in drug addicts. Less common organisms that typically involve the choroid are *Pneumocystis carinii, Cryptococcus,* and *Mycobacterium avium-intracellulare.* Choroidal infection is blood-borne and portends imminent demise.

Herpes zoster ophthalmicus is a rare presenting feature of HIV infection and may be very severe, with anterior segment necrosis and ophthalmoplegia. Similarly, syphilis in association with HIV infection produces a severe blinding uveitis. Herpes simplex, molluscum contagiosum, and Kaposi's sarcoma frequently affect the eyelids and surrounding tissues.

Neuro-ophthalmologic problems are divided into those related directly to HIV infection of the brain, such as optic neuropathy and intranuclear ophthalmoplegia, and those caused by cerebral abscesses or encephalitis, commonly due to *Cryptococcus,* lymphoma, or toxoplasmosis.

MULTISYSTEM AUTOIMMUNE DISEASES

SYSTEMIC LUPUS ERYTHEMATOSUS

Systemic or disseminated lupus erythematosus is a multisystem disease manifested by facial "butterfly skin lesions," pericarditis, Raynaud's phenomenon, renal involvement, arthritis, anemia, and central nervous system signs. Ocular findings include episcleritis and scleritis and keratoconjunctivitis sicca (in 25% of cases). Uveitis rarely occurs, and retinal involvement produces signs of arteriolar occlusion as a result of immune complex deposition with associated choroidal vasculitis. The fundus picture may be complicated by a hypertensive retinopathy, which in severe cases can cause capillary occlusion or even proliferative retinopathy.

Pathogenesis & Diagnosis

The disease is an immunologic disorder marked by the presence of circulating immune complexes. Diagnostic tests include anti-DNA antibodies and mitochondrial type V antibodies. Active disease is associated with raised circulating immune complexes and reduced fractions of complement.

Treatment

Systemic steroids and pulsed intravenous cyclophosphamide are most effective.

DERMATOMYOSITIS

In this rare disease, there is characteristically a degenerative subacute inflammation of the muscles, sometimes including the extraocular muscles. The lids are commonly a part of the generalized dermal involvement and may show marked swelling and erythema. Retinopathy with cotton wool spots and hemorrhages may occur. High doses of systemic corticosteroids will frequently effect a remission that continues even after cessation of therapy. The ultimate prognosis is poor, however.

SCLERODERMA

This rare chronic disease is characterized by widespread alterations in the collagenous tissues of the mucosa, bones, muscles, skin, and internal organs. Individuals of both sexes between 15 and 45 years of age are affected. The skin in local areas becomes tense and leathery, and the process may spread to involve large areas of the limbs, rendering them virtually immobile.

The skin of the eyelids is often involved. Iritis and cataract occur less frequently. Retinopathy similar to that which occurs in lupus erythematosus and dermatomyositis may be present. Systemic corticosteroid treatment improves the prognosis.

POLYARTERITIS NODOSA

This collagen disease affects the medium-sized arteries, most commonly in men. There is intense inflammation of all the muscle layers of the arteries, with fibrinoid necrosis and a peripheral eosinophilia. The main clinical features include nephritis, hypertension, asthma, peripheral neuropathy, muscle pain with wasting, and peripheral eosinophilia. Cardiac involvement is common, though death is usually caused by renal dysfunction.

Ocular changes are seen in 20% of cases and consist of episcleritis and scleritis, which is often painless. (see Chapter 7). When the limbal vessels are involved, guttering of the peripheral cornea may occur. A retinal microvasculopathy is common. Sudden dramatic visual loss may be due to ischemic optic neuropathy reflecting the severity of the vasculitis in the ciliary vessels or to a central retinal artery occlusion. Ophthalmoplegia may result from arteritis of the vasa nervorum (Fig-

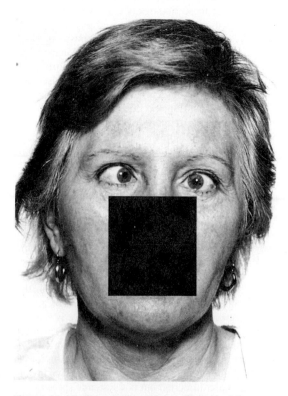

Figure 15–32. Polyarteritis nodosa. Bilateral sixth nerve palsies.

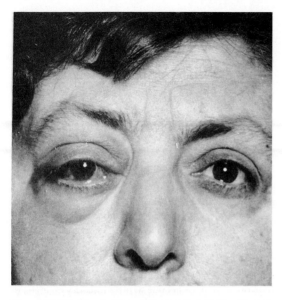

Figure 15–33. Classic Wegener's granulomatosis with proptosis, ptosis, and ophthalmoplegia. The condition has remained static for 10 years with use of corticosteroids and cyclophosphamide.

ure 15–32). Systemic corticosteroids and cyclophosphamide are of some value, but the long-term prognosis is uniformly bad.

WEGENER'S GRANULOMATOSIS

This granulomatous process shares certain clinical features with polyarteritis nodosa. The three diagnostic criteria are (1) necrotizing granulomatous lesions of the respiratory tract, (2) generalized necrotizing arteritis, and (3) renal involvement with necrotizing glomerulitis.

Ocular complications occur in 50% of cases, and proptosis resulting from orbital granulomatous formation occurs with associated ocular muscle or optic nerve involvement (Figure 15–33). If the vasculitis affects the eye, conjunctivitis, peripheral corneal ulceration, episcleritis, scleritis, uveitis, and retinal vasculitis may occur. Nasolacrimal duct obstruction is a rare complication.

Antineutrophil cytoplasmic antibodies are present in most cases and have both diagnostic and prognostic value. Combined corticosteroids and immunosuppressives (particularly cyclophosphamide) often produce a satisfactory response.

RHEUMATOID ARTHRITIS

Rheumatoid arthritis, a disease that is more common in women than in men, rarely presents with uveitis, but scleritis and episcleritis are comparatively common.

The scleritis may herald exacerbation of the systemic disease, tends to occur with widespread vasculitis and may lead to scleromalacia perforans (see Chapter 7).

Corticosteroid drops are helpful in episcleritis or anterior uveitis, but systemic treatment (nonsteroidal anti-inflammatory agents and corticosteroids) is necessary for scleritis. Keratoconjunctivitis sicca is present in 15% of cases (see Chapter 4). Peripheral corneal melting may occur in more severe cases.

JUVENILE RHEUMATOID ARTHRITIS (Still's Disease)

Ocular complications of Still's disease occur three times more frequently in girls with pauciarticular disease. The systemic disease appears to be disproportionately mild in children with severe visual loss, and diagnosis and treatment may therefore be delayed. Ocular involvement may occur before joint involvement. A chronic insidious uveitis with a high incidence of anterior segment complications develops (eg, posterior synechiae, cataract, secondary glaucoma, band-shaped keratopathy). Antinuclear antibodies are positive in 88% of patients with juvenile rheumatoid arthritis who develop uveitis, whereas they are positive in only 30% of the group as a whole.

SJÖGREN'S SYNDROME

Sjögren's syndrome is a systemic disorder with diverse features. The disease is characterized by the clinical triad of keratoconjunctivitis sicca, xerostomia (dryness of the mouth), and a connective tissue disease, usually rheumatoid arthritis. It is more common in females. The onset of ocular symptoms occurs most frequently during the fourth, fifth, and sixth decades. Lymphoid proliferation is a prominent feature of Sjögren's syndrome and may involve the kidneys, the lungs, or the liver, causing renal tubular acidosis, pulmonary fibrosis, or cirrhosis. Lymphoreticular malignant disease such as reticulum cell sarcoma may complicate the benign course of Sjögren's syndrome many years after its onset.

The histopathologic changes in the lacrimal gland consist of infiltration of lymphocytes, histiocytes, and occasional plasma cells leading to atrophy and destruction of the glandular structures. These changes are part of the generalized polyglandular involvement in Sjögren's syndrome, which results in dryness of the eyes, mouth, skin, and mucous membranes.

Because of the relative inaccessibility of the lacrimal gland, the labial salivary gland biopsy serves as an important diagnostic procedure in patients with suspected Sjögren's syndrome.

Tear lysozyme and lactoferrin levels are absent or reduced in over 90% of patients, and very high titers of nuclear antibodies are present.

GIANT CELL ARTERITIS (Including Temporal or Cranial Arteritis)

This is a disease of elderly patients (mostly women over age 60). Medium-sized arteries are involved, particularly the intima of the vessels. Branches of the external carotid system are frequently involved, though pathologic studies have shown more diffuse arterial involvement. Polymyalgia rheumatica may precede or accompany the disease. Patients feel ill and have excruciating pain over the temporal or occipital arteries. Visual loss due to an ischemic optic neuropathy is frequent, and a few cases have a central retinal artery occlusion. Visual loss may also be due to cortical blindness. Other central nervous system signs include cranial nerve palsies and signs referable to brain stem lesions. The diagnosis is confirmed by a high erythrocyte sedimentation rate (ESR) and a positive temporal artery biopsy. In early stages of the disease, the ESR may be normal, but usually it is 80–100 mm in the first hour. It is important to make the diagnosis early, because immediate systemic corticosteroid administration produces dramatic relief of pain and prevents further ischemic episodes. The disease activity is monitored by the erythrocyte sedimentation rate and the clinical state. The corticosteroid dose may have to be maintained for several years and should be kept below 5 mg prednisolone daily if possible, since with higher doses toxic effects develop.

IDIOPATHIC ARTERITIS OF TAKAYASU (Pulseless Disease)

This disease, found most frequently in young women and occasionally in children, is a polyarteritis of unknown cause with increased predilection for the aorta and its branches. Manifestations may include evidence of cerebrovascular insufficiency, syncope, absence of pulsations in the upper extremities, and ophthalmologic changes compatible with chronic hypoxia of the ocular structures. Ophthalmodynamometry may be of value by demonstrating decreased carotid blood flow on one or both sides.

Thromboendarterectomy, prosthetic graft, and systemic corticosteroid therapy have been reported to be successful.

ANKYLOSING SPONDYLITIS

Ankylosing spondylitis occurs mainly in males 16–40 years of age. In most cases, an intermittent anterior uveitis is seen, but in a minority anterior and posterior uveitis exists with glaucoma and cataracts developing in the long term. In a few cases, aortic valve disease is also seen (see Chapter 7). There is a strong association with HLA-B27. Antigenic cross-reactivity is present between HLA-B27 and *Klebsiella pneumoniae,* but the etiology remains poorly understood.

REITER'S DISEASE

The diagnosis of Reiter's disease is based on a triad of signs that includes urethritis, conjunctivitis, and arthritis (see Chapter 16). Scleritis, keratitis, and uveitis may also be seen in addition to conjunctivitis.

BEHÇET'S DISEASE

Behçet's disease consists of the clinical triad of relapsing uveitis and aphthous and genital ulceration (Figure 15–34). Ocular signs occur in 75% of cases; the uveitis is severe, occasionally associated with hypopyon. Visual loss is due to inflammatory changes in the retinal vessels and retina, and there is a propensity to microvascular venous occlusions and retinal infiltrates. Treatment often involves multiple immunosuppression (eg, steroids, cyclosporine, azathioprine), but despite manipulation with these drugs the visual outcome is bad in 25% of cases. Ocular involvement is associated with the HLA-B5 haplotype.

HERITABLE CONNECTIVE TISSUE DISEASES

MARFAN'S SYNDROME (Arachnodactyly) (Figure 15–35)

The most striking feature of this rare syndrome is increased length of the long bones, particularly of the fingers and toes. Other characteristics include scanty subcutaneous fat, relaxed ligaments, and, less commonly, other associated developmental anomalies, including congenital heart disease and deformities of the spine and joints. Ocular complications are often seen—in particular, dislocation of the lenses, usually superiorly and nasally. Less common ocular anomalies include severe refractive errors, megalocornea, cataract, uveal colobomas, and secondary glaucoma. There is a high infant mortality rate. Removal of a dislocated lens may be necessary. The disease is genetically determined, nearly always autosomal dominant, often with incomplete expression, so that mild, incomplete forms of the syndrome are seen. Several reports have correlated cytogenetic changes with Marfan's syndrome.

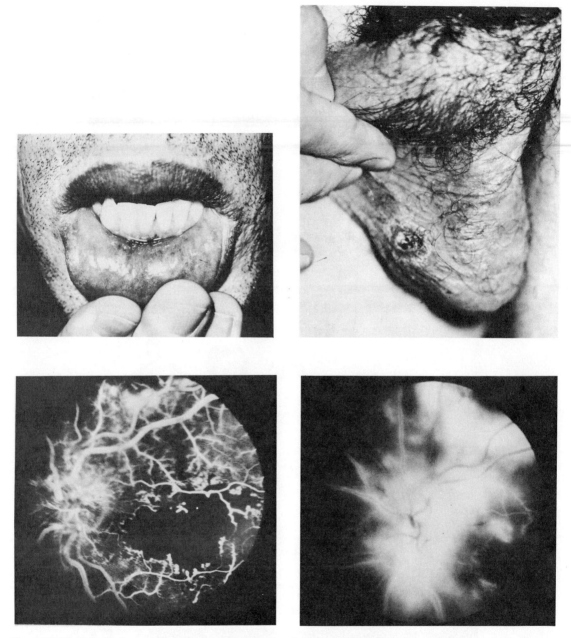

Figure 15–34. Behçet's disease. Clinical features include oral and genital ulcers. Ocular features include increased capillary permeability and areas of retinal ischemia and infiltration. Marked leakage of capillaries is seen in the late stages of fluorescein angiography (bottom right).

OSTEOGENESIS IMPERFECTA
(Brittle Bones & Blue Scleras)

This rare autosomal dominant syndrome is characterized by multiple fractures, blue scleras, and, less commonly, deafness. The disease is usually manifest soon after birth. The long bones are very fragile, fracturing easily and often healing with fibrous bony union. The bones become more fragile with age. The very thin sclera allows the blue color imparted by the underlying uveal tract to show through. There is usually no visual impairment. Occasionally, abnormalities such as keratoconus, megalocornea, and corneal or lenticular opacities are also present.

Ophthalmologic treatment is seldom necessary.

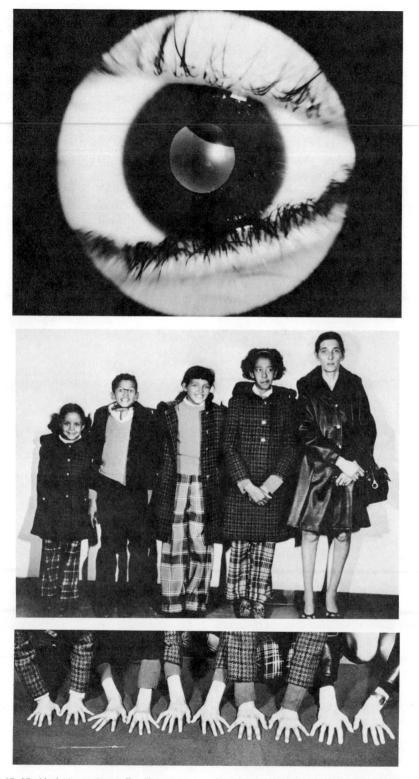

Figure 15–35. Marfan's syndrome. Familial expression of arachnodactyly and upward dislocation of the lens.

HEREDITARY METABOLIC DISORDERS

HEPATOLENTICULAR DEGENERATION
(Wilson's Disease)

This rare autosomal recessive disease of young adults—characterized by abnormal copper metabolism—causes changes in the basal nuclei, cirrhosis of the liver, and a pathognomonic corneal pigmentation called the Kayser-Fleischer ring. The ring appears as a green or brown band peripherally and deep in the stroma near Descemet's membrane and may only be visible with a slitlamp. The disease is progressive and often results in death by age 40. Treatment with penicillamine has resulted in sustained clinical improvement in some cases.

CYSTINOSIS

This rare autosomal recessive derangement of amino acid metabolism causes widespread deposition of cystine crystals throughout the body. Dwarfism, nephropathy, and death in childhood from renal failure are the rule. Cystine crystals can be readily seen in the conjunctiva and cornea, where fine particles are seen predominantly in the outer third of the corneal stroma.

There is no treatment.

ALBINISM

Generalized albinism is a disease affecting the metabolism of melanin and is inherited as an autosomal recessive trait. The skin and hair are white, and there is a generalized lack of pigment throughout the body that is apparent from birth. The eyebrows and lashes are white. The irides appear reddish, and the pupils appear red. The fundus is red, with a prominent choroidal vessel pattern, since the pigment epithelium of the retina is deficient. Photophobia is a prominent symptom. Macular hyperplasia and nystagmus are frequently present, with visual acuity being reduced to about 20/200.

GALACTOSEMIA

Galactosemia is a rare autosomal recessive disorder of carbohydrate metabolism clinically manifested soon after birth by feeding problems, vomiting, diarrhea, abdominal distention, hepatomegaly, jaundice, ascites, cataracts, mental retardation, and elevated blood and urine galactose levels. Dietary exclusion of milk and all foods containing galactose and lactose for the first

3 years of life will prevent the clinical manifestations and will result in improvement of existing abnormalities. Even the cataract changes, which are characterized by vacuoles of the cortex, are reversible in the early stage.

Identification of the carrier state is possible by finding a 50% reduction of galactose 6-phosphatase.

MISCELLANEOUS SYSTEMIC DISEASES WITH OCULAR MANIFESTATIONS

VOGT-KOYANAGI-HARADA SYNDROME
(Figure 15–36)

Bilateral uveitis associated with alopecia, poliosis, vitiligo, and hearing defects, usually in young adults, has been termed Vogt-Koyanagi disease. When the choroiditis is more exudative, serous retinal detachment occurs, and the complex is known as Harada's syndrome. There is a tendency toward recovery of visual function, but this is not always complete. Initial treatment is with local steroids and mydriatics, but systemic steroids in high doses are frequently required to prevent permanent visual loss.

ERYTHEMA MULTIFORME
(Stevens-Johnson Syndrome)

Erythema multiforme is a serious mucocutaneous disease that occurs as a hypersensitivity reaction to drugs or food. Children are most susceptible. The manifestations consist of generalized maculopapular rash, severe stomatitis, and purulent conjunctivitis, sometimes leading to symblepharon and occlusion of the lacrimal gland ducts (**dry eye syndrome**). In severe cases, corneal ulcers, perforations, and panophthalmitis can destroy all visual function. Systemic corticosteroid treatment often favorably influences the course of the disease and usually preserves useful visual function. Secondary infection with *Staphylococcus aureus* is common and must be vigorously treated with local antibiotics instilled into the conjunctival sac. Frequently there is marked reduction of tear formation that can be helped by instillation of artificial tears.

LAURENCE-MOON-BIEDL SYNDROME

Obesity, mental deficiency, polydactyly, hypogonadism, and retinitis pigmentosa form the complete syndrome. The retinal changes are not always typical

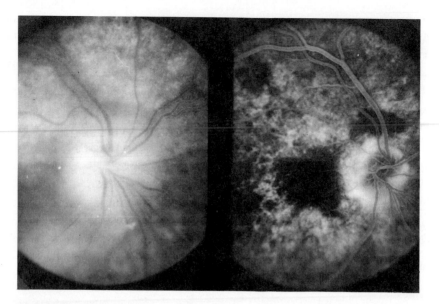

Figure 15–36. Vogt-Koyanagi-Harada syndrome. Acute pigment epithelial disease with disk swelling and cells in the vitreous *(left).* Three months later, disk swelling has subsided and pigment epithelial damage is seen *(right).*

of retinitis pigmentosa and may be present soon after birth or develop during adolescence. This rare syndrome is genetically determined and follows an autosomal recessive pattern with a high rate of consanguinity. The heterozygous state may be identified by mild incomplete evidence of the disease. It is interesting that a single abnormal gene can account for such a multiplicity of clinical findings.

ROSACEA
(Acne Rosacea)

This disease of unknown cause is primarily dermatologic, beginning as hyperemia of the face associated with acneiform lesions and eventually causing hypertrophy of tissues (such as rhinophyma). Chronic blepharitis due to staphylococcal infection or seborrhea is often present. Rosacea keratitis develops in about 5% of cases. Episcleritis, scleritis, and nongranulomatous iridocyclitis are rare ocular complications.

Topical corticosteroids help in controlling keratitis or iridocyclitis, but there is no specific therapy. Long-term systemic tetracycline therapy is often beneficial.

LYME DISEASE

Lyme disease is a vector-mediated multisystem illness caused by the spirochete *Borrelia burgdorferi.* The usual vectors are small ixodid ticks that have a complex three-host life cycle involving multiple mammalian and avian species.

The disease has three major stages. Initially, in the area of the tick bite, there develops the characteristic

skin lesion of erythema chronicum migrans, often accompanied by regional lymphadenopathy, malaise, fever, headache, myalgia, and arthralgia. Several weeks to months later there is a period of neurologic and cardiac abnormalities. After a few more weeks or even years, rheumatologic abnormalities develop—initially, migratory musculoskeletal discomfort, but later a frank arthritis that may recur over several years.

Conjunctivitis is a frequent finding in the first stage. Cranial nerve palsies—particularly of the seventh but also of the third, fourth, or sixth cranial nerves—often occur in the neurologic phase. Other ophthalmologic abnormalities that have been reported include uveitis, ischemic optic neuropathy, optic disk edema, bilateral keratitis, and choroiditis with exudative retinal detachments.

Laboratory diagnosis is by demonstration of specific IgM and IgG antibodies in serum or cerebrospinal fluid. The spirochetes may also be isolated from these sources.

Doxycycline and ampicillin are effective in curing the initial infection but unfortunately may not prevent late complications.

IMMUNOSUPPRESSIVE AGENTS USED IN MANAGEMENT OF EYE DISEASE

Immunosuppressive agents are used to suppress inflammatory reactions within the eye, particularly those affecting the uveal tract but also the sclera, retina, and optic nerve. Frequently, the cause of inflammation is not known, and the use of these drugs is therefore empirical. All patients must have a full medical examination before treatment is started. Special consideration must be given to patients with infections and blood diseases, and regular blood counts must be performed during the course of treatment.

Corticosteroids (eg, prednisolone) are the mainstay of immunosuppressive treatment in ophthalmology. High doses (eg, 60 mg of prednisolone daily) may be required to control inflammation, and there is a high incidence of side effects. Weight gain, acne, and hirsutism are common; peptic ulceration, myopathy, osteoporosis, and avascular necrosis are less frequently encountered. Alternate-day regimens produce fewer side effects in some patients. Azathioprine may be added as a corticosteroid-sparing drug; 2.5 mg/kg daily is an effective dose, and the total course should not last longer than 18 months. Intravenous methylprednisolone (1 g/d given over 3 hours in dextrose saline for 3 days) is an effective method of controlling exacerbations in patients already taking high doses of corticosteroids.

Cyclosporine is an immunosuppressive agent isolated from the fermentation products of a fungus that was recovered from Norwegian soil. It has an effective immunomodulating action and causes suppression of T helper cells. It is a useful alternative drug for refractory sight-threatening noninfectious inflammatory eye disease in patients who have not responded to corticosteroids or in whom the optimal therapeutic dose of corticosteroids is associated with intolerable side effects. The recommended dose is 5 mg/kg orally daily. The most important side effect is renal toxicity, but liver toxicity may also occur. Close surveillance and monitoring of kidney and liver function are mandatory on every patient receiving cyclosporine therapy. The drug should not be given to hypertensive patients. Reduction of the daily dose may be associated with troublesome rebound of the ocular inflammation.

Fortunately, **cytotoxic agents** are rarely indicated in the management of inflammatory eye disease except in severe cases of Behçet's syndrome and Wegener's granulomatosis. These drugs and their important side effects are listed in Table 15–3. Cytotoxic agents are sometimes used in the treatment of myasthenia gravis (see Figure 15–37 and Chapter 15).

OCULAR COMPLICATIONS OF CERTAIN SYSTEMICALLY ADMINISTERED DRUGS (See Also Chapter 3.)

AMIODARONE

Amiodarone is a benzofuran derivative used to treat cardiac dysrhythmias, particularly Wolff-Parkinson-White syndrome, and angina pectoris. Most patients develop small punctate deposits with a vortex pattern in the basal cell layer of the corneal epithelium (Figure 15–38). The severity of keratopathy is related to the total daily dose and is mild at a dose of less than 200 mg daily. The deposits rarely interfere with vision, and although they progress with continued treatment, even in low dosage, they always resolve completely when treatment is stopped. A small percentage of patients develop thyroid ophthalmopathy, though the mechanism is not fully understood.

ANTICHOLINERGICS (Atropine & Related Synthetic Drugs)

All of these drugs, when given preoperatively or for gastrointestinal disorders, may cause blurred vision in presbyopic patients because of a direct action on accommodation. They also tend to dilate the pupils, so

Table 15–3. Cytotoxic agents used in the management of inflammatory eye disease.

Drug	Daily Dose (mg/kg)	Maximum Length of Treatment	Side Effects
Azathioprine	2.5–3	18 months	Bone marrow depression (usually leukopenia, but may be anemia, thrombocytopenia, and bleeding) (irreversible in elderly patients). Skin rashes, drug fever, nausea and vomiting, sometimes diarrhea. Hepatic dysfunction (raised liver enzymes, mild jaundice). Lymphoma.
Chlorambucil	0.05–0.2	2½ years (4 g)	Moderate depression of peripheral blood count. Excessive doses produce severe bone marrow depression with leukopenia, thrombocytopenia, and bleeding. Lymphoma. Prevent cystitis with adequate hydration. Chlorambucil: Leukemia may occur. Large doses near puberty may cause infertility. Cyclophosphamide: Nausea and vomiting acutely. Alopecia and hemorrhagic cystitis occasionally. Infertility may occur.
Cyclophosphamide	1.25–2.5	3 years	
Colchicine	0.01–0.03	5 years	Occasionally nausea, vomiting, abdominal pain, diarrhea. Rarely, hair loss, bone marrow depression, peripheral neuritis, myopathy.

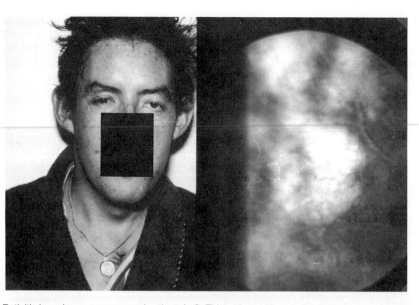

Figure 15–37. Retinitis in an immunosuppressed patient. *Left:* This patient with myasthenia gravis underwent thymectomy and received long-term immunosuppression with cytotoxic agents. *Right:* He developed retinal necrosis and Ramsay Hunt syndrome following infection with herpes zoster.

that in patients with narrow anterior chamber angles there is the added threat of angle-closure glaucoma. This is the cause of angle-closure glaucoma (frequently attributed to "nervousness") occasionally seen in patients hospitalized for general surgery.

ANTIDEPRESSANTS

Tricyclic antidepressants and monoamine oxidase inhibitors have an anticholinergic effect and theoretically may exacerbate open-angle glaucoma or provoke an attack of angle-closure glaucoma. However, these side effects are rare in clinical practice.

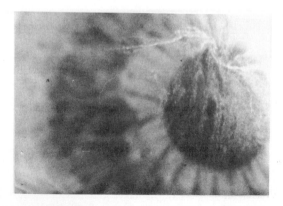

Figure 15–38. Amiodarone keratopathy. (Courtesy of DJ Spalton.)

CHLORAMPHENICOL

Chloramphenicol, in addition to the possibility of causing severe blood dyscrasias, hepatic and renal disease, and gastrointestinal disturbances, can sometimes cause optic neuritis. This is especially true in children. Bilateral blurred vision with central scotomas occurs. Stopping the drug does not always restore vision.

Despite the possibility of toxic optic neuropathy, chloramphenicol may still be required for the treatment of bacterial endophthalmitis. The drug is generally not administered for more than 1 week.

CHLOROQUINE

Chloroquine is an effective antimalarial drug. With high dosage—often 250–750 mg daily administered for months or years—serious ocular toxicity has occurred. Corneal changes were described first and consisted of diffuse haziness of the epithelium and subepithelial area, occasionally sufficient to simulate an epithelial dystrophy. These changes cause only mild blurring of vision and are reversible upon drug withdrawal. Similar changes have been described in patients receiving quinacrine. Minimal corneal involvement is not necessarily an indication for discontinuance of chloroquine therapy.

A less common but more serious ocular complication of long-term chloroquine therapy is retinal damage, causing loss of central vision as well as constriction of peripheral visual fields. Pigmentary changes and edema of the macula, marked alteration of the retinal vessels, and in some cases peripheral pigmentary changes can be seen ophthalmoscopically. Hydroxychloroquine is a derivative of chloroquine that is regularly used in the treatment of collagen diseases (especially systemic lupus erythematosus), rheumatoid arthritis, and chronic skin disease, including discoid lupus and sarcoidosis. The range of ocular complications is the same as with chloroquine, but both their incidence and their severity are greatly reduced.

CHLOROTHIAZIDE

Xanthopsia (yellow vision) has been reported in patients taking this oral diuretic.

CONTRACEPTIVES, ORAL

Although numerous reports suggest that in predisposed individuals oral contraceptives can provoke or precipitate ophthalmic vascular occlusive disease or optic nerve damage, it is difficult to establish a definite cause and effect relationship. Optic neuritis, retinal arterial or venous thrombosis, and pseudotumor cerebri have been described in patients taking oral contraceptives. Since there is some uncertainty regarding the possibility of such ocular complications, oral contraceptives should be used only by healthy women with no history of vascular, neurologic, or ocular disease.

CORTICOSTEROIDS

It has been clearly demonstrated that long-term systemic corticosteroid therapy can cause chronic open-angle glaucoma and cataracts and can provoke and worsen attacks of herpes simplex keratitis. Locally administered corticosteroids are much more potent in this respect and have the added disadvantage of causing fungal overgrowth if the corneal epithelium is not intact. Steroid-induced subcapsular lens opacities cause some impairment of visual function but usually do not progress to advanced cataract. Cessation of therapy will arrest progression of the lenticular opacities, but the changes are irreversible.

OXYGEN

Premature infants who are given any concentration of oxygen in excess of that in the air may develop retinopathy of prematurity (retrolental fibroplasia). These infants should receive only the amount of oxygen necessary for survival. The incidence of the condition was considerably reduced in the 1960s with rigid restriction of oxygen, but despite continued restriction, the incidence has recently risen again. This may be due

to prematurity itself (with advanced medical techniques, smaller infants are surviving); the condition is found in 40–77% of infants weighing less than 1 kg.

In adults, administration of hyperbaric oxygen (3 atm) can cause constriction of the retinal arterioles.

PHENOBARBITAL & PHENYTOIN

Ocular complications relate to oculomotor involvement, producing nystagmus and weakness of convergence and accommodation. The nystagmus may persist for many months after cessation of the drug, and the degree of oculomotor abnormality is related to drug dosage. Early abnormalities include disturbance of smooth pursuit.

PHENOTHIAZINES

The phenothiazines usually exert an atropine-like effect on the eye so that the pupils may be dilated, especially with large doses. Of greater clinical significance, however, are the pigmentary ocular changes, which include pigmentary retinopathy and pigment deposits on the corneal endothelium and anterior lens capsule. The corneal and lens pigmentation may cause blurring of vision, but the pigment deposits usually disappear several months after the drug is discontinued. In pigmentary retinopathy, there is a diminution of central vision, night blindness, diffuse narrowing of the retinal arteries, and occasionally severe blindness.

The piperidine group (eg, thioridazine) has a higher risk of causing pigmentary retinopathy, and the maximum daily dose should not exceed 600 mg. The retinal changes are partly reversible under normal circumstances, but in some patients more severe irreversible changes occur at the "safe" dosage level.

The dimethylamine group (eg, chlorpromazine) rarely produces retinal pigmentary changes.

The piperazine group (eg, trifluoperazine) does not produce these retinal complications.

All of these drugs can produce an extrapyramidal syndrome that may involve eye movements. Large doses can provoke profound hypotension, which may produce ischemic optic neuropathy.

Patients receiving large doses or prolonged treatment with phenothiazines should be questioned regarding visual disturbances and should have periodic ophthalmoscopic examinations.

QUININE & QUINACRINE

Quinine and quinacrine, when used in the treatment of malaria, may cause bilateral blurred vision, sometimes following a single dose. There is constriction of the visual field and, rarely, total blindness. The tendency is toward partial recovery, though usually there are permanent peripheral field defects. The ganglion cells of the retina are affected first, presumably as a result of vasoconstriction of the retinal arterioles. Varying degrees of retinal edema occur early. Optic atrophy is a late finding.

SEDATIVE TRANQUILIZERS

When taken regularly, the so-called minor tranquilizers can decrease tear production by the lacrimal gland, thus resulting in ocular irritation because of dry eyes. Tear production returns to normal when the tranquilizers are discontinued.

The principal drugs in this group are meprobamate, chlordiazepoxide, and diazepam.

TAMOXIFEN

Asymptomatic intraretinal crystals are observed in 1–5% of patients who take 20 mg of tamoxifen twice daily. Corneal crystals and optic neuropathy have been reported in patients receiving 80–120 mg daily.

RADIATION

Both optic neuropathy and retinopathy may occur months or years after radiation treatment to the head and neck, particularly to the sinuses or the chiasm. The retinal endothelial cells are damaged, and ischemic retinopathy develops with cotton wool spots, hemorrhages, and capillary closure. Patients with optic neuropathy present with arcuate field defects, and gadolinium-enhanced MRI reveals characteristic sharply demarcated lesions in the optic nerve. Both conditions progress slowly, and although there is no treatment, anticoagulation or aspirin may halt the process.

FETAL EFFECTS OF DRUGS

The visual pathways of the fetus are occasionally affected by drugs taken by the mother during pregnancy.

Phenytoin may cause optic nerve hypoplasia.

Pigmentary retinopathy has been reported in a child of a mother taking **busulfan** for acute myeloid leukemia.

Warfarin is teratogenic and may produce a hypoplastic nose, stippled epiphyses, and skeletal abnormalities. Affected children may present with recurrent sticky eyes from obstruction of the nasolacrimal duct secondary to malformation of the nose. Other ocular abnormalities include optic atrophy, microphthalmia, and lens opacities.

REFERENCES

Acheson JF, Sanders MD: Coagulation abnormalities in ischaemic optic neuropathy. Eye 1994;8:89.

Aiello PD et al: Visual prognosis in giant cell arteritis. Ophthalmology 1993;100:550.

Akova YA, Jabbur NR, Foster CS: Ocular presentation of polyarteritis nodosa. Ophthalmology 1993;100:1775.

Arruga J, Sanders MD: Ophthalmologic findings in 70 patients with evidence of retinal embolism. Ophthalmology 1982;89:1336.

Bahn RJ, Heufelder AE: Pathogenesis of Graves ophthalmopathy. N Engl J Med 1993;11:1468.

Bergsma D, Bron AJ, Cotlier E (editors): *The Eye and Inborn Errors of Metabolism.* AR Liss, 1976.

Cogan DG: *Ophthalmic Manifestations of Systemic Vascular Disease.* Saunders, 1974.

de Boer JH et al: Detection of intraocular antibody production to herpesviruses in acute retinal necrosis syndrome. Am J Ophthalmol 1994;117:201.

Dhillon B: The management of cytomegalovirus retinitis in AIDS. Br J Ophthalmol 1994;78:66.

Edwards JE Jr et al: Ocular manifestations of *Candida* septicemia: Review of seventy-six cases of hematogenous Candida endophthalmitis. Medicine 1974;53:47.

Elman MJ et al: The risk of systemic vascular disease and mortality in patients with central retinal vein occlusion. Ophthalmology 1990;97:1543.

Eva PR, Pascoe PT, Vaughan DG: Refractive change in hyperglycaemia: Hyperopia, not myopia. Br J Ophthalmol 1982;66:500.

Feltkamp TEW: Ophthalmological significance of HLA associated uveitis. EYE 1990;4:839.

Ferry AP, Font RL: Carcinoma metastatic to the eye and orbit. Arch Ophthalmol 1975;93:472.

Fong ACO, Schatz H: Central retinal vein occlusion in young adults. Surv Ophthalmol 1993;37:393.

Fraunfelder FT: *Drug-Induced Ocular Side-Effects and Drug Interactions.* Lea & Febiger, 1976.

Gass JDM, Olson CL: Sarcoidosis with optic nerve and retinal involvement. Arch Ophthalmol 1976;94:945.

Gold DH, Weingeist TA (editors): *The Eye in Systemic Disease.* Lippincott, 1990.

Goldberg RA, Rootman J, Clive RA: Tumours metastatic to the orbit: A changing picture. Surv Ophthalmol 1990;35:1.

Graham EM: The investigation of patients with retinal vascular occlusion. Eye 1990;4:464.

Hardy RA: Paraneoplastic syndromes in ophthalmology. In: *Year Book of Ophthalmology.* Ernest JT, Deutsch TA (editors): Year Book, 1988.

Holland GN: Acquired immunodeficiency syndrome and ophthalmology: The first decade. Am J Ophthalmol 1992;114:86.

Holland GN et al: Ocular toxoplasmosis in patients with the acquired immunodeficiency syndrome. Am J Ophthalmol 1988;106:653.

Jabs DA: Treatment of cytomegalovirus retinitis—1992. (Editorial.) Arch Ophthalmol 1992;110:185.

Jabs DA, Johns CJ: Ocular involvement in chronic sarcoidosis. Am J Ophthalmol 1986;102:297.

Kaplan HJ, Waldrep JC: Immunologic insights into uveitis and retinitis: The immunoregulatory circuit. Ophthalmology 1984;91:655.

Katz B (editor): Neuro-ophthalmology in systemic disease. Ophthalmol Clin North Am 1992;5:3.

Keltner JL: Giant-cell arteritis: Signs and symptoms. Ophthalmology 1982;89:1101.

Keltner JL et al: Dural and carotid cavernous sinus fistulas: Diagnosis, management, and complications. Ophthalmology 1987;94:1585.

Leonard TJ, Moseley IF, Sanders MD: Ophthalmoplegia in carotid cavernous sinus fistula. Br J Ophthalmol 1984;68:128.

Marsh RJ, Cooper M: Ophthalmic herpes zoster. Eye 1993;7:350.

McDonnell PJ et al: Ocular involvement in patients with fungal infections. Ophthalmology 1985;92:706.

Morinelli EN et al: Infectious multifocal choroiditis in patients with acquired immune deficiency syndrome. Ophthalmology. 1993;100:1014.

Nussenblatt RB, Palestine AG: *Uveitis: Fundamental and Clinical Practice.* Year Book, 1989.

O'Connor GR: Factors related to the initiation and recurrence of uveitis. Am J Ophthalmol 1983;96:577.

Orcutt JC, Page NGR, Sanders MD: Factors affecting visual loss in benign intracranial hypertension. Ophthalmology 1984;92:1303.

Rahi AHS, Barner A: *Immunopathology of the Eye.* Blackwell, 1976.

Rose FC (editor): *The Eye in General Medicine.* Chapman & Hall, 1983.

Rothova A: Ocular involvement in toxoplasmosis. Br J Ophthalmol 1993;77:371.

Sadun AA: The efficacy of optic nerve sheath decompression for anterior ischemia and other optic neuropathies. Am J Ophthalmol 1993;115:384.

Sanders MD, Hoyt WF: Hypoxic ocular sequelae of carotid-cavernous fistulae. Br J Ophthalmol 1969;53:82.

Tamesis RR, Roster CS: Ocular syphilis. Ophthalmology 1990;97:1281.

Wall M, George D: Idiopathic intracranial hypertension: A prospective study of 50 cases. Brain 1991;114:155.

Walsh JB: Hypertensive retinopathy: Description, classification, and prognosis. Ophthalmology 1982;89:1127.

Watson PG, Hazleman BL (editors): *The Sclera and Systemic Disorders.* Saunders, 1976.

Weinberg DV, Murphy R, Naughton K: Combined daily therapy with intravenous ganciclovir and foscarnet for patients with recurrent cytomegalovirus retinitis. Am J Ophthalmol 1994;117:776.

Whitcup SM et al: Intraocular lymphoma: Clinical and histological diagnosis. Ophthalmology 1993;100:1399.

Winkward KE, Hamed LM, Glaser JS: The spectrum of optic nerve disease in human immunodeficiency virus infection. Am J Ophthalmol 1989;107:373.

Winterkorn JMS: Lyme disease: Neurologic and ophthalmic manifestations. Surv Ophthalmol 1990;35:191.

Yohai RA et al: Survival factors in rhino-orbital-cerebral mucormycosis. Surv Ophthalmol 1994;39:3.

16

Immunologic Diseases of the Eye

William G. Hodge, MD, FRCS(C)

The eye is frequently considered to be a special target of immunologic disease processes, but proof of the causative role of these processes is lacking in some disorders. In this sense, the immunopathology of the eye is less clearly delineated than that of the kidney, the testis, or the thyroid gland. Because the eye is a highly vascularized organ and because the rather labile vessels of the conjunctiva are embedded in a nearly transparent medium, inflammatory eye disorders are more obvious (and often more painful) than those of other organs such as the thyroid or the kidney. The iris, ciliary body, and choroid are the most highly vascularized tissues of the eye. The similarity of the vascular supply of the uvea to that of the kidney and the choroid plexus of the brain has given rise to justified speculation concerning the selection of these three tissues, among others, as targets of immune complex diseases (eg, serum sickness).

Immunologic diseases of the eye can be grossly divided into two major categories: antibody-mediated and cell-mediated diseases. As is the case in other organs, there is ample opportunity for the interaction of these two systems in the eye.

ANTIBODY-DEPENDENT & ANTIBODY-MEDIATED DISEASES

Before it can be concluded that a disease of the eye is antibody-dependent, the following criteria must be satisfied:

(1) There must be evidence of specific antibody in the patient's serum or plasma cells.

(2) The antigen must be identified and, if feasible, characterized.

(3) The same antigen must be shown to produce an immunologic response in the eye of an experimental animal, and the pathologic changes produced in the experimental animal must be similar to those observed in the human disease.

(4) It must be possible to produce similar lesions in animals passively sensitized with serum from an affected animal upon challenge with the specific antigen.

Unless all of the above criteria are satisfied, the disease may be thought of as *possibly* antibody-dependent. In such circumstances, the disease can be regarded as antibody-mediated if only one of the following criteria is met:

(1) If antibody to an antigen is present in higher quantities in the ocular fluids than in the serum (after adjustments have been made for the total amounts of immunoglobulins in each fluid).

(2) If abnormal accumulations of plasma cells are present in the ocular lesion.

(3) If abnormal accumulations of immunoglobins are present at the site of the disease.

(4) If complement is fixed by immunoglobulins at the site of the disease.

(5) If an accumulation of eosinophils is present at the site of the disease.

(6) If the ocular disease is associated with an inflammatory disease elsewhere in the body for which antibody dependency has been proved or strongly suggested.

HAY FEVER CONJUNCTIVITIS
(See also Chapter 5.)

This disease is characterized by edema and hyperemia of the conjunctiva and lids (Figure 16–1) and by itching and watering of the eyes. There is often an associated itching sensation in the nose as well as rhinorrhea. The conjunctiva appears pale and boggy because of the intense edema, which is often rapid in onset. There is a distinct seasonal incidence, some patients being able to establish the onset of their symptoms at precisely the same time each year. These times usually correspond to the release of pollens by specific grasses, trees, or weeds.

Immunologic Pathogenesis

Hay fever conjunctivitis is one of the few inflammatory eye disorders for which antibody dependence has been definitely established. It is recognized as a form of atopic disease with an implied hereditary sus-

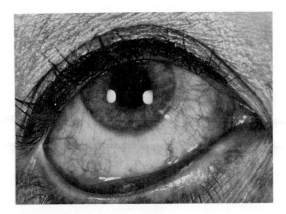

Figure 16–1. Hay fever conjunctivitis. Note edema and hyperemia of the conjunctiva. (Courtesy of M. allansmith and B. McClellan.)

ceptibility. IgE (reaginic antibody) is believed to be attached to mast cells lying beneath the conjunctival epithelium. Contact of the offending antigen with IgE triggers the release of vasoactive substances, principally leukotrienes and histamine, in this area, and this in turn results in vasodilation and chemosis.

The role of circulating antibody to ragweed pollen in the pathogenesis of hay fever conjunctivitis has been demonstrated by passively transferring serum from a hypersensitive person to a nonsensitive one. When exposed to the offending pollen, the previously nonsensitive individual reacted with the typical signs of hay fever conjunctivitis.

Immunologic Diagnosis

Victims of hay fever conjunctivitis show many eosinophils in Giemsa-stained scrapings of conjunctival epithelium. They show the immediate type of response, with wheal and flare, when tested by scratch tests of the skin with extracts of pollen or other offending antigens. Biopsies of the skin test sites have occasionally shown the full-blown picture of an Arthus reaction, with deposition of immune complexes in the walls of the dermal vessels. Passive cutaneous anaphylaxis can also be used to demonstrate the presence of circulating antibody.

Immunologic Treatment

Immunotherapy with gradually increasing doses of subcutaneously injected pollen extracts or other suspected allergens appears to reduce the severity of the disease in some individuals if started well in advance of the season. The mechanism is presumed to be production of blocking antibodies in response to the injection of small, graded doses of the antigen. This procedure cannot be recommended routinely, however, in view of the generally good results and relatively few complications of antihistamine therapy. Acute anaphylactoid reactions have occasionally resulted from overzealous immunotherapy. Antihistamine therapy is also often beneficial.

Other forms of treatment are discussed in Chapter 5.

VERNAL CONJUNCTIVITIS & ATOPIC KERATOCONJUNCTIVITIS (See also Chapter 5.)

These two diseases also belong to the group of atopic disorders. Both are characterized by itching and lacrimation of the eyes but are more chronic than hay fever conjunctivitis. Furthermore, both ultimately result in structural modifications of the lids and conjunctiva.

Vernal conjunctivitis characteristically affects children and adolescents; the incidence decreases sharply after the second decade of life. Like hay fever conjunctivitis, vernal conjunctivitis occurs only in the warm months of the year. Most of its victims live in hot, dry climates. The disease characteristically produces giant ("cobblestone") papillae of the tarsal conjunctiva (Figure 16–2). The keratinized epithelium from these papillae may abrade the underlying cornea, giving rise to complaints of foreign body sensation.

Atopic keratoconjunctivitis affects individuals of all ages and has no specific seasonal incidence. The skin of the lids has a characteristic dry, scaly appearance. The conjunctiva is pale and boggy. Both the conjunctiva and the cornea may develop scarring in the later stages of the disease. Atopic cataract has also been described. Staphylococcal blepharitis, manifested by scales and crusts on the lids, commonly complicates this disease. These patients are also more prone to herpes simplex ocular infections.

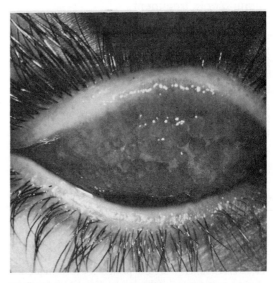

Figure 16–2. Giant papillae ("cobblestones") in the tarsal conjunctiva of a patient with vernal conjunctivitis.

Although vernal and atopic disease may lie along a disease spectrum, often the two disorders can be differentiated. Atopic disease tends to occur in older patients, and there is little or no seasonal exacerbation. The papillae in atopic disease are smaller than in vernal disease and are as often found on the lower palpebral conjunctiva as the upper. Furthermore, corneal vascularization and conjunctival scarring are much more common in atopic disease. Finally, in atopic disease eosinophils on smears are less numerous and less often degranulated.

Immunologic Pathogenesis

Reaginic antibody (IgE) is fixed to subepithelial mast cells in both of these conditions. Contact between the offending antigen and IgE is thought to trigger degranulation of the mast cell, which in turn allows for the release of vasoactive amines in the tissues. It is unlikely, however, that antibody action alone is responsible, since—at least in the case of papillae of vernal conjunctivitis—there is heavy papillary infiltration by mononuclear cells. Hay fever and asthma occur much more frequently in patients with vernal conjunctivitis and atopic keratoconjunctivitis than in the general population. Of the criteria outlined above for demonstration of *possibly* antibody-dependent diseases, (2), (5), and (6) have been met by atopic keratoconjunctivitis.

Immunologic Diagnosis

Patients with atopic keratoconjunctivitis and vernal conjunctivitis generally show large numbers of eosinophils in conjunctival scrapings. Skin testing with food extracts, pollens, and various other antigens reveals a wheal-and-flare type of reaction within 1 hour after testing, but the significance of these reactions is not established.

Immunologic Treatment

Avoidance of known allergens is helpful; such objects as duck feathers, animal danders, and certain food proteins (egg albumin and others) are common offenders. Specific allergens have been much more difficult to demonstrate in the case of vernal disease, though some workers feel that such substances as rye grass pollens may play a causative role. Installation of air conditioning in the home or relocation to a cool, moist climate is useful in vernal conjunctivitis.

Other treatments are discussed in Chapter 5.

JOINT DISEASES AFFECTING THE EYE

The diseases in this category vary greatly in their clinical manifestations depending upon the specific disease entity and the age of the patient. **Uveitis** and **scleritis** (Chapter 7) are the principal ocular manifestations associated with joint diseases. **Juvenile**

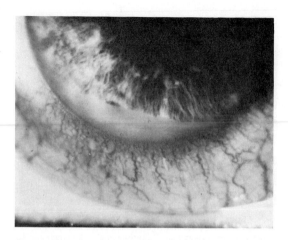

Figure 16–3. Acute iridocyclitis in a patient with ankylosing spondylitis. Note fibrin clot in anterior chamber.

rheumatoid arthritis affects females more frequently than males and is commonly accompanied by iridocyclitis of one or both eyes (see Chapter 17).

Ankylosing spondylitis affects males more frequently than females, and the onset is in the second to sixth decades. It may be accompanied by iridocyclitis of acute onset, often with fibrin in the anterior chamber (Figure 16–3).

Reiter's disease affects men more frequently than women. The first attack of ocular inflammation usually consists of a self-limited papillary conjunctivitis. It follows, at a highly variable interval, the onset of nonspecific urethritis and the appearance of inflammation in one or more of the weight-bearing joints. Subsequent attacks of ocular inflammation may consist of acute iridocyclitis of one or both eyes, occasionally with hypopyon (Figure 16–4). **Rheumatoid**

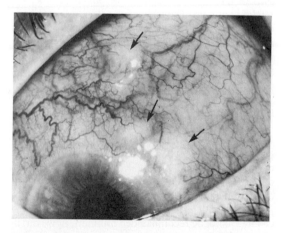

Figure 16–4. Acute iridocyclitis with hypopyon in a patient with Reiter's disease.

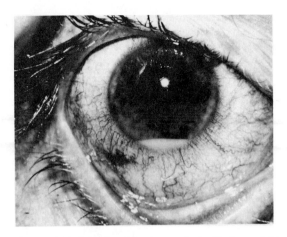

Figure 16–5. Scleral nodules in a patient with rheumatoid arthritis. (Courtesy of S Kimura.)

arthritis of adult onset may be accompanied by acute scleritis or episcleritis (Figure 16–5). (See also Chapter 7.)

Immunologic Pathogenesis

Rheumatoid factor, an IgM autoantibody directed against the patient's own IgG, may play a major role in the pathogenesis of rheumatoid arthritis. The union of IgM antibody with IgG is followed by fixation of complement at the tissue site and the attraction of leukocytes and platelets to this area. An occlusive vasculitis, resulting from this chain of events, is thought to be the cause of rheumatoid nodule formation in the sclera as well as elsewhere in the body. The occlusion of vessels supplying nutrients to the sclera is thought to be responsible for the "melting away" of the scleral collagen that is so characteristic of rheumatoid arthritis (Figure 16–6).

While this explanation may suffice for rheumatoid

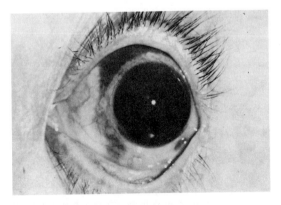

Figure 16–6. Scleral thinning in a patient with rheumatoid arthritis. Note dark color of the underlying uvea.

arthritis, patients with the ocular complications of juvenile rheumatoid arthritis, ankylosing spondylitis, and Reiter's syndrome usually have negative tests for rheumatoid factor, so other explanations must be sought.

Outside the eyeball itself, the lacrimal gland has been shown to be under attack by circulating antibodies. Destruction of acinar cells within the gland and invasion of the lacrimal gland (as well as the salivary glands) by mononuclear cells result in decreased tear secretion. The combination of dry eyes (keratoconjunctivitis sicca), dry mouth (xerostomia), and rheumatoid arthritis is known as Sjögren's syndrome (see Chapter 15).

A growing body of evidence indicates that the immunogenetic background of certain patients accounts for the expression of their ocular inflammatory disease in specific ways. Analysis of the HLA antigen system shows that the incidence of HLA-B27 is significantly greater in patients with ankylosing spondylitis and Reiter's syndrome than could be expected by chance alone. It is not known how this antigen controls specific inflammatory responses. Other well-established HLA disease associations include HLA-A11 in sympathetic ophthalmia, HLA-A29 in birdshot choroidopathy, HLA-B51 in Behçet's syndrome, and HLA-B7 in macular histoplasmosis.

Immunologic Diagnosis

Rheumatoid factor can be detected in the serum by a number of standard tests involving the agglutination of IgG-coated erythrocytes or latex particles. Unfortunately, the test for rheumatoid factor is not positive in the majority of isolated rheumatoid afflictions of the eye.

The HLA types of individuals suspected of having ankylosing spondylitis and related diseases can be determined. HLA-B27 is associated with ankylosing spondylitis and Reiter's syndrome. X-ray of the sacroiliac area is a valuable screening procedure that may show evidence of spondylitis prior to the onset of low back pain in patients with the characteristic form of iridocyclitis.

OTHER ANTIBODY-MEDIATED EYE DISEASES (See also Chapter 15.)

The following antibody-mediated diseases are infrequently encountered by the practicing ophthalmologist.

Systemic lupus erythematosus, associated with the presence of circulating antibodies to DNA, produces an occlusive vasculitis of the nerve fiber layer of the retina. Such infarcts result in cytoid bodies or "cotton wool" spots in the retina (Figure 16–7).

Pemphigus vulgaris produces painful intraepithe-

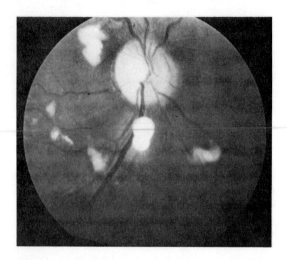

Figure 16–7. "Cotton wool" spots in the retina of a patient with lupus erythematosus.

lial bullae of the conjunctiva. It is associated with the presence of circulating antibodies to an intercellular antigen located between the deeper cells of the conjunctival epithelium.

Cicatricial pemphigoid is characterized by subepithelial bullae of the conjunctiva. In the chronic stages of this disease, cicatricial contraction of the conjunctiva may result in severe scarring of the cornea, dryness of the eyes, and ultimate blindness. Pemphigoid is associated with local deposits of tissue antibodies directed against one or more antigens located in the basement membrane of the epithelium. Immunosuppressive treatment is often needed in the progressive stages of this disease. Immunosuppressive treatment is often needed in the progressive stages of this disease.

Lens-induced uveitis is a rare condition that may be associated with circulating antibodies to lens proteins. It is seen in individuals whose lens capsules have become permeable to these proteins as a result of trauma or other disease (see Chapter 7). Interest in this field dates back to Uhlenhuth (1903), who first demonstrated the organ-specific nature of antibodies to the lens. Witmer showed in 1962 that antibody to lens tissue may be produced by lymphoid cells of the ciliary body.

CELL-MEDIATED DISEASES

This group of diseases appears to be associated with cell-mediated immunity or delayed hypersensitivity.

Various structures of the eye are invaded by mononuclear cells, principally lymphocytes and macrophages, in response to one or more chronic antigenic stimuli. In the case of chronic infections such as tuberculosis, leprosy, toxoplasmosis, and herpes simplex, the antigenic stimulus has clearly been identified as an infectious agent in the ocular tissue. Such infections are often associated with delayed skin test reactivity following the intradermal injection of an extract of the organism.

More intriguing but less well understood are the granulomatous diseases of the eye for which no infectious cause has been found. Such diseases are thought to represent cell-mediated, possibly autoimmune processes, but their origin remains obscure.

OCULAR SARCOIDOSIS

Ocular sarcoidosis is characterized by a panuveitis with occasional inflammatory involvement of the optic nerve and retinal blood vessels (see Chapter 7).

Immunologic Pathogenesis

Although many infectious or allergic causes of sarcoidosis have been suggested, none has been confirmed. Noncaseating granulomas are seen in the uvea, optic nerve, and adnexal structures of the eye as well as elsewhere in the body. The presence of macrophages and giant cells suggests that particulate matter is being phagocytosed, but this material has not been identified.

Patients with sarcoidosis are usually anergic to extracts of the common microbial antigens such as those of mumps, *Trichophyton, Candida,* and *Mycobacterium tuberculosis.* As in other lymphoproliferative disorders such as Hodgkin's disease and chronic lymphocytic leukemia, this may represent suppression of T cell activity such that the normal delayed hypersensitivity responses to common antigens cannot take place. Meanwhile, circulating immunoglobins are usually detectable in the serum at higher than normal levels.

Immunologic Diagnosis

The diagnosis is largely inferential. Negative skin tests to a battery of antigens to which the patient is known to have been exposed are highly suggestive, and the same is true of the elevation of serum immunoglobulins. Biopsy of a conjunctival nodule or scalene lymph node may provide positive histologic evidence of the disease. X-rays of the chest reveal hilar adenopathy in many cases. Elevated levels of serum lysozyme, serum angiotensin-converting enzyme, or serum calcium may be detected.

Treatment

See Chapter 15.

SYMPATHETIC OPHTHALMIA & VOGT-KOYANAGI-HARADA SYNDROME

These two disorders are discussed together because they have certain common clinical features. Both are thought to represent autoimmune phenomena affecting pigmented structures of the eye and skin, and both may give rise to meningeal symptoms.

Clinical Features

Sympathetic ophthalmia is an inflammation in the second eye after the other has been damaged by penetrating injury. In most cases, some portion of the uvea of the injured eye has been exposed to the atmosphere for at least 1 hour. The uninjured or "sympathizing" eye develops minor signs of anterior uveitis after a period ranging from 2 weeks to many years. However, the vast majority of cases occur within 1 year. Floating spots and loss of the power of accommodation are among the earliest symptoms. The disease may progress to severe iridocyclitis with pain and photophobia. Usually, however, the eye remains relatively quiet and painless while the inflammatory disease spreads around the entire uvea. Despite the presence of panuveitis, the retina usually remains uninvolved except for perivascular cuffing of the retinal vessels with inflammatory cells. Papilledema and secondary glaucoma may occur. The disease may be accompanied by vitiligo (patchy depigmentation of the skin) and poliosis (whitening) of the eyelashes.

Vogt-Koyanagi-Harada syndrome consists of inflammation of the uvea of one or both eyes characterized by acute iridocyclitis, patchy choroiditis, and serous detachment of the retina (see Chapter 15). It usually begins with an acute febrile episode with headache, dysacusis, and occasionally vertigo. Patchy loss or whitening of scalp hair is described in the first few months of the disease. Vitiligo and poliosis are commonly present but are not essential for the diagnosis. Although the initial iridocyclitis may subside quickly, the course of the posterior disease is often indolent, with long-standing serous detachment of the retina and significant visual impairment.

Immunologic Pathogenesis

In both sympathetic ophthalmia and Vogt-Koyanagi-Harada syndrome, delayed hypersensitivity to melanin-containing structures is thought to occur. Although a viral cause has been suggested for both of these disorders, there is no convincing evidence of an infectious origin. It is postulated that some insult, infectious or otherwise, alters the pigmented structures of the eye, skin, and hair in such a way as to provoke delayed hypersensitivity responses to them. Soluble materials from the outer segments of the photoreceptor layer of the retina (retinal S-antigens) have recently been incriminated as possible autoantigens. Patients with Vogt-Koyanagi-Harada syndrome are usually Orientals, which suggests an immunogenetic predisposition to the disease.

Histologic sections of the traumatized eye from a patient with sympathetic ophthalmia may show uniform infiltration of most of the uvea by lymphocytes, epithelioid cells, and giant cells. The overlying retina is characteristically intact, but nests of epithelioid cells may protrude through the pigment epithelium of the retina, giving rise to **Dalen-Fuchs nodules.** The inflammation may destroy the architecture of the entire uvea, leaving an atrophic, shrunken globe.

Immunologic Diagnosis

Skin tests with soluble extracts of human or bovine uveal tissue are said to elicit delayed hypersensitivity responses in these patients. Several investigators have recently shown that cultured lymphocytes from patients with these two diseases undergo transformation to lymphoblasts in vitro when extracts of uvea or rod outer segments are added to the culture medium. Circulating antibodies to uveal antigens have been found in patients with these diseases, but such antibodies are to be found in any patient with long-standing uveitis, including those suffering from several infectious entities. The spinal fluid of patients with Vogt-Koyanagi-Harada syndrome may show increased numbers of mononuclear cells and elevated protein in the early stages.

OTHER DISEASES OF CELL-MEDIATED IMMUNITY

Giant cell arteritis (temporal arteritis) (see Chapter 16) may have disastrous effects on the eye, particularly in elderly individuals. The condition is manifested by temporal arteritis and polymyalgia rheumatica. Ocular complications include anterior ischemic optic neuropathy and central retinal artery occlusion. Such patients have an elevated sedimentation rate. Biopsy of the temporal artery reveals extensive infiltration of the vessel wall with giant cells and mononuclear cells.

Polyarteritis nodosa (see Chapter 15) is a vasculitis which predominantly affects small to medium-sized vessels. It can affect both the anterior and posterior segments of the eye. The corneas of such patients may show peripheral thinning and cellular infiltration. The retinal vessels reveal extensive necrotizing inflammation characterized by eosinophil, plasma cell, and lymphocyte infiltration.

Behçet's disease (see Chapter 15) has an uncertain place in the classification of immunologic disorders. It is characterized by recurrent iridocyclitis with hy-

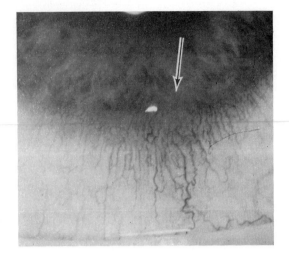

Figure 16–8. Phlyctenule (arrow) at the margin of the cornea. (Courtesy of P Thygeson.)

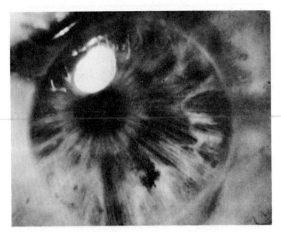

Figure 16–9. A cornea severely scarred by chronic atopic keratoconjunctivitis into which a central graft of clear cornea has been placed. Note how distinctly the iris landmarks are seen through the transparent graft. (Reproduced, with permission, from Stites DP, Terr AI [editors]: *Basic & Clinical immunology,* 7th ed. Appleton & Lange, 1991.)

popyon and occlusive vasculitis of the retinal vessels. Although it has many of the features of a delayed hypersensitivity disease, dramatic alterations of serum complement levels at the very beginning of an attack suggest an immune complex disorder. Furthermore, high levels of circulating immune complexes have recently been detected in patients with this disease. Most patients with eye symptoms are positive for HLA-B51, a subtype of HLA-B5.

Contact dermatitis of the eyelids represents a significant though minor disease caused by delayed hypersensitivity. Atropine, perfumed cosmetics, materials contained in plastic spectacle frames, and other locally applied agents may act as the sensitizing hapten. The lower lid is more extensively involved than the upper lid when the sensitizing agent is applied in drop form. Periorbital involvement with erythematous, vesicular, pruritic lesions of the skin is characteristic.

Phlyctenular keratoconjunctivitis (Figure 16–8) represents a delayed hypersensitivity response to certain microbial antigens, principally those of *M tuberculosis* and *Staphylococcus aureus* (see Chapter 5 and 6).

CORNEAL GRAFT REACTIONS
(Figure 16–9)

Blindness due to opacity or distortion of the central portion of the cornea is a remediable disease. If all other structures of the eye are intact, a patient whose vision is impaired solely by corneal opacity can expect great improvement from a graft of clear cornea into the diseased area (see Chapter 6). Trauma, including chemical burns, is one of the most common causes of central corneal opacity. Others include scars from herpetic keratitis, endothelial cell dysfunction with chronic corneal edema (including pseudophakic bullous keratopathy and Fuchs's dystrophy), keratoconus, and opacities from previous graft failures. All of these conditions represent indications for penetrating corneal grafts, provided the patient's eye is no longer inflamed and the opacity has been allowed maximal time to undergo spontaneous resolution (usually 6–12 months). It is estimated that approximately 10,000 corneal grafts are performed in the USA annually. Of these, about 90% can be expected to produce a beneficial result.

The cornea was one of the first human tissues to be successfully grafted. The fact that recipients of corneal grafts generally tolerate them well can be attributed to (1) the absence of blood vessels or lymphatics in the normal cornea, (2) the lack of presensitization to tissue-specific antigens in most recipients, and (3) anterior chamber acquired immune deviation (ACAID). This is a series of unique immunologic properties of the anterior chamber, the most important of which is delayed hypersensitivity. Reactions to corneal grafts do occur, however, particularly in individuals whose own corneas have been damaged by previous inflammatory disease. Such corneas may have developed both lymphatics and blood vessels, providing afferent and efferent channels for immunologic reactions in the engrafted cornea.

Although attempts have been made to transplant

corneas from other species into human eyes (xenografts), particularly in countries where human material is not available for religious reasons, most corneal grafts have been taken from human eyes (allografts). Except in the case of identical twins, such grafts always represent the implantation of foreign tissue into a donor site; thus, the chance for a graft rejection due to an immune response to foreign antigens is virtually always present.

The cornea is a three-layered structure composed of a surface epithelium, an oligocellular collagenous stroma, and a single-layered endothelium. Although the surface epithelium may be sloughed and later replaced by the recipient's epithelium, certain elements of the stroma and all of the donor's endothelium remain in place for the rest of the patient's life. This has been firmly established by sex chromosome markers in corneal cells when donor and recipient were of opposite sexes. The endothelium must remain healthy in order for the cornea to remain transparent, and an energy-dependent pump mechanism is required to keep the cornea from swelling with water. Since the recipient's endothelium is in most cases diseased, the central corneal endothelium must be replaced by healthy donor tissue.

A number of foreign elements exist in corneal grafts that might stimulate the immune system of the host to reject this tissue. In addition to those mentioned above, the corneal stroma is regularly perfused with IgG and serum albumin from the donor, although none of the other blood proteins are present—or only small amounts. While these serum proteins of donor origin rapidly diffuse into the recipient stroma and are thus removed from the graft site, they are theoretically immunogenic. The HLA antigen system may play a significant role in graft reactions. HLA incompatibility between donor and recipient has been shown by several authors to be significant in determining graft survival, particularly when the corneal bed is vascularized. It is known that most cells of the body possess these HLA antigens, including the endothelial cells of the corneal graft as well as certain stromal cells (keratocytes). The epithelium has been shown by Hall and others to possess a non-HLA antigen that diffuses into the anterior third of the stroma. Thus, while much foreign antigen may be eliminated by purposeful removal of the epithelium at the time of grafting, that amount of antigen which has already diffused into the stroma is automatically carried over into the recipient.

Despite numerous analytic studies supporting the role of HLA incompatibility in corneal graft rejection, a recent multicenter clinical trial found no use in HLA typing high risk grafts. In this study, ABO blood typing did provide a slight protective effect in high-risk cases. These surprising findings are leading many investigators to restudy the role of major and minor antigens in corneal graft rejection.

Both humoral and cellular mechanisms have been implicated in corneal graft reactions. It is likely that early graft rejections (2–4 weeks from surgery) are cell-mediated reactions. Cytotoxic lymphocytes have been found in the limbal area and stroma of affected individuals, and phase microscopy in vivo has revealed an actual attack on the grafted endothelial cells by these lymphocytes. Such lymphocytes generally move inward from the periphery of the cornea, making what is known as a "rejection line" as they move centrally. The donor cornea becomes edematous as the endothelium becomes compromised by an accumulation of lymphoid cells.

Late rejection of a corneal graft may occur several weeks to many months after implantation of donor tissue into the recipient eye. Such reactions may be antibody-mediated, since cytotoxic antibodies have been isolated from the serum of patients with a history of multiple graft reactions in vascularized corneal beds. These antibody reactions are complement-dependent and attract polymorphonuclear leukocytes, which may form dense rings in the cornea at the sites of maximum deposition of immune complexes. In experimental animals, similar reactions have been produced by corneal xenografts, but the intensity of the reaction can be markedly reduced either by decomplementing the animal or by reducing its leukocyte population through mechlorethamine therapy.

Treatment

The mainstay of the treatment of corneal graft reactions is corticosteroid therapy. This medication is generally given in the form of frequently applied eye drops (eg, 1% prednisolone acetate every hour) until the clinical signs abate. These clinical signs consist of conjunctival hyperemia in the perilimbal region, a cloudy cornea, cells and protein in the anterior chamber, and keratic precipitates on the corneal endothelium. The earlier treatment is applied, the more effective it is likely to be. Neglected cases may require systemic or periocular corticosteroids in addition to local eye drop therapy. Occasionally, vascularization and opacification of the cornea occur so rapidly as to make corticosteroid therapy useless, but even the most hopeless-appearing graft reactions have occasionally been reversed by corticosteroid therapy. Oral cyclosporine has been used successfully in the treatment of corneal graft rejection, and some benefit has also been derived from cyclosporine eye drops.

Patients known to have rejected many previous corneal grafts are managed somewhat differently, particularly if disease affects their only remaining eye. Some surgeons may choose to find a close HLA match between donor and recipient, but conflicting analytic studies make doing so of questionable use. An attempt is made to find a close HLA match between donor and recipient. Pretreatment of the recipient with immunosuppressive agents such as azathioprine has also been resorted to in some cases.

REFERENCES

Boisjoly HM et al: Risk factors of corneal graft failure. Ophthalmology 1993;100:1728.

Chandler JW, Gillette TE: Immunologic defense mechanisms of the ocular surface. Ophthalmology 1983;90:585.

Foulks GN et al: Histocompatibility testing for keratoplasty in high-risk patients. Ophthalmology 1983;90:239.

Friedlaender MH, O'Connor GR: *Eye diseases.* In: *Basic & Clinical Immunology,* 8th ed. Stites DP, Terr AI (editors). Appleton & Lange, 1994.

Froebel KS et al: An investigation of the general immune status and specific immune responsiveness to retinal-(S)-antigen in patients with chronic posterior uveitis. Eye 1989;3:263.

Hylkema HA et al: Circulating immune complexes in uveitis patients. Int Ophthalmol 1989;13:253.

Jakobiec FA, Lefkowitch J, Knowles DM II: B- and T-lymphocytes in ocular disease. Ophthalmology 1984;91:635.

Kanski JJ: Juvenile arthritis and uveitis. Surv Ophthalmol 1990;34:253.

Kaplan HJ, Waldrep JC: Immunologic insights into uveitis and retinitis: The immunoregulatory circuit. Ophthalmology 1984;91:655.

Klok AM et al: Antibodies against ocular and oral antigens in Behçet's disease associated with uveitis. Curr Eye Res 1989;8:957.

Mizuno K, Clark AF, Streilein JW: Anterior chamber-associated immune deviation induced by soluble antigens. Invest Ophthalmol Vis Sci 1989;30:1112.

Nichols CW et al: Conjunctival biopsy as an aid in evaluation of the patient with suspected sarcoidosis. Ophthalmology 1980;87:287.

Nussenblatt RB: HLA and ocular disease. Proceedings of the Immunology of the Eye Workshop 1. Steinberg GM, Gery I, Nussenblatt RB (editors). Immunology Abstracts 1980;Spring Suppl:25.

Nussenblatt RB: Immunoregulation of uveitis. Int Ophthalmol 1990;14:13.

Nussenblatt RB, Palestine AG: *Uveitis: Fundamentals and Clinical Practice.* Year Book, 1989.

O'Connor GR, Chandler JW (editors): *Advances in Immunology and Immunopathology of the Eye.* Masson, 1985.

Rahi AHS, Garner A: *Immunopathology of the Eye.* Blackwell, 1976.

Rosenbaum JT: An algorithm for the systemic evaluation of patients with uveitis: Guidelines for the consultant. Semin Arthritis Rheum 1990;19:248.

Sacks EH et al: Lymphocytic subpopulations in the normal human conjunctiva: A monoclonal antibody study. Ophthalmology 1986;93:1276.

Salisbury JD, Gebhardt BM: Suppression of corneal allograft rejection by cyclosporin A. Arch Ophthalmol 1981; 99:1640.

Smolin G, O'Connor GR: *Ocular Immunology,* 2nd ed. Lea & Febiger, 1986.

Theodore FH, Bloomfield SE, Mondino BJ: *Clinical Allergy and Immunology of the Eye.* Williams & Wilkins, 1983.

Special Subjects of Pediatric Interest

17

Douglas R. Fredrick, MD

Pediatric ophthalmology offers particular challenges to the ophthalmologist, pediatrician, and family physician. Symptoms are often nonspecific, and the usual examination techniques require modification. Development of the visual system is still occurring during the first decade of life, with the potential for amblyopia even in response to relatively mild ocular disease. Because the development of the eye often reflects organ and tissue development of the body as a whole, many congenital somatic defects are mirrored in the eye. Collaboration with pediatricians, neurologists, and other health workers is essential in managing these conditions. Similar collaboration is required in assessing the educational needs of any child with poor vision.

Details of the embryology and the normal postnatal growth and development of the eye are discussed in Chapter 1.

NEONATAL OCULAR EXAMINATION

A careful eye examination soon after birth may reveal congenital abnormalities that suggest the presence of abnormalities elsewhere in the body and the need for further investigations. Recent demonstration of the value of retinal cryotherapy in the treatment of retinopathy of prematurity has highlighted the need for careful retinal examination of at-risk preterm babies.

The instruments required for the ocular examination of the newborn are a good hand light, direct and indirect ophthalmoscopes, a loupe for magnification, and occasionally a portable slitlamp. Phenylephrine 2.5% and cyclopentolate 1% or tropicamide 1% are generally safe for pupillary dilation in full-term neonates, though even these concentrations may have adverse effects on blood pressure and gastrointestinal function. The combination of cyclopentolate 0.2% and phenylephrine 1% (Cyclomydril) should be used to dilate the pupils of low-weight neonates.

Subjective response testing is limited to observing the following response to a visual target, of which the most effective is a human face—particularly the mother's face. Visual fixation and following movements can be demonstrated in most newborn babies. Following movements in this age group are usually coarse and jerky and should not be expected to resem-

---

PEDIATRIC EYE EXAMINATION SCHEDULE

Neonatal Examination
External eye examination and ophthalmoscopic examination through dilated pupils as outlined in the text. Two drops of sterile 2.5% phenylephrine and 1% cyclopentolate or 1% tropicamide in each eye are instilled 1 hour prior to examination. (Cyclopentolate 0.2% and phenylephrine 1% combination [Cyclomydril] may be sufficient in babies with lightly pigmented eyes and low-weight neonates.) Special emphasis should be placed on the optic disks and maculas; detailed examination of the peripheral retinas is not necessary unless the baby is at risk for retinopathy of prematurity.

Age 6 Months
Test ocular fixation and ocular movement. Look for strabismus.

Age 4 years
Test visual acuity with illiterate "E" chart or HOTV matching optotypes, and stereopsis by the random dot "E" test or Titmus stereo test. Visual acuity should be normal 20/20–20/30.

Age 5–16 years
Test visual acuity at age 5. If normal, test visual acuity with the Snellen chart every 2 years until age 16. Color vision should be tested at ages 8–12. No other routine eye examination (eg, ophthalmoscopy) is necessary if visual acuity is normal and the eyes appear normal upon inspection.

---

ble the smooth pursuit movements of older children and adults. The characteristics of the nystagmus induced by whole body rotation can be quite valuable in assessment of both the visual pathways and the control of eye movements in neonates, but their evaluation is complex.

External Inspection

The eyelids are inspected for growths, deformities, lid notches, and symmetric movement with opening and closing of the eyes. The absolute and relative size of the eyeballs is noted, as well as position and alignment. The size and luster of the corneas are noted, and the anterior chambers are examined for clarity and iris configuration. The size, position, and light reaction of the pupils are also noted. The pupils are normally relatively dilated until 29 weeks of gestation, at which time the pupillary light response first becomes apparent. The light response is not a reliable test until 32 weeks of gestation. Anisocoria of 0.5 mm can be seen in as many as 20% of neonates.

Ophthalmoscopic Examination

With undilated pupils, some information can be obtained by use of the ophthalmoscope in a dimly lighted room. Ideally, however, all newborns should be examined with an ophthalmoscope through dilated pupils. Ophthalmoscopic examination will demonstrate any corneal, lens, or vitreous opacities as well as abnormalities in the fundus. In premature infants, remnants of the tunica vasculosa lentis are frequently visible, either in front of the lens, behind the lens, or in both positions. The remnants are usually absorbed by the time the infant has reached term, but rarely they remain permanently and appear as a complete or partial "cobweb" in the pupil. At other times, remnants of the primitive hyaloid system fail to absorb completely, leaving a cone on the optic disk that projects into the vitreous and is called Bergmeister's papilla.

Physiologic cupping of the disk is usually not seen in premature infants and is rarely seen at term; if seen then, it is usually very slight. In such cases the optic disk will appear gray, resembling optic nerve atrophy. This relative pallor, however, gradually changes to the normal adult pink color at about 2 years of age. Preretinal and intraretinal hemorrhages have been reported in 30–45% of newborns, usually clearing completely within a few weeks and leaving no permanent visual dysfunction.

OCULAR EXAMINATION OF INFANTS & YOUNG CHILDREN

Tests for Visual Acuity

In the early years, visual acuity should be appraised as part of each general "well child" examination. It is best not to wait until the child is old enough to respond to visual charts, since these may not furnish accurate information until school age.

During the first 3–4 years, estimations of vision rely greatly on observation and reports about the child's behavior both at play and during interactions with parents and with other children. Unfortunately, at this age seemingly normal visual performance is possible with relatively poor vision, and obviously abnormal performance probably reflects extremely poor acuity. The influence of visual impairment on motor and social development must always be borne in mind. The pupillary responses to light are a gross test of visual function and are reliable only for ruling out complete dysfunction of the anterior visual or efferent pupillary pathways. The ability to fixate and follow a target is much more informative. The target must be appropriate to the age of the child. Binocular following and converging reflexes are best examined first to establish the child's cooperation. Each eye should then be tested

separately, preferably with occlusion of the fellow eye by an adhesive patch. Comparison of the performance of the two eyes will give useful information about their relative acuities. Resistance to occlusion of one eye strongly suggests it is the preferred eye and therefore that the fellow eye must have comparatively poor vision. In cases of latent nystagmus—nystagmus increasing with occlusion of one eye—the child is likely to resent occlusion of each eye because of the effect such nystagmus has on visual acuity. Manifest nystagmus is indicative of an anterior visual pathway disorder or other central nervous system disease until these have been excluded. (Further discussion of the assessment of nystagmus is given in Chapter 14).

After 3 months of age, the presence of strabismus, detected by examining the relative position of the corneal light reflections, must also be regarded as indicative of poor vision in the deviated eye, particularly if this eye does not take up or is slow to take up fixation of a light upon occlusion of the fellow eye. (Further discussion of the assessment of strabismus is given in Chapter 12.)

These inferences about the status of the developing sensory systems can now be augmented by the quantitative techniques of optokinetic nystagmus, forced-choice preferential looking methods, and visually evoked responses (see Chapter 2). Although visually evoked potentials have suggested that normal adult visual acuity is attained before 2 years of age, this is probably an overestimate and it is likely that 3–4 years of age is a more accurate estimate (Table 17–1). Forced-choice preferential looking methods have gained increasing popularity as a reliable and relatively easy assessment of visual acuity in preverbal children, even in the very young. They do, however, have a tendency to overestimate visual acuity in amblyopes.

From about age 4 on, it becomes possible to elicit subjective responses by use of the illiterate "E" chart. Usually, at the first- or second-grade level, the regular Snellen chart may be employed. Stereoacuity can be shown to develop in most infants beginning at 3 months of age, but clinical testing is not generally possible until 3–4 years of age. Absence of stereopsis, as judged with the random dot "E" test or the Titmus stereo test, is suggestive of strabismus or amblyopia and the need for further investigation.

Refraction

Objective refraction is an important part of the pediatric ophthalmic examination, especially if there is

Table 17–1. Development of visual acuity (approximate).

Age	Visual Acuity
2 months	20/400
6 months	20/100
1 year	20/50
3 years	20/20

any suggestion of poor vision or strabismus. In young children, this should be performed under cycloplegia in order to overcome the child's tendency to accommodate. In many circumstances, 1% cyclopentolate drops applied twice—separated by an interval of 5 minutes—30 minutes prior to examination will provide sufficient cycloplegia, but atropine is recommended if convergent strabismus is present or the eyes are heavily pigmented. Because atropine drops are commonly associated with systemic side effects, 1% atropine ointment applied 2–3 times a day for 2 or 3 days prior to examination is the recommended regimen. The parents should be warned of the symptoms of atropine toxicity—fever, flushed face, and rapid pulse—and the necessity for discontinuing treatment, cooling the child with sponge bathing, and, in severe cases, seeking urgent medical assistance. Cycloplegic refraction provides the additional advantage of good mydriasis to facilitate fundal examination.

About 80% of children between the ages of 2 and 6 years are hyperopic, 5% are myopic, and 15% are emmetropic. About 10% have refractive errors that require correction before age 7 or 8. Hyperopia remains relatively static or gradually diminishes until 19 or 20 years of age. Myopia often develops between ages 6 and 9 and increases throughout adolescence, with the greatest change at the time of puberty. Astigmatism is relatively common in babies but decreases in prevalence during the first few years of life. Thereafter, it remains relatively constant in prevalence and degree throughout life.

Anterior & Posterior Segment Examination

Further examination needs to be tailored to each child's age and ability to cooperate. Anterior segment examination in the young child relies mainly upon the use of a hand light and magnifying loupe, but slitlamp examination is often possible in babies with the cooperation of the mother—and in young children with appropriate encouragement. Measurement of intraocular pressure and gonioscopy are more of a problem and frequently necessitate examination under anesthetic. Fundal examination relies upon good mydriasis. It is generally easier in neonates and babies than in young children because they can be restrained easily by being wrapped in a blanket.

The foveal light reflection is absent in infants. Instead, the macula has a bright "mother-of-pearl" appearance with a suggestion of elevation. This is more pronounced in black infants. At 3–4 months of age, the macula becomes slightly concave and the foveal light reflection appears.

The peripheral fundus in the infant is gray, in contrast to the orange-red fundus of the adult. In white infants, the pigmentation is more pronounced near the posterior pole and gradually fades to almost white at the periphery. In black infants, there is more pigment in the fundus, and a gray-blue sheen is seen through-

out the periphery. In white infants, a white periphery is normal and should not be confused with retinoblastoma. During the next several months, pigment continues to be deposited in the retina, and usually at about 2 years of age the adult color is evident.

CONGENITAL OCULAR ABNORMALITIES

Congenital defects of the ocular structures fall into two main categories: (1) developmental anomalies, of which genetic defects are an important cause; and (2) tissue reactions to intrauterine insults (infections, drugs, etc).

Congenital Abnormalities of the Globe

Failure of formation of the optic vesicle results in **anophthalmos.** Failure of invagination leads to a **congenital cystic eye.** Failure of closure produces **colobomas of the iris, retina, and choroid. Cryptophthalmos** occurs when the eyelids fail to separate.

Abnormally small eyes can be divided into **nanophthalmos,** in which function is normal, and **microphthalmos,** in which function is abnormal and there may be other ocular abnormalities such as cataract, coloboma, or congenital cyst.

Lid Abnormalities

Congenital ptosis is commonly due to dystrophy of the levator muscle of the upper lid. Other causes are congenital Horner's syndrome and congenital third nerve palsy.

Palpebral coloboma is a cleft of usually the upper lid, due to incomplete fusion of fetal maxillary processes. Large defects require early repair to avoid corneal ulceration due to exposure.

Corneal Defects

There may be partial or complete opacity of the corneas such as is found in congenital glaucoma, forceps injuries at birth, faulty development of the corneal endothelium, developmental anterior segment abnormalities with persistent corneal-lens attachments, intrauterine inflammation, interstitial keratitis, and mucopolysaccharide depositions of the cornea as in Hurler's syndrome. The most frequent cause of opaque corneas in infants and young children is congenital glaucoma, in which the eye is often larger than normal (buphthalmos). Forceps injuries at birth may cause extensive corneal opacities with edema as a result of rupture of Descemet's membrane. These usually clear spontaneously.

Megalocornea is an enlarged cornea with normal clarity and function, usually transmitted as an X-linked recessive trait. It must be differentiated from congenital glaucoma. There are usually no associated defects.

Iris & Pupillary Defects

Misplaced or ectopic pupils (corectopia) are frequently observed. The usual displacement is upward and laterally (temporally) from the center of the cornea. Such displacement is occasionally associated with ectopic lens, congenital glaucoma, or microcornea. Multiple pupils are known as **polycoria.** **Coloboma of the iris** indicates incomplete closure of the fetal ocular cleft and usually occurs inferiorly and nasally. It may be associated with coloboma of the lens, choroid, and optic nerve. **Aniridia** (absence of the iris) is a rare abnormality, frequently associated with secondary glaucoma and usually due to an autosomal dominant hereditary pattern. There is a significant association between sporadic aniridia and Wilms' tumor. Frequent abdominal examinations with periodic renal ultrasonography should be performed to detect Wilms' tumor at an early treatable stage.

The color of the iris is determined largely by heredity. Abnormalities in color include **albinism,** due to the absence of normal pigmentation of the ocular structures and frequently associated with poor visual acuity and nystagmus; and **heterochromia,** which is a difference in color in the two eyes that may be a primary developmental defect with no functional loss, due to congenital Horner's syndrome or secondary to an inflammatory process.

Lens Abnormalities

The lens abnormalities most frequently noted are cataracts, though there may be faulty development, forming colobomas, or subluxation, as seen in Marfan's syndrome.

Any lens opacity that is present at birth is a congenital cataract, regardless of whether or not it interferes with visual acuity. Congenital cataracts are often associated with other conditions. Maternal rubella during the first trimester of pregnancy is a common cause of congenital cataract. Other congenital cataracts have a hereditary background.

Congenital opacities may occur at any time during formation of the lens, and the stage during which the opacity started to develop is often measurable by the depth of the opacity. The innermost fetal nucleus of the lens forms early in embryonic life and is surrounded by the embryonic nucleus. During adult life, further growth in the lens is peripheral and subcapsular.

If the opacity is small enough so that it does not occlude the pupil, adequate visual acuity is attained by focusing around the opacity. If the pupillary opening is entirely occluded, however, normal sight does not develop, and the poor fixation may lead to nystagmus and amblyopia. Good visual results have been reported with both unilateral and bilateral cataracts treated by early surgery. Aphakic correction is then achieved usually with extended-wear contact lenses that need to be changed frequently to maintain optimal correction.

A major management problem in congenital cataracts is the associated amblyopia. Whether this can be dealt with adequately is a major determinant in deciding whether early surgery for monocular congenital cataract is justified. In the case of bilateral congenital cataracts, the time interval between operating on the two eyes must be as short as possible if amblyopia in the second eye is to be avoided. If early surgery is to be undertaken for congenital cataracts, it is best done within the first few weeks of life, and early referral to an ophthalmologist thus is essential. Surgery for congenital cataracts is discussed in Chapter 8.

Developmental Anomalies of the Anterior Segment

Failure of migration or subsequent development of neural crest cells produces abnormalities involving the anterior chamber angle, iris, cornea, and lens. Axenfeld's syndrome, Rieger's syndrome, and Peter's anomaly are examples. Glaucoma is a major clinical problem. The associated extraocular abnormalities are probably also manifestations of abnormal neural crest development.

Vitreous Abnormalities

Remnants of the hyaloid artery may be seen on the posterior surface of the lens (Mittendorf's dot) or on the optic disk (Bergmeister's papilla).

Persistent hyperplastic primary vitreous is an important cause of leukocoria that must be differentiated from retinoblastoma, congenital cataract, and retinopathy of prematurity.

Choroid & Retina

Gross defects of the choroid and retina are visible with the ophthalmoscope. The choroidal structures may show congenital colobomas, usually in the lower nasal region, which may also include the iris and all or part of the optic nerve. Choroidal colobomas are often associated with syndromes such as CHARGE association,* Aicardi's syndrome, and Goldenhar's syndrome. Posterior polar chorioretinal scarring is a pigmentary disturbance often caused by intrauterine toxoplasmosis.

Optic Nerve

Congenital anomalies of the optic nerve are relatively common. They are usually benign, such as minor abnormalities of the retinal vessels at the nerve head and tilted disks due to an oblique entrance of the nerve into the globe, but they may be associated with severe visual loss in the case of optic nerve hypoplasia or the rare central coloboma of the disk (morning glory syndrome).

Optic nerve hypoplasia is a nonprogressive congenital abnormality of one or both optic nerves in which

---

*CHARGE = *c*oloboma, *h*eart disease, choanal *a*tresia, *re*tarded *g*rowth, *g*enital anomalies, and *e*ar anomalies.

the number of axons in the involved nerve is reduced. Previously regarded as rare, it is now understood to be a major cause of visual loss in children. The degree of visual impairment varies from normal acuity with a wide variety of visual field defects to no perception of light. Clinical diagnosis is hampered by the difficulties of examining young children and the subtlety of the clinical signs. In more marked cases, the optic disk is obviously small and the circumpapillary halo of the normal-sized scleral canal produces the characteristic "double ring sign." In other cases, the hypoplasia may be only segmental and much more difficult to detect.

Optic nerve hypoplasia is frequently associated with midline deformities, including absence of the septum pellucidum, agenesis of the corpus callosum, dysplasia of the third ventricle, pituitary and hypothalamic dysfunction, and midline facial abnormalities. Jaundice and hypoglycemia in the neonatal period and growth retardation, hypothyroidism, and diabetes insipidus during childhood are important clinical effects of the resultant endocrine disturbances. More severe intracranial abnormalities such as anencephaly and porencephaly also occur. Endocrine and neuroradiographic investigations should be undertaken in all patients with optic nerve hypoplasia except perhaps those with unilateral segmental hypoplasia who are developing normally and have no other clinically evident congenital abnormalities.

Visual performance in children with optic nerve hypoplasia may be improved by occlusion therapy. Conversely, optic nerve hypoplasia is an important cause of poor vision that does not normalize with occlusion therapy in children with or without strabismus. A number of patients with optic nerve hypoplasia are not diagnosed until adult life because of the subtlety of the optic nerve abnormality.

Extraocular Dermoids

Congenital rests of surface ectodermal tissues may lead to formation of dermoids that occur frequently in the extraocular structures. These dermoids occur most commonly superolaterally, arising from the frontozygomatic suture.

Congenital Nasolacrimal Duct Obstruction

Canalization of the distal nasolacrimal duct normally occurs before birth or during the first month of life. As many as 30% of babies will have epiphora during this time. Approximately 6% have more prolonged symptoms, of which the majority will also resolve aided by lacrimal sac massage and treatment of episodes of conjunctivitis with topical antibiotics. Nasolacrimal probing is usually curative in the remainder and is best left until about 1 year of age. In the event of acute dacryocystitis, earlier probing is often indicated. The possibility of more extensive congenital nasolacrimal anomalies should be born in mind in patients with craniofacial anomalies. Epiphora may also

be due to inflammatory anterior segment disease, lid abnormalities, and congenital glaucoma.

Orbital Abnormalities

Craniofacial dysostosis (Crouzon's disease) is a rare hereditary deformity due to an autosomal dominant gene, characterized by exophthalmos, atrophy of the maxilla, enlargement of the nasal bones, abnormal increase in the space between the eyes (ocular hypertelorism), optic atrophy, and bony abnormalities of the region of the perilongitudinal sinus. The palpebral fissures slant downward (in contrast to the upward slant of Down's syndrome). Strabismus and nystagmus are also present. The strabismus is secondary to both structural anomalies of the muscles and orbital angle anomalies.

Various congenital abnormalities of skull development—due to premature closure of the skull sutures—are associated with deformities of the orbits and ocular complications resembling those associated with Crouzon's disease. Examples are oxycephaly and acrobrachycephaly.

INVESTIGATION OF THE BLIND BABY WITH NORMAL OCULAR & NEUROLOGIC EXAMINATION

An important part of pediatric ophthalmology is the investigation of babies with poor visual performance for which clinical examination reveals no ocular or neurologic cause. The important conditions to be considered are Leber's congenital amaurosis, cortical blindness, cone dystrophy, oculomotor apraxia, and delayed visual maturation. This presumes that subtle defects such as optic nerve hypoplasia, albinism, and high refractive errors have been excluded.

Leber's congenital amaurosis—as distinct from Leber's hereditary optic neuropathy—and cone dystrophy are congenital retinal dystrophies detectable by electroretinography. Visual evoked responses and neuroimaging studies are used to diagnose cortical blindness. In oculomotor apraxia, a defect in initiation of horizontal saccades gives the impression of visual unresponsiveness, though the visual pathways are normal. Affected children develop characteristic compensatory head movements to overcome the eye movement disorder. Delayed visual maturation is a rare condition in which vision does not develop until after 3 months of age. In some cases, there may be associated ocular and neurologic abnormalities that limit final visual performance, but normal vision is attained in those in which it is an isolated condition.

POSTNATAL PROBLEMS

The most common ocular disorders of children are external infections of the conjunctiva and eyelids (bacterial conjunctivitis, hordeola, blepharitis), strabismus, ocular foreign bodies, allergic reactions of the conjunctiva and eyelids, refractive errors (particularly myopia), and congenital defects. Since it is more difficult to elicit an accurate history of causative factors and subjective complaints in children, it is not uncommon to overlook significant ocular disorders (especially in very young children). Aside from the altered frequency of occurrence of the types of ocular disorders, the causes, manifestations, and treatment of eye disorders are about the same for children as for adults. Certain special problems encountered more frequently in infants and children are discussed below.

Ophthalmia Neonatorum (Conjunctivitis of the Newborn)

Conjunctivitis of the newborn may be of chemical, bacterial, chlamydial, or viral origin. Differentiation is sometimes possible according to the timing of presentation, but appropriate smears and cultures are essential. Antenatal diagnosis and treatment of maternal genital infections should prevent many cases of neonatal conjunctivitis. The presence of active maternal genital herpes at the time of delivery is an indication for elective cesarean section.

A. Conjunctivitis Due to Chlamydial Infection: *Chlamydia* is now the commonest identifiable infectious cause of neonatal conjunctivitis in the USA. Inclusion blennorrhea due to chlamydial infection has its onset between the fifth and fourteenth days; the presence of typical inclusion bodies in the epithelial cells of a conjunctival smear confirms this diagnosis. Direct immunofluorescent antibody staining of conjunctival scrapings is a highly sensitive and specific diagnostic test. Systemic therapy with erythromycin is more effective than topical therapy and aids in the eradication of concurrent nasopharyngeal carriage, which may predispose to the development of pneumonitis.

B. Conjunctivitis Due to Chemical Trauma: Chemical conjunctivitis caused by the silver nitrate drops instilled into the conjunctival sac at birth is most apparent during the first or second day of life. Silver nitrate conjunctivitis is usually self-limited. Silver nitrate solution (1%) should be contained in sealed single-use disposable containers. Because of the possibility of chemical conjunctivitis, some authorities advocate use of topical erythromycin or tetracycline instead for prophylaxis. Instillation of silver nitrate or an antibiotic is still required by statute in most states in the USA.

C. Conjunctivitis Due to Bacterial Infection: Bacterial conjunctivitis, usually due to *Staphylococcus aureus*, *Haemophilus* species, *Streptococcus pneumoniae*, *Streptococcus faecalis*, *Neisseria gonorrhoeae*, or *Pseudomonas* species (the last two being the most serious because of potential corneal damage), presents between the second and fifth days after birth. Provisional identification of the causative organism may be made from conjunctival smears. Gonococcal conjunctivitis necessitates parenteral therapy with aqueous penicillin G procaine given intravenously for penicillin-sensitive strains and ceftriaxone given intravenously with topical erythromycin for penicillinase-producing strains. In all cases due to chlamydial or gonococcal infection, both parents should also be given systemic treatment. Other types of bacterial conjunctivitis require topical instillation of antibacterial agents, such as sodium sulfacetamide, bacitracin, or tetracycline, as soon as results of smears are known.

D. Conjunctivitis Due to Viral Infection: Herpes simplex virus produces characteristic giant cells and viral inclusions on cytologic examination. Herpetic keratoconjunctivitis usually resolves spontaneously but may require antiviral therapy, particularly when associated with disseminated infection that occurs chiefly in atopic individuals.

Uveitis in Childhood

Inflammatory eye disease is relatively uncommon in children, but there are a number of important syndromes. The conditions that are seen in the same form as in adults are acute nongranulomatous anterior uveitis associated with the HLA-B27 spondylarthritides, intermediate uveitis, Fuchs' heterochromic cyclitis, and idiopathic anterior uveitis. These are treated in the same way as in adults but with care in the use of systemic steroids because of their effects on growth. Uveitis in association with juvenile rheumatoid arthritis is generally asymptomatic in its early stages and often remains undetected until severe loss of vision due to glaucoma, cataract, or band keratopathy, has already occurred. Regular ophthalmic screening of children with juvenile rheumatoid arthritis is essential. Girls with a pauciarticular onset of juvenile rheumatoid arthritis, especially if they have circulating antinuclear antibody, are at particularly high risk for developing uveitis. Long-term use of topical steroids and mydriatics is effective in controlling the uveitis associated with juvenile rheumatoid arthritis. (Further discussion of uveitis in children is included in Chapter 7).

Retinopathy of Prematurity

Retinopathy of prematurity, previously called retrolental fibroplasia, has been estimated to result in 550 new cases of infant blindness each year in the United States. Improved neonatal care may reduce the percentage of babies affected but has also greatly increased the total number at risk. Retinal cryotherapy is now recommended treatment for babies with severe active disease.

Retinal vascularization proceeds centrifugally from the optic nerve, beginning at the fourth month of gestation. Retinal vessels normally reach the nasal ora serrata at 8 months and the temporal ora serrata at 9 months. Retinopathy of prematurity develops if this process is disturbed. It is usually bilateral but often asymmetric. The active phase involves changes at the junction of vascularized and avascular retina, initially as an obvious demarcation line (stage 1), followed by formation of a distinct ridge (stage 2), then extraretinal fibrovascular proliferation (stage 3). Even among patients with stage 3 disease, there is a very high incidence of spontaneous regression. Consideration is also given to the location of the changes with respect to distance from the optic disk, the extent of the disease in clock hours, and the presence of venous dilation and arterial tortuosity in the posterior segment ("plus" disease). The cicatricial phase (stages 4 and 5) is manifested by increasingly severe retinal detachment.

The major risk factors for retinopathy of prematurity are decreasing gestational age and decreasing birth weight. Although recognition of the causative role of supplemental oxygen and its restriction seems to have reduced the incidence of retinopathy of prematurity, other factors must also be important. Associated risk factors include acidosis, apnea, patent ductus arteriosus, septicemia, blood transfusions, and intraventricular hemorrhage.

It is recommended that all babies with a birth weight of 1500 g or less and those that receive prolonged supplemental oxygen therapy should undergo repeated screening for retinopathy of prematurity. As many as 60% of such babies will develop the disease, even if only in its early stages. Screening should begin at 2–4 weeks after birth and continue until the retina is fully vascularized, until the changes of retinopathy of prematurity have undergone spontaneous resolution, or until appropriate treatment has been given. Pupillary dilation is achieved with Cyclomydril (cyclopentolate 0.2% and phenylephrine 1%). In eyes with five contiguous or eight cumulative clock hours of stage 3 "plus" disease, it is recommended that retinal cryotherapy or photocoagulation be applied to the entire avascular retina anterior to the ridge in order to reduce the risk of subsequent cicatricial disease. Whether treatment should be given to both eyes if they both fulfill the criteria has not been determined. Such treatment should be carried out with the assistance of an experienced neonatologist and under careful monitoring because of the risks of serious systemic complications including respiratory and cardiorespiratory arrest.

Vitrectomy and lensectomy may be beneficial in cicatricial disease but probably should be reserved for babies with severe disease in both eyes.

See also Chapter 10 and discussion of oxygen toxicity in Chapter 15.

Congenital Glaucoma

Congenital glaucoma (see Chapter 11) may occur alone or in association with many other congenital lesions. Early recognition is essential to prevent permanent blindness. Involvement is often bilateral. The most striking symptom is extreme photophobia. Early signs are corneal haze or opacity, increased corneal diameter, and increased intraocular pressure. Since the outer coats of the eyeball are not as rigid in the child, the increased intraocular pressure expands the corneal and scleral tissues, producing an eye that is larger than normal (buph-

thalmos). The major differential diagnoses are forceps injuries at birth, developmental anomalies of the cornea or anterior segment, and mucopolysaccharidoses such as Hurler's syndrome. All of these cause corneal clouding but none produce enlargement of the globe. Useful vision may be preserved by early diagnosis and medical and surgical treatment by an ophthalmologist.

Leukocoria
(White Pupil)

Parents will occasionally see a white spot through the infant's pupil (leukocoria). Although retinoblastoma must be ruled out, the opacity is more often due to cataract, retinopathy of prematurity, or persistent hyperplastic primary vitreous.

Retinoblastoma

This rare malignant tumor of childhood is fatal if untreated. In 90% of cases, the diagnosis is made before the end of the third year. In about 30% of cases, retinoblastoma is bilateral. Development of the tumor is thought to occur because of the loss—from both members of the chromosome pair—of the normally protective dominant allele at a single locus within chromosomal band 13q14 (see Chapter 18). This gene is normally responsible for production of a nuclear phosphoprotein with DNA binding activity. Loss of the allele is caused by mutations, either in the somatic retinal cells alone (nonheritable retinoblastoma) or in the germ line cells as well (heritable retinoblastoma). In heritable retinoblastoma, the genetic predisposition is inherited as an autosomal dominant trait; children of survivors have a nearly 50% chance of having the disease; and the tumor is more apt to be bilateral and multifocal. Parents who have produced one child with retinoblastoma run a 4–7% risk of having a subsequent child with the disease. Recent sequencing of the retinoblastoma gene locus now allows more specific genetic counseling and identification of individuals carrying the mutation. In sporadic cases, the tumor is usually not discovered until it has advanced far enough to produce an opaque pupil. Infants and children with presenting symptoms of strabismus should be examined carefully to rule out retinoblastoma, since a deviating eye may be the first sign of the tumor. In children of families affected by familial retinoblastoma, regular screening is important in the early detection of tumors.

Enucleation is the treatment of choice in nearly all extensive unilateral cases of retinoblastoma. In bilateral cases, conservative therapy with radiotherapy, either with episcleral plaques or external beam, and photocoagulation techniques are used increasingly to preserve the less severely affected eye.

Strabismus

Strabismus is present in about 2% of children. Its early recognition is often the responsibility of the pediatrician or the family physician. Occasionally, childhood strabismus has neurologic significance. The idea that a child may outgrow crossed eyes should be discouraged. Any child with evidence of strabismus after 3 months of age must be referred as soon as possible for ophthalmologic assessment. Neglect in the treatment of strabismus may lead to undesirable cosmetic effects, psychic trauma, and amblyopia (see below) in the deviating eye. Strabismus is covered in Chapter 12.

Amblyopia

Amblyopia is decreased visual acuity of one eye (uncorrectable with lenses) in the absence of organic eye disease. Organic eye disease may be present but insufficient to explain the level of vision.

Normal development of the physiologic mechanisms of the retina and visual cortex is determined by postnatal visual experience. Visual deprivation due to any cause, congenital or acquired, during the critical period of development (probably lasting up to age 8 in humans) prevents the establishment of normal vision in the involved eye. Reversal of this effect becomes increasingly difficult with increasing age of the child. Early suspicion and prompt referral for treatment of the underlying condition are important in preventing amblyopia.

The most common causes of amblyopia are strabismus, in which the image from the deviated eye is suppressed to prevent diplopia, and anisometropia, in which an inability to focus the eyes simultaneously causes suppression of the image of one eye and high hypermetropia, in which both eyes may become amblyopic because of failure to form a focused image in either eye. All of these conditions are treatable.

Since poor visual function in a young child may go unnoticed, routine screening is advocated to detect amblyogenic factors (eg, by photorefraction of babies for refractive errors and strabismus) or established amblyopia (by testing visual acuity at age 4).

Child Abuse
(Shaken Baby Syndrome)

Child abuse is an increasingly recognized cause of childhood trauma. Making the diagnosis is essential if affected children are to be given the protection they must have, but wrong diagnosis must also be avoided if families are not to be unjustly treated.

In the shaken baby syndrome, external signs of head injury are absent, but intraretinal, preretinal, and vitreous hemorrhages are common. They are often accompanied by intracranial hemorrhage and may be indicative of the presence of subdural hemorrhage even if a CT scan is normal. Unexplained retinal hemorrhages in children less than 3 years of age without external evidence of head injury is strongly suggestive of child abuse.

Blunt trauma to the head and eyes is a more readily recognized form of child abuse. Ocular manifestations include subconjunctival hemorrhage, hyphema, cataract, lens subluxation, glaucoma; retinal, vitreous, intrascleral, and optic nerve hemorrhages; and papilledema.

Victims of child abuse may present initially to ophthalmologists, and the diagnosis must be kept in mind. Ophthalmologists may also provide evidence of injuries to the head and eyes in children presenting with unexplained injuries to other parts of the body.

Learning Disabilities
& Dyslexia

Ophthalmologists are often asked to evaluate children with suspected learning disabilities in order to rule out ocular disorders. Dyslexia is the most common type of learning disability and is characterized by the inability to develop good reading and writing skills. Affected children are usually of normal intelligence and have no associated physical or visual abnormalities. Parents and educators sometimes attribute learning disabilities to visual perceptual abnormalities, but most of these affected children have no visual or ocular impairment. It is believed that dyslexia is caused by a specific defect of information processing in the central nervous system. The diagnosis of learning disabilities can be readily made by education specialists, and treatment is often effective in ameliorating this condition. When asked to evaluate a child with a learning disorder, the ophthalmologist should perform a complete examination and treat any refractive, strabismic, or amblyopic conditions identified. It is important to advise the parents that ocular or visual abnormalities generally do not lead to learning disabilities, and special educational programs may be necessary to treat these children. "Vision training," "visual therapy," and "perceptual training" programs have not been evaluated in a scientifically controlled, randomized, or prospective fashion, and thus their efficacy has not been proved. Ophthalmologists should provide indicated care of ocular problems and refer patients to appropriate educational programs for diagnosis and treatment of learning disabilities.

REFERENCES

Bradford GM, Keech KV, Scott WE: Factors affecting visual outcome after surgery for bilateral congenital cataracts. Am J Ophthalmol 1994;117:58.

Brown DR, Biglan AW, Stretavsky MAM: Screening criteria for the detection of retinopathy of prematurity in patients in a neonatal intensive care unit. J Paed Ophthalmol Strab 1987;24:212.

Brown GC, et al: Systemic complications associated with retinal cryoablation for retinopathy of prematurity. Ophthalmology 1990;97:855.

Committee for the Classification of Retinopathy of Prematurity: An international classification of retinopathy of prematurity. Arch Ophthalmol 1984;102:1130.

Cryotherapy for Retinopathy of Prematurity Cooperative Group: Multicenter trial of cryotherapy for retinopathy of prematurity. Preliminary results. Arch Ophthalmol 1988;106:471.

Cryotherapy for Retinopathy of Prematurity Cooperative Group: Multicenter trial of cryotherapy for retinopathy of prematurity. One-year outcome—structure and function. Arch Ophthalmol 1990;108:1408.

Drummond GT, Scott WE, Keech RV: Management of monocular congenital cataracts. Arch Ophthalmol 1989;107:45.

Elner SG, et al: Ocular and associated systemic findings in suspected child abuse: A necropsy study. Arch Ophthalmol 1990;108:1094.

Friendly DS, Jaafar MS, Morillo DL: A comparative study of grating and recognition visual acuity testing in children with anisometropic amblyopia without strabismus. Am J Ophthalmol 1990;110:293.

Fries PD, Katowitz JA: Congenital craniofacial anomalies of ophthalmic importance. Surv Ophthalmol 1990;35:87.

Gallie BL, Phillips RA: Retinoblastoma: A model of oncogenesis. Ophthalmology 1984;91:667.

Gaynon MW, et al: Retinal folds in the shaken baby syndrome. Am J Ophthalmol 1988;106:423.

Giangiacomo J, et al: Sequential cranial computed tomography in infants with retinal hemorrhages. Ophthalmology 1988;95:295.

Good WV et al: Cortical visual impairment in children. Surv Ophthalmol 1994;38:351.

Halloran SL et al: Accuracy of detection of the retinoblastoma gene by esterase D linkage. Arch Ophthalmol 1985;103:1329.

Hammerschlag MR et al: Efficacy of neonatal ocular prophylaxis for the prevention of chlamydial and gonococcal conjunctivitis. N Engl J Med 1989;320:769.

Harley RD (editor): *Pediatric Ophthalmology,* 2nd ed. Saunders, 1983.

Helveston EM: *Management of Dyslexia and Related Learning Disabilities.* Focal Points 1985, *Clinical Modules for Ophthalmologists,* Vol 3, Module 1. American Academy of Ophthalmology, 1985.

Kalina RE: Treatment of retinal detachment due to retinopathy of prematurity: Documented disappointment. (Editorial.) Ophthalmology 1991;98:3.

Katowitz JA, Welsh MG: Timing of initial probing and irrigation in congenital nasolacrimal duct obstruction. Ophthalmology 1987;94:698.

Lambert S, Hoyt CS, Narahara MH: Optic nerve hypoplasia. Surv Ophthalmol 1987;32:1.

Lambert SR, Taylor D, Kriss A: The infant with nystagmus, normal appearing fundi, but an abnormal ERG. Surv Ophthalmol 1989;34:173.

Levin AV et al: Extended-wear contact lenses for the treatment of pediatric aphakia. Ophthalmology 1988;95:1107.

Mets MB: Drops, drops, drops in pediatric ophthalmology. In: *Year Book of Ophthalmology 1988.* Deutsch E (editor). Year Book, 1988.

Nussenblatt RB: Immunoregulation of uveitis. Int Ophthalmol 1990;14:13.

Nussenblatt RB, Palestine AG: *Uveitis: Fundamentals and Clinical Practice.* Year Book, 1989.

Pagon RA et al: Coloboma, congenital heart disease, and choanal atresia with multiple anomalies: CHARGE association. J Pediatr 1981;99:223.

Pediatric ophthalmology. Pediatr Clin North Am 1987;34:1.

Prendiville A, Schulenberg WE: Clinical factors associated with retinopathy of prematurity. Arch Dis Child 1988;63:522.

Strömland K, Miller M, Cook C: Ocular teratology. Surv Ophthalmol 1991;35:429.

Taylor D: Monocular infantile cataract, intraocular lenses, and amblyopia. (Editorial.) Br J Ophthalmol 1989;73:857.

Taylor D: *Pediatric Ophthalmology.* Blackwell, 1990.

Turleau C et al: Del 11/P aniridia complex: Report of three patients and review of 37 observations from the literature. Clin Genet 1984;26:356.

Wiggs JL, Dryja TP: Predicting the risk in hereditary retinoblastoma. Am J Ophthalmol 1988;106:346.

Winceslaus J et al: Diagnosis of ophthalmia neonatorum. Br Med J 1987;6610:1377.

18

Genetic Aspects

Taylor Asbury, MD, & Paul Riordan-Eva, FRCS, FRCOphth

Genetic influences are being described in an increasing number of diseases, and a primary causative role for genetic defects is being more clearly defined in many instances. Thus, it becomes increasingly important to understand the principles of genetic transmission. Much of the background work in clinical genetics has been done in ophthalmology. The eye seems to be unusually prone to genetically determined disease, and an accurate diagnosis of ocular disease can usually be arrived at on the basis of careful clinical examination.

Clinicians can estimate the risk of occurrence of many genetically determined diseases (usually the rare but severe ones), but the familial incidence of many other diseases also known to be genetically determined still cannot be accurately predicted.

Mechanisms of Inheritance

An individual's genetic identity (**genotype**) is carried in the DNA found in the cell nucleus and mitochondria. The DNA in the nucleus of the normal human somatic cell is organized into 23 pairs of **chromosomes.** Twenty-two of these pairs are somewhat similar (homologous) and are therefore termed **autosomal.** The twenty-third pair is composed of the **sex chromosomes** (X and Y). In the female, this pair is homologous (XX), whereas in the male it is heterologous (XY). A number of agents (quinacrine mustard, trypsin, Giemsa's stain) produce morphologic banding of human chromosomes that permits their identification and classification into a number of groups. Mitochondrial DNA is a double-stranded circular molecule of which each mitochondrion has several copies.

The genotype is composed of many small functional units termed **genes,** which are situated at specific sites (**loci**) along the length of the DNA. Genes are thus also arranged in pairs. The alternate forms of a gene at a locus controlling a particular characteristic are known as **alleles.** There are commonly two alternate forms, but there may be more. When the alleles at a particular locus are the same, the individual is said to be homozygous, and when they are different, heterozygous.

Genes exert their effects by controlling the production of proteins within the cell. Complementary copies of the DNA constituting specific genes are formed with

RNA, and these are used to direct protein synthesis. The mechanisms regulating gene expression are complex.

DNA recombinant technology using isolated human DNA fragments inserted into bacterial cells has led to the identification of the DNA sequences and protein products of specific genes. Linkage studies and DNA probes have identified the position of specific gene loci and carriers for certain mutant genes.

The **gametes** (spermatozoon and ovum) are produced by a special type of cell division called **reduction-division meiosis,** in which the 23 pairs of chromosomes dissociate, each daughter cell receiving one chromosome of each pair. One of each pair passes into each daughter cell as a random occurrence. Exchange of chromosomal material (**translocation**) between the members of each pair also occurs. At fertilization, each chromosome of the spermatozoon joins its corresponding chromosome of the ovum to produce a cell with 46 chromosomes of unique genetic constitution. Mitochondrial DNA is derived entirely from the ovum. All cell divisions after fertilization (**mitosis**) involve duplication and separation of all the chromosomes to produce cells with the constant number of 46 chromosomes and identical genetic constitution.

The expression of the genotype in physical characteristics is known as the **phenotype.** The inheritance of certain characteristics of the human phenotype, such as eye color, can be explained on the basis of interaction between the two alleles at a single chromosomal locus. Each allele determines the development of one form of the particular characteristic. In the homozygous individual, this form is correspondingly expressed. In the heterozygous individual, one allele is said to be **dominant** because it determines the phenotype, while the other is **recessive** (not expressed). This is the basis of **mendelian inheritance,** from which are derived many of the terms used to describe patterns of inheritance. The inheritance of many phenotypic characteristics, however, cannot easily be classified in this way. This has led to modifications of the original mendelian concepts, including variable expression and variable penetration of genes. Recent improvements in the understanding of gene regulation and expression, as well as recognition of the role of environmental factors, have demonstrated why this model breaks down. Nevertheless, the framework of mendelian inheritance is still of immense value in clinical genetics as a means of describing modes of inheritance and estimating the risk of transmission of certain genetically determined abnormalities. The major alternative patterns of inheritance are those due to chromosomal abnormalities and those described as multifactorial, involving multiple genes or major environmental influences and maternal inheritance due to defects of mitochondrial DNA.

MENDELIAN INHERITANCE

Mendelian inheritance can be divided into three main patterns: autosomal dominant, autosomal recessive, and X-linked recessive.

Autosomal Dominant Inheritance

An abnormal dominant gene produces its specific abnormality even though its paired gene (allele) is normal. Males and females are affected alike and—being heterozygous—have a theoretic 50% chance of passing along the affected gene (and therefore the abnormality) to each of their offspring even when mated to genotypically normal individuals (Figure 18–1).

Given a particular group of pedigrees, autosomal dominant inheritance is established if the following conditions are met: (1) Males and females are equally affected. (2) Direct transmission has occurred over two or more generations. (3) About 50% of individuals in the pedigrees are affected.

Quite a large number of uncommon but serious diseases with ocular manifestations are transmitted in this way: forms of juvenile glaucoma, Marfan's syndrome, congenital stationary night blindness (Figure 18–2), osteogenesis imperfecta, neurofibromatosis types 1 and 2, Lindau-Von Hippel disease, and tuberous sclerosis. The process of natural selection tends to keep most of these serious diseases at a low incidence since many of these persons do not or cannot reproduce.

Dominant disease may be more or less severe from generation to generation depending upon its **expression;** a disease with "variable expression" is one that can occur in a mild or severe form. An example is neurofibromatosis type 1, in which genotypically affected individuals may have merely café au lait spots or may have many serious manifestations. One cannot predict if or when the disease will be more serious (with central nervous system tumors or optic nerve gliomas) in a succeeding generation. If the genetic pattern is present but there is no evidence of the disease, one says that its **penetrance** is reduced. It may be quite difficult to differentiate dominant inheritance with reduced penetrance from recessive inheritance (see below).

In certain diseases such as hemoglobin S disease, there is a clearly defined intermediate phenotype that corresponds to the heterozygous individual. This is known as **codominant inheritance.**

Autosomal Recessive Inheritance

Abnormal recessive genes must lie in pairs (duplex state) to produce manifest abnormality. Thus, each parent must contribute one recessive abnormal gene. Each parent is clinically unaffected (genotypically affected but phenotypically normal), since a normal dominant gene makes the abnormal gene recessive (Figure 18–3).

It is difficult to establish that a given disease results from autosomal recessive inheritance. Some of the criteria used to establish recessive inheritance are the following:

(1) Occurrence of the same disease in collateral branches of the family.

(2) History of consanguinity. The higher the rate of consanguinity in the pedigrees of a given disease, the more likely the disease is to be recessive. Consanguinity creates greater opportunities for the genes to lie in the duplex state, inasmuch as an individual with two related parents can receive the same affected gene from each, a common ancestor having originally passed on the affected gene.

(3) The occurrence of the disease in about 25% of siblings. This only holds for groups of pedigrees. There is a 25% chance that the two abnormal genes will be passed on to one individual. There is a 50% chance that a normal gene will modify the affected gene. In this case, the individual is a carrier of the disease (just like the parents) but is not affected with the disease (ie,

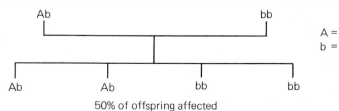

50% of offspring affected

A = Abnormal dominant gene
b = Normal gene lying at same position in the paired chromosome cells

Figure 18–1. Autosomal dominant inheritance.

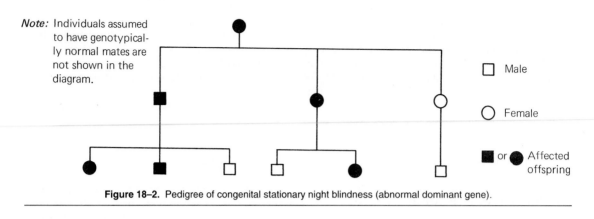

Note: Individuals assumed to have genotypically normal mates are not shown in the diagram.

☐ Male

○ Female

■ or ● Affected offspring

Figure 18–2. Pedigree of congenital stationary night blindness (abnormal dominant gene).

genotypically affected but phenotypically normal). In the remaining 25% of siblings, two normal genes lie together and the abnormal gene is completely lost (ie, the individual is genotypically normal). Although a number of pedigrees are required to definitely establish recessive inheritance, even a single pedigree is suggestive if more than one sibling is similarly affected without an antecedent history.

Many disease processes have been definitely established as resulting from autosomal recessive inheritance, and many others are suspected of having such a genetic background. Included among the definite cases are Laurence-Moon-Biedl syndrome and inborn errors of metabolism such as oculocutaneous albinism (Figure 18–4), galactokinase deficiency, and Tay-Sachs disease.

X-Linked (Sex-Linked) Recessive Inheritance

Many of the genes of the X chromosome are unopposed by a gene of the Y chromosome. Abnormalities of these genes cause disease in the male, whereas in the female an abnormal recessive gene of the sex chromosome is masked by its normal allele. Therefore, nearly all of the X-linked diseases are manifested in males, whereas the disease is passed through the female. A

male and his maternal grandfather are affected, and the intervening female is the carrier.

The criteria for X-linked inheritance are (1) that only males are affected, (2) that the disease is transmitted through carrier females to half of the sons, and (3) that there is no father-to-son transmission.

Among the important eye diseases with an X-linked genetic pattern are color blindness (Figure 18–5), ocular albinism, and one type of retinitis pigmentosa.

Females have a mosaic of somatic cells consisting of cell groups with one X chromosome functioning and cell groups with the other X chromosome functioning (Lyon hypothesis). When the female is a carrier of an X-linked disease, this mosaicism is occasionally detectable. Such is the case in female carriers of ocular albinism, in whom groups of pigmented and albino retinal pigment epithelial cells are visible ophthalmoscopically.

MATERNAL INHERITANCE

Maternal inheritance, in which a condition is inherited only from the mother, does not obey the accepted rules of any form of mendelian inheritance. It has particular relevance to ophthalmology because its exis-

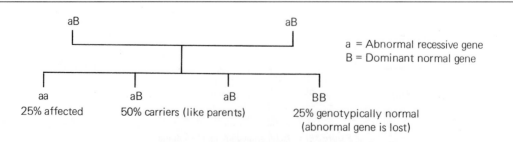

aB   aB

a = Abnormal recessive gene
B = Dominant normal gene

aa   aB   aB   BB
25% affected   50% carriers (like parents)   25% genotypically normal
(abnormal gene is lost)

Figure 18–3. Autosomal recessive inheritance. Mating of two carriers.

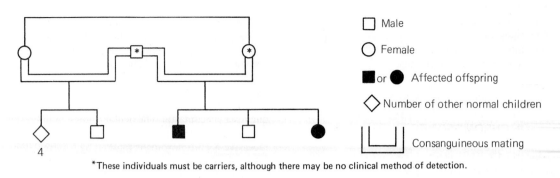

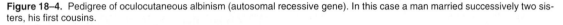

*These individuals must be carriers, although there may be no clinical method of detection.

Figure 18–4. Pedigree of oculocutaneous albinism (autosomal recessive gene). In this case a man married successively two sisters, his first cousins.

tence was recognized through the study of inheritance patterns in Leber's hereditary optic neuropathy, which causes severe bilateral optic neuropathy in young adults. The explanation for maternal inheritance is a defect in mitochondrial DNA, which is derived entirely from the individual's mother.

Maternal inheritance should produce a genetic abnormality that is transmitted only through the female line and then potentially to all offspring, that is never found in the offspring of an affected male, and that is detectable in every generation, with males and females being equally affected.

In almost all families affected by Leber's hereditary optic neuropathy, a mitochondrial DNA point mutation involving a gene responsible for the production of a protein involved in oxidative phosphorylation can be identified. The most frequent mutation, known as the Wallace mutation, is at base pair 11778. The inheritance pattern of Leber's hereditary optic neuropathy does not in fact fulfill all the features outlined above, which suggests the presence of other influences. The

significant anomaly is a marked male gender bias in clinical expression of the disease.

CHROMOSOMAL ABNORMALITIES

When mitosis is interrupted in metaphase, the chromosomes can be spread on a slide, counted, and photographed. These cytogenetic studies have made possible the classification of chromosomes into seven groups based upon characteristics such as size and the position of the centromere. The groups contain as few as two or as many as seven chromosomes, with the chromosomes of any group being indistinguishable from each other. The study of cytogenetics has also established that some clinical states can be correlated with an abnormal number of chromosomes, most frequently one more (trisomy) or occasionally one less (monosomy) than the normal number of 46. A few of the more common syndromes are summarized briefly below. Since the addition or subtraction of an entire

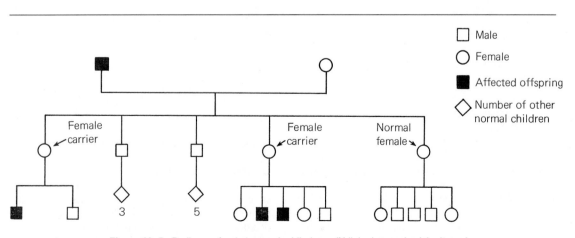

Figure 18–5. Pedigree of red-green color blindness (X-linked recessive inheritance).

gene is obviously a major genetic abnormality, these syndromes are characterized by many and extensive deformities. Many such abnormal fertilizations result in early abortions and stillbirths.

1. SYNDROMES ASSOCIATED WITH AN ABNORMAL NUMBER OF CHROMOSOMES

Trisomy 13 (Patau's Syndrome)

Anophthalmos, microphthalmos, retinal dysplasia, optic atrophy, coloboma of the uvea, and cataracts are the major eye anomalies; cerebral defects, cleft palate, heart lesions, polydactyly, and hemangiomas are the more severe nonophthalmic changes. Death by age 6 months is the rule.

Trisomy 18 (Edwards' Syndrome)

The main features of this rare syndrome are mental and physical retardation, congenital heart defects, and renal abnormalities. Corneal and lenticular opacities, unilateral ptosis, and optic atrophy have been described.

Trisomy 21 (Down's Syndrome)

Although Down's syndrome is a fairly common and well-known entity, the hereditary pattern was long ill-defined. Waardenburg originally suggested that Down's syndrome was a chromosomal problem in 1932. Cytogenetic studies in 1958 revealed an extra chromosome indistinguishable from chromosome 21. The principal manifestations are small stature, a flattened, round, mongoloid facies, saddle nose, thick lower lip, large tongue, soft, seborrheic skin, smooth hair, obesity, small genitalia, short fingers, a simian fold, congenital heart anomalies, mental retardation, and frequent psychic disturbances. The ocular signs include hyperplasia of the iris, narrow palpebral fissures with Oriental slant, strabismus, epicanthus, cataract, high myopia (33%), keratoconus, and Brushfield (silver-gray) spots on the iris.

The incidence of Down's syndrome is significantly increased in children born to older women, particularly those past age 35.

2. ABNORMALITIES INVOLVING SEX CHROMOSOMES

Turner's syndrome is a monosomy (45 chromosomes). For some reason, the affected female receives only one X chromosome. Clinically, growth retardation, rudimentary ovaries and female genitalia, amenorrhea, pterygium colli, epicanthus, cubitus valgus, and ptosis occur. Of particular ophthalmic interest is the high incidence of color blindness (8%). This is the same frequency as for males (the female incidence is 0.4%) and is read-

ily explained by the fact that the normally recessive gene is unopposed and is expressed just as in the male.

Klinefelter's syndrome is a trisomy involving the X chromosomes. These phenotypical males have 47 chromosomes: the normal 44 autosomes and three sex chromosomes, XXY. These individuals are sterile, with small testes, a eunuchoid physique, and frequently gynecomastia. The ocular finding of interest is the very rare occurrence of color blindness, since the recessive X chromosome is masked by a normal dominant (as in the normal female).

OTHER GENETIC CONSIDERATIONS

Genetic Counseling

Valuable advice can often be given to families concerned with the percentage risk of transmitting serious disease to future generations. This entails a working knowledge of basic genetic principles and sensitive counseling skills. A careful history of the pedigree in question is very important, since a single disease may have more than one mode of transmission (eg, retinitis pigmentosa has three or more basic patterns). On the other hand, careful inquiries about maternal health during pregnancy may suggest that the anomaly—eg, congenital cataracts—is developmental and therefore unrelated to the genes.

Consanguineous mating increases the prevalence of autosomal recessive traits, and the most likely explanation for two individuals' having the same recessive gene is the fact that they are related.

Prenatal Diagnosis

In some cases it is possible to offer families at risk for a specific hereditary disease the option of prenatal diagnosis. This may involve searching for chromosomal abnormalities or specific structural protein defects such as enzyme deficiencies. Currently, techniques are being devised to identify abnormalities at the gene level using DNA linkage studies (eg, in X-linked retinitis pigmentosa) or DNA probes. Prenatal diagnosis by testing amniotic fluid cells obtained by amniocentesis at 14–16 gestational weeks has become a safe and practical procedure. The list of hereditary diseases that can be diagnosed with this method is rapidly increasing. There is, however, a 3-week delay before results of cytogenetic analysis become available. Chorionic villus sampling has certain advantages: It can be undertaken at 8–12 gestational weeks, and results are known within 24 hours. Its overall safety is still being determined.

Genetic Carrier State

Recognition of the genetic carrier state makes possible more accurate prediction of possible disease transmission and helps to establish the genetic nature of a disease by providing an occasion for examination of relatives of affected individuals. Detection is possible in many diseases. There are three types:

(1) Autosomal dominant diseases in which the disease appears in a mild or subclinical form (low expression). Because the offspring of such individuals still have the theoretic 50% chance of passing on the disease process, the recognition of this carrier state is important in genetic counseling.

(2) Autosomal recessive diseases with heterozygous manifestations. Affected genes that are normally balanced by a normal allele may cause minor subclinical abnormalities that disclose the presence of the abnormal gene. One can predict the 25% possibility of occurrence of some autosomal recessive diseases if the carrier state can be recognized in both potential mates.

(3) Female carrier in X-linked recessive disease. Subclinical evidence of the disease in daughters of affected fathers differentiates carriers from noncarriers in a number of X-linked recessive diseases (often quite obvious in tapetoretinal degenerative conditions).

Mutation

Mutation occurs when a gene undergoes alteration in the germ cell as a result of spontaneous chemical change within the gene and the change is manifested by a new characteristic. The causes of the change are not well understood, but such extrinsic environmental factors as heat, x-rays, and exposure to radioactive materials may induce it. Most often, the new characteristic is unfavorable (ie, disease-producing), but some mutations are favorable and account for the evolution of species (Darwin).

Certain mutations occur repeatedly in specific genes and cause specific disease. Hemophilia, which follows an X-linked pattern, and retinoblastoma, in which a single locus on chromosome 13 is involved, are examples of disease occurring as a result of mutation. Very few individuals with severe abnormalities reproduce, so that the incidence of such diseases is dependent very highly upon mutation. Mutations causing less severe diseases are inherited as dominant, recessive, or X-linked traits depending upon the type of mutated gene. Research into the genetics of retinitis pigmentosa has demonstrated that clinically identical patterns of disease may be caused by many different mutations.

Retinoblastoma

Recent advances in our understanding of the genetic basis of retinoblastoma illustrate many of the points discussed above. Retinoblastoma is a malignant tumor of retinal photoreceptors seen in childhood. Most cases are sporadic, without transmission to subsequent generations, but a significant proportion are familial. The "two-hit" hypothesis of oncogenesis for this and other hereditary cancers proposes that tumor development is a recessive trait at the cellular level and that two separate mutations are necessary to produce the required homozygous state. In retinoblastoma, the relevant mutation is deletion at the chromosomal locus 13q14. In sporadic cases, both mutations occur in the somatic cells of the retina, and for that reason the disease is not genetically transmissible. In familial cases, the first mutation is present in the germ cells, and the second develops in retinal cells.

In familial cases, predisposition for tumor development is inherited as an autosomal dominant trait, being present in 50% of children of retinoblastoma patients. Nine out of ten individuals who inherit the germ cell mutation develop the tumor. Familial cases tend to be bilateral and multifocal and to have onset at an early age, whereas sporadic cases are unilateral, unifocal, and appear later. Individuals who inherit the germ cell mutation are also known to have a greatly increased risk for development of independent second primary tumors—particularly osteosarcoma—in later life.

Present practice consists of regular screening of all siblings and children of retinoblastoma patients for the development of retinoblastoma. This necessitates frequent general anesthesia for ophthalmoscopy. It would be advantageous to be able to restrict the screening procedure to individuals truly at risk, ie, those who have inherited the germ cell mutation.

All bilateral cases and those with a family history can be assumed to be familial; unilateral cases may be familial or sporadic. Cases without a family history may be sporadic or may be the first of a series of familial cases following de novo mutation in the germ line. However, these features are not sufficient to reliably identify only those with the germ line mutation.

Fortunately, the necessary process of gene tracking is now becoming possible both by gene linkage studies, using the esterase-D protein, which has a gene locus close to that of the retinoblastoma gene; and by DNA probes for the esterase-D and retinoblastoma genes. These techniques are also applicable to prenatal diagnosis, using chorionic villus sampling. Consequently, it is theoretically possible to identify exactly which retinoblastoma cases are familial and to determine even before birth which siblings or children also possess the germ cell mutation, thus allowing termination of the pregnancy or a much more specific childhood screening program.

GLOSSARY OF GENETIC TERMS*

Abiotrophic disease: Genetically determined disease which is not evident at birth but which becomes manifest later in life.

Acquired: Contracted after birth or in utero.

---

*Modified from Krupp MA et al: *Physician's Handbook,* 21st ed. Lange, 1985.

Alleles: Alternative forms of an individual gene.

Autosomes: The chromosomes (22 pairs of autosomes in humans) other than the sex chromosomes.

Chromosome: A small thread-like or rod-like structure into which the nuclear chromatin separates during mitosis. The number of chromosomes is constant for any given species (23 pairs in humans: 22 pairs of autosomes and one pair of sex chromosomes).

Codominant inheritance: Inheritance pattern in which the individuals heterozygous for the abnormality have a phenotype distinguishable from that of the homozygote.

Congenital: Existing at or before birth; not necessarily hereditary.

DNA probes: DNA fragments used to locate specific gene sequences to which they are complementary.

Dominant: Designating a gene whose phenotypic effect largely or entirely obscures that of its allele.

Expressivity: Variability of phenotype amongst genotypically identical individuals.

Familial: Pertaining to traits, either hereditary or acquired, which tend to occur in families.

Gamete (germ cell): A cell that is capable of uniting with another cell in sexual reproduction (ie, the ovum and spermatozoon).

Gene: A unit of heredity which occupies a specific locus in the chromosome which, either alone or in combination, produces a single characteristic. It is usually a single unit that is capable of self-duplication or mutation.

Genetic carrier state: A condition wherein a given hereditary characteristic is not manifest in one individual but may be genetically transmitted to the offspring of that individual.

Genotype: The hereditary constitution, or combination of genes, that characterizes a given individual or a group of genetically identical organisms.

Germ cell: See Gamete, above.

Hereditary: Transmitted from ancestor to offspring through the germ plasm.

Heterozygous: Having two members of a given hereditary factor pair that are dissimilar, ie, the two genes of an allelic pair are not the same.

Homozygous: Having two members of a given hereditary factor pair that are similar, ie, the two genes of an allelic pair are identical.

Linkage studies: Statistical analysis of frequency of association of genetic abnormalities to estimate the proximity of the gene loci.

Lyon hypothesis: Inactivation of one X chromosome in each somatic cell of the female, the inactivated chromosome forming the sex chromatin (Barr) body.

Meiosis: A special type of cell division occurring during the maturation of sex cells, by which the normal diploid set of chromosomes is reduced to a single (haploid) set, two successive nuclear divisions occurring, while the chromosomes divide only once.

Mitosis: Cell division in which daughter nuclei receive identical components of the number of chromosomes characteristic of the species.

Monosomy: The existence of one chromosome of one variety, rather than the normal pair of chromosomes.

Mosaicism: The presence of cells of functionally different genetic constitution within the same individual. Normally present in the female in respect of the X chromosome (Lyon hypothesis).

Mutation: A transformation of a gene, often sudden and dramatic, with or without known cause, into a different gene occupying the same locus as the original gene on a particular chromosome; the new gene is allelic to the normal gene from which it has arisen.

Penetrance: The likelihood or probability that a gene will become morphologically (phenotypically) expressed. The degree of penetrance may depend upon acquired as well as genetic factors.

Phenotype: The visible characteristics of an individual or those which are common to a group of apparently identical individuals.

Recessive: Designating a gene whose phenotypic effect is largely or entirely obscured by the effect of its allele.

Sex chromosome: The chromosome or pair of chromosomes that determines the sex of the individual. (In the human female, the sex chromosome pair is homologous, XX; in the male, heterologous, XY.)

Sex linkage: See X linkage, below.

Somatic cells: Cells incapable of reproducing the organism.

Translocation: Exchange of DNA fragments between chromosomes at the time of meiosis.

Trisomy: The existence of three chromosomes of one variety, rather than the normal pair of chromosomes.

X linkage: The pattern of inheritance of genes located on the X chromosome.

Zygote: The cell formed by the union of two gametes in sexual reproduction.

REFERENCES

Charles SJ et al: Genetic counselling in X-linked ocular albinism: Clinical features of the carrier state. Eye 1992;6:75.

Dryja TP: Doyne Lecture: Rhodpsin and autosomal dominant retinitis pigmentosa. Eye 1992;6:1.

Farber dB (moderator): Molecular genetics of retinitis pigmentosa. West J Med 1991;155:388.

Fullwood P et al: X linked exudative vitreoretinopathy: Clinical features and genetic linkage analysis. Br J Ophthalmol 1993;77:168.

Harper PS: *Practical Genetic Counselling,* 3rd ed. Wright, 1988.

Jay B: New light on visual pigment genes. Br J Ophthalmol 1990;74:238.

Johnson AT et al: Clinical features and linkage analysis of a family with autosomal dominant juvenile glaucoma. Ophthalmology 1993;100:524.

Jones KL: *Smith's Recognizable Patterns of Human Malformation,* 4th ed. Saunders, 1988.

Keith CG: *Genetics and Ophthalmology.* Churchill Livingstone, 1978.

Kinnear PE, Jay B, Witkop CJ Jr: Albinism. Surv Ophthalmol 1985;30:75.

Maumenee IH, Nelson LB (editors): Ocular genetics. In: Duane TD, Jaeger EA (editors): *Biomedical Foundations of Ophthalmology,* vol 3. Lippincott, 1988.

McKusick VA: The defect in Marfan syndrome. Nature 1991;352:279.

McKusick VA: *Mendelian Inheritance in Man,* 8th ed. Johns Hopkins Univ Press, 1988.

Musarella MA: Gene mapping of ocular diseases. Surv Ophthalmol 1992;36:285.

Newman NJ: Mitochondrial disease and the eye. Ophthalmol Clin North Am 1992;5:405.

Pagon RA: Retinitis pigmentosa. Surv Ophthalmol 1988;33:137.

Pyeritz RE: Medical genetics. In: *Current Medical Diagnosis & Treatment 1995.* Tierney LM Jr, McPhee SJ, Papadakis MA (editors). Appleton & Lange, 1995.

Ragge NK: Clinical and genetic patterns of neurofibromatosis 1 and 2. Br J Ophthalmol 1993;77:662.

Rennie WA (editor): *Goldberg's Genetic and Metabolic Eye Diseases,* 2nd ed. Little, Brown, 1986.

Russell P: *Essential Genetics,* 2nd ed. Blackwell Scientific, 1987.

Scriver CR et al (editors): *The Metabolic Basis of Inherited Disease,* 6th ed. McGraw-Hill, 1989.

Ullman S, Nelson LB, Jackson LG: Prenatal diagnostic techniques: Chorionic villus sampling. Surv Ophthalmol 1985;30:33.

Wiggs J et al: Prediction of the risk of hereditary retinoblastoma using DNA polymorphisms within the retinoblastoma gene. N Engl J Med 1988;318:151.

Taylor Asbury, MD, & James J. Sanitato, MD

Ocular trauma is a common cause of unilateral blindness in children and young adults; persons in these age groups sustain the majority of severe ocular injuries. Young adults—especially men—are the most likely victims of penetrating ocular injuries. Domestic accidents, violent assaults, exploding batteries, sports-related injuries, and motor vehicle accidents are the most common circumstances in which ocular trauma occurs.

INITIAL EXAMINATION OF OCULAR TRAUMA

The history should include an estimate of visual acuity prior to and immediately following the injury. It should be noted whether any visual loss was slowly progressive or sudden in onset. An intraocular foreign body must be suspected if there is a history of hammering, grinding, or explosions. Injuries in a child with a history that is not appropriate for the injury sustained should raise a suspicion of child abuse (see Chapter 17).

Physical examination begins with the measurement and documentation of visual acuity. If visual loss is severe, check for light projection, two-point discrimination, and the presence of an afferent pupillary defect. Test ocular motility and periorbital skin sensation, and palpate for defects in the bony orbital rim. At the bedside, the presence of enophthalmos can be determined by viewing the profiles of the corneas from over the brow. If a slitlamp is not available in the emergency room, a penlight, loupe, or direct ophthalmoscope set on +10 (black numbers) can be used to examine the tarsal surfaces of the lids and the anterior segment for injury.

The corneal surface is examined for foreign bodies, wounds, and abrasions. The bulbar conjunctiva is inspected for hemorrhage, foreign material, or lacerations. The depth and clarity of the anterior chamber are noted. The size, shape, and light reaction of the pupil should be compared with the other eye to ascertain if an afferent pupillary defect is present in the injured eye. If the eyeball is undamaged, the lids, palpebral conjunctiva, and fornices can be more thoroughly examined, including inspection after eversion of the upper lid. The direct and indirect ophthalmoscopes are used to view the lens, vitreous, optic disk, and retina. Photographic documentation is useful for medicolegal purposes in all cases of external trauma. In all cases of ocular trauma, the apparently uninjured eye should also be carefully examined.

Immediate Management of Ocular Trauma

If there is obvious rupture of the globe, one should avoid further manipulation until the patient has been given general anesthesia. No cycloplegic agents or topical antibiotics should be applied prior to surgery because of potential toxicity to exposed intraocular tissues. A Fox shield (or the bottom third of a paper cup) is taped over the eye, and parenteral broad-spectrum antibiotics are started. Analgesics, antiemetics, and tetanus antitoxin are given as needed, with restriction of food and fluids. Induction of general anesthesia should not include the use of depolarizing neuromuscular blocking agents, because these transiently increase pressure on the globe and thus increase any tendency to herniation of intraocular contents. Small children may also be better examined initially with the aid of a short-acting general anesthetic.

In severe injuries, it is important for the nonophthalmologist to bear in mind the possibility of causing further damage by unnecessary manipulation while attempting to do a complete ocular examination.

Caution: Topical anesthetics, dyes, and other medications placed in an injured eye *must be sterile.* Both tetracaine and fluorescein are available in sterile, individual dose units.

ABRASIONS & LACERATIONS OF THE LIDS

Particulate matter should be removed from abrasions of the lids to reduce skin tattooing. The wound is then irrigated with saline and covered with an antibiotic ointment and sterile dressing. Avulsed tissue is cleaned and reattached. Because of the excellent vascularity of the lids, there is a good chance that ischemic necrosis will not occur.

Partial-thickness lacerations of the lids not involv-

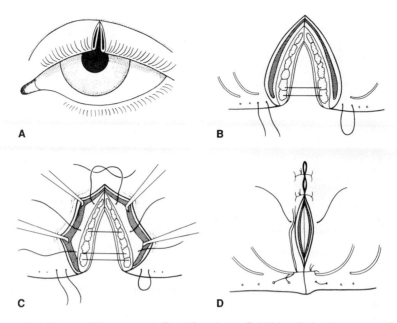

Figure 19–1. Repair of full-thickness lid laceration. **A:** The defect shown. **B:** Initial vertical mattress suture through tarsal plate. **C:** Interrupted suture closure of tarsal plate. **D:** Interrupted suture closure of skin. (Reproduced, with permission, from Phelps C: *Manual of Common Ophthalmic Surgical Procedures.* Churchill Livingstone, 1986.)

ing the lid margin may be surgically repaired in the same way as other skin lacerations. Full-thickness lid lacerations involving the lid margin, however, must be repaired carefully to prevent marginal lid notching and trichiasis (Figure 19–1).

Correct lid repair requires precise approximation of the lacerated lid margin, tarsal plate, and skin (Figure 19–1A). This is initiated by placing a double-armed 6-0 silk suture in mattress fashion through the edge of the tarsal plate. The needle is first passed through corresponding edges of the tarsal plate before exiting the meibomian gland orifice on the opposing side. The other needle with 6-0 silk is then passed similarly with a 3–4 mm spacing (Figure 19–1B). A second 6-0 silk suture is preplaced through lash follicles 2 mm equidistant on either side of the laceration. These sutures are not tied until the tarsus has been repaired with interrupted absorbable 5-0 sutures (Figure 19–1C). Finally, the skin is closed with interrupted 6-0 nylon sutures (Figure 19–1D). Antibiotic ointment is then applied to the repaired lid tissue.

If primary repair is not effected within 24 hours, edema may necessitate delayed closure. The wound should be cleaned thoroughly and antibiotics administered. After swelling has subsided, repair may be performed. Debridement should be minimized, especially if the skin is not lax.

Lacerations near the inner canthus frequently involve the canaliculi. Early repair is desirable, since the tissue becomes more difficult to identify and repair when swollen. It is always preferable to repair lacerations of the canaliculi to prevent stricture.

Sharp lacerations through the distal canaliculus can be repaired with a Veirs rod stent or other modifications. Avulsions or proximal canalicular lacerations require silicone nasocanalicular intubation with Quickert probes. Various methods of intubating a single canaliculus have been described that serve to avoid the risky and traumatic use of pigtail probes.

FOREIGN BODIES ON THE SURFACE OF THE EYE & CORNEAL ABRASIONS

Corneal foreign bodies and abrasion cause pain and irritation that can be felt during eye and lid movement, and corneal epithelial defects may cause a similar sensation. Fluorescein will stain the exposed basement membrane of an epithelial defect and can highlight aqueous leakage from penetrating wounds (positive Seidel test). A pattern of vertical scratch marks on the cornea indicates foreign bodies embedded on the tarsal conjunctival surface of the upper lid. Contact lens overwear produces corneal edema.

Simple corneal epithelial defects are treated with antibiotic ointment and a pressure patch to immobilize the lids. For removal of foreign matter, a topical anesthetic can be given and a spud or fine-gauge needle used to remove the material during slitlamp examination. A cotton-tipped applicator should not be used because it rubs off a large area of epithelium, often without removing the foreign body. Metallic rings surrounding copper or iron fragments (Figure 19–2)

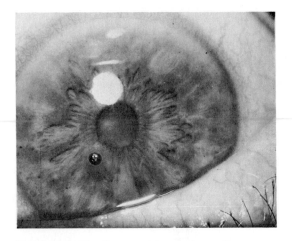

Figure 19–2. Metallic corneal foreign body. (Courtesy of A Rosenberg.)

can be removed with a battery-operated drill with a burr tip. Deeply embedded inert materials (eg, glass, carbon) may be allowed to remain in the cornea. If removal of deeply embedded fragments is necessary or if there is an aqueous leak requiring sutures or cyanoacrylate glue, the procedure should be undertaken by microsurgical technique in an operating room, where the anterior chamber can be re-formed, if necessary, with or without viscoelastics under sterile conditions.

Following removal of a foreign body, antibiotic ointment should be instilled and the eye patched. The wound should be examined daily for evidence of infection until it is completely healed.

Never give a topical anesthetic solution to the patient for repeated use after a corneal injury, as this delays healing, masks further damage, and can lead to permanent corneal scarring. In addition, chronic anesthetic use can cause corneal infiltrates and ulceration which clinically can mimic the appearance of an infectious ulcer. Steroids should be avoided while an epithelial defect exists. Because corneal abrasions are a frequent complication of general anesthesia, care should be taken to avoid this injury during induction and throughout the procedure by taping the lids closed or instilling a lubricating ophthalmic ointment in the conjunctival fornices. Recurrent epithelial erosions sometimes follow corneal injuries and are treated with patching or a bandage contact lens.

PENETRATING INJURIES & CONTUSIONS OF THE EYEBALL

Rupture of the eyeball can occur as a result of sharp penetrating injury or blunt contusive force. Blunt trauma produces a rise in orbital and intraocular pressure, with deformation of the globe. Rapid decompression occurs when the eye wall ruptures or the or-

bital contents herniate into adjacent sinuses (blowout fracture; see below). The superonasal limbus is the most common site of globe rupture (contrecoup effect—the lower temporal quadrant being most exposed to trauma). Generally, blunt traumatic injuries have a worse prognosis than penetrating injuries because of the increased incidence of retinal detachment and intraocular tissue avulsion and herniation.

While most penetrating injuries cause a marked loss of vision, injuries due to small high-velocity particles generated by grinding or hammering might present with only mild pain and blurring. Other signs include hemorrhagic chemosis, conjunctival laceration, a shallow anterior chamber with or without an eccentrically placed pupil, hyphema, or vitreous hemorrhage. The intraocular pressure can be low, normal, or, rarely, slightly elevated.

In addition to rupture of the scleral wall, contusive forces to the eyeball can result in motility disorders, subconjunctival hemorrhage, corneal edema, iritis, hyphema, angle-recession glaucoma, traumatic mydriasis, rupture of the iris sphincter, iridodialysis, paralysis of accommodation, lens dislocation, and cataract. Injuries sustained by posterior structures include vitreal and retinal hemorrhages, retinal edema (commotio retinae, or Berlin's edema), retinal holes, vitreous base avulsions, retinal detachment, choroidal rupture, and optic nerve contusion or avulsion (Figures 19–3 and 19–4).

Many of these injuries cannot be seen upon external examination. Some, such as cataract, may not develop until days or weeks after the injury.

Treatment

Except for injuries involving rupture of the eyeball itself, most of the effects of contusion of the eye do not require immediate surgical treatment. However, any

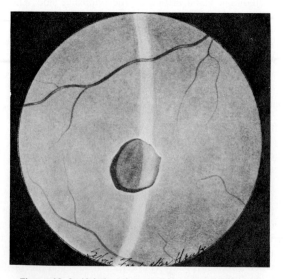

Figure 19–3. Hole in retina, macular area, posttraumatic.

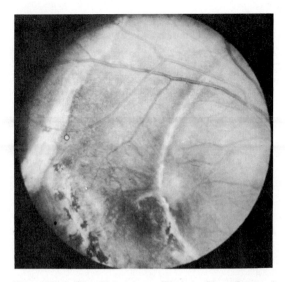

Figure 19–4. Choroidal ruptures. (Photo by Diane Beeston.)

injury severe enough to cause intraocular hemorrhage increases the risk of delayed secondary hemorrhage and possible intractable glaucoma and permanent damage to the eyeball. The further management of these cases is described in the section below on hyphema.

In the closure of anterior segment wounds, microsurgical techniques should be used. Corneal lacerations are repaired with 10-0 nylon sutures to form a watertight closure. An incarcerated iris or ciliary body exposed for less than 24 hours can be reposited in the globe with viscoelastics or by introducing a cyclodialysis spatula through a limbal stab incision and sweeping the tissue out of the wound. If this cannot be achieved, if the tissue has been exposed for more than 24 hours, or if it is ischemic and severely damaged, then the prolapsing tissue should be excised at the level of the wound lip. Any excised tissue should be sent for pathologic examination. Cultures are taken for investigation of possible bacterial or fungal infection. Lens remnants and blood are removed with mechanical irrigation and aspiration or vitrectomy or vitrectomy equipment. Anterior chamber reformation during repair is achieved with viscoelastics, air, or physiologic intraocular fluids.

Scleral wounds are closed with interrupted 8-0 or 9-0 nonabsorbable sutures. The rectus muscles may be temporarily disinserted to provide better exposure. Posterior scleral exit wounds in a double penetrating injury are self-sealing, and generally no attempt is made at closure.

The prognosis for traumatic retinal detachments is poor because of macular injury, giant retinal tears, and formation of intravitreal fibrovascular membranes that occur with penetrating injury. Such intravitreal membranes generate sufficient contractile force to detach the retina. Vitrectomy is effective in their treatment, but the timing of this procedure remains controversial.

Early vitrectomy with intravitreal antibiotics is indicated for endophthalmitis. In noninfected cases, delaying surgery for 10–14 days may decrease the risk of intraoperative hemorrhage and permit a posterior vitreous detachment to develop, making surgery technically easier.

Vitreoretinal surgery in the presence of large corneal wounds can be done through a temporary Landers-Foulks keratoprosthesis prior to corneal grafting. Primary enucleation or evisceration should only be considered when the globe is completely disorganized. The fellow eye is susceptible to sympathetic ophthalmia whenever penetrating ocular trauma occurs, particularly if there has been damage to the uveal tissues; fortunately, this complication occurs very rarely.

INTRAOCULAR FOREIGN BODIES (Figure 19–5)

A complaint of discomfort or blurred vision in an eye with a history of striking metal upon metal, explosion, or high-velocity projectile injury should arouse a strong suspicion of intraocular foreign body. The anterior portion of the eye should be inspected with a loupe or slitlamp in an attempt to localize the wound of entry. Direct and indirect ophthalmoscopic visualization of an intraocular foreign body should be attempted. An orbital soft tissue x-ray or CT scan must be taken to verify the presence of a radiopaque foreign body as well as for medicolegal reasons.

Foreign bodies that have been identified and localized within the eye must be removed whenever possible. Particles of iron or copper must be removed to prevent later disorganization of ocular tissues from toxic degenerative changes (siderosis from iron and chalcosis from copper). Some of the newer alloys are more inert and may be tolerated. Other kinds of particles, such as glass or porcelain, may be tolerated indefinitely and are usually better left alone.

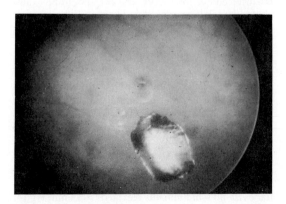

Figure 19–5. Ophthalmoscopic view of intraocular metallic (iron) foreign body in vitreous.

Localization of intraocular foreign bodies includes the geometric method of Sweet, the Comberg contact lens (containing a post and ring), ultrasonography, and coronal CT scan of the orbits. MRI is contraindicated in localizing intraocular metallic foreign bodies because the magnetic field produced during scanning can cause the foreign bodies to become high-velocity intraocular projectiles with catastrophic ocular effects.

Treatment

If the foreign body is anterior to the lens zonules, it should be removed through a limbal incision from the anterior chamber. If it is located behind the lens and anterior to the equator, it should be removed through the area of pars plana that is nearest to the foreign body because less retinal damage is caused in that manner. If the foreign body is posterior to the equator, it is best removed via the pars plana by vitrectomy and intraocular forceps, thus avoiding major choroidal hemorrhages from incisions of the posterior wall of the eyeball. This method is used for both magnetic and nonmagnetic foreign bodies. Special forceps are available for grasping spherical pellets.

Any damaged area of the retina must be treated with diathermy, photocoagulation, or endolaser coagulation to prevent retinal detachment.

HYPHEMA

Contusive forces will frequently tear the iris vessels and damage the anterior chamber angle. Blood in the aqueous may settle out in a visible layer (hyphema). Acute glaucoma occurs if the trabecular meshwork is blocked by fibrin and cells or if clot formation produces pupillary block.

Treatment

Patients with visible hyphema filling more than 5% of the anterior chamber should be placed at bed rest, and steroid and cycloplegic drops should be instilled in the affected eye for 5 days. The eye should be examined frequently for secondary bleeding, glaucoma, or corneal blood staining from iron pigment. Rebleeding occurs in 16–20% of cases within 2–3 days. This complication carries a high risk of glaucoma and corneal staining. Several studies indicate that the use of oral aminocaproic acid to stabilize clot formation reduces the risk of rebleeding. A dose of 100 mg/kg every 4 hours up to a maximum of 30 g/d for 5 days is a good regimen. If glaucoma occurs, management includes the use of ocular timolol 0.25% or 0.5.% applied twice a day; acetazolamide, 250 mg orally four times a day; and hyperosmotic agents (mannitol, glycerol, and sorbitol).

The hyphema must be surgically evacuated if the intraocular pressure remains elevated (> 35 mm Hg for 7 days or 50 mm Hg for 5 days) to avoid optic nerve damage and corneal staining. If the patient has a hemoglobinopathy, glaucomatous optic atrophy is likely to develop much more readily, and surgical evacuation of the clot should be considered much earlier. Vitrectomy instruments are used to remove the central clot and lavage the anterior chamber. The mechanized probe and irrigation port are introduced anterior to the limbus through clear cornea to avoid damage to the iris and lens. No attempt is made to extract the clot from the anterior chamber angle or from iris tissue. A peripheral iridectomy is then performed. Another means of clearing the anterior chamber is by viscoelastic evacuation. A small limbal incision is made to inject the viscoelastic, and a larger incision 180 degrees away allows the hyphema to be pushed out.

Late-onset glaucoma may follow months to years later as a result of angle recession. With rare exceptions, corneal blood staining clears slowly over a period of up to 1 year.

BURNS OF THE EYE

Chemical Burns

All chemical burns must be treated as ophthalmic emergencies. Immediate tap-water lavage should be started at the site of injury before the patient is transported. Any obvious foreign bodies should also be irrigated away if possible. In the emergency room, a brief history and examination precedes copious irrigation of the ocular surfaces, including the conjunctival fornices. Sterile isotonic saline (several liters per injured eye) is instilled with standard intravenous tubing. A lid speculum and local anesthetic infiltration of the lids may be necessary to overcome blepharospasm. Analgesics and topical anesthetic and cycloplegic agents are nearly always indicated. Use a moistened cotton-tipped applicator and jeweler's forceps to remove particulate matter from the fornices. Watch for respiratory distress due to soft tissue swelling of the upper airways. The pH of the ocular surface is checked by placing a strip of indicator paper in the fornix; resume irrigation if the pH is not between 7.3 and 7.7. After lavage, apply an antibiotic ointment and a pressure dressing.

Since alkali rapidly penetrates through ocular tissues and will continue to cause damage long after the injury is sustained, prolonged lavage and repeated pH checks are needed. Acids form a barrier of precipitated necrotic tissue that tends to limit further penetration and damage. Alkali burns cause an immediate rise in intraocular pressure owing to contraction of the sclera and trabecular meshwork damage. A secondary pressure rise occurs 2–4 hours later from the release of prostaglandins, which potentiate an intense uveitis. This is difficult to monitor through the opaque cornea. Treatment is with topical steroids, antiglaucoma agents, and cycloplegics during the first 2 weeks. Beyond 2 weeks, steroids must be used with caution because they inhibit reepithelialization. Corneal melting and possible perforation from continued collagenase activity can then occur. Ascorbate (vitamin C) and citrate drops are minimally effective for preventing corneal melting in patients with severe burns or persistent corneal epithelial defects. A trial with collagenase inhibitors (acetylcysteine) may prove beneficial. Corneal exposure and persistent epithelial defects are treated with artificial lubricants, tarsorrhaphy, or a bandage contact lens.

Long-term complications of chemical burns include angle-closure glaucoma, corneal scarring, symblepharon, entropion, and keratitis sicca. Competency of the conjunctival and scleral vasculature has been shown to be of prognostic value. A greater loss of perilimbal epithelium and conjunctival and scleral vasculature indicates a poorer prognosis.

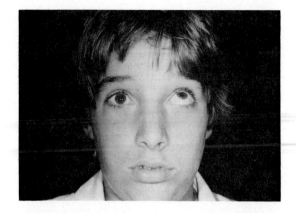

Figure 19–6. Right orbital blowout fracture in upgaze.

Thermal Burns

Thermal burns of the lids are treated with topical antibiotics and sterile dressings. If corneal damage is sustained, the extensive lid swelling initially makes pressure patching unnecessary. After 2–3 days, ectropion and lid retraction begin. Tarsorrhaphies and moisture chambers fashioned from plastic wrap then protect the cornea. Full-thickness skin grafts are delayed until skin contraction is no longer progressing.

Ultraviolet irradiation, even in moderate doses, often produces a painful superficial keratitis. Pain often begins 6–12 hours after exposure. This keratitis follows exposure to an electric welding arc without the protection of a filter, short circuits in high-voltage lines, or exposure to the reflections from snow without protective sunglasses ("snow blindness").

In severe cases of "flash burn," instillation of a sterile topical anesthetic may be necessary for examination. Treatment consists of pressure patching with an antibiotic ointment. A mydriatic is instilled if there is iritis.

Infrared exposure rarely produces an ocular reaction. ("Glassblower's cataract" is rare today but once was common among workers who were required to watch the color changes in molten glass in furnaces without proper filters.) Radiant energy from viewing the sun or an eclipse of the sun without an adequate filter, however, may produce a serious burn of the macula, resulting in permanent impairment of vision.

Excessive exposure to radiation (x-ray) produces cataractous changes that may not appear for many months after the exposure. The same risk is inherent with exposure to nuclear radiation.

INJURIES INVOLVING THE ORBIT & ITS CONTENTS

Orbital Fractures
(Figure 19–6)

Orbital fractures commonly occur with facial trauma. Fractures of the maxilla are classified by the

Le Fort system: type I is below the orbital floor; type II passes through the nasal and lacrimal bones in addition to the maxilla forming the medial orbital floor; and type III involves the medial and lateral walls and the orbital floor in the presence of separation of the facial skeleton from the cranium. Orbital roof fractures are rare and are generally caused by penetrating injuries. If visual loss is progressing in the presence of an optic canal fracture, steroids and surgical decompression may be necessary. When visual loss is sudden and complete, however, recovery is less likely. Carotid-cavernous sinus fistulas are associated with orbital apex fractures, and the orbit should therefore be auscultated for bruits.

Tripod fractures of the zygoma involve the orbital floor but in the absence of dislocation may not need surgical repair. Zygomatic arch fractures do not involve the orbit. Telescoping fractures of the frontal process of the maxilla and the lacrimal and ethmoid bones produce a saddle-nose deformity with telecanthus and lacrimal system obstruction.

When the orbital entrance receives a blow, the compressive forces can fracture the thin medial and inferior walls, with prolapse and possible entrapment of soft tissues. There may be associated intraocular injury, including hyphema, angle recession, and retinal detachment. If the blowout is large, enophthalmos of the globe may develop immediately. Enophthalmos can occur later after the swelling subsides and atrophy or scarring of the soft tissues develops.

Diplopia can be caused by direct neuromuscular damage or swelling of orbital contents. This must be differentiated from entrapment of the inferior rectus and oblique muscle or adjacent tissue within the fracture. When entrapment is present, passive movement of the eye with forceps (forced ductions test) is restricted. Sufficient time should pass to allow for spontaneous improvement in eye movements with the resolution of swelling. Sensation is tested in the distribution of the infraorbital nerve. Hypesthesia is present with orbital floor fractures. A series of plain x-ray films of the bony orbit should include a Waters view x-ray to show the maxillary sinus (antral) roof. These x-rays may reveal bony defects, an air-fluid level in the sinus, or herniated soft tissues. When interpretation of these films is equivocal, CT scan should be performed.

The indications for surgical repair of the blowout fracture are (1) persistent diplopia within 30 degrees of the primary position of gaze in the presence of entrapment; (2) enophthalmos of 2 mm or more; or (3) a large fracture (half the orbital floor), which is likely to cause late enophthalmos. Delaying surgery for 1–2 weeks helps the surgeon to assess whether the diplopia will resolve without intervention. Longer delays decrease the likelihood of successful repair of enophthalmos and strabismus because of progressive scarring.

Surgical repair is usually accomplished via an infraciliary or transconjunctival route, though transantral and infraorbital approaches are also done. The periorbita is incised and elevated to expose the fracture site in the floor and medial walls. Herniated tissue is pulled back into the orbit, and the defect is covered by an alloplastic implant, with care being taken not to damage the infraorbital neurovascular bundle. Complications include blindness, diplopia, extrusion of the implant, or migration of the implant to press against the lacrimal sac, causing obstruction and dacryocystitis. Other complications include hemorrhage, infection, lower eyelid retraction, and infraorbital anesthesia. Subsequent procedures for strabismus and ptosis may be needed.

Penetrating Injury of the Orbit

Penetrating injuries of the orbital tissue may be produced by high-velocity projectiles or sharp instruments. Radiopaque foreign bodies can be localized by methods similar to those used in locating intraocular foreign bodies within the eye.

Contusions of the Orbit

Contusion injuries to the orbital contents may result in hemorrhage or subsequent atrophy of the tissue, with enophthalmos. Traumatic paresis of the extraocular muscles occasionally occurs but is usually transient.

Pulsating Exophthalmos Following Orbital Injury

Pulsating exophthalmos occasionally follows a penetrating or contusion injury to the orbital contents due to the formation of an arteriovenous shunt. A common site of involvement is a bone fracture into the cavernous sinus. Pulsating exophthalmos occasionally requires ligation of the carotid artery on the side of the fistula.

PREVENTION OF INJURIES TO THE EYE (See also Chapter 21.)

Persons engaging in industrial or athletic activities while wearing prescription lenses made of glass or plastic are at increased risk from shattered lens fragments. The eyewear most effective in preventing injuries consists of polycarbonate lenses in polyamide frames with a posterior retention rim. Solid wraparound frames should be used (rather than hinged frames) because they better withstand lateral blows. In athletic or high-risk recreational activities (eg, air or paint-pellet gun "war games"), guards without lenses do not always protect the eye adequately. Proper eye protection is particularly indicated for those playing racquetball, handball, and squash. The sight of many eyes has been lost in these sports, particularly from ocular contusion trauma in the absence of adequate eye protection.

REFERENCES

Aiello LP, Iwamoto M, Guyer DR: Penetrating ocular fishhook injuries. Surgical management and long-term visual outcome. Ophthalmology 1992;99:862.

Beare JD: Eye injuries from assault with chemicals. Br J Ophthalmol 1990;74:514.

Bloom SM, Gittinger JW Jr, Kazarian EL: Management of corneal contact thermal burns. Am J Ophthalmol 1986; 102:536.

Bolling JP, Wesley RE: Conservative treatment of orbital roof blow-in fracture. Ann Ophthalmol 1987;19:75.

Brackup AB et al: Long-term follow-up of severely injured eyes following globe rupture. Ophthal Plast Reconstr Surg 1991;7:194.

Braverman DE, Brown RE Jr: Externalized silicone tube in single canalicular intubation. Am J Ophthalmol 1987;103:335.

Dannenberg AL, Parver LM, Fowler CJ: Penetrating eye injuries related to assault. The National Eye Trauma System Registry. Arch Ophthalmol 1992;110:849.

Dannenberg AL et al: Penetration eye injuries in the workplace. The National Eye Trauma System Registry. Arch Ophthalmol 1992;110:843.

DeBustros S, Michels RG, Glaser BM: Evolving concepts in the management of posterior segment penetrating ocular injuries. Retina 1990;10(Suppl 1):S72.

Dhir SP et al: Ocular fireworks injuries in children. J Pediatr Ophthalmol Strabismus 1991;28:354.

Farber MD, Fiscella R, Goldberg MF: Aminocaproic acid versus prednisone for the treatment of traumatic hyphema: A randomized clinical trial. Ophthalmology 1991;98:279.

Fuller DG, Hutton WL: Prediction of postoperative vision in eyes with severe trauma. Retina 1990;10(Suppl 1):20.

Goldfarb MS, Hoffman DS, Rosenberg S: Orbital cellulitis and orbital fractures. Ann Ophthalmol 1987;19:97.

Groessl S, Nanda SK, Mieler WF: Assault-related penetrating ocular injury. Am J Ophthalmol 1993;116:26.

Harris GJ, Fuerste FH: Lacrimal intubation in the primary repair of midfacial fractures. Ophthalmology 1987;94:242.

Jain BK, Talbot EM: Bungee jumping and intraocular haemorrhage. Br J Ophthalmol 1994;78:236.

Kearns P: Traumatic hyphaema: A retrospective study of 314 cases. Br J Ophthalmol 1991;75:137.

Kersten RC: Blowout fracture of the orbital floor with entrapment caused by isolated trauma to the orbital rim. Am J Ophthalmol 1987;103:215.

Klopfer J et al: Ocular trauma in the United States. Eye injuries resulting in hospitalization, 1984 through 1987. Arch Ophthalmol 1992;110:838.

Kutner B et al: Aminocaproic acid reduces the risk of secondary hemorrhage in patients with traumatic hyphema. Arch Ophthalmol 1987;105:206.

Lawrence T, Wilison D, Harvey J: The incidence of secondary hemorrhage after traumatic hyphema. Ann Ophthalmol 1990;22:276.

Macewen CJ: Eye injuries: A prospective survey of 5671 cases. Br J Ophthalmol 1989;73:888.

Mamalis N et al: Blunt ocular trauma secondary to "war games." Ann Ophthalmol 1990;22:416.

Meredith TA, Gordon PA: Pars plana vitrectomy for severe penetrating injury with posterior segment involvement. Am J Ophthalmol 1987;103:549.

Mitchell GC et al: A two-year prospective study of penetrating ocular trauma at the Wilmer Ophthalmological Institute. Ann Ophthalmol 1987;19:104.

Ng CS et al: Factors related to the incidence of secondary haemorrhage in 462 patients with traumatic hyphema. Eye 1992;6:308.

Nichols CJ et al: Ocular injuries caused by elastic cords. Arch Ophthalmol 1991;109:371. [Published erratum appears in Arch Ophthalmol 1991;109:878.]

Punnonen E, Laatikainen L: Prognosis of perforating eye injuries with intraocular foreign bodies. Acta Ophthalmol 1989;67:483.

Sharif KW, McGhee CN, Tomlinson RC: Ocular trauma caused by air-gun pellets: A ten year survey. Eye 1990;4:855.

Spaulding SC, Sternberg P Jr: Controversies in the management of posterior segment ocular trauma. Retina 1990;10(Suppl 1):S76.

Spoor TC et al: Traumatic hyphema in an urban population. Am J Ophthalmol 1990;109:23.

Steinsapir KD, Goldberg RA: Traumatic optic neuropathy. Surv Ophthalmol 1994;38:487.

Strahlman E et al: Causes of pediatric eye injuries. A population-based study. Arch Ophthalmol 1990;108:603.

Thompson JT et al: Infectious endophthalmitis after penetrating injuries with retained intraocular foreign bodies. Ophthalmology 1993;100:1468.

Uusitalo RJ, Ranta-Kemppainen L, Tarkkanen A: Management of traumatic hyphema in children: An analysis of 340 cases. Arch Ophthalmol 1988;106:1207.

Volpe NJ et al: Secondary hemorrhage in traumatic hyphema. Am J Ophthalmol 1991;112:507.

Williams C et al: Outpatient management of small traumatic hyphaemas: Is it safe? Eye 1993;7:155.

Wilson TW, Jeffers JB, Nelson LB: Aminocaproic acid prophylaxis in traumatic hyphema. Ophthalmic Surg 1990;21:807.

Wilson WB et al: Magnetic resonance imaging of nonmetallic orbital foreign bodies. Am J Ophthalmol 1988;105:612.

Zheutlin JD, Thompson JT, Shafner RS: The safety of magnetic resonance imaging with intraorbital metallic objects after retinal re-attachment or trauma. Am J Ophthalmol 1987;103:831.

Optics & Refraction

Paul Riordan-Eva, FRCS, FRCOphth, & Orson W. White, MD*

The correct interpretation of visual information depends on the eye's ability to focus incoming rays of light on the retina. An understanding of this process and how it is influenced by normal variations or ocular disease is essential to the successful use of any optical aid, eg, glasses, contact lenses, intraocular lenses, or low-vision aids. To achieve this understanding, it is necessary to master the concepts of geometric optics, which define the effect on light rays as they pass through different surfaces and media.

GEOMETRIC OPTICS

Speed, Frequency, & Wavelength of Light

Speed, frequency, and wavelength of light are related by the following expression:

$$\text{Frequency} = \frac{\text{Speed}}{\text{Wavelength}}$$

In different optical media, speed and wavelength of light change, but frequency is constant. Color depends on frequency, so that the color of a ray of light is not altered as it passes through optical media except by selective nontransmittance or fluorescence. The optical characteristics of a substance can only be defined with respect to clearly specified frequencies of light. A substance to be used for lenses to refract visible light is usually tested with the yellow sodium light (D line) and the blue (F line) and the red (C line) of a rarefied hydrogen discharge tube.

In a vacuum, the speed of all frequencies of light is the same, ie, 299,792.46 kilometers per second (186,282.40 statute miles per second). Since the frequency of the yellow D line is approximately 5.085×10^{14} Hz, the wavelength of this line in a vacuum is 0.5896 μm. Similarly, the wavelengths in a vacuum of the blue F and red C lines are 0.4861 μm and 0.6563 μm, respectively.

Index of Refraction

If the speed of a light ray is altered by a change in the optical medium, refraction of the ray will also oc-

cur (Figure 20–1). The effect of an optical substance on the speed of light is expressed as its index of refraction, n. The higher the index, the slower the speed and the greater the effect on refraction.

In a vacuum, n has the value of 1.00000. The **absolute index of refraction** of a substance is the ratio of the speed of light in a vacuum to the speed of light in the substance. The **relative index of refraction** of a substance is calculated with reference to the speed of light in air. The absolute index of refraction of air varies with the temperature, pressure, and humidity of the air and the frequency of the light, but it is about 1.00032. In optics, n is assumed to be relative to air unless specified as absolute.

Thermal Coefficient of Index of Refraction

The index of refraction changes with the temperature of the medium—it is higher when the substance is colder. This lability of n to temperature is different for different substances. The change in n per degree Celsius for the following substances (all to be multiplied by 10^{-7}) is as follows: glass, 1; fluorite, 10; plastic, 140;

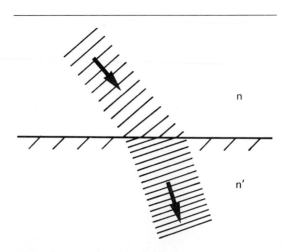

Figure 20–1. Refraction of light as it enters a transparent medium of higher refractive index n .

*Deceased.

water, aqueous, and vitreous, 185. This makes plastic undesirable for precision optical devices. (Plastic also has eight times the thermal expansion of glass.) Water lenses date back to antiquity but are not practical, because of problems with thermal instability, evaporation, freezing, and susceptibility to contamination. It is interesting that in the eye, these objections all but disappear, making the fluid lenses of the eye acceptable.

Dispersion of Light

In a vacuum, the speed of all frequencies of light is the same; thus, the index of refraction is also the same for all colors (1.00000). In all substances, n is different for each color or frequency, being larger at the blue end and smaller at the red end of the spectrum. This difference can be quantified as the dispersion value, V:

$$V = \frac{n_D - 1}{n_F - n_C}$$

where n_D, n_F, and n_C are the indices of refraction for the yellow sodium line and the blue and the red hydrogen lines.

The higher the value of V, the less the dispersion of colors. Table 20–1 gives the indices of refraction and some dispersion values for substances of ophthalmologic interest.

Table 20–1. Indices of refraction and dispersion values of some substances of ophthalmologic interest.

Substance (20 °C unless noted)	Indices of Refraction (n_D)	Dispersion Values (V)
Water	1.33299	
Water 37 °C	1.33093	55.6
Sea water	1.344	
Sea water, 11,000 meters' depth	1.361	
Polymethylmethacrylate	1.49166	57.37
Polymethylmethacrylate 37 °C	1.48928	
Acrylonitrile styrene copolymer	1.56735	34.87
Polystyrene	1.59027	30.92
Fluorite	1.4338	95.2
Spectacle crown glass	1.523	58.8
Flint glass	1.617	36.6
Aqueous and vitreous 37 °C	1.3337	55.6
Hydroxyethylmethacrylate (HEMA)	1.43	
Cellulose acetate butyrate (CAB)	1.47	
Silicone	1.439	

Transmittance of Light

Optical materials vary in their transmittance or transparency to different frequencies. Some "transparent" materials such as glass are almost opaque to ultraviolet light. Red glass would be almost opaque to the green frequency. Optical media must be selected according to the specific wavelength of light with which they are to be used.

Laws of Reflection & Refraction

The laws of reflection and refraction were formulated in 1621 by the Dutch astronomer and mathematician Willebrod Snell at the University of Leyden. These laws, together with Fermat's principle, form the basis of applied geometric optics. They can all be stated as follows (Figure 20–2).

(1) Incident, reflected, and refracted rays all reside in a plane known as the plane of incidence, which is normal (at a right angle) to the interface.

(2) The angle of incidence equals the angle of reflection but has the opposite sign: $I = -I'$.

(3) The product of the index of refraction of the medium of the incident ray and the sine of the angle of incidence of the incident ray is equal to the product of the same terms of the refracted ray. The refracted ray is designated by a prime: $n \sin I = n' \sin I'$ (**Snell's law**).

(4) A ray of light passing from one point to another follows the path that takes the least time to negotiate (**Fermat's principle**). Optical path length is the index of refraction times the actual path length.

Critical Angle & Total Reflection

In Figure 20–2, consider the ray in the more dense medium as the arriving ray. We see that it is refracted

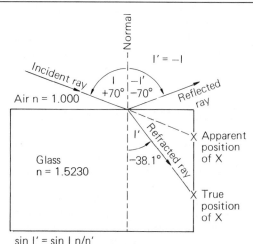

Figure 20–2. Example of the laws of reflection and refraction.

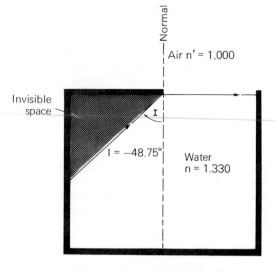

Figure 20–3. Example of the critical angle.

into the less dense medium away from the normal. If we gradually increase the angle of incidence (Figure 20–3) in the denser medium until we reach the critical angle, a startling event takes place: None of the light escapes, but all is suddenly, totally, and perfectly reflected (total internal reflection). This angle is reached as the sine of the incident ray in the denser medium reaches the value $-n'/n$. This is one method used to determine the index of refraction. For water, with an index of refraction of 1.330, the critical angle has the sine of –1/1.330, or –48.75 degrees.

Total reflection obeys the laws of regular reflection, ie, $I = -I'$. This allows perfect reflection without coatings and is used extensively in prisms and fiberoptics.

In Figure 20–3, the shaded area is not visible from the surface. This is why the angle of the eye cannot be inspected except with the gonioscopic lens (see Chapter 2). The index of refraction of the *aqueous*—and not the index of refraction of the tears or cornea, as is frequently stated—is the determining factor in this context.

CALCULATIONS USED IN OPTICS

There are two approaches to the application of the principles of geometric optics to single lenses or to compound lens systems. **Trigonometric ray tracing** is the more valid and exact approach, as it makes no assumptions other than those already determined by the laws of refraction. The **algebraic method** is a system based on a number of assumptions that greatly simplify calculation of the effects of various lens systems but also limit accuracy to an ever-increasing extent as

the lens systems become more complex. The algebraic method cannot be relied on for accurate results, particularly in the assessment of the optical effects of contact lenses, intraocular lenses, and keratorefractive procedures—all of which are becoming more frequently used in the practice of ophthalmology.

Certain considerations are universal to optical calculations whatever method is used. For any optical system, the object and its image are said to lie in **conjugate planes.** If the object were to be placed in the plane of its own image, the optical system would produce its new image in the original object plane. Thus, the effects of any optical system will be the same for whichever direction light travels through the system. Each optical system has an infinite number of pairs of conjugate planes. Corresponding points on conjugate planes are known as **conjugate points.**

Trigonometric Ray Tracing

The trigonometric method of ray tracing consists of mathematically plotting the course of certain specified rays through the lens systems. The three rays most frequently traced are shown in Figure 20–4. They are named according to their positions relative to the first refracting surface. The marginal ray enters at the margin of the lens, the paraxial ray very near the optical axis (center of the lens), and the zonal ray in the portion of the lens where the average luminous flux of light passes through the lens. At each refracting surface, the change in direction of each of these rays is calculated according to the principles of Snell's law. This requires knowledge of the radius of curvature of the surface, the index of refraction of the medium on each side of the refracting surface, and the distance to the next surface. Elementary trigonometry is the only mathematical skill necessary for such calculations, though a programma-

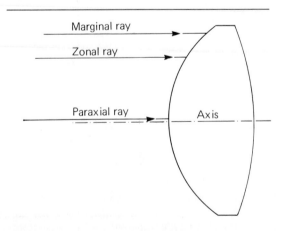

Figure 20–4. Illustration of three rays traced in trigonometric ray tracing.

ble calculator greatly assists with the number of such calculations that have to be carried out.*

Trigonometric ray tracing provides an exact determination of the point of focus and information on the quality of the image formed by a lens system. The difference between the back focal lengths (distance along the optical axis from the last refracting surface to the point of focus) of the marginal and paraxial rays is a measure of the "spread of focus," thus indicating the degree of **spherical aberration** (see below). Similarly, if rays of different color (frequency), with their different indices of refraction in each medium, are traced through the system, the degree of **chromatic aberration** (see below) will be determined. The optical pathway is the sum of the actual distance a ray passes through the substances multiplied by the index of refraction in the various substances through which it passes. How closely the optical pathways of the marginal and paraxial rays match determines the brightness and contrast of the final image.

Trigonometric ray tracing permits determination of the performance of each refracting surface relative to the contribution to the final image. For example, it is easily shown that a planoconvex intraocular lens gives a better image with the convex surface forward and the flat surface closer to the retina. The point of focus often requires—and is easily adjusted by—postoperative refraction. *However, the distorted image caused by selecting an intraocular lens of improper shape cannot be repaired by refraction. Suitability in this respect must be achieved by proper preoperative lens design, and this can only be achieved by calculation using the trigonometric method of ray tracing.*

Graphic ray tracing is a system comparable to trigonometric ray tracing that uses drawings to deter-

mine the optical properties of lens systems; it should not be confused with the method of "ray tracing" described in several books, in which tracings of an image are based on nodal points and focal planes (a derivation of the algebraic method of optical calculations discussed below).

Algebraic Method

Karl Friedrich Gauss (1777–1855) is responsible for refining a method of optical calculations that dispensed with the sines and cosines of the trigonometric method. This assumed that the lenses are "infinitely thin," placed close together, and of small diameter, such that any angle will be so small that the size of the angle measured in radians will have the same value as the sine of the angle and that the sine and the tangent of the angle can be assumed to be the same. The results are the **thin lens equations** used by opticians to calculate curves for lenses. "Fudge factors" derived from experience are then necessary to correct for the inaccuracies of these equations.

Use of the algebraic method depends on certain definitions. The position of the lens, reduced to a single line, is the **principal plane**, which intersects the optical axis at the **nodal point** (optical center). The **primary focal point (F)** is that point along the optical axis where an object must be placed to form an image at infinity. The **secondary focal point (F′)** is that point along the optical axis where parallel incident rays are brought to a focus. If the medium on either side of the lens is of the same refractive index, the distance between the nodal point and each of the focal points, the **focal length,** is the same.

Figure 20–5 shows some of the important thin lens equations.

The **diopter (D)** is a measure of lens power derived from the algebraic method of optical calculations. It is defined as the reciprocal of the focal length of a lens in air measured in meters. Diopters are additive, but only for low-power lenses. The result of combining lenses of high power varies greatly with their thickness and the separation distance. High-power lenses must

---

*Further explanation of the calculations involved in trigonometric ray tracing may be found in Dr Orson White's chapter on optics and refraction in the 11th edition of this book.

$$\text{Diopters} \cong \frac{1}{\text{Focal length}} \cong \frac{1}{\text{Distance of image}} - \frac{1}{\text{Distance of object}}$$

$$\text{Diopters} \cong (n-1)\ \frac{1}{\text{Radius}_1} - \frac{1}{\text{Radius}_2}$$

$$\frac{\text{Size of image}}{\text{Distance of image}} \cong \frac{\text{Size of object}}{\text{Distance of object}}$$

$$\text{Magnification} = \frac{\text{Size of image}}{\text{Size of object}} \cong \frac{\text{Distance of image}}{\text{Distance of object}}$$

Power for Several Lenses Combined

$$\text{Diopters total} \cong \text{Dio}_1 + \text{Dio}_2 + \text{Dio}_3,\ \text{etc}$$

Figure 20–5. Algebraic thin lens approximations. All lengths in meters.

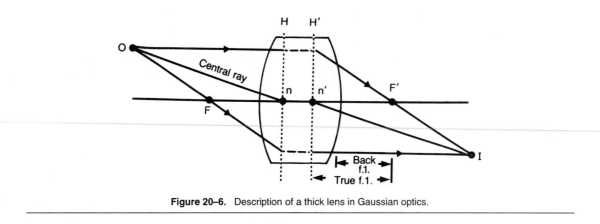

Figure 20–6. Description of a thick lens in Gaussian optics.

be described by three values: (1) radii of curvature, (2) index of refraction, and (3) thickness.

In Gaussian optics, a thick lens is treated as if there are two nodal points and two principal planes (n and n′ and H and H′ in Figure 20–6). The nodal points lie on the principal planes only if the refractive medium is the same on either side of the lens. The true focal lengths are measured from the principal planes to the focal points, but the front and back focal lengths—essential to the prescription of corrective lenses—are measured from the respective surfaces of the lens to the focal points. The reciprocal of the back focal length corresponds to the back vertex power as measured with a lensometer.

For making high plus contact lenses or thick spectacle lenses, the equation for dioptric power according to the algebraic method is as follows:

$$\text{Dio} \cong \frac{1}{F} \cong (n-1)\left[\frac{1}{r_1} - \frac{1}{r_2} - \frac{(n-1)d}{nr_1r_2}\right]$$

where F = focal length, r = radius, and d = thickness of lens, all measured in meters, and n = refractive index.

For contact lenses, a derivation of the thin lens equations is presently used to relate dioptric power to radius of curvature:

$$\text{Dio} \approx \frac{(n-1)}{r} \approx \frac{1.3375 - 1}{r} \approx \frac{337.5}{\text{rmm}} \text{ and rmm} \approx \frac{337.5}{\text{Dio}}$$

n of "cornea" is for this purpose assumed to be 1.3375. rmm = radius in millimeters. These equations are only approximations.

The ray tracing method commonly described in ophthalmic optics texts is a graphic representation of the algebraic system of optical calculations—in comparison to true graphic ray tracing, which is a graphic representation of the trigonometric system. Rays are traced through the optical system to connect conjugate points. The positions of the conjugate planes are derived mathematically from the thin lens equations. The size and orientation of the object are then determined by tracing the central ray, which passes straight through the tip of the image, the nodal point of the lens (without being refracted), and the tip of the object. The rays that traverse the focal points of the lens are derived by extrapolation (Figure 20–7).

For multiple lens systems, the conjugate planes and the path of the central ray are determined for each lens in succession, producing an image that becomes the object for the next lens until the size and orientation of the final image is located. In the case of a thick lens, refraction occurs at the principal planes of the lens, the position of rays being translated from one principal plane to another without any change in their vertical separation from the optical axis (Figure 20–6). The central ray passes from the tip of the object to the first nodal point and then emerges from the second nodal point parallel to its original direction to reach the tip of the image. When the media on either side of the lens have different refractive indices, the nodal points do not coincide with the principal planes.

Magnification

Linear magnification is the ratio of the height of the image to the height of the object. For an infinitely thin lens in air—as assumed by the algebraic method of optical calculation—this ratio is equal to the ratio of the distance of the image to the distance of the object. For real lens systems, such as those of the eye, a more complex equation including the index of refraction of the initial and final media must be used. Trigonometric ray tracing quickly provides other information necessary for the calculation.

Change of Vertex Distance

If the vertex distance (the distance from the eye) of a lens of given power is altered, the effective power of the lens will also change. To calculate a new lens that

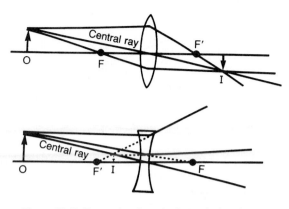

Figure 20–7. Ray tracing through plus and minus lenses.

will have the same effect at the new distance, a derivation of the thin lens equations can be used:

(Dio = power in diopters)

$$Dio_2 \approx \frac{1}{\dfrac{1}{Dio_1} - (Dist_1 - Dist_2)}$$

Example 1 : A + 13 diopter lens at 11mm (0.011 m) is to be replaced by a lens at 9 mm (0.009 m)

$$Dio_2 \cong \frac{1}{\dfrac{1}{13} - (0.011 - 0.009)} \cong 13.347 \text{ diopters}$$

Example 2 : Same lens to be replaced by a contact lens

$$Dist_2 = 0$$

$$Dio_2 \cong \frac{1}{\dfrac{1}{13} - (0.011)} \cong 15.169 \text{ diopters}$$

This vertex equation is also an approximation and should not be used for intraocular lens calculations, but it is useful for conversion from spectacle to contact lens powers.

Aberrations of Spherical Lenses

Spherical lenses are subject to a number of aberrations that reduce the quality of image produced. The variation of refractive index with frequency of light (dispersion) results in greater refraction of blue than red light (**chromatic aberration**) (Figure 20–8). Marginal rays are refracted more than paraxial rays, producing **spherical aberration** (Figure 20–9). **Coma,** a characteristic comet-shaped blur, is the re-

sult of spherical aberration of light originating away from the optical axis of the lens. When light traverses a spherical lens obliquely, there is an additional cylindrical lens effect—**astigmatism of oblique incidence. Curvature of field** is the production of a curved image from a flat object. Prismatic effects of the lens periphery also cause image distortion. Achromatic lenses may be made by cementing together plus and minus lenses of different refractive indices. The nonchromatic aberrations are overcome by combining or shaping lenses to reduce the power of the lens periphery, by restricting the area of the lens used to the paraxial zones, and by use of meniscus lenses.

Cylindrical Lenses

A **planocylindrical lens** (Figure 20–10) has one flat surface and one cylindrical surface, producing a lens with no optical power in the meridian of its axis and maximum power in the meridian 90 degrees away from the axis meridian. The total effect is the formation of a line image, parallel to the axis of the lens, from a point object. The orientation of a planocylindrical lens is specified by the meridian of its axis. The ophthalmic convention for specifying the orientation of the axis of a cylindrical lens is shown in Figure 20–11. Zero begins nasally in the right lens and temporally in the left lens and proceeds in a counterclockwise direction to 180 degrees.

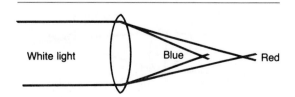

Figure 20–8. Chromatic aberration of lenses.

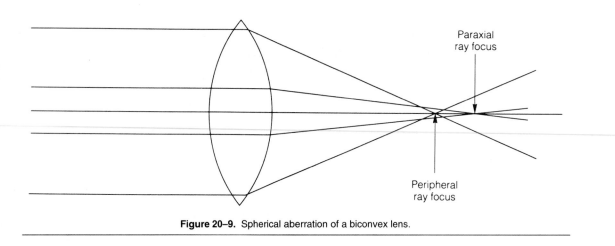

Figure 20–9. Spherical aberration of a biconvex lens.

In a **spherocylindrical lens,** the cylindrical surface is curved in two meridians but not to the same extent. In ophthalmic lenses, these principal meridians are at 90 degrees to each other. The effect of a spherocylindrical lens on a point object is to produce a geometric figure known as the **conoid of Sturm** (Figure 20–12), consisting of two focal lines separated by the interval of Sturm. The position of the focal lines relative to the lens is determined by the power of the two meridians and their orientation by the angle between the meridians. Cross-sections through the conoid of Sturm reveal lines at the focal lines and generally ellipses elsewhere. In one position, the cross-section will be a circle that represents the **circle of least confusion.**

A spherocylindrical lens can be thought of as a combination of a spherical lens and a planocylindrical lens. It can then be specified by the orientation of principal meridians and the power acting in each (Figure 20–13). In a cross diagram, the arms are drawn parallel to the principal meridians and labeled with the relevant power. In longhand notation, the cylinder is specified by the orientation of its axis, which is 90 degrees away from the meridian of maximum power.

Writing prescriptions for spherocylindrical lenses uses longhand notation, and the lens can be specified in either plus or minus cylinder form (Figure 20–13). The procedure for transposing between these forms is as follows: (1) algebraically sum the original sphere and cylinder; (2) reverse the sign of the cylinder; and (3) change the axis of the cylinder by 90 degrees.

If their principal meridians correspond, combinations of spherocylindrical lenses can be summed mathematically. Otherwise, trigonometric formulas are required. Alternatively, the power of such combinations can be determined by placing them together in a lensometer. The principal meridians of any such combination will be 90 degrees apart.

Prisms

A prism consists of a transparent material with nonparallel flat surfaces. In cross-section, it has an apex and a base. The prism is specified by its power and the orientation of its base.

A prism refracts light toward its base, whereas an object seen through a prism appears deviated toward the apex of the prism. The amount of deviation varies according to the tilt of the prism, ie, the angle of incidence of the light. For glass prisms, calibration is performed in the **Prentice position,** in which the incident light is perpendicular to the face of the prism (Figure 20–14). For plastic prisms and in general optics, a prism is calibrated in the **position of minimum deviation,** in which the amount of refraction at the two surfaces of the prisms is equal (Figure 20–14). When prisms are used in clinical practice, these orientations must be adhered to for accurate results.

For a glass prism in the Prentice position, the incident ray is not refracted at the first surface because the surfaces are perpendicular to one another (Figure 20–15). At the second surface, the angle of incidence is the same as the apex angle of the prism (A). If I´ is the angle of the final refracted ray, from Snell's law, sin I´ = (n/n´) sin A, n being the refractive index of the prism and n´ the refractive index of the surrounding medium. For example, if the prism is of glass with n = 1.523 and A = 30 degrees, then sin I´ is 1.523 × 0.5, or 0.7615. I´ is 49.6 degrees. The angle of deviation is I´ −A, or 19.6 degrees.

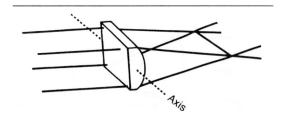

Figure 20–10. A planocylindrical lens with axis in the horizontal meridian.

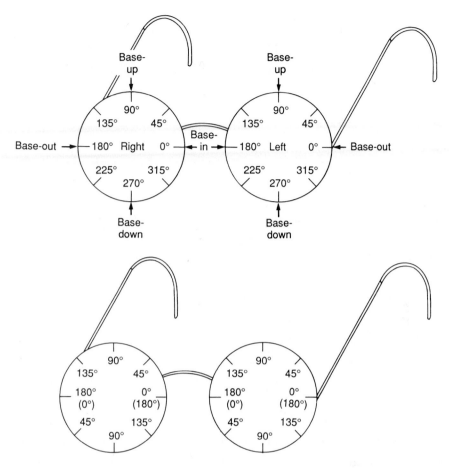

Figure 20–11. ***Top:*** Illustration of prism base notation. ***Bottom:*** Illustration of cylinder axis notation.

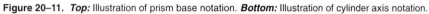

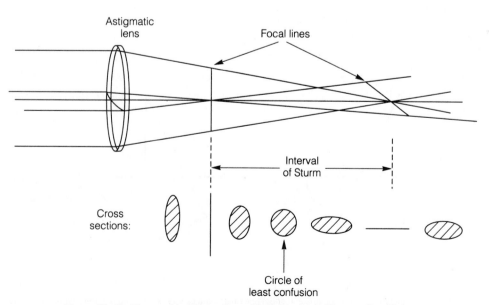

Figure 20–12. The conoid of Sturm, formed by light refracted by an astigmatic lens.

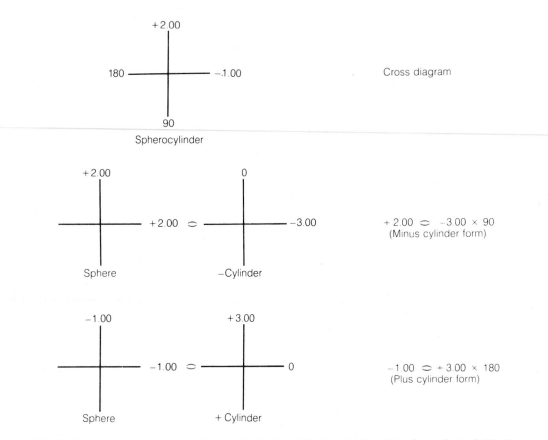

Figure 20–13. Cross diagram and equivalent combinations, including longhand notations, for a spherocylindrical lens.

The power of a prism is measured in prism diopters (Δ). One prism diopter deviates an image 1 cm at 1 m (Figure 20–16). The arc tangent of 1/100 is 0.57 degrees. So 1^Δ produces an angle of deviation of almost one-half degree. The "rule of thumb" is that a prism of 2^Δ produces an angle of deviation of 1 degree, but this cannot be applied to prisms of more than 100^Δ.

Prisms are used in ophthalmology both to measure

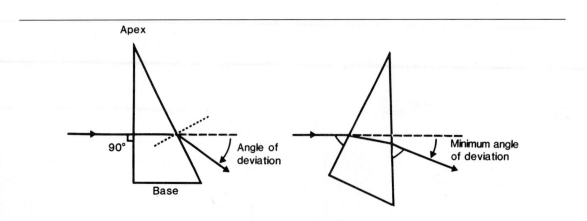

Figure 20–14. Calibration of prisms. Glass prisms and spectacle prisms are calibrated according to the Prentice position, whereas plastic prisms are calibrated according to the position of minimum deviation.

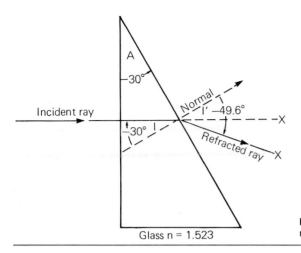

Figure 20–15. Example of the prism as used in ophthalmology.

and to treat heterotropia and heterophoria. The orientation of a prism's base is indicated by its direction, usually descriptively, ie, "base-up right eye," "base-down left eye," "base-in" or "base-out," or occasionally by a mathematical system (Figure 20–11).

Fresnel prisms are lightweight plastic prisms consisting of narrow, parallel strips of prism with the same apex angle as the desired single prism (Figure 20–17). They are available as press-on prisms for attachment to the back of spectacle lenses, providing an easily adjusted temporary prismatic correction that is less heavy than conventional glass prisms. Their disadvantages are the image degradation due to light scatter and dirt within the grooves.

Prismatic Effect of Spherical Lenses

Spherical lenses have increasing prismatic power as the light path moves away from the optical center of the lens. The amount of prism power can be calculated from Prentice's rule, which states that the prism power in prism diopters is equal to the dioptric power of the lens in diopters multiplied by the displacement from the optical center in centimeters. For example, at 0.5 cm away from the optical center of a 6^Δ lens, the prismatic power is 3^Δ. Plus lenses produce prism power with the base orientated toward the optical center of the lens, and minus lenses produce prism power with the base orientated away from their optical center.

The prismatic effect of spherical lenses is an important consideration in the correction of anisometropia. Appropriate spectacle lenses may produce significant vertical prismatic deviation when the peripheral portions of the lenses are used. This occurs mainly when the patient attempts to read. The prismatic effect can be overcome by adopting a chin-down position, thus using the optical centers of the lenses once again, by grinding of a compensatory prism into the reading segment of the glasses **(slab-off prism),** or by changing to contact lenses.

If a prism needs to be incorporated into a patient's spectacle correction, such as in the control of hypertropia, it may be achieved by decentration of the spherical lens rather than by addition of a prism to the spherical component.

Rapid Detection of Lens Characteristics

The nature of a spherical lens may be rapidly detected by looking through it 0.5 m (19 inches) or so from the eye and moving the lens at right angles to the visual axis. The image seen through a minus (concave) lens will tend to move *with* the lens. The same test with a plus (convex) lens causes the image to tend to move *away from* the direction of motion. This effect is due to the prismatic effect of the periphery of the lens. The power of the lens can be approximated by neutralization of these movements by lenses of known power. A cylindrical lens shows changing distortion of the image when the lens is rotated about the visual axis. (Spherical lenses do not.) The orientations of the lens in which the image is clearest indicate the principal meridians. The power in each of the principal meridians can then be determined by the method described above for

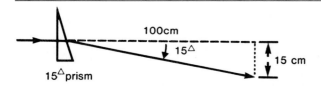

Figure 20–16. Power of a prism in prism diopters.

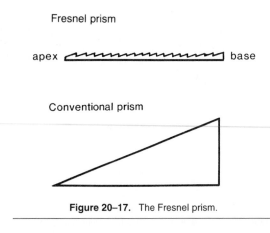

Figure 20–17. The Fresnel prism.

spherical lenses. A prism is recognized by deviation of the image as the static lens is viewed through its center.

OPTICS & THE EYE

Many attempts have been made to simplify the optical system of the human eye, particularly using the thick lens equations of the algebraic method of optical calculations. Much has been made of the concept that the image on the retina is formed by two lens elements, the cornea contributing about 43 D and the lens the remaining 19 D, but this is a gross oversimplification. The **schematic eye of Gullstrand** and its reduced form (Figure 20–18) are models from which mathematical values for the optical characteristics of the eye were derived. For instance, in the reduced schematic eye, the cornea is assumed to be the only refracting surface, the principal plane (H) being placed at its apex and a single nodal point (n) at its center of curvature. The globe has an axial length of 22.5 mm, and the refractive index of the eye is said to be 1.33. Unfortunately, these numbers have become accepted by many as true physiologic values rather than as the convenient mathematically derived values they really are. The refractive index of aqueous is about 1.3337 (for the sodium D line at 37 °C).

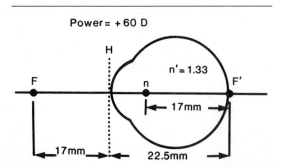

Figure 20–18. The reduced schematic eye.

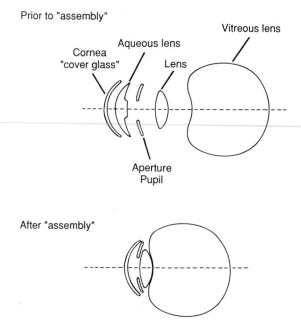

Figure 20–19. The optical system of the eye, illustrating the three-lens concept.

Trigonometric ray tracing demonstrates that the optical system of the human eye is more accurately conceptualized as a three-lens system: the aqueous lens, the lens lens, and the vitreous lens (Figure 20–19). Contrary to popular belief, the cornea itself has almost no power of refraction in the optical system but is important only in shaping the anterior curve of the aqueous lens. The crystalline lens is an interesting optical component because its index of refraction varies throughout its thickness rather than being constant, as assumed in most optical calculations. The vitreous lens is particularly important because of its major effect on magnification.*

Reassessment of models for the optical system of the human eye is essential now that much of ophthalmic surgery, whether it be cataract surgery, keratorefractive procedures, or vitreous surgery, produces profound effects on individual components of the system. Gullstrand's models, in which the system is assumed to function as an integrated unit, cannot be applied under such circumstances.

Accommodation

The eye changes refractive power to focus on near objects by a process called accommodation. Study of Purkinje images, which are reflections from various optical surfaces in the eye, has shown that accommo-

---

*Further discussion of the three-lens concept may be found in Dr Orson White's chapter on optics and refraction in the 11th edition of this book.

dation results from changes in the crystalline lens. Contraction of the ciliary muscle results in thickening and increased curvature of the lens, probably due to relaxation of the lens capsule.

Visual Acuity

Assessment of visual acuity with the Snellen chart is described in Chapter 2. The average resolving power of the normal human eye is 1 minute of arc. Since the Snellen letters are made from squares of 5 × 5 units (Figure 20–20), the 20/20 size letter has a visual angle of 5 minutes of arc at 20 feet. This is equivalent to 8.7 mm (0.35 inch) width and height. The eye minifies an image at 20 feet by about 350 times. Therefore, the size of the 20/20 letter on the retina is 0.025 mm high and wide. This is equivalent to a resolution capacity of 100 lines per millimeter. For a 6-mm pupil and light of wavelength 0.56 μm (in air), the absolute theoretic limit would be 345 lines per millimeter.

REFRACTIVE ERRORS

Emmetropia is absence of refractive error and **ametropia** is the presence of refractive error.

Presbyopia

The loss of accommodation that comes with aging to all people is called presbyopia (Table 20–2). A person with emmetropic eyes (no refractive error) will begin to notice inability to read small print or discriminate fine close objects at about age 44–46. This is worse in dim light and usually worse early in the morning or when the subject is fatigued. Many people complain of a feeling of sleepiness when reading. These symptoms increase until about age 55, when they stabilize but persist.

Presbyopia is corrected by use of a plus lens to make up for the lost automatic focusing power of the lens. The

Table 20–2. Table of accommodation.

Age (Years)	Mean Accommodation (Diopters)
8	13.8
25	9.9
35	7.3
40	5.8
45	3.6
50	1.9
55	1.3

plus lens may be used in several ways. Reading glasses have the near correction in the entire aperture of the glasses, making them fine for reading but blurred for distant objects. Half-glasses can be worn to abate this nuisance by leaving the top open and uncorrected for distance vision. Bifocals do the same but allow correction of other refractive errors. Trifocals correct for distance vision by the top segment, the middle distance by the middle section, and the near distance by the lower segment. Progressive power lenses similarly correct for far, middle, and near distances but by progressive change in lens power rather than stepped changes.

Myopia

When the image of distant objects focuses in front of the retina in the unaccommodated eye, the eye is myopic, or nearsighted (Figure 20–21). If the eye is longer than average, the error is called axial myopia. (For each additional millimeter of axial length, the eye is approximately 3 diopters more myopic.) If the refractive elements are more refractive than average, the error is called curvature myopia or refractive myopia. As the object is brought closer than 6 meters, the image moves closer to the retina and comes into sharper focus. The point reached where the image is most sharply focused on the retina is called the "far point." One may estimate the extent of myopia by calculating the reciprocal of the far point. Thus, a far point of 0.25 m would suggest a 4-diopter minus lens correction for distance. The myopic person has the advantage of being able to read at the far point without glasses even at the age of presbyopia. A high degree of myopia results in greater susceptibility to degenerative retinal changes, including retinal detachment.

Concave spherical (minus) lenses are used to correct the image in myopia. These lenses move the image back to the retina.

Hyperopia

Hyperopia (hypermetropia, farsightedness) is the state in which the unaccommodated eye would focus the image behind the retina (Figure 20–21). It may be due to reduced axial length (axial hyperopia), as occurs in certain congenital disorders, or reduced refractive

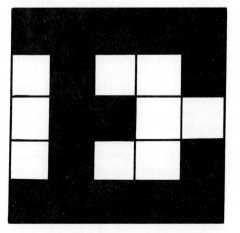

Figure 20–20. Snellen block E.

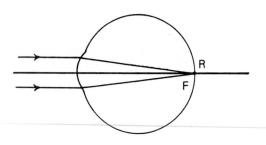

Emmetropia

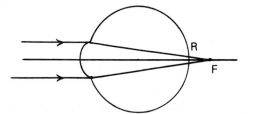

Hyperopia

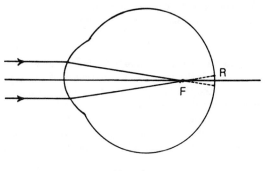

Myopia

Figure 20–21. Spherical refractive errors as determined by the position of the secondary focal point with respect to the retina.

error (refractive hyperopia), as exemplified by aphakia.

Hyperopia is a more difficult concept to explain than myopia. The term "farsighted" contributes to the difficulty, as does the prevalent misconception among laymen that presbyopia is farsightedness and that one who sees well far away is farsighted. If hyperopia is not too great, a young person may obtain a sharp distant image by accommodating, as a normal eye would to read. The young hyperopic person may also make a sharp near image by accommodating more—or much more than one without hyperopia. This extra effort may result in eye fatigue that is more severe for near work. The degree of hyperopia a person may have without symptoms is—like most clinical conditions—variable.

However, the amount decreases with age as presbyopia (decrease in ability to accommodate) increases. Three diopters of hyperopia might be tolerated in a teenager but will require glasses later, even though the hyperopia has not increased. If the hyperopia is too high, the eye may be unable to correct the image by accommodation. The hyperopia that cannot be corrected by accommodation is termed manifest hyperopia. This is one of the causes of deprivation amblyopia in children and can be bilateral. There is a reflex correlation between accommodation and convergence of the two eyes. Hyperopia is therefore a frequent cause of esotropia (crossed eyes) and monocular amblyopia (see Chapter 12).

Latent Hyperopia

As explained above, a prepresbyopic person with hyperopia may obtain a clear retinal image by accommodation. The degree of hyperopia overcome by accommodation is known as latent hyperopia. It is detected by refraction after instillation of cycloplegic drops, which determines the sum of both manifest and latent hyperopia. Refraction with a cycloplegic is very important in young patients who complain of eyestrain when reading and is vital in esotropia, where full correction of hyperopia may achieve a cure.

Remember that a moderately "farsighted" person may see well for near or far when young. However, as presbyopia comes on, the hyperope first has trouble with close work—and at an earlier age than the nonhyperope. Finally, the hyperope has blurred vision for near *and far* and requires glasses for both near and far.

Astigmatism

In astigmatism, the eye produces an image with multiple focal points or lines. In **regular astigmatism,** there are two principal meridians, with constant power and orientation across the pupillary aperture, resulting in two focal lines. The astigmatism is then further defined according to the position of these focal lines with respect to the retina (Figure 20–22). When the principal meridians are at right angles and their axes lie within 20 degrees of the horizontal and vertical, the astigmatism is subdivided into **astigmatism with the rule,** in which the greater refractive power is in the vertical meridian; and **astigmatism against the rule,** in which the greater refractive power is in the horizontal meridian. Astigmatism with the rule is more commonly found in younger patients and astigmatism against the rule more commonly in older patients (Figure 20–23). **Oblique astigmatism** is regular astigmatism in which the principal meridians do not lie within 20 degrees of the horizontal and vertical. In **irregular astigmatism,** the power or orientation of the principal meridians changes across the pupillary aperture.

The usual cause of astigmatism is abnormalities of corneal shape. The crystalline lens may also contribute. In contact lens terminology, lenticular astigmatism is called residual astigmatism because it is not corrected

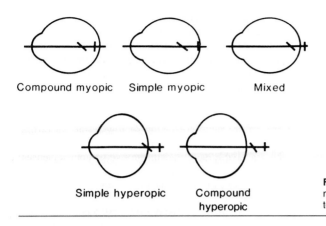

Compound myopic   Simple myopic   Mixed

Simple hyperopic   Compound hyperopic

Figure 20–22. Types of regular astigmatism as determined by the positions of the two focal lines with respect to the retina.

by a spherical hard contact lens, which does correct corneal astigmatism.

Astigmatic errors can be corrected with cylindrical lenses, frequently in combination with spherical lenses. Because the brain is capable of adapting to the visual distortion of an uncorrected astigmatic error, new glasses that do correct the error may cause temporary disorientation, particularly an apparent slanting of images.

Natural History of Refractive Errors

Most babies are slightly hyperopic at birth. The hyperopia slowly decreases, with a slight acceleration in the teens, to approach emmetropia. The corneal curvature is much steeper (6.59 mm radius) at birth and flattens to nearly the adult curvature (7.71 mm) by about 1 year. The lens is much more spherical at birth and reaches adult conformation at about 6 years. The axial length is short at birth (17.3 mm), lengthens rapidly in the first 2 or 3 years (to 24.1 mm), then moderately (0.4 mm per year) until age 6, and then slowly (about 1 mm total) to stability at about 10 or 15 years. Presbyopia becomes manifest in the fifth decade.

Refractive errors are inherited. The mode of inheritance is complex, as it involves so many variables. Refractive error, though inherited, need not be present at birth any more than tallness, which is also inherited, need be present at birth. For example, a child who reaches emmetropia at age 10 years will probably soon become myopic. Myopia usually increases during the teens. This should be expected, just as the need for larger shoes is expected, and not looked on with alarm by the patient and parents. In a similar way, hyperopia usually decreases slightly during the teens. Myopia does not generally decrease with age, as is popularly believed, nor does farsightedness come with aging.

Anisometropia

Anisometropia is a difference in refractive error between the two eyes. It is a major cause of amblyopia because the eyes cannot accommodate indepen-

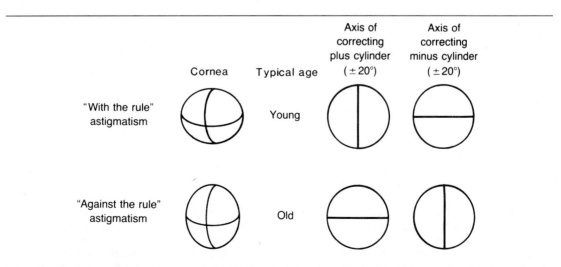

Figure 20–23. Types of astigmatism as determined by the orientation of the principal meridians and the orientation of the correcting cylinder axis.

dently and the more hyperopic eye is chronically blurred. Refractive correction of anisometropia is complicated by differences in size of the retinal images **(aniseikonia)** and oculomotor imbalance due to the different degree of prismatic power of the periphery of the two corrective lenses. Aniseikonia is predominantly a problem of monocular aphakia. Spectacle correction produces a difference in retinal image size of approximately 25%, which is rarely tolerable. Contact lens correction reduces the difference in image size to approximately 6%, which can be tolerated. Intraocular lenses produce a difference of less than 1%.

Correction of Refractive Errors

A. Spectacle Lenses: Spectacles continue to be the safest method of refractive correction. To reduce nonchromatic aberrations, the lenses are made in meniscus form (corrected curves) and tilted forward (pantascopic tilt).

B. Contact Lenses: The first contact lenses were glass fluid-filled scleral lenses. These were difficult to wear for extended periods and caused corneal edema and much ocular discomfort. Hard corneal lenses, made of polymethylmethacrylate, were the first really successful contact lenses and gained wide acceptance for cosmetic replacement of glasses. Subsequent developments include gas-permeable rigid lenses, made of cellulose acetate butyrate, silicone, or various silicone and plastic polymers, and soft contact lenses, made of various hydrogel plastics, all of which provide increased comfort but greater risk of serious complications.

Hard and gas-permeable lenses correct refractive errors by changing the curvature of the anterior surface of the eye. The total refractive power consists of the power induced by the back curvature of the lens, the base curve, together with the actual power of the lens due to the difference between its front and back curvatures. Only the second is dependent on the refractive index of the contact lens material. Hard and gas-permeable lenses overcome corneal astigmatism by modifying the anterior surface of the eye into a truly spherical shape.

Soft contact lenses, particularly the more flexible forms, adopt the shape of the patient's cornea. Thus, their refractive power resides only in the difference between their front and back curvature, and they correct little corneal astigmatism unless a cylindrical correction is incorporated.

Contact lens base curves are selected according to corneal curvature, as determined by keratometry or trial fittings. The front curvature is then calculated from the results of overrefraction with a trial contact lens, or from the patient's spectacle refraction as corrected for the corneal plane.

Hard contact lenses are specifically indicated for the correction of irregular astigmatism, such as in kerato-

conus. Soft contact lenses are used for the treatment of corneal surface disorders, but for control of symptoms rather than for refractive reasons. All forms of contact lenses are used in the refractive correction of aphakia, particularly in overcoming the aniseikonia of monocular aphakia, and the correction of high myopia, in which they produce a much better visual image than spectacles. But the vast majority of contact lenses worn are for cosmetic correction of low refractive errors. This has important implications for the risks that can be reasonably accepted in the use of contact lenses. (Further discussion of therapeutic and cosmetic contact lens use, and the associated complications, is given in Chapter 6.)

C. Keratorefractive Surgery: Keratorefractive surgery encompasses a range of methods for changing the curvature of the anterior surface of the eye. The expected refractive effect is generally derived from empirical results of similar procedures in other patients and not based upon mathematical optical calculations. Further discussion of the methods and outcome of keratorefractive procedures is included in Chapter 6.

D. Intraocular Lenses: Implantation of an intraocular lens has become the preferred method of refractive correction for aphakia. A large number of designs are available, most commonly consisting of an optic made of polymethylmethacrylate and loops (haptics) made of the same material or polypropylene. Foldable lenses made of hydrogel plastics are being developed to reduce the size of wound required for cataract extraction. The safest position for an intraocular lens appears to be within the capsular bag following extracapsular surgery.

The most popular method of determining the necessary intraocular lens power is the empirical regression method of analyzing experience with lenses of one style in many patients, from which is derived a mathematical formula based on a constant for the particular lens *(A)*, average keratometer readings *(K)*, and axial length in millimeters *(L)*. An example is the **SRK (Sanders-Retzlaff-Kraff) equation:**

$$\text{Power IOL} = A - 2.5 L - 0.9 K$$

This formula gives clinically satisfactory results in most cases. When the eye is not of average dimensions, such as in high myopia, the results are less good, and various modifications have been derived.

Certain theoretic formulas are also available, also utilizing a lens constant, keratometer readings, and axial length, together with estimated anterior chamber depth following surgery. Unfortunately, none of these formulas are based on trigonometric ray tracing methods, which do accurately predict the correct power of intraocular lens for an individual patient.

E. Clear Lens Extraction for Myopia: Extraction of noncataractous lenses has been advocated for the refractive correction of myopia. For the process to have any success, the eye must be highly myopic, and the surgery is then sufficiently likely to have an adverse result that it is rarely justifiable.

METHODS OF REFRACTION

Determination of a patient's refractive correction can be achieved by objective or subjective means and is best accomplished by a combination of the two methods where possible.

Objective Refraction

Objective refraction is performed by retinoscopy, in which a streak of light, known as the **intercept,** is projected into the patient's eye to produce a similarly shaped reflex, the **retinoscopic reflex,** in the pupil (Figure 20–24). Parallel alignment of the intercept and the retinoscopic reflex indicates the presence of only a spherical error, or an additional cylindrical error in which the intercept coincides with one of the principal meridians. Rotation of the projected streak will determine which of these applies and the location of the other principal meridian in the case of a cylindrical error.

The intercept is then swept across the patient's pupil, and the effect on the retinoscopic reflex is noted (Figure 20–25). If it moves in the same direction **(with movement),** plus lenses are placed before the patient's eye; and if it moves in the opposite direction **(against movement),** minus lenses are added—until the pupillary reflex fills the whole pupillary aperture and no movement is detected **(point of neutralization).** When the point of neutralization has been reached, the patient's refractive error has been corrected with an additional correction related to the distance between the patient and examiner **(working distance).** Spherical power equal to the reciprocal of the working distance (measured in meters) is subtracted to compensate for this additional correction and obtain the patient's refractive correction. The working distance is usually ⅔ m, and thecorrection to be subtracted for the working distance thus is usually 1.5 D.

Automated refractors are available to rapidly determine the objective refraction, but they are not useful in children or in adults with significant anterior segment disease.

Subjective Refraction

In cooperative patients, subjective refraction produces more accurate results than objective refraction. It relies on the patient's response to alterations in lens power and orientation, using objective refraction or the patient's current refractive correction as the starting point.

The spherical correction is checked by small changes, initially increasing the plus power so as to overcome any accommodative effort, until the clearest image is obtained. The duochrome test of black letters on red and green backgrounds uses the normal chromatic aberration of the eye to refine spherical correction. When the black letters of the two halves of the chart are equally clear, the end point has been reached.

A **cross cylinder** consists of two planocylindrical lenses of equal power but opposite sign superimposed such that their axes of refractive power lie at right angles to one another. This is equivalent to a spherocylindrical lens in which the power of the cylinder is twice the power of the sphere and of the opposite sign. The cross cylinder allows rapid small changes in the axis and power of a cylindrical correction.

Cycloplegic Refraction

In the determination of full hyperopic refractive correction, either in the management of childhood esotropia or the assessment of eyestrain in adult hyperopes, it is necessary to overcome accommodation. This can usually be achieved in adults by fogging techniques in which plus lenses are used to overcome accommodative effort. But otherwise—and always in children—accommodation has to be relaxed by cycloplegic drugs. Cyclopentolate 1%, 1 drop instilled

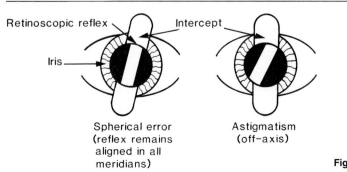

Spherical error
(reflex remains
aligned in all
meridians)

Astigmatism
(off-axis)

Figure 20–24. The retinoscopic reflex.

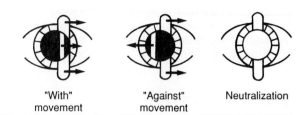

"With" movement   "Against" movement   Neutralization

Figure 20–25. Movement of the retinoscopic reflex.

twice 30 minutes prior to refraction, may be sufficient, but atropine 0.5% or 1% ointment, applied twice a day for 3 days, may be necessary in children with dark irides and in the initial assessment of accommmodative esotropia. Parents should be warned of the symptoms of atropine toxicity (fever, flushed face, and rapid pulse) and the necessity for discontinuing treatment, cooling the child with sponge bathing, and—in severe cases—seeking urgent medical assistance.

REFERENCES

*Conrady AE: *Applied and Optical Design.* Vol 1: Oxford Univ Press, 1929; Dover, 1957. Vol 2 (edited and completed by Kingslake R): Dover, 1960.

Duke-Elder S (editor): *System of Ophthalmology.* Vol 5: *Ophthalmic Optics and Refraction.* Mosby, 1970.

Gordon RA, Donzis PB: Refractive development of the human eye. Arch Ophthalmol 1985;103:785.

Hales RH: *Contact Lenses: A Clinical Approach to Fitting,* 2nd ed. Williams & Wilkins, 1983.

Helmholtz H: *Helmholtz' Treatise on Physiological Optics,* 1910. Optical Society of America, 1925. [English language edition.]

*Kingslake R: *Lens Design Fundamentals.* Academic Press, 1978.

Meyer-Arendt JR: *Introduction to Classical and Modern Optics,* 2nd ed. Prentice-Hall, 1984.

Michaels DD: *Visual Optics and Refraction: A Clinical Approach.* Mosby, 1980.

Smith WJ: *Modern Optical Engineering.* McGraw-Hill, 1966.

White O: Spectacle addition and spectacle subtraction. Trans Pac Coast Otoophthalmol Soc 1980;61:7.

Wyld J: The design of refractor objectives by ray tracing. In: *Amateur Telescope Making,* vol 3. Ingalls AG (editor). Kingsport Press/Scientific American, 1974.

*Ray tracing references.

Preventive Ophthalmology

John P. Whitcher, MD, MPH

Preventive medicine is increasingly important in attempts to fulfill society's expectations of modern medicine with the resources available. Although prevention is a logical approach to the solution of many problems in all branches of medicine, in practice there are a number of hurdles to be overcome. For any particular condition, it is essential that individuals at risk be easily identified. If their identification requires population screening, the screening process should be easy to perform, accurate, and reliable. Preventive measures must be both effective and acceptable to the target population. Unwarranted interference with the at-risk individual's lifestyle only leads to poor compliance. Legislation may be required for certain measures but may engender resentment when it is felt to infringe on personal liberty. For preventive medicine to be successful, there must be cooperation among all segments of society—not just the medical community—in identifying problem areas, establishing workable solutions, and disseminating information. The successes that have been achieved in occupational health are an example of what can be accomplished if a consensus of opinion is established.

In ophthalmology, the major avenues for preventive medicine are ocular injuries and infections, genetic and systemic diseases with ocular involvement, and ocular diseases in which the early treatable stages are often unrecognized or ignored.

PREVENTION OF OCULAR INJURIES

Approximately 1 million Americans have visual loss due to trauma, of which 75% are blind in one eye, and approximately 50,000 suffer serious sight-threatening injuries each year. Young men and children are particularly prone to suffer major ocular trauma. Simple measures are available for preventing many injuries to the eye.

Occupational Injuries

Many manufacturing processes pose a particular threat to the eye. Grinding or drilling commonly propels small fragments of metal into the environment at high velocity, and these missiles can easily lodge on the cornea or penetrate the globe through the cornea or sclera. Tools with sharp ends, such as screwdrivers, are also commonly involved in producing penetrating ocular injuries. Welding arcs produce ultraviolet radiation that may cause epithelial keratitis ("arc eye"). Industrial chemicals—particularly those containing high concentrations of alkali or acid—can rapidly produce severe ocular damage that is often bilateral and associated with a poor visual outcome.

Workers must be properly trained in the use of tools, machinery, and chemicals. Safety guards must be fitted to all machinery, and safety goggles must be worn whenever the worker is doing hazardous work or is in the workplace area where such hazards exist. It is surprising how many workers assume that they are no longer at risk of injury when they are not themselves performing hazardous tasks even though they are in the vicinity of work being performed by others.

The growing interest in "do-it-yourself" projects in the home exposes many more individuals to the risks of ocular injury from machinery, tools, and chemicals. Education of the public about these matters is particularly important, since the risks involved may not be obvious to the ordinary householder or hobbyist.

Early recognition and urgent expert ophthalmologic assessment of any injuries sustained is essential. In the case of chemical injuries, immediate copious lavage of the eyes with sterile water, saline if available, or tap water for at least 5 minutes is the most important method of limiting the damage incurred. Neglect of penetrating injuries or corneal foreign bodies markedly increases the potential for long-term morbidity. Obtaining an accurate history is crucial in identifying the possibility of a penetrating injury. This is particularly true when medical help is sought some time after the injury and the patient may not realize the importance of a seemingly minor episode of trauma. Any worker who presents with unexplained visual loss or intraocular inflammation must be carefully questioned about the possibility of recent ocular injuries and the possibility of an occult intraocular foreign body borne in mind.

Chronic exposure to some industrial processes may lead to ocular damage. For example, improperly screened nuclear materials can lead to early and rapid cataract formation in exposed workers.

Nonoccupational Injuries

The marked reduction in the incidence of severe ocular and facial damage associated with car windshield injuries as a result of legislation requiring the wearing of seat belts is a testament to the effectiveness of such legislation. Similar attempts to reduce the incidence of injuries from fireworks by limiting their availability have not yet been as successful.

Various sports are notorious for the high incidence of severe injuries to the eye, eg, blunt injuries such as in racquetball or penetrating injuries such as in ice hockey. The availability of toughened plastic protective glasses—which can be fitted with refractive correction if required—is a major advance in preventing such injuries.

A large number of ocular injuries are suffered in the home. Corks from bottles of champagne or other sparkling wines can produce severe blunt injuries, and explosion of any bottle containing carbonated beverages may lead to penetrating eye injuries from glass fragments. Unless adequately supervised, children using pencils, scissors, or airguns may sustain or cause serious penetrating injuries.

Unfortunately, a significant proportion of serious ocular trauma results from violent assaults, notably those involving firearms. Prevention requires a reduction in the frequency of such incidents.

Acute keratitis from **ultraviolet irradiation** as seen after exposure to a welding arc may also occur during skiing if protective goggles are not worn. The role of long-term exposure to ultraviolet light in the etiology of cataract and age-related macular degeneration is still debated. Since the cornea and crystalline lens are effective barriers to the transmission of ultraviolet light—becoming even more effective with age in the case of the crystalline lens—it is hardly surprising that the development of age-related macular degeneration in phakic individuals has not been shown to be related to ultraviolet exposure and thus is not preventable by the use of sunglasses. The effect of ultraviolet light on the maculas of the increasing numbers of aphakic and pseudophakic individuals has yet to be fully assessed. Largely on empirical grounds, ultraviolet filters have been incorporated into many of the intraocular lenses implanted. And individuals without such filters in their intraocular lenses or who are aphakic have been encouraged to incorporate ultraviolet filters in their spectacle lenses or wear appropriate sunglasses whenever possible. There is substantial evidence linking ultraviolet exposure to the development of cataract. But since ultraviolet exposure occurs from the time of birth, advocating the regular use of ultraviolet filters in spectacle lenses or sunglasses as a preventive measure is unlikely to be workable or effective. The role of ultraviolet light exposure in the etiology of certain corneal disorders—particularly pterygium—and of basal cell carcinoma and melanoma of the eyelids is much more widely accepted. Education of the public about the dangers of skin cancer following prolonged sun exposure is very important. Ultraviolet-blocking skin creams should not be used around the eyes, and for that reason reliance must be placed on avoiding unnecessary exposure to the sun or the use of sunglasses. In patients with xeroderma pigmentosum, the eyelids and bulbar conjunctiva frequently develop carcinomas and melanomas, and their development can be minimized, if not prevented entirely, by protective lenses.

Solar retinitis (eclipse retinopathy) is a specific type of radiation injury that usually occurs after solar eclipses as a result of direct observation of the sun without an adequate filter. Under normal circumstances, sun-gazing is difficult because of the glare, but cases have been reported in young people who have suffered self-inflicted macular damage by deliberate sun-gazing, perhaps while under the influence of drugs.

The optical system of the eye behaves as a strong magnifying lens, focusing the light onto a small spot on the macula, usually in one eye only, and producing a thermal burn. The resulting edema of the retinal tissue may clear with minimal loss of function, or it may cause significant atrophy of the tissue and produce a defect that is visible ophthalmoscopically as a macular hole. In the latter event, a permanent central scotoma results. Eclipse retinopathy can easily be prevented by the use of adequate filters when observing eclipses, but the surest way to prevent it is to watch the eclipse on television.

Similar to eclipse retinopathy is the iatrogenic retinal damage that may occur from use of the operating microscope and indirect ophthalmoscope. The risk of damage from the operating microscope can be reduced by the use of filters to block both ultraviolet light and the blue portion of the visible spectrum, light barriers such as an opaque disk placed on the cornea, or air injected into the anterior chamber.

PREVENTION OF ACQUIRED OCULAR INFECTION

Infections are a major cause of preventable ocular morbidity. Preventive measures are based on maintenance of the integrity of the normal barriers to infection and the avoidance of inoculation with pathogenic organisms. The pathogenicity of various organisms and the size of the inoculum required to establish infection vary enormously according to the state of the eye. A compromised eye is highly susceptible to infection.

The major barrier to exogenous ocular infection is the epithelium of the cornea and conjunctiva. This can be damaged directly by trauma, including surgical trauma and contact lens wear, or by the secondary effects of other abnormalities of the outer eye, such as lid abnormalities or tear deficiency. In all such situations, particular care must be taken to avoid or recognize secondary infection in its earliest stages.

In the presence of a corneal or conjunctival epithelial defect, particularly when there is an associated full-thickness wound of the cornea or sclera—eg, following penetrating trauma or intraocular surgery—it is essential to use prophylactic antibiotic therapy and most importantly to make certain that any drops or ointments are sterile. Accidental epithelial injury should be avoided whenever possible, particularly in compromised eyes, eg, dry eyes, eyes with corneal exposure due to exophthalmos or abnormal eyelid function such as produced by facial nerve paralysis or ectropion, and eyes with reduced corneal sensation. The classic situation is the combination of fifth and seventh nerve dysfunction such as occurs with cerebellopontine angle tumors, producing a dry, anesthetic eye with poor eyelid closure. Any comatose patient is also at risk of corneal exposure, and prophylactic eyelid taping should be undertaken.

Any unnecessary exposure of the eye to pathogenic organisms should be avoided, but it becomes critical in certain situations. During intraocular surgery, the normal barriers to infection are circumvented, and meticulous attention must be paid to avoiding contamination of the eye with organisms. The ocular environment must be assessed preoperatively to identify and treat any sources of pathogenic organisms. These include colonization or infection of the lacrimal sac, the lid margins, the conjunctiva, and the cornea. In emergency situations, it may only be possible to identify such sources and use prophylactic antibiotic therapy to reduce the chances of subsequent infection, whereas for elective surgery more definitive therapy to eradicate or minimize the pathogenic organisms should be possible. There is much debate about the value of preoperative and perioperative prophylactic antibiotics in patients with no identifiable external ocular disease. It is important to recognize that one of the major causes of endophthalmitis after cataract surgery is *Staphylococcus epidermidis,* which frequently colonizes normal eyelids. Considerations may need to be given to other sites of bacterial colonization or infection such as the bladder, throat, nose, and skin. Sterility must be ensured of the operative field, instruments, intraocular and topical medications, and other fluids introduced into the eye. During the postoperative period, sterile medications must be used and contact with other patients with established ocular infections avoided.

Contact lens wear is strongly associated with suppurative keratitis due to the combination of an abnormal load of pathogenic organisms and probable recurrent minor trauma to the corneal epithelium. The incidence of suppurative keratitis is particularly high with soft lenses, especially with extended wear. It is apparent that many people wearing contact lenses for cosmetic reasons are not aware of the risks involved. Whereas it may be reasonable to face the risks of infection with extended-wear soft lenses in elderly aphakes who are dependent on contact lenses for refractive correction and cannot cope with daily-wear lenses—or in patients with highly compromised eyes that are symptomatic from bullous keratopathy—the arguments in favor of extended-wear soft lenses for refractive correction in patients with low refractive errors are less strong. A number of patients in this latter group start off their contact lens career using extended-wear disposable lenses, which is of course an attractive arrangement because it dispenses with the need for lens cleaning and the associated paraphernalia, but this practice is likely to require an unwelcome sacrifice of safety for convenience. Contact lens wear exposes the eye to an abnormal load of pathogenic organisms, which have been shown to adhere with particular tenacity to soft lenses, unless the user is absolutely meticulous about contact lens hygiene. The development of toxic reactions to preservatives within the contact lens solutions with the necessary dependence on preservative-free solutions increases the chances of suppurative keratitis from organisms capable of surviving in such solutions, eg, *Pseudomonas* and *Acanthamoeba.*

All contact lens wearers must be apprised of the relative risk of suppurative keratitis and the need for meticulous contact lens hygiene. They should be advised to keep a pair of spectacles available so that contact lens wear be discontinued immediately whenever an eye becomes uncomfortable or inflamed. If ocular discomfort or inflammation persists, the wearer should seek ophthalmologic advice without delay.

Neonatal conjunctivitis (see Chapter 17) is a good example of exposure to a heavy load of pathogenic organisms with the added inherent susceptibility of the poorly developed immune mechanisms of the neonatal eye. The major organisms that may produce neonatal conjunctivitis are *Neisseria gonorrhoeae,* chlamydiae, herpes simplex, *Staphylococcus aureus, Haemophilus* species, and *Streptococcus pneumoniae.* Exposure to these organisms occurs during passage down the birth canal. It should be possible to prevent neonatal conjunctivitis by treating mothers harboring these organisms prior to delivery, and this has been achieved for the bacteria, including *Chlamydia.* The alternative approach is the routine ocular prophylaxis of neonates. This started with the silver nitrate prophylaxis of Credé and has been superseded in a number of centers by topical erythromycin in view of the predominance of chlamydial neonatal conjunctivitis.

Shedding of herpes simplex virus by the expectant mother is not necessarily associated with clinically obvious lesions, and shedding may occur in mothers who do not have any history of such lesions. Identification of mothers likely to infect their babies would require routine viral cultures from all women prior to delivery, and even then it would not be possible to identify specifically those actually shedding virus at the time of delivery. In the presence of frank clinical lesions at the time of delivery, elective cesarean section may be advisable.

PREVENTION OF IATROGENIC OCULAR INFECTION

Ophthalmologists have been clearly implicated in the transmission of infectious eye disease. Outbreaks of **epidemic keratoconjunctivitis** have been traced to contamination in the ophthalmologist's office. The adenovirus is transmitted via the ophthalmologist's hands, a tonometer, or solutions contaminated by droppers accidentally rubbed against the infected conjunctiva or lid margin of a patient. Contaminated ophthalmic solutions have also been the source of infection in bacterial corneal ulcers and endophthalmitis following intraocular surgery. *Pseudomonas aeruginosa* used to be a common contaminant of ophthalmic solutions, particularly fluorescein. Instillation of contaminated fluorescein solution to delineate corneal epithelial defects (eg, after removal of a corneal foreign body) may result in severe pseudomonal keratitis and, frequently, loss of the eye.

Other infections can be similarly spread, but their occurrence is not generally recognized. The ophthalmologist should be alert to the possibility that if ophthalmic instruments are improperly sterilized (as by cold sterilization), they may be contaminated with hepatitis B virus. Recent identification of the AIDS virus in tears has suggested a small possibility of transmission by ophthalmologists. To date, no such incident has occurred.

There is good experimental evidence that applanation tonometer tips can be adequately sterilized, particularly with respect to human immunodeficiency virus type 1, herpes simplex virus, and adenovirus, by wiping with 70% isopropyl alcohol swabs and then allowing the instrument to evaporate dry. It is imperative that the tonometer tip be completely dry before use on the next patient or corneal epithelial damage will result. This method of sterilization is more practical than immersion in alcohol, hypochlorite, or hydrogen peroxide and less likely to damage the tonometer tip, though immersion in such disinfectant solutions at the end of each working day and after examination of high-risk patients is probably advisable. In this case, the tonometer tip should be rinsed in tap water and dried before use. Goldmann three-mirror and similar contact lenses used for patient examination are also susceptible to damage from immersion in disinfectants and should be treated in a similar manner to tonometer tips. The Schiotz tonometer needs to be immersed in disinfectant, autoclaved, or exposed to ethylene oxide for effective sterilization. The noncontact tonometer is recommended for reducing the risks of disease transmission, but it may generate an aerosol spray that endangers the individual operating the tonometer.

Ophthalmologists and their staffs must maintain the highest level of personal hygiene at all times and must use standard sterile technique when appropriate, keeping in mind the possibility of contamination of any solution brought into contact with the eye.

Hands play a major role in the transmission of infection. They should be washed or disinfected (eg, with isopropyl alcohol) before and after the examination of every patient, especially if an ocular infection is thought to be present.

PREVENTION OF OCULAR DAMAGE DUE TO CONGENITAL INFECTIONS

Viral disease of the mother with resultant embryopathy may lead to such ocular anomalies in the offspring as retinopathy, infantile glaucoma, cataract, uveal tract coloboma, etc, and prevention may in some cases be possible. Two viruses, rubella and cytomegalovirus, can be extremely damaging to the infant, and one of them—rubella virus—can be prevented by vaccination. Once a common childhood disease, rubella led to lifelong immunity, but vaccination is now indicated for susceptible young women approaching childbearing age. Susceptibility can be determined by assessing the antibody content of the young woman's blood. If a mother contracts rubella during early pregnancy, she should be informed of the likelihood of ocular and other abnormalities in her baby, and the arguments for and against abortion should be presented.

Unfortunately, cytomegalovirus (the other virus causing a high incidence of congenital anomalies) continues to be a serious and unsolved threat. No protective vaccine is currently available, though one is currently under study.

Toxoplasmosis is another important cause of congenital infection, leading to (1) chorioretinitis, which may be apparent at birth or may remain subclinical until reactivation occurs later in life; (2) cerebral or cerebellar calcification; (3) hydrocephalus; and occasionally (4) more severe central nervous system abnormalities. Unless the mother is immunocompromised, fetal infection occurs only if she acquires primary infection during pregnancy. This can be prevented by eating only meat that is well cooked, by washing vegetables and fruits, and by wearing gloves when disposing of cat litter or working in the garden so that contact with viable oocysts and tissue cysts is avoided. It has been shown that if acute maternal infection during pregnancy can be identified—such as with the serial serologic tests that are required by law in France and Austria—appropriate antibiotic treatment in those pregnancies allowed to proceed, with adjustments according to whether fetal infection is also present, reduces the incidence of congenital infection and improves the clinical outcome in fetuses that are infected.

PREVENTION OF GENETIC DISEASES WITH OCULAR INVOLVEMENT

Until recently, the prevention of genetic disorders received little attention. Now, however, there are genetic counseling centers in many medical centers, and the genetic nature of many disorders that affect the eye is recognized and their transmission better understood than formerly. In conference with internists and pediatricians, it is up to the ophthalmologist to recommend genetic counseling for patients contemplating marriage and children. Patients with histories of childhood diabetes, retinitis pigmentosa, consanguineous mating, retinoblastoma, neurofibromatosis, etc, need genetic counseling to prevent disaster for their offspring.

Some clinical conditions, eg, Down's syndrome (trisomy 21), are associated with an abnormal number of chromosomes or with abnormalities of the sex chromosomes. Prenatal diagnosis can now be made by testing amniotic fluid cells obtained by amniocentesis (a safe and practical procedure), and a positive diagnosis gives the patient the option of abortion.

EARLY DETECTION OF TREATABLE OCULAR DISEASE

A number of primary ocular diseases are treatable only during their early stages or are more effectively treated at that time. Detection of such diseases may be possible through the timely recognition of relevant symptoms or may require specific vigilance on the part of medical workers because of the absence of symptoms.

Age-Related Macular Degeneration

Age-related macular degeneration is the leading cause of permanent visual loss in the elderly in industrialized countries, and its incidence is increasing with each decade over age 50. There are two major forms of the disease: (1) atrophic ("dry") degeneration, in which there is progressive degeneration of the outer retina, retinal pigment epithelium, Bruch's membrane, and choriocapillaris; and (2) exudative ("wet") degeneration, in which there is a sudden onset of visual loss due to leakage of serous fluid or blood into the retina followed by new vessel formation under the retinal pigment epithelium (subretinal neovascular membrane).

Laser photocoagulation of subretinal neovascular membranes may delay the onset of central visual loss but only when the membrane is far enough away from the fovea to permit treatment. Elderly patients developing sudden visual loss due to macular disease—particularly paracentral distortion or scotoma, with preservation of central acuity—should undergo urgent ophthalmic assessment, including fluorescein angiography, to determine their suitability for laser treatment. There is no effective treatment for the atrophic form of macular degeneration except for the provision of low vision aids.

Primary Open-Angle Glaucoma

Primary open-angle glaucoma is a major cause of preventable blindness worldwide, particularly among individuals of African racial origin. About two million Americans have the disease, though half are undiagnosed. The prevalence of primary open-angle glaucoma increases from 0.1% for those aged 40–49 to 3% for those over age 70. Symptoms do not usually occur until there is advanced visual field loss. For treatment to be effective, the disease must be detected at a much earlier stage. Specific screening programs are hampered by the high prevalence of raised intraocular pressure in the absence of glaucomatous visual field loss (ocular hypertension), which is ten times more common than primary open-angle glaucoma, the high frequency of normal intraocular pressure on a single reading in untreated open-angle glaucoma, and the complexities of screening for optic disk or visual field abnormalities.

The best means of detecting primary open-angle glaucoma early is performance of tonometry and direct ophthalmoscopy of the optic disk on all adult patients every 3 years and whenever they undergo a routine medical examination, with referral to ophthalmologists of all those with relevant abnormalities. In the case of patients at high risk of developing primary open-angle glaucoma, such as first degree relatives of affected individuals, formal ophthalmic assessment should take place every year.

PREVENTION OF AMBYLOPIA ("Lazy Eye")

Amblyopia can be defined for the purposes of this discussion as diminished visual acuity in one eye in the absence of organic eye disease. Central vision develops from birth to age 6 or 7; if vision has not developed by then, there is little or no chance that it will develop later. In the absence of eye disease, the two main abnormalities that will prevent a child from acquiring binocular vision are strabismus and anisometropia.

Strabismus

Esotropia or exotropia in a young child causes double vision. The child quickly learns to suppress the image in the deviating eye and learns to see normally with one eye. Unfortunately, vision does not develop in the unused eye; unless the good eye is patched, thus forcing the child to use the deviating eye, sight will never develop in that eye. The child will grow up with one perfectly normal eye that is essentially blind, since it has never developed a functional connection with the visual centers of the brain. This is more likely to occur with esotropia than with exotropia.

Anisometropia

Young children are more concerned with the perception of near objects than with those at a distance. If one eye is nearsighted (myopic) and the other farsighted (hyperopic), the child will favor the nearsighted eye. Thus, the farsighted eye will not be used even though it is straight. The result will be the same as in untreated strabismus, ie, monocular blindness due to failure of visual development in an unused eye. The incidence of anisometropia is about 0.75–1%.

Early Diagnosis

The best way to prevent amblyopia is to test the visual acuity of all preschool children. By the time a child reaches school, it is usually too late for occlusion therapy. The parents can perform the test at home with the illiterate "E" chart. This is sometimes known as the "Home Eye Test." Pediatricians and others responsible for the care of small children should test visual acuity no later than age 4.

Photorefraction is said to be useful in screening for anisometropia, ametropia, astigmatism, and strabismus in preschool children. Any child observed to have strabismus after the age of 3 months should be seen by an ophthalmologist.

PREVENTION OF OCULAR DAMAGE DUE TO SYSTEMIC DISEASES

It is important for nonophthalmologic practitioners, particularly internists, general practitioners, and pediatricians, to be aware of the systemic diseases that have an ophthalmic component which may produce asymptomatic ocular damage.

Diabetic retinopathy is the most common cause of blindness developing between ages 20 and 64. Treatment is available to prevent such blindness, but for best effect it must be administered before visual loss has occurred, ie, diabetics must undergo regular fundal examination and be referred whenever treatment is indicated. The major abnormalities that must be recognized are new vessel formation on the optic disk and exudates around the macula. Any diabetic developing visual loss should also be referred for ophthalmic assessment. (The management of diabetic retinopathy is discussed further in Chapter 15.)

Uveitis associated with juvenile rheumatoid arthritis is generally asymptomatic in its early stages and often remains undetected until severe loss of vision due to glaucoma, cataract, or band keratopathy has already occurred. Regular ophthalmic screening should take place, particularly of girls with a pauciarticular onset of the disease and circulating antinuclear antibody.

Even in the USA, where it should now be all but unknown, occasional cases of xerophthalmia still occur, and in the underdeveloped areas the world over, where nutrition is often poor, it is still common. Vitamin A deficiency disease, in which the eye changes (xerophthalmia and keratomalacia) are the most damaging and often cause blindness (see Chapter 23), is usually the result of a deficient diet associated with poverty. It should be borne in mind, however, that it may also be associated with chronic alcoholism, weight-reducing diets, dietary management of food allergy, or poor absorption from the gastrointestinal tract due to the use of mineral oil or gastrointestinal disease such as chronic diarrhea.

In vitamin A-deficient children, measles may result in severe corneal disease. Because of the eye signs (ie, night blindness, Bitot's spots, or a lackluster corneal epithelium), the ophthalmologist may be the first to recognize vitamin A deficiency. Early recognition and treatment can prevent loss of vision or blindness due to secondary infection and corneal perforation. Treatment of the acute condition may require large intramuscular doses of vitamin A followed by corrective diet and careful analysis of all possible causes.

PREVENTION OF VISUAL LOSS DUE TO DRUGS

All drugs can cause adverse reactions. It is the ophthalmologist's responsibility to prevent visual loss or major ocular disability from drugs used to treat eye diseases.

Ophthalmic drugs should be packaged and labeled so that mistakes are not made by elderly or poorly sighted patients. Atropine and other strong medications may call for color-labeling. On the first visit to a new ophthalmologist, the patient should be asked to bring along any previously prescribed medications in order to avoid duplication and possible overdosage.

Certain ophthalmic drugs have such frequently occurring and damaging side effects that their use requires special monitoring and special warnings to the patient. Atropine and scopolamine, used to dilate the pupil in iridocyclitis, may precipitate acute glaucoma in certain patients with narrow anterior chamber angles. After prolonged use, they can also lead to conjunctivitis and allergic eczema of the eyelids. Many antiglaucoma drugs can produce stenosis of the puncta and shrinkage of the conjunctiva. Topical anesthetics should never be prescribed or made available for long-term use because severe corneal ulceration and scarring may result.

Corticosteroids used locally in drop or ointment forms may depress the local defense mechanisms and precipitate corneal ulceration, often fungal. They may also worsen herpetic keratitis and other corneal infections and on prolonged use may lead to open-angle glaucoma and to posterior subcapsular cataract. Much of the severity of both herpes simplex virus and varicella-zoster virus corneal infections can be blamed on the unwise use of topical corticosteroids. In this situation, short-term improvement has been traded for long-term disaster.

Many drugs used **systemically** have serious ocular side effects, eg, keratopathy, retrobulbar neuritis, retinopathy, and Stevens-Johnson syndrome (erythema multiforme). For this reason, the ophthalmologist must take a careful history of the patient's use of drugs as part of the initial examination. Of special interest are the keratopathy and retinopathy that often follow the use of chloroquine in discoid lupus erythematosus. It is the function of the consulting ophthalmologist to detect any early ocular changes and to inform the dermatologist of them so that he can substitute another medication.

REFERENCES

Aswad MI et al: Bacterial adherence to extended wear soft contact lenses. Ophthalmology 1990;97:296.

Bochow T et al: Ultraviolet light exposure and risk of posterior subcapsular cataracts. Arch Ophthalmol 1989; 107:814.

Chandler JW: Controversies in ocular prophylaxis of newborns. (Editorial.) Arch Ophthalmol 1989;107:814.

Daffos F et al: Prenatal management of 746 pregnancies at risk for congenital toxoplasmosis. N Engl J Med 1988;318:271.

De Respinis PA et al: Survey of severe eye injuries in children. Am J Dis Child 1989;143:711.

Dunn JP et al: Corneal ulcers associated with disposable hydrogel contact lenses. Am J Ophthalmol 1989;108:113.

Duttner LR et al: Potential bacterial contamination in fluorescein-anesthetic solutions. Am J Ophthalmol 1990; 110:426.

Fraunfelder FT: National Registry of Drug-Induced Ocular Side-Effects. (Editorial.) Am J Ophthalmol 1990;110:426.

Friedlander MH (editor): *Prevention of Eye Disease*. Mary Ann Liebert, Inc., 1988.

Givens KT et al: Congenital rubella syndrome: Ophthalmic manifestations and associated systemic disorders. Br J Ophthalmol 1993;77:358.

Gordon YJ et al: Prolonged recovery of desiccated adenoviral serotypes 5, 8, and 19 from plastic and metal surfaces in vitro. Ophthalmology 1993;100:1835.

Hoyt CS: Photorefraction: A technique for preschool visual screening. (Editorial.) Arch Ophthalmol 1987;105:1497.

Jordan DR: The potential damaging effects of light on the eye. Part 1. Can J Ophthalmol 1986;21:216.

Kanski JJ: Screening for uveitis in juvenile chronic arthritis. Br J Ophthalmol 1989;73:225.

Kattan HM et al: Nosocomial endophthalmitis survey: Current incidence of infection after intraocular surgery. Ophthalmology 1991;98:227.

Larrison WI et al: Sports related ocular trauma. Ophthalmology 1990;97:1265.

Liggett PE et al: Ocular trauma in an urban population. Review of 1132 cases. Ophthalmology 1990;97:581.

Meredith TA: Prevention of postoperative infection. (Editorial.) Arch Ophthalmol 1991;109:944.

Michels M, Sternberg P: Operating microscope-induced retinal phototoxicity: Pathophysiology, clinical manifestation and prevention. Surv Ophthalmol 1990;34:237.

Murrah WF: Epidemic keratoconjunctivitis. Ann Ophthalmol 1988;20:36.

Palmberg R et al: Potential bacterial contamination of eyedrops Pepose JS et al: Disinfection of Goldman tonometers against human immunodeficiency virus type 1. Arch Ophthalmol 1989;107:983.

Poggio EC et al: The incidence of ulcerative keratitis among users of daily-wear and extended-wear soft contact lenses. N Engl J Med 1989;321:779.

Rosenwasser GOD et al: Topical anesthetic abuse. Ophthalmology 1990;97:962.

Schein OD et al: The relative risk of ulcerative keratitis among users of daily-wear and extended-wear soft contact lenses: A case-control study. N Engl J Med 1989;321:773.

Speaker MG et al: Role of external bacterial flora in the pathogenesis of acute postoperative endophthalmitis. Ophthalmology 1991;98:639.

Taylor HR et al: Corneal changes associated with chronic UV-irradiation. Arch Ophthalmol 1989;107:1481.

Threlkeld AB et al: Efficacy of a disinfectant wipe method for the removal of adenovirus 8 from tonometer tips. Ophthalmology 1993;100:1841.

West SK et al: Exposure to sunlight and other risk factors for age-related macular degeneration. Arch Ophthalmol 1989;107:875.

Young RW: Solar radiation and age-related macular degeneration. Surv Ophthalmol 1988;32:252.

22

Low Vision

Eleanor E. Faye, MD

In all subspecialties of eye care, patients with irreversible or temporary reduction of vision present a challenge in effective management—not only by medical and surgical treatment but also by helping patients to overcome their disabilities.

Patients with impaired visual performance owing to reduced visual acuity uncorrectable by conventional spectacles or contact lenses or to restricted visual field are commonly called **low-vision patients.** There may be additional complaints of increased glare sensitivity and abnormalities of color perception, contrast sensitivity, dark adaptation, ocular motility, and fusion.

The many optical and other devices used to improve visual performance in low-vision patients are called **low-vision aids.** In this chapter, discussion will center on assessment of low vision and provision of low-vision aids. Ophthalmologic details about specific entities mentioned will not be discussed.

Since levels of visual performance are most realistically judged according to individual requirements, the term "low vision" may actually denote a wide range of visual impairment from nearly normal to profound loss. In the United States, over six million persons are visually impaired but not classified as legally blind.* Over 75% of patients seeking treatment for low vision are age 65 or over. Macular degeneration accounts for over 50% of all cases. Complicated cataract, glaucoma, diabetic retinopathy, optic atrophy, degenerative myopia, and retinitis pigmentosa are other major causes.

Effective low-vision management does not place artificial definitions in the way of visual rehabilitation but considers each individual's level of function, visual objectives, and the available low-vision aids. Low-vision treatment should be started at whatever stage a patient experiences difficulty with customary visual tasks. Although progression of impaired vision is the rule, early intervention allows the patient time to adjust to new techniques. An uncertain prognosis is not sufficient reason to delay treatment.

Management of the patient with low vision includes (1) taking a history that incorporates questions about customary activities; (2) examining the patient for changes in visual acuity, visual field, contrast sensitivity, color perception, and glare sensitivity; (3) evaluating near vision and reading skills; (4) selection and prescription (or lending) of aids that help achieve visual objectives, with the necessary instruction in their use; and (5) follow-up to ensure adjustment and correct use of the aids or to answer further questions.

HISTORY TAKING

Patients should be asked about the nature of their visual impairment, its duration, and its rapidity of onset. Customary activities that have become tedious or impossible should be specifically discussed. Table 22–1 lists a number of activities that are adversely affected by substandard vision. Individual activities can usually be matched with specific optical and nonoptical aids so that realistic objectives based upon the patient's expectations can be established. Patients should be encouraged to understand the effects of their condition on the visual system. Fears of eventual blindness must be aired and set to rest.

EXAMINATION

Standard refraction may reveal unsuspected refractive errors and is important in prescribing high-add bifocals and in following patients with retinal disease who have intraocular lens implants. Best corrected acuity is measured at 4 m, 2 m, or 1 m with the Lighthouse Ferris-Bailey ETDRS chart, which has lines (each with five letters) of 0.1 log unit difference and a convenient Snellen conversion table (Figure 22–1). The 4 m test distance is used for acuity from 20/20 to 20/200; the 2 m test distance for acuities less than 20/200; and the 1 m test distance for acuities less than 20/400. Standard Snellen charts may be used at test distances of 10 ft or less, but projector charts are not recommended for testing low vision.

One should determine the dominant eye and the preferred eye.

---

*Legal blindness—defined as a best corrected visual acuity of 20/200 or less in the better eye or a visual field of 20 degrees or less–affects 1 million individuals in the USA (see Chapter 23).

Table 22–1. Common activities that are adversely affected by visual impairment are listed with suggestions for low vision aids.

Activity	Optical Aids	Nonoptical Aids
Shopping	Hand magnifier	Lighting, color cues
Fixing a snack	Bifocals	Color cues, consistent storage plan
Eating out	Hand magnifier	Flashlight, portable lamp
Identifying money	Bifocal, hand magnifier	Arrange wallet in compartments
Reading print	High power spectacle, bifocal, hand magnifier, stand magnifier, closed circuit television	Lighting, high-contrast print, large print, reading slit
Writing	Intermediate add hand magnifier, focusable telescope, closed circuit television	Lighting, bold tip pen, black ink
Dialing a telephone	Hand magnifier	Large print dial, hand-printed directory
Crossing streets	Telescope	Cane, ask directions
Finding taxis and bus signs	Telescope	
Reading medication labels	Hand magnifier	Color codes, large print
Reading stove dials	Hand magnifier	Color codes
Thermostat adjustment	Hand magnifier	Enlarged print model
Using a computer	Intermediate add spectacles	High-contrast color, large print program
Reading signs	Spectacle	Move closer
Watching sporting event	Telescope	Sit in front rows

Amsler grids are used to locate central scotomas and to chart their position and density and areas of distortion. Note is made of whether the patient sees less distortion monocularly or binocularly. If less distortion is noted binocularly, the patient may be a candidate for reading lenses that correct both eyes rather that the customary monocular lens. Central scotomas may also be charted on a tangent screen. Peripheral fields are best tested on a tangent screen in patients with retinitis pigmentosa and on a Goldmann perimeter in patients with glaucoma and neurologic deficits.

Contrast sensitivity may be assessed both monocularly and binocularly with the Vistech Contrast Sensitivity Vision Test (See Chapter 2). Loss of high-frequency and mid-frequency targets is a predictor of difficulty reading print with low-vision optical devices. Superior binocular performance suggests selection of an aid that is used binocularly, eg, base-in prism glasses or binocular reading telescopes. Glare tests are used if lens or corneal opacities complicate other disorders such as glaucoma or macular degeneration to determine whether cataract extraction or keratoplasty might improve acuity. Color identification tests identify difficulty with color cues.

NEAR VISION

Near vision may be evaluated using a combination of single-letter tests (Figure 22–2) and graded text of various sizes. Single letters serve to establish near acuity, graded text to establish reading skills with a selected optical aid. The reciprocal of **distance acuity** may be used to determine the approximate strength of the initial trial lens for near vision—eg, 20/160 suggests a trial of 8 D of add to read 10-point print.

SELECTION OF AIDS & PATIENT INSTRUCTION

When the dioptric range has been established for the task objectives (the range may be from +3 D to +68 D), the type of low-vision device best suited to the task and degree of vision loss is selected.

The patient uses various devices under the supervision of a trained instructor until proficiency and efficacy have been established. The mechanics of the aids are reviewed, questions are answered, goals are clarified, and the patient is allowed ample time in a quiet setting to explore the new skills. This may involve one or more sessions and ideally culminates in providing a loaner lens in doubtful cases or prescription of one or more devices. Some patients require home or job trial of an aid before they can be secure. Older patients usually need more adaptation time than younger or congenitally visually impaired persons.

Proper patient instruction is the key to success in management of low-vision patients. Prescription of lenses without instruction is successful in only 50% of cases, whereas with instruction the success rate rises to over 90%.

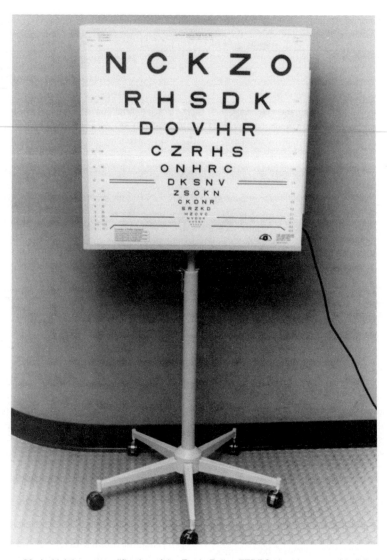

Figure 22–1. Lighthouse modification of the Ferris-Bailey ETDRS chart in a movable light box.

The patient's progress is reviewed after two or three weeks. Patients are encouraged to call if there are unforeseen problems. Many minor technical difficulties can be solved over the phone.

LOW-VISION AIDS

There are three basic types of low-vision optical aids: (1) convex lens aids such as spectacles, hand magnifiers, and stand magnifiers; and (2) telescopic systems such as spectacle telescopes, clip-on telescopic loupes, and handheld devices. Nonoptical aids include writing aids, large-print publications, improved lighting, yellow filters, and reading stands. Antireflective lenses that absorb specific wavelengths are used to protect eyes from ultraviolet light and glare. (3) Electronic reading systems include closed-circuit television reading machines and computers with large print capability.

The practitioner must be familiar with the devices available and the advantages and disadvantages of each in order to provide proper guidance to the instructor and the patient. Prescribing low-vision devices requires that both the physician and the instructor also understand how the symptoms of the disorder and acuity affect the indications for spectacles, contact lenses, telescopes, intraocular lenses, and low-vision magnifying devices.

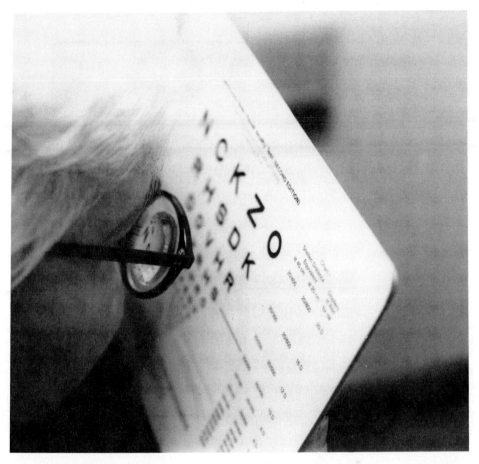

Figure 22–2. Low-vision spectacle aid. Patient demonstrates close reading distance (with lenticular spectacle) but with both hands free to hold reading material.

CONVEX LENS AIDS

Spectacles and hand and stand magnifiers are the mainstays of the low-vision practitioner. Various mountings for lenses have inherent advantages and disadvantages. If the patient uses a convex lens in a spectacle frame, reading material must be held at the focal distance of the lens, eg, 10 cm for a 10-D lens (Figure 22–2). The closer distances obstruct light, but for a reader the advantage of having both hands free to hold the material outweighs the unfamiliar close reading distance, while lamps can be adjusted to provide sufficient illumination.

Spectacles up to 12 D may be used binocularly (with base-in prisms to aid convergence). From 14 to 60 D, a monocular aspheric lenticular or doublet lens should be prescribed.

Hand magnifiers are convenient lenses for short-term tasks such as shopping, reading dials and labels, and identifying paper money (Figure 22–3). The advantage of a convex lens held by hand is that a greater working distance is achieved by holding lens and read-

ing material away from the eye. Holding the lens and reading material may be a disadvantage for some patients with neurologic or orthopedic handicaps. Hand magnifiers span a dioptric range of 4–68 D. The image from a hand magnifier is preferably viewed with best corrected distance vision. (Since the image is coming from infinity, the parallel rays exiting the lens may be viewed without accommodative effort.)

Stand magnifiers are much like hand magnifiers except that the lens is mounted on a base of predetermined height (Figure 22–4). Because a lens mounting may block light, a lens in an illuminating handle may be the best choice for most patients. Presbyopic patients generally must wear a conventional reading add in conjunction with a fixed-focus stand magnifier.

TELESCOPE SYSTEMS

The telescopic systems generally preferred by patients for distance or intermediate range are hand-held monoculars from 2× to 10× power (Figure 22–5). For

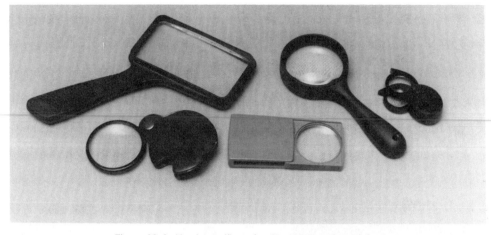

Figure 22–3. Hand magnifiers of various types and strengths.

patients with vocational or hobby requirements, focusable Galilean or Keplerian (internal prism) systems in a spectacle frame are the best choice. The power range for spectacle telescopes is 2× to 8×. High powers (6× to 8×) are heavy.

All optical devices limit the field of vision—spectacles the least and telescopes the most. Therefore, preexisting field limitations of the patient with large central or peripheral scotomas must always be a consideration when prescribing telescopes.

Electric Reading Systems

Electronic devices, which are more expensive than the average simple reading aid, are worth a trial for persons who have special needs. Closed circuit television (CCTV) machines have been designed for the varied visual needs of visually impaired students, working adults, and older persons who require a more versatile low-vision reading device than optical devices can provide. High plus reading lenses and tele-

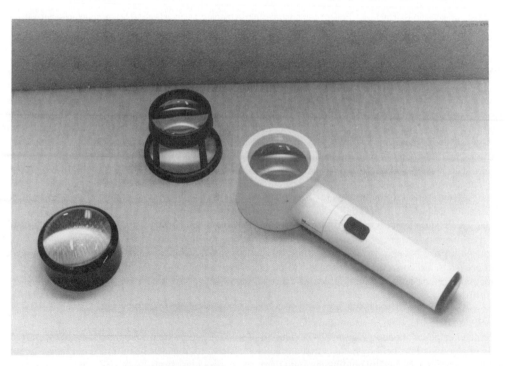

Figure 22–4. Stand magnifiers with and without illumination handle.

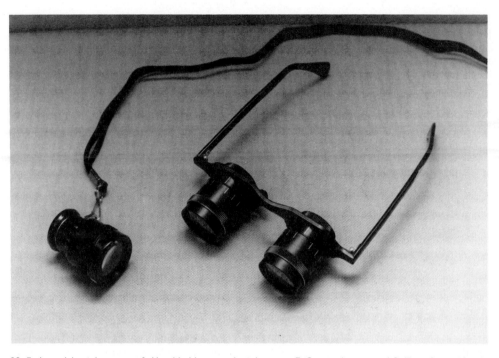

Figure 22–5. Low vision telescopes. **A:** Hand-held monocular telescope. **B:** Spectacle-mounted Galilean focusable telescope.

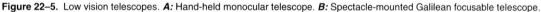

scopes have optical limitations of power, visual field, and reading distance. Their advantages are portability and availability. The advantage of CCN is a more normal reading posture.

The television reading machine through use of a zoom lens provides a range of magnification from 1.5× to 45× or higher and a comfortable reading distance with full field. Although not truly portable nor available everywhere, CCTV is useful in situations that require variable magnification with a variety of reading material.

The machine consists of a high-resolution television monitor with a built-in camera (some models feature a hand-held camera), a zoom lens, an accessory lamp, and a special X-Y reading table. Models for the classroom have an independent swivel camera that can be focused on the blackboard or typewriter. Other models have a split screen for typing, writing, or computer access. Large-print software is available that makes it possible to view enlarged computer print on the same screen as the camera material.

TINTS & COATINGS

In addition to providing magnifying lenses for reading and telescopes for all ranges of vision from distance to near, the practitioner must consider the effect of glare and low contrast on performance. As a rule, lenses that cut out ultraviolet light below 400 nm are coated with an antireflective multilayer coating and tinted gray to reduce light intensity or amber-yellow to improve contrast.

MANAGEMENT OF LOW-VISION PATIENTS

Treatment plans must take into account the effect of the eye disorder on both visual acuity and visual field. Symptoms of glare, blur, and central or peripheral visual deficits may vary, but they do directly affect the strength of the aid required and to some extent the type of aid that can be prescribed as well as the adjustment to the aid.

Low-vision problems can be classified in four categories: (1) blurred or hazy central and peripheral vision, characteristic of cloudy media (cornea, lens, lens capsule, vitreous); (2) impaired focal resolution without central scotomas and with normal peripheral acuity, characteristic of macular edema or albinism; (3)

central scotomas, characteristic of degenerative or inflammatory macular disorders and optic nerve disease; and (4) peripheral scotomas, characteristic of advanced glaucoma, retinitis pigmentosa, and other peripheral retinal disorders.

BLURRED, HAZY VISION

Generalized blurring or haziness of vision may be produced by abnormalities of the ocular media, including a variety of corneal stromal, epithelial, and endothelial disorders, lens opacities, posterior capsular opacification, vitreous opacities, abnormalities of pupillary size from miosis to aniridia, and retinal edema. Patients also experience reduction of acuity from glare with or without photophobia and note reduced contrast perception for stairs, curbs, and objects.

Useful tests of visual function include Snellen visual acuity, glare sensitivity tests, and contrast sensitivity tests. A potential acuity meter (PAM) may help differentiate pathologic processes involving the media from those involving the retina.

Treatment

Visual acuity varies markedly with lighting and image contrast. Modification of illumination and attention to details of image enhancement have high priority in treatment. Antireflective lens coatings and neutral gray lenses reduce light intensity, and yellow-amber lenses enhance contrast. Ultraviolet filters should be used, particularly for pseudophakic patients.

Magnification may not be effective, because a magnified image may still be indistinct. Large, bold print may be a better choice—or reading slits of matte plastic or cardboard to reduce glare and outline the text. Contact lenses or keratoplasty for corneal disorders, cataract extraction with or without intraocular lens implantation for lens opacities, and posterior capsulotomy for posterior capsular opacification may also be indicated.

IMPAIRED FOCAL RESOLUTION

Macular edema from a variety of disorders and congenital foveal aplasia characteristic of albinism cause impaired focal resolution with normal peripheral acuity. As a rule, visual acuity is in the higher range from 20/50 to 20/200.

Useful tests of visual function include Snellen visual acuity, Amsler grid, and PAM.

Treatment

These patients should have careful refraction for best possible foveal vision. Characteristically, they respond to reading adds of +4 to +10 D and are proficient readers at the relatively normal reading distances such

lenses require. Bifocals or contact lenses should be considered for stable conditions.

Magnifying hand and stand glasses are useful. Amber and antireflective sunglasses improve contrast and reduce glare. Albinos adapt well to hand-held and spectacle-mounted telescopes.

CENTRAL SCOTOMAS

The two commonest causes of central scotomas are atrophic and exudative (hemorrhagic) age-related macular degeneration, both of which are increasingly common in today's aging society. Other causes are macular holes, myopic macular degeneration, optic nerve disease, and congenital macular disorders.

Patients most often report blurred or distorted central vision (peripheral vision is clear unless cataracts complicate the picture). Difficulty in reading and in discerning facial features are the most common complaints in early stages of macular disease. Dense scotomas are characteristic of the disciform stage of exudative macular disease and of optic nerve disease. In the early stages, contrast perception is generally not affected. Travel ability remains relatively normal even in advanced disease.

Useful tests of visual function include Snellen visual acuity, Amsler grid, and contrast sensitivity. Reduced contrast suggests the need for more magnification than predicted from the Snellen visual acuity test.

Treatment

Patients may use eccentric head positions to place images in healthier retinal areas. This technique may be demonstrated to the patient during visual acuity tests or on an Amsler grid.

Magnifying lenses are of benefit. The strength of the prescription is related directly to near visual acuity and contrast as well as to position and density of the scotoma. Patients may use several types of lenses for various tasks, eg, spectacles for reading, and a hand magnifier for shopping. Most patients with macular degeneration learn to use low-vision aids successfully, particularly after supportive instruction sessions. Older patients may require more reinforcement and additional time to adjust. They particularly need reassurance about the remote possibility of blindness.

PERIPHERAL SCOTOMA

Peripheral field loss is characteristic of end-stage glaucoma, retinitis pigmentosa, other peripheral retinal diseases, and cerebral vascular disease. While central vision is essential for details, the peripheral field of vision is essential for locating oneself in space, for traveling about safely, and for awareness of potential hazards and objects in the periphery. A person with advanced retinitis pigmentosa may be able to read small print yet need a guide to get around.

Adequate lighting is essential for patients with residual foveal fields. Most patients' photophobia is relieved by amber-orange lenses that block ultraviolet and visible blue light below 527 nm. When contrast perception is reduced by cataract, a combination of contrast sensitivity and glare tests may indicate the best timing for cataract surgery.

When central fields are less than 7 degrees, magnification of an image is not perceived by such a patient as advantageous. Telescopes are therefore not useful, and hand magnifiers and closed-circuit television may be the devices of choice because the amount of magnification can be regulated by the patient. A posterior chamber intraocular lens implant for patients undergoing cataract extraction is *essential* to maintain normal image size.

TRAINING PROGRAMS

Many practitioners and staff benefit from joint training programs to learn the role of each person in management of low-vision patients in a private practice or clinic. Basic setups for a low-vision practice are reviewed in a number of publications.

No patient with impaired vision should have to search far and wide for low-vision care. Such care should be integrated into every ophthalmologic practice, and practitioners should offer referral of patients with complex requirements to low-vision centers for rehabilitation.

REFERENCES

Faye EE (editor). *Clinical Low Vision,* 2nd ed. Little, Brown, 1984.

Freeman P, Jose, R: *The Art and Practice of Low Vision.* Butterworth, 1991.

Goodrich GL et al: Training and practice effects in performance with low-vision aids: A preliminary study. Am J Optom Physiol Opt 1977;54:312.

Jose RT (editor): *Understanding Low Vision.* American Foundation for the Blind, 1983.

Kwitko ML, Weinstock FJ: *Geriatric Ophthalmology.* Grune & Stratton, 1985.

Legge G, Rubin G, Leubker A: Psychophysics of reading. V. The role of contrast in normal vision. Vision Research 1987;27:1165.

Tielsch JM et al: Blindness and visual impairment in an American urban population: The Baltimore eye survey. Arch Ophthalmol 1990;108:286.

Additional Resources

American Foundation for the Blind (1994). Directory of Agencies Serving the Visually Handicapped in the US: American Foundation for the Blind, 1994.

Journal of Visual Impairment and Blindness. American Foundation for the Blind. [Monthly periodical.]

The Journal of Visual Rehabilitation. Lincoln, Nebraska. [Quarterly.]

The Lighthouse, Inc.: *Catalogue of Low Vision Products.* [Complete stock of low-vision aids and products.]

The Lighthouse Training and Continuing Program for the Center for Vision and Aging. The Lighthouse, Inc. [Professional education programs.]

National Center for Vision and Aging. The New York Lighthouse. [Information and pamphlets.]

23

Blindness

John P. Whitcher, MD, MPH

In this chapter we shall discuss blindness as a world-wide health problem, summarizing information about its epidemiology, emphasizing the value of community-based methods to prevent or treat its causes, and outlining resources available in more developed countries for rehabilitation of the blind. All of the disorders that may cause blindness are discussed more fully in other parts of this book.

DEFINITION OF BLINDNESS

The World Health Organization defines visual impairment as shown in Table 23–1. WHO officials encourage investigators and reporting agencies in all countries to report blindness and near blindness according to the categories defined in this table.

In the USA, the most widely used definition of partial blindness is that used by the Internal Revenue Service for the purpose of determining who is eligible for tax deductions on that basis: *central visual acuity 20/200 or less in the better eye with best correction, or widest diameter of visual field subtending an angle of no greater than 20 degrees.* An alternative functional definition is *loss of vision sufficient to prevent one from being self-supporting in an occupation, making the individual dependent on other persons, agencies, or devices in order to live.*

"Industrial blindness" is said to be present when a worker can no longer pursue an occupation because of poor vision; "automobile blindness" when vision is so poor that the responsible licensing agency in that state will not issue a driver's license. The term color blindness is a misnomer since this genetically transmitted disorder is not blindness as that term is generally understood and is only a minor handicap to a few people. Loss of vision may affect only the central fields, only the peripheral fields, or only specific portions of the peripheral fields in one or both eyes. Total loss of vision in one eye is said to reduce visual capacity by only 10%, though it makes the other eye infinitely more valuable.

Table 23–1. Categories of visual impairment. (Adapted from the International Classification of Diseases, World Health Organization, 1977.)

Category of Visual Impairment		Visual Acuity (Best Corrected)
Low vision	1	6/18 3/10 (0.3) 20/70
	2	6/60 1/10 (0.1) 20/200
Blindness	3	3/60 (finger counting at 3m) 1/20 (0.05) 20/400
	4	1/60 (finger counting at 1m) 1/50 (0.02) 5/300
	5	No light perception

Visual Field

Patients with a visual field radius no greater than 10 degrees but greater than 5 degrees around central fixation should be placed in category 3 and patients with a field no greater than 5 degrees around central fixation in category 4—even if the central acuity is not impaired.

PREVALENCE OF BLINDNESS THROUGHOUT THE WORLD

WHO estimates that there are between 27 and 35 million blind people in the world today. This figure rises to at least 42 million if the criterion is extended to visual acuity of 20/200 or worse. Even where health statistics are most reliable, the methods of counting the blind are often crude and may be applied according to different criteria in different places and at different times within any extensive geographic area. Furthermore, extrapolations are often made from small sample studies to large populations. Ninety percent of the world's blind live in developing countries, mostly in Asia (approximately 20 million) and Africa (approximately 6 million), clustered largely in disadvantaged communities in rural areas and urban slums. The risk of blindness in many of these neglected communities is 10–40 times higher than in the industrially developed regions of Europe and America.

Table 23–2 lists some countries where fairly reliable data are available about the prevalence of blindness.

Table 23–2. Approximate prevalence of blindness (%) (Estimates based on WHO surveys.)[1]

Chad	3.2–5	Malawi	1
Liberia	3.2	Brazil	0.3
Egypt	2.6	Mexico	0.3
Phillipines	2.1	Australia	0.2
Afghanistan	2	Japan	0.2
Bangladesh	2	USA	0.2
Pakistan	2	UK	0.18
Saudi Arabia	2	Canada	0.15
India	1.5	USSR	0.12
Indonesia	1.3	China	0.1
Chile	1	Germany	0.1

[1]Based on available data, 1969–1980. Some data were only rough estimates when obtained and may have changed markedly since then. In some cases, the survey criteria used did not correspond to WHO definitions. Data taken from Maitchouk IF: Data on blindness: Prevalence and causes throughout the world. In: Lim ASM, Jones BR (editors): World's major blinding conditions. *Vision* 1982;1:99. (International Agency for the Prevention of Blindness.)

CAUSES OF BLINDNESS & METHODS OF PREVENTION & TREATMENT

The relative importance of various causes of blindness differs according to the level of social development in the geographic area being studied. In developing countries, cataract is the leading cause, with trachoma, leprosy, onchocerciasis, and xerophthalmia also being important. In more developed countries, blindness is to a a great extent related to the aging process. Cataract is still important despite the availability of facilities for its treatment, along with age-related macular degeneration and glaucoma. Other causes are diabetic retinopathy, herpes simplex keratitis, retinal detachment, and inherited retinal degenerative disorders.

In terms of the worldwide prevalence of blindness, the vastly greater number of people in the developing world and the greater likelihood of their being affected mean that the causes of blindness in those areas are numerically more important. Cataract is responsible for an estimated 17 million cases of blindness, trachoma between 6 and 9 million, leprosy at least 1 million, and onchocerciasis 1 million. Xerophthalmia is estimated to affect 5 million children each year; 500,000 develop active corneal involvement, and half of these go blind.

WHO estimates that up to 80% of cases of blindness in developing countries are avoidable, ie, preventable or treatable. The recent worldwide eradication of smallpox demonstrates what can be achieved in the area of infectious disease and the superiority of prevention over treatment. Similar efforts are being made to prevent the infectious diseases trachoma, leprosy, and onchocerciasis as well as the noninfectious xerophthalmia. The sheer numbers of individuals blinded by cataract continues to overwhelm the resources available. In all programs to reduce blindness in the developing world, cooperation between governments and nongovernmental charitable organizations has proved to be essential. The WHO Prevention of Blindness Programme has established centers in about 60 developing countries to undertake collaborative studies, particularly generating epidemiologically sound information to form the basis for rational planning, implementation, and proper evaluation of programs for prevention of blindness.

In more developed countries, the causes of blindness are less amenable to prevention. In general, it is necessary to rely on recognition and treatment of the early stages of the disease. This depends on education of ophthalmologists, nonophthalmologic medical personnel, and lay people about the necessity for screening for glaucoma and diabetic retinopathy and about the importance of the early symptoms of retinal detachment, age-related macular degeneration, and herpes simplex keratitis. The inherited conditions are amenable to prevention by genetic counseling.

Cataract

Cataract accounts for at least 50% of cases of blindness worldwide. As life expectancy increases, there is a continuing rise in the total number of people affected. In many parts of the developing world, the facilities available for treating cataract are grossly inadequate, hardly sufficient to cope with the new cases arising and completely inadequate for dealing with the backlog of existing cases, which is conservatively estimated to be 10 million worldwide.

It is not clearly understood why the frequency of cataract in different geographic areas varies so greatly, though exposure to ultraviolet radiation and recurrent episodes of dehydration, such as occur in severe diarrheal diseases, are thought to be important. If medical means could be found to delay the development of cataract by 10 years, it is estimated that this would reduce the number of individuals requiring surgery by 45%.

Mobile eye camps have aided in management, but there are too few to control the disorder. Many more cataract surgeons are needed in countries such as India and Pakistan. In a number of blindness surveys, the problem of uncorrected aphakia is particularly apparent. It has been suggested that intraocular lens implantation at the time of surgery, though requiring greater expertise, may be a better solution than relying on the subsequent provision of spectacles.

Trachoma

Trachoma causes bilateral keratoconjunctivitis, generally in childhood, that leads in adulthood to corneal scarring, which, when severe, causes blindness. About 400 million people have trachoma, most of them in Africa, the Middle East, and Asia. Trachoma can be treated with sulfonamides or tetracycline drugs, and an estimated 60 million individuals currently require treatment. But prevention of spread of infection by provision of proper sanitary facilities, including clean water for drinking and washing, is more effective in eliminating the disease.

Leprosy

Leprosy (Hansen's disease) affects 15–16 million people in the world and has a higher percentage of ocular involvement than any other systemic disease. Up to 10% of leprosy patients are blind from the disease. The social stigma attached to leprosy has greatly hindered its treatment, but there are effective chemotherapeutic agents and the possibility of a vaccine.

Onchocerciasis

Onchocerciasis is transmitted by bites of the blackfly, which breeds in clear running streams (hence the name river blindness). It is endemic in the greater part of tropical Africa and Central and South America. The most heavily infested zone is the Volta River basin, which extends over parts of Dahomey, Ghana, Ivory Coast, Mali, Niger, Togo, and Upper Volta. Worldwide, 28 million people are affected by onchocerciasis, with 20% of individuals in endemic areas being blind from the disease.

The major ophthalmic manifestations of onchocerciasis are keratitis, uveitis, retinochoroiditis, and optic atrophy. The disease is prevented by insect eradication and personal protection by screening. Treatment is with ivermectin.

Xerophthalmia

Xerophthalmia is due to hypovitaminosis A. Clinically, there is xerosis of the conjunctiva with characteristic Bitot's spots and softening of the cornea (keratomalacia), which may lead to corneal perforation. Protein malnutrition exacerbates the condition and renders it refractory to treatment. Xerophthalmia is a common cause of blindness in infants, particularly in India, Bangladesh, Indonesia, and the Philippines. Affected infants often do not reach adulthood, dying from malnutrition, pneumonia, or diarrhea.

Xerophthalmia can be prevented by general dietary improvement or vitamin A supplementation. If the problems of distribution and administration were solved, the cost of a quantity of the vitamin sufficient to prevent blindness in 1000 infants would be only about $25.00.

Other Causes

Glaucoma, retinal detachment, diabetic retinopathy, and herpes simplex keratitis are discussed in greater detail elsewhere in this text. The incidence of blindness due to glaucoma has decreased in recent years as a result of earlier detection, improved medical and surgical treatment, and a greater awareness and understanding of the disorder by the lay population.

Diabetic retinopathy is an increasingly more common cause of blindness everywhere in the world. Recent advances in surgical treatment (vitrectomy, laser therapy) are of some help, but many patients still suffer from proliferative retinopathy, recurrent vitreous hemorrhages, and eventual bilateral blindness. A vast research effort directed at all aspects of diabetes is in progress, and there is justification for hoping that the next generation of diabetics will benefit greatly from what is being done now.

Hereditary conditions are important causes of blindness but should gradually decrease in incidence in response to the efforts of genetic counselors to increase public awareness of the preventable nature of these disorders.

As is true also in other countries where medical care and social services are widely available, blindness in the USA is to a great extent related to the aging process, and about half of the legally blind people in this country are over age 65. The leading causes of blindness in this age group are degenerative retinal disorders, glaucoma, diabetes, and vascular diseases.

COSTS OF AVOIDING BLINDNESS

Some examples of what can be achieved for modest outlays of scarce funds are as follows:

(1) To cure one person of trachoma in Saudi Arabia: $1.25.

(2) To restore vision to one person in Pakistan blinded by cataracts: $25.00.

(3) To prevent blindness due to xerophthalmia in one infant in Java: 27 cents.

On the advice of WHO experts, the World Council for the Welfare of the Blind and several international professional ophthalmic societies and agencies agreed to take the initiative, which led to the establishment in 1974 of the International Agency for Prevention of Blindness (Vision International), with Sir John Wilson, a blind barrister, as president. The aim of this agency is to work with groups formed for the purpose of preventing blindness. Its theme, Foresight Prevents Blindness, was brought into prominent display when WHO celebrated the first World Health Day on April 7, 1976. Its goal was stated as follows: "In every donor country during 1976, every family should be asked—in thanksgiving for sight—to give $10.00 to save the sight of its fellow countrymen or of the millions in the third world. If we can raise this campaign to that degree of universal appeal, the result could be spectacular."

REHABILITATION OF THE BLIND

Although no completely reliable statistics are available, the most widely used estimates place the legally blind population of the USA at 2.24 per thousand (ie, approximately 500,000). Approximately 50,000 become legally blind annually, and many others have enough visual loss to constitute a serious employment problem.

Blindness does not necessarily imply helplessness. Individual adjustment to marked visual impairment or total blindness varies with age at onset, temperament, education, economic resources, and many other factors. The older patient, for example, may accept blindness quite stoically, whereas for the younger patient the vocational or social impact of blindness is often catastrophic. Blindness is accepted more easily by persons who are born blind and by persons of any age who lose their vision gradually rather than suddenly.

The aim of rehabilitation is to enable the patient to lead as nearly normal a life as possible. Approximately 5000 blind persons in the USA are rehabilitated and obtain paid employment each year. An additional larger number of blind homemakers are able to perform their household duties without assistance or are able to live independently of others.

Rehabilitation must be individualized. Many special services (see Appendix III) and increasingly complex optical and nonoptical aids (see Chapter 22) are available, but they are not universally helpful. Different categories of the blind have different needs, and some blind people simply cannot benefit from a number of services or aids available. It has been said that over half of the blind people in the USA are over age 65. The elderly widowed housewife may need or want no more than mobility training in home care and a steady supply of Talking Books. A young person facing blindness in later life due to retinitis pigmentosa requires the full range of social services, including educational assessment, job rehabilitation, and psychologic counseling as well as a number of sophisticated aids.

The responsibility of the physician clearly does not end with the diagnosis, prevention, and treatment of ocular disorders that might result in blindness. The physician caring for the patient who is suddenly faced with actual or imminent blindness is in a position to be of great assistance. When blindness is a possibility but is not inevitable (eg, during acute ocular inflammation), optimism and reassurance are warranted. However, it is unwise to offer false hope or to delay "breaking the news" when blindness is inevitable. If it is certain that blindness will occur, it is important to extend to the distraught patient as well as to the patient's family the warmth, understanding, encouragement, and assistance so desperately needed. The physician should be alert to the severe depressive reactions that may occur.

It is especially important to assist the patient in making the adjustment to blindness while some vision is still present. Early referral to rehabilitation agencies is essential for recently blinded adults and those with irreversible progressive visual loss. Training programs or reeducation for the many changes involved in daily living and employment are greatly simplified if the patient has the partial support provided by even limited vision.

The physician should work actively with both the patient and the family and with other professional people concerned with rendering services to the blind. The physician must know what referral sources are available and how to use them skillfully. Medical social workers, public health nurses, and counseling services and agencies serving the blind and visually handicapped are common sources of reliable information. It may be valuable to have the patient talk with a blind person who has made a satisfactory adjustment to blindness.

Mobility Training & Guide Dogs

Mobility training is most important in rehabilitation of the blind. Many state commissions for the blind offer a wide variety of mobility training courses, either directly or in cooperation with private agencies. The courses are offered on an outpatient and residential basis and have varied objectives according to the special needs of the people who apply for help. The curriculum commonly includes self-care, home functions, and mobility within the community. Several universities* have undergraduate and postgraduate programs in mobility training for the blind.

The usefulness of guide dogs is limited by their daily care needs and the physical strength required to hold them in check. They are most useful for students and professional men and women in good health who lead fairly well organized lives. At this time, less than 2% of blind people in the USA use guide dogs. Sonar sensor canes may ultimately be a better answer to the mobility problem even for those who are now using a dog successfully.

Braille

This remarkably effective system of reading for the blind was introduced in 1825. The braille characters consist of raised dots arranged in two columns of three. The system is so simple that a blind child can quickly learn to read braille, and proficient readers can learn to read braille as fast as they can talk. The system has been adapted to musical notation and technical and scientific uses also. An international braille code was introduced in 1951.

Braille is used less commonly now than formerly, since many blind people prefer auditory aids both for informational and recreational purposes. But the recent availability of portable data storage systems with braille-encoded input and conventional or braille form printed output has brought about a resurgence of interest. Braille continues to be essential on tags attached

---

*Undergraduate level programs are at Cleveland State University in Ohio, Florida State University in Florida, and Stephen F. Austin University in Texas. Graduate programs are available at Boston University, California State University (Los Angeles), Northern Colorado University, San Francisco State University, University of Arkansas, University of Wisconsin, and Western Michigan State University.

to items in common personal use even for people who do not wish to use it for reading.

All paper money in the Netherlands and Switzerland is braille-printed to show the denomination.

Electronic Devices

Optacon is an electronic device that converts visual images of letters into tactile forms. It is easily portable and can be used with almost any kind of reading matter. Auditory aids are becoming increasingly important (eg, talking calculators, clocks, paper money identifiers).

FINANCIAL ASSISTANCE PROGRAMS

It is unfortunate that over half of the blind people in the USA are essentially dependent upon Social Security and whatever local supplemental aid may be available to them. For the younger blind population, rehabilitation programs are commonly administered at the state level by a division of the department of education specifically set up to serve blind people in the state.

Some of these programs are better than others, and all physicians should support efforts to increase the effectiveness of such programs in their geographic area of influence. The programs are of wide scope and offer preliminary counseling followed by academic or vocational training as the circumstances warrant. Once a realistic vocational objective has been established, full financial support is commonly available. This single resource is probably the most crucial referral available to the ophthalmologist, particularly in the case of young patients. Counseling services are available as early as the junior high school years to ensure compliance with a curriculum consistent with measured aptitudes and interests. In many states, such rehabilitation programs as mobility training are administered under state auspices but contracted to private agencies for operational purposes.

In many countries, the blind receive no financial or other support from their governments and are either cared for by their families or left to manage by themselves in any way they can.

Special services available to the blind in the USA are listed and discussed in Appendix III.

REFERENCES

Abiose A et al: Distribution and aetiology of blindness and visual impairment in mesoendemic onchocercal communities, Kaduna State, Nigeria. Br J Ophthalmol 1994;78:8.

Courtright P et al: Trachoma and blindness in the Nile Delta: Current patterns and projection to the future in the mid-Egyptian population. Br J Ophthalmol 1989;73:536.

Dawson CR, Jones BR, Tarizzo ML: *Guide to Trachoma Control in Programmes for the Prevention of Blindness.* World Health Organization, 1981.

Faye EE (editor): *Clinical Low Vision,* 2nd ed. Little, Brown, 1984.

Ffytche TJ: The continuing challenge of ocular leprosy. Br J Ophthalmol 1991;75:123.

Fielder AR, Best AB, Bax MCO: The management of visual impairment in childhood. Clin Dev Med 1993;128:1.

Foster A, Gilbert C: Epidemiology of childhood blindness. Eye 1992;6:173.

Global scale of avoidable blindness. Lancet 1990;336:1038.

Kupfer C (editor): *World Blindness and its Prevention,* vol 3, Oxford Univ Press, 1988.

Lim ASM, Jones BR (editors): World's major blinding conditions. Vision 1982;1:1. [Entire issue.]

Minassian DC: Epidemiological methods in prevention of blindness. Eye 1988;2(Suppl):S3.

Minassian DC, Mehra V: 3.8 million blinded by cataract each year; projections from the first epidemiological study of incidence of cataract blindness in India. Br J Ophthalmol 1990;74:341.

Moll AC et al: Prevalence of blindness and low vision of people over 30 years in the Wenchi District, Ghana, in relation to eye care programmes. Br J Ophthalmol 1994;78:275.

Phillips CI et al: Blindness in schoolchildren: Importance of heredity, congenital cataract, and prematurity. Br J Ophthalmol 1987;71:578.

The Prevention of Blindness: Report of a WHO Study Group. World Health Organization Technical Report Series 518, 1973. [Entire issue.]

Robinson GC, Jan JE: Acquired ocular visual impairment in children 1960–1989. Am J Dis Child 1993;147:325.

Roy FH: World blindness: Definition, incidence and major treatable causes. Ann Ophthalmol 1974;6:1049.

Smith RJH: Blindness in two worlds. (Editorial.) Br J Ophthalmol 1989;73:81.

Sommer A: *Nutritional Blindness: Xerophthalmia and Keratomalacia.* Oxford Univ Press, 1982.

Sommer A: Organizing to prevent third world blindness. (Editorial.) Am J Ophthalmol 1989;107:544.

Sommer A et al: Racial differences in the cause-specific prevalence of blindness in East Baltimore. N Engl J Med 1991;325:1412.

Strategies for the Prevention of Blindness in National Programmes: A Primary Health Care Approach. World Health Organization, 1984.

Taylor HR, Sommer A: Cataract surgery: A global perspective. (Editorial.) Arch Ophthalmol 1990;108:797.

Taylor HR et al: Hygiene factors and increased risk of trachoma in central Tanzania. Arch Ophthalmol 1989;107:1821.

Taylor HR et al: Increase in mortality associated with blindness in rural Africa. Bull WHO 1991;69:335.

Taylor HR et al: Treatment of onchocerciasis: The ocular effects of ivermectin and diethylcarbamazine. Arch Ophthalmol 1986;104:863.

Lasers in Ophthalmology

24

James B. Wise, MD

Ophthalmology was the first medical specialty to utilize laser energy in patient treatment, and it still accounts for more laser operations than any other specialty. The transparency of the optical media allows laser light to be focused upon the intraocular structures without the need for endoscopy. Laser therapy has made the treatment of a number of serious ocular diseases much safer and more effective. Because lasers can cause harm as well as benefit, ocular laser surgery should be performed only by ophthalmologists with laser experience. Low-energy scanning laser systems are useful for diagnostic imaging of ocular structures and for measuring blood flow by interferometry.

OCULAR LASER SYSTEMS

A laser consists of a transparent crystal rod (solid-state laser) or a gas- or liquid-filled cavity (gas or fluid laser) constructed with a fully reflective mirror at one end and a partially reflective mirror at the other. Surrounding the rod or cavity is an optical or electrical source of energy that will raise the energy level of the atoms within the rod or cavity to a high and unstable level, a process known as population inversion. When the excited atoms spontaneously decay back to a lower energy level, their excess energy is released in the form of light. This light can be emitted in any direction. In the laser cavity, however, light emitted in the long axis of the cavity can bounce back and forth between the mirrors, setting up a standing wave that stimulates the remaining excited atoms to release their energy into the standing wave, producing an intense beam of light which exits the cavity through the partially reflective mirror (Figure 24–1). The light beam produced is all of the same wavelength (monochromatic), with all of the light waves in phase with each other (coherent). The light waves follow very closely parallel courses, with almost no tendency to spread out. These unique properties of laser light allow the beam to be focused down to extremely small spots, resulting in very high-energy densities. In some lasers, such as the Q-switched Nd:YAG laser, all the light energy is released in a few nanoseconds to produce temperatures in excess of 10,000 °K at the point of focus.

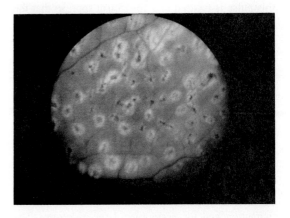

Figure 24–1. Argon laser burn scars in retina after destruction of diabetic retinopathy.

MECHANISMS OF LASER EFFECTS

Photocoagulation

The principal lasers used in ophthalmic therapy are the thermal lasers, which depend upon absorption of the laser light by tissue pigments. The absorbed light is converted into heat, thus raising the target tissue temperature enough to coagulate and denature the cellular components. These lasers are used for retinal photocoagulation, for treatment of diabetic retinopathy and sealing of retinal holes, and for photocoagulation of the trabecular meshwork, iris, and ciliary body in the treatment of glaucoma. They can be used at higher energy levels to evaporate tissue, as in laser iridotomy. These laser photocoagulators operate in continuous mode or very rapidly pulsed (thermal) mode. The blue-green argon laser is the workhorse of this class. Others include the krypton red laser; the solid-state diode laser, producing a near infrared wavelength; the tunable dye laser, producing wavelengths from green to red; the frequency-doubled Nd:YAG laser, producing green light; and the thermal Nd:YAG laser, producing infrared light. Because laser light is monochromatic, selective absorption into specific tissues by specific wavelengths is possible, while adjacent tissues are spared. An example is the yellow wavelength of the tunable dye laser, which can be used to treat neovascularization near the macula, because the yellow light is absorbed by hemoglobin but not by the yellow xanthophyll pigment of the macula. Absorption of laser light by specific tissues can be enhanced by intravenous injection of absorbing dyes such as fluorescein or indocyanine green.

Photodisruption

Photodisruption lasers release a giant pulse of energy with a pulse duration of a few nanoseconds. When this pulse is focused to a 15–25 μm spot, so that the nearly instantaneous light pulse exceeds a critical level of energy density, "optical breakdown" occurs in which the temperature rises so high (about 10,000 °K) that electrons are stripped from atoms, resulting in a physical state known as a plasma. This plasma expands with momentary pressures as high as 10 kilobars (150,000 psi), producing a cutting effect on the ocular tissues. Because the initial plasma size is so small, it has little total energy and produces little effect away from the point of focus. Though a significant shock wave is produced, studies on polyethylene membranes indicate that direct contact with the plasma is required for cutting tissue. Photodisruptors are used principally for perforating cloudy posterior capsules after cataract extraction and for performing laser iridotomy. The principal laser of this class is the Q-switched neodymium:YAG laser.

Photo-evaporation

The prototype of this class is the carbon dioxide laser, which produces a long-wavelength infrared heat beam. The beam is absorbed by water and therefore will not enter the interior of the eye. This laser can evaporate away surface lesions such as lid tumors and can be used for bloodless incisions in skin or sclera, but it causes too much scarring to be useful for ocular plastic surgery. The carbon dioxide laser beam can also be delivered through probes for contact photoincision and photocoagulation within the eye. The holmium:YAG and erbium:YAG lasers produce shorter-wavelength infrared, which is absorbed within a few micrometers by water. They cut tissues with little coagulation.

Photodecomposition

Photodecomposition lasers produce very short wavelength ultraviolet light that interacts with the chemical bonds of biologic materials, breaking the bonds and converting biologic polymers into small molecules that diffuse away. These lasers collectively are called excimer ("excited dimer") lasers because the cavity contains two gases, such as argon and fluorine, that react into unstable molecules which then emit the laser light. At present restricted by the government to experimental protocols in the USA but widely used in Europe and Asia, they can precisely recontour the corneal surface by computer-controlled ablation of successive thin layers of the cornea, correcting refractive errors such as myopia and astigmatism. Photodecomposition lasers can also remove shallow corneal opacities resulting from injuries or dystrophies.

THERAPEUTIC APPLICATIONS OF LASERS

DIABETIC RETINOPATHY

Many patients with long-term diabetes mellitus will gradually develop diffuse obliteration of the retinal microcirculation, especially of the capillaries, resulting in generalized retinal ischemia. This ischemic state leads to retinal and iridal neovascularization, at least partly mediated by diffusible vasoproliferative factors released from the ischemic retina into the ocular fluids. Untreated retinal neovascularization leads to vitreous hemorrhages and traction retinal detachment. Iris neovascularization produces neovascular glaucoma. In nonproliferative diabetic retinopathy, vision is impaired by macular edema and exudates resulting from breakdown of the inner blood-retinal barriers at the level of the retinal capillary endothelium. (The clinical features of diabetic retinopathy are more fully discussed in Chapter 10.)

Laser treatment for diabetic retinopathy is performed in two ways. Focal and diffuse (grid pattern) photocoagulation of the macula reestablishes the competence of the inner blood-retinal barrier with a consequent reduction in edema and exudates. Burns 50–100 μm in diameter are applied, avoiding the foveal avascular zone, which is approximately 300 μm in diameter. The areas to be treated are identified by fluorescein angiography (areas of discrete or diffuse fluorescein leakage, and areas of capillary nonperfusion associated with retinal thickening) or by clinical examination (zones of retinal thickening). Focal treatment of neovascularization is not sufficient by itself because of recurrence and inability to treat elevated areas. Retinal or iris neovascularization is treated by panretinal photocoagulation (PRP). This consists of peppering the entire retina, except for the area within the temporal vascular arcades, with 500 μm diameter burns placed one or two burn widths apart. PRP uses 1000–2000 burns, usually delivered over two to four sessions, with the sessions given about 2 weeks apart. Treatment is staged to reduce the incidence of uveitis, macular edema, exudative retinal detachment, and even shallowing of the anterior chamber with secondary angle closure. In the presence of significant macular edema, focal macular photocoagulation should be performed prior to or together with the PRP to avoid exacerbation of the edema.

PRP causes the neovascular areas to wither away so that the retinopathy becomes inactive and new vessels cease to appear. While the exact mechanism of action is unproved, reduction in volume of ischemic tissue and reduced production of the diffusible vasostimulative substances are thought to be important. Direct treatment of neovascularization is not necessary. PRP is effective even when performed with the krypton red or diode red lasers, which do not directly close vessels because of poor absorption of the red light by hemoglobin.

PRP properly used is highly effective in producing regression of neovascularization, but associated fibrosis will remain and can continue to produce retinal traction. Vitreous hemorrhage can prevent retinal laser treatment. Therefore, PRP should be used as soon as high-risk characteristics are noted and before irreversible changes have occurred. High-risk characteristics are disk neovascularization and any neovascularization at other retinal sites associated with vitreous hemorrhage. The value of earlier treatment—at the time of preproliferative retinopathy—is being investigated. Laser therapy for nonproliferative retinopathy is most effective when given before visual loss has occurred. Because timely laser therapy is so effective in preventing blindness in diabetes, any diabetic with retinopathy greater than scattered microaneurysms should be seen on a regular basis by an ophthalmologist with laser experience.

CENTRAL RETINAL VEIN THROMBOSIS

Thrombosis involving the central retinal vein produces the classic fundus appearance of disk swelling, marked venous dilation, and almost confluent retinal hemorrhages (see Chapter 10). While these changes can progress to retinal neovascularization, vitreous hemorrhage, and fibrosis, a more common complication is the development of neovascular glaucoma. If severe retinal ischemia is present on fluorescein angiography, there is a 60% chance of this complication. In neovascular glaucoma, substances produced by the ischemic retina diffuse forward and stimulate formation of a fibrovascular membrane that grows across the iris surface and covers the trabecular meshwork, resulting in glaucoma characterized by very high pressures, pain, and marked resistance to medical and surgical therapy, so that enucleation of the blind and painful eye may be required. Panretinal photocoagulation as described above for treatment of proliferative diabetic retinopathy—preferably with the krypton red or diode red laser to avoid preretinal fibrosis caused by heat absorption in the hemorrhages—can greatly reduce the incidence of neovascular glaucoma in ischemic central retinal vein thrombosis.

Once neovascular glaucoma is present, adequate panretinal photocoagulation will usually cause regression of anterior segment neovascularization, allowing the glaucoma to be controlled medically or by filtering surgery. Unfortunately, established neovascular glaucoma is often associated with corneal edema, miosis, or hyphema, so that laser therapy cannot be performed and only cyclodestructive procedures or enucleation can be used. Because established neovascular glaucoma is so resistant to treatment, prophylactic krypton red laser photocoagulation is advised in all cases of ischemic central retinal vein thrombosis. A relative afferent pupillary defect, vision of 20/200 or less, and multiple retinal cotton wool spots are highly suggestive of ischemia severe enough to warrant prophylactic panretinal photocoagulation. Electroretinography and fluorescein angiography provide further evidence when needed.

BRANCH RETINAL VEIN THROMBOSIS

This condition varies from tiny localized areas of venous congestion and hemorrhage to hemiretinal involvement from thrombosis of the superior or inferior division of the central retinal vein. The principal complications are chronic macular edema (with or without exudates) and retinal neovascularization followed by vitreous hemorrhage and traction retinal detachment. Prophylactic scatter photocoagulation of the ischemic retina, when demonstrated by fluorescein angiography to exceed five disk diameters in extent, reduces the chance of neovascularization. If significant retinal neovascularization does develop, prompt laser treatment should be performed before vitreous hemorrhage occurs and blocks access of the laser light to the bleeding vessels. Once again, krypton red laser is preferable in the presence of retinal hemorrhages. Focal and grid-pattern argon laser photocoagulation are used to treat macular edema and exudates by obliteration of areas of retinal leakage as demonstrated by fluorescein angiography.

RETINAL TEARS

When a peripheral retinal tear occurs—usually due to senile vitreous degeneration causing vitreous traction—the patient often notices the sudden appearance of floaters. The tear can cause retinal detachment, but if detected prior to the accumulation of subretinal fluid it can be walled off by applying a double ring of laser burns around it to cause adhesion of the adjacent attached retina to the pigment epithelium. Once retinal detachment has occurred, surgery is required. Prompt retinal examination through a dilated pupil is therefore indicated in any eye with floaters of sudden onset.

MACULAR DEGENERATION
& RELATED DISEASES

Bruch's membrane forms a barrier layer between the pigment epithelium and the choriocapillaris, which is the capillary layer of the choroid. If Bruch's membrane deteriorates or is damaged, capillary nets can grow through the break beneath the pigment epithelium, at first causing exudative pigment epithelial detachment with distortion and edema of the overlying retina and then later causing hemorrhage and fibrosis with destruction of the retinal function in that area. The macular retina is particularly likely to develop Bruch's membrane breaks and neovascularization, though these changes can occur anywhere in the fundus. The most frequent cause is age-related macular degeneration, which begins as asymptomatic yellowish deposits (drusen) in the macular area. As the years advance, pigment epithelial atrophy and clumping are seen, and finally Bruch's membrane breaks appear, leading to fluid leaks, neovascularization, fibrosis, and loss of central vision. This condition is the leading cause of legal blindness in the older population. Bruch's membrane breaks and neovascular nets can occur at sites of old chorioretinitis from childhood histoplasmosis, toxoplasmosis, and various other inflammations. They can develop from traumatic choroidal ruptures even in children, and can occur in a host of hereditary diseases involving the retina. If sub-pigment epithelial neovascular nets are located away from the central foveal area, they can be destroyed by careful laser photocoagulation to preserve central vision. The yellow macular pigment (xanthophyll) avidly absorbs blue light, weakly absorbs green light, and does not absorb yellow, orange, or red light. Hemoglobin avidly absorbs blue, green, yellow, and orange light but very weakly absorbs red light. Melanin absorbs all visible wavelengths. Selective absorption of laser energy is therefore possible. If the neovascular net has melanin pigment in it or is bleeding, then krypton red laser light allows deep penetration to the choriocapillaris without hemoglobin or xanthophyll absorption. If the net does not have much melanin and has not bled, then argon green or dye laser yellow or orange will be absorbed by hemoglobin to coagulate the net, but the scattered light will not be absorbed by xanthophyll. The entire neovascular net must be heavily treated for control. Unfortunately, in many cases the net is already under the fovea at the time of diagnosis, or bleeding is already so extensive that laser treatment is not possible. Early diagnosis is therefore of utmost importance in this group of diseases, and patients at risk must diligently look for and report the small blurs and distortions of vision which are the first signs of neovascular growth. Fluorescein angiography can then be used to demonstrate the retinal circulation, including areas of neovascularization and abnormal vascular permeability. Laser treatment of subfoveal neovascular membranes produces an immediate reduction in central acuity but may lead to a better long-term outcome than can be expected without treatment. Intravenous indocyanine green localizes in the neovascular membranes and selectively absorbs 805-nm diode laser light, allowing more certain destruction of the membranes with perhaps less foveal damage.

GLAUCOMA

Treatment of open-angle glaucoma, angle-closure glaucoma, and glaucoma resistant to surgery has been radically altered by availability of effective laser techniques.

Angle-Closure Glaucoma

In primary angle-closure glaucoma, aqueous flow through the pupil is blocked by contact of the lens with the posterior surface of the iris. The resulting pressure in the posterior chamber forces the peripheral iris forward into contact with the trabecular meshwork, blocking outflow and increasing intraocular pressure. While the classic, dramatic acute glaucoma attack is usually considered the prototype of angle-closure glaucoma, acute attacks are actually very rare. Creeping or subacute angle-closure glaucoma is far more common, especially in darkly pigmented eyes of Southeast Asians, and can occur with a normal central anterior chamber depth. Angle closure can be determined only by examining the angle, which is usually done by slitlamp gonioscopy through a gonioscopy contact lens containing a mirror.

Surgical iridectomy was the standard treatment for angle-closure glaucoma for decades but carried the risks of hemorrhage, infection, anesthetic accidents, and even sympathetic ophthalmia. Studies of ruby laser iridotomy began in animals in 1964, but not until 1975 was an effective argon laser technique developed for human eyes. In 1979, laser iridotomy was made more effective by the Abraham contact lens, whose 66-diopter focusing button increased iris energy density. The more recent Wise iridotomy-sphincterotomy lens has a 103-diopter button that gives the highest energy density possible with a practical contact lens. With these high-energy densities, laser iridotomy is nearly 100% successful with either the argon laser or the Q-switched Nd:YAG laser, failing only when the cornea is so cloudy that the laser cannot be focused upon the iris. With the argon laser, the beam is focused through the Wise lens upon the far peripheral iris fibers, which are cut in a line parallel to the limbus by multiple shots at 0.01- or 0.02-second exposures and energy levels of 1–2 W. With the Nd:YAG laser, iridotomy can be done through the Wise lens by a high-power single-point method using about 8 mJ per shot in a single shot or a two- or three-shot burst (Figure 24–2), or it can be done by cutting the far peripheral iris fibers in a line parallel to the limbus with multiple shots at 1.0–1.5 mJ. The argon laser is preferable for dark brown, thick irides,

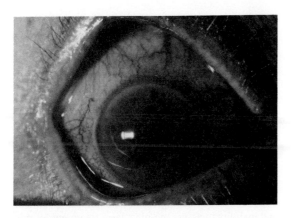

Figure 24–2. Laser iridotomy for angle closure glaucoma.

which tend to bleed with the Nd:YAG laser, while light blue irides do not absorb argon laser energy well and are more easily perforated with the Nd:YAG laser. If both lasers are available, a very efficient method for thick brown irides is to cut the thick stroma with the argon laser and then remove strands and pigment with a few low-power Nd:YAG laser bursts. Because of its safety, laser iridotomy should be done not only for established angle-closure glaucoma but whenever progressive pupillary block is occurring, before irreversible damage from angle closure has occurred.

Primary Open-Angle Glaucoma

This is the most common type of glaucoma in Western countries and is characterized by painless, gradual reduction in trabecular meshwork function with decreasing outflow, increasing intraocular pressure, progressive cupping of the optic nerve, and insidious loss of visual field, leading ultimately to blindness. Prior to 1979, treatment consisted of medical therapy, followed by fistulizing surgery if necessary. At that time, surgery had a significant risk of complications, and so patients were subjected to very heavy medical therapy and often developed severe glaucomatous field loss before the risks of surgery were accepted. In 1979, Wise and Witter published a new concept of laser glaucoma therapy—laser trabeculoplasty—which consists of spacing 100 or more nonperforating argon laser burns 360 degrees around the trabecular meshwork, to shrink the collagen in the tissues of the trabecular ring, reducing the circumference and therefore the diameter of the trabecular ring, pulling the trabecular layers apart with reopening of the intertrabecular spaces and of Schlemm's canal. Growth of new trabecular cells may also occur. Trabeculoplasty increases outflow and has no influence upon aqueous secretion. Though in some eyes the abnormal meshwork can continue to deteriorate, with late failure requiring filtration surgery, 10-year control of glaucoma has been reported, and this author has three eyes controlled for 18 years. Most eyes continue to require some medical therapy. The value of

trabeculoplasty lies in reducing medical therapy and in postponing or avoiding the risks of filtration surgery. The only significant side effects are a rise in pressure for 1–4 hours in about one-third of eyes (preventable by apraclonidine drops) and a rise in pressure for 1–3 weeks in about 4% of treated eyes. To reduce the severity of these pressure rises, many laser surgeons do trabeculoplasty in 180 degrees of the trabecular meshwork, treating the other 180 degrees later if necessary. Trabeculoplasty with other laser wavelengths, such as krypton red, diode infrared, and cw.Nd:YAG (cw = "continuous wave") infrared, is also effective. In a large randomized trial, primary argon laser trabeculoplasty plus medical therapy (if needed) gave better control of intraocular pressure than did primary medical therapy alone.

Cyclophotocoagulation

Glaucoma refractory to the usual surgeries can often be controlled by direct destruction of the ciliary processes, usually by cryosurgery. Cyclophotocoagulation through intact conjunctiva and sclera was originated by Beckman, using a high-energy ruby laser, but is currently performed by air or contact delivery with the thermal-mode Nd:YAG laser and by contact delivery with the diode laser. Good results have been reported, but multiple treatments may be required. The side effects, such as pain, inflammation, and reduction of vision, are similar to cryosurgery but are significantly less severe. By using a fiberoptic probe passed through the pars plana during vitrectomy, argon laser cyclophotocoagulation gave good results in one series.

Laser Suture Lysis

Trabeculectomy is currently the procedure of choice for glaucoma drainage surgery (see Chapter 11) because the partial-thickness scleral flap reduces the incidence of complications caused by early postoperative hypotony. In order to increase the degree of drainage and perhaps achieve greater long-term reduction in intraocular pressure similar to that obtained with the older full-thickness drainage procedures, laser lysis of the scleral flap sutures can be carried out 7–14 days after standard trabeculectomy and 3–8 weeks after trabeculectomy augmented by antifibrotic therapy with mitomycin. The sutures are cut by focusing short laser pulses upon them through the transparent conjunctiva, aided by compressing the overlying tissues with the Hoskins suture lens. The argon laser may be used, but the krypton red or diode infrared lasers are preferred to avoid flap perforation by hemoglobin absorption of argon blue laser wavelengths.

LASER PHOTOMYDRIASIS
& LASER SPHINCTEROTOMY

For a variety of reasons, but most frequently because of long-term miotic therapy, the pupil can become fixed at a very small size, reducing vision and interfering with pupillary dilation for retinal examination or treatment. Multiple laser burns of 200 μm diameter placed in a ring outside the pupil will produce temporary enlargement, but marked uveitis and intraocular pressure rises can occur, and the dilating effect disappears over time. A better method is argon laser sphincterotomy, in which one or more linear cuts across the iris sphincter are made by focusing the argon laser through the Wise iridotomy-sphincterotomy lens and using numerous shots at 0.01-second exposure and about 1 W energy. This produces permanent enlargement of the pupil with less irritation. Energy levels must be kept low to avoid lens burns. The Nd:YAG laser at very low energy levels can be used to cut persistent nonpigmented bridging strands.

POSTERIOR CAPSULOTOMY AFTER CATARACT SURGERY

Modern cataract surgery uses extracapsular extraction or phacoemulsification followed by posterior chamber intraocular lens implantation (see Chapter 8). If the residual posterior capsule later opacifies, vision can be restored by focusing Q-switched Nd:YAG laser pulses just posterior to the capsule to produce a central capsulotomy (thus avoiding further intraocular surgery). Careful focus through a condensing contact lens is necessary to avoid damage to the intraocular lens. A small increase in the risk of retinal holes and retinal detachment is present after capsulotomy. At the present time opacification of the capsule is not preventable, so that some eyes will require capsulotomy for useful vision. However, the risk of retinal detachment from delaying capsulotomy until vision is impaired is almost certainly less than the risk from primary capsulotomy during the cataract surgery, which also carries the additional risks of implant lens malposition and vitreous complications.

CUTTING VITREOUS BANDS & OPACITIES

Incomplete clearance of vitreous from the anterior chamber during the management of vitreous loss secondary to trauma or surgery may result in pupillary distortion, chronic uveitis, and cystoid macular edema. These bands can be cut with the Q-switched Nd:YAG laser, either directly though the cornea by focusing on the band through a condensing contact lens such as the Wise lens, or in the angle by focusing through the mirror of a condensing goniolens such as the Trokel lens or the Lasag CGA lens. Multiple shots at minimal optical breakdown levels should be used to minimize concussion to cornea and iris. Eyes with chronic cystoid

macular edema have improved after cutting of vitreocorneal bands.

Localized opacities and bands in the anterior vitreous can be cut with the Nd:YAG laser to clear the visual axis or reduce traction upon the retina. Most of the time, however, the vitreous abnormalities are widespread, and surgical vitrectomy is required.

VAPORIZATION OF LID TUMORS

The carbon dioxide laser has been used to bloodlessly remove both benign and malignant lid tumors. However, because of scarring, lack of a histologic specimen, and inability to assess margins, laser treatment for this purpose appears inferior to other methods in most cases.

LASER SCLEROSTOMY

Hoping to avoid the surgical and anesthetic hazards of filtering surgery for glaucoma, numerous investigators have attempted to achieve scleral perforation by laser light energy. In 1969, L'Esperance injected colloidal carbon (India ink) into the peripheral cornea and then perforated that area by directing the argon laser across the anterior chamber with a mirrored goniolens. None of the attempts at gonioscopic sclerostomy have produced adequate openings in humans.

L'Esperance and Beckman used the carbon dioxide laser to bloodlessly perforate sclera and iris during filtering surgery for neovascular glaucoma. Gaasterland, among others, has perforated the sclera in animals with excimer, visible, and infrared laser energy by contact intraocular delivery through optical fibers passed across the anterior chamber or by contact extraocular delivery by passing the fibers beneath the conjunctiva. Iwach et al have performed human sclerostomy with the holmium:YAG laser. With all of these methods, a surgical or laser iridectomy is often necessary to prevent iris from occluding the sclerostomy. Because of frequent fistula closure and the complications caused by the immediate hypotony, none of these methods have so far produced results equal to standard surgical trabeculectomy.

REFRACTIVE SURGERY

The excimer lasers, particularly the 193-nm wavelength argon fluoride laser, can evaporate tissue very cleanly with almost no damage to cells adjacent to or under the cut. By using multiple pulses and progressively changing spot size to evaporate successive thin layers of the cornea, computer-controlled recontouring of the cornea can precisely and apparently permanently correct moderate myopic and astigmatic refractive errors. Initial difficulties with superficial corneal haze appear to have been overcome. High hyperopic and high myopic (over 6 diopters) errors do not respond as well. Many thousands of eyes have been successfully treated for myopia in Europe and in Asia, but so far these instruments remain under government restriction to investigational protocols in the USA. Where available, refractive surgery with the excimer laser has largely replaced surgical radial keratotomy, which is less predictable and which has complications, such as deep scarring, ocular perforation, intraocular infection, and late hyperopic shift, which do not occur with the laser.

LASER DIAGNOSTIC IMAGING

Confocal imaging is a video method that uses a rapidly scanning tiny laser spot, whose reflected light is imaged through a pinhole upon a detector, thus suppressing all reflections except those from the focal plane. By scanning at multiple levels and then combining the images by computer processing, precise and reproducible three-dimensional images of ocular structures can be produced (Figure 24–3). The principal use of these instruments is to evaluate and follow glau-

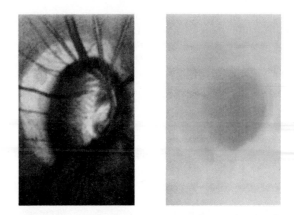

Figure 24–3. *Left:* Scanning laser ophthalmoscope image of disk with glaucomatous damage. *Right:* Computed contour map of same disk. Darker areas are depressed, as in the enlarged cup.

coma-induced changes in the optic nerve head, but other uses include macular, lens, and corneal imaging. Laser interferometry is used to measure blood flow in the ciliary body and retinal blood vessels.

REFERENCES

The Branch Vein Occlusion Study Group: Argon laser scatter photocoagulation for prevention of neovascularization and vitreous hemorrhage in branch vein occlusion: A randomized clinical trial. Arch Ophthalmol 1982;104:34.

Cioffi BA, Rovin AL, Eastman RD: Confocal laser scanning ophthalmoscope: Reproducibility of optic nerve head topographic measurements with the confocal scanning laser ophthalmoscope. Ophthalmology 1993;100:57.

Gaasterland DE et al: Ab interno and ab externo filtering operation by laser contact surgery. Ophthalmic Surg 1987;18:254.

Gartry D, Kerr Muir M, Marshall J: Excimer laser treatment of corneal surface pathology: A laboratory and clinical study. Br J Ophthalmol 1991;75:258.

Glaucoma Laser Trial Research Group: The glaucoma laser trial (GLT). 2. Results of argon laser trabeculoplasty versus topical medications. Ophthalmology 1990;97:1403.

Goldberg MF, Jampol LM: Knowledge of diabetic retinopathy before and 18 years after the Airlie House Symposium on Treatment of Diabetic Retinopathy. Ophthalmology 1988;94:741.

Iwach AG et al: Update of the subconjunctival THC:YAG (holmium) laser sclerostomy ab externo clinical trial: 30-month report. Ophthalmic Surg 1994;25:13.

Klapper RM et al: Transscleral neodymium:YAG thermal cyclophotocoagulation in refractory glaucoma. Ophthalmology 1988;95:719.

L'Esperance FA Jr: Laser trabeculosclerostomy. In: *Ophthalmic Lasers: Photocoagulation, Photoradiation, and Surgery,* 2nd ed. Mosby, 1983.

Macular Photocoagulation Study Group: Argon laser photocoagulation for neovascular maculopathy: Five-year results from randomized clinical trials. Arch Ophthalmol 1991;109:1109.

Macular Photocoagulation Study Group: Laser photocoagulation of subfoveal neovascular lesions in age-related macular degeneration: Results of a randomized clinical trial. Arch Ophthalmol 1991;109:1220.

Magargal LE et al: Neovascular glaucoma following central retinal vein obstruction. Ophthalmology 1981;88:1095.

Michelson G, Groh MJM: Dipivefrin reduces blood flow in the ciliary body of humans. Ophthalmology 1994;101:659.

Patel A et al: Endolaser treatment of the ciliary body for uncontrolled glaucoma. Ophthalmology 1986;93:831.

Reichel E et al: Indocyanine green dye-enhanced diode laser photocoagulation of poorly defined subfoveal choroidal neovascularization. Ophthalmic Surg 1994;25:195.

Seiler T, Wollensack J: Myopic photorefractive keratectomy with the excimer laser. One-year follow-up. Ophthalmology 1991;98:1156.

Tengroth B et al: Excimer laser photrefractive keratectomy for myopia: Clinical results in sighted eyes. Ophthalmology 1993;100:739.

Vogel A et al: Cavitation bubble dynamics and acoustic transient generation in ocular surgery with pulsed neodymium:YAG lasers. Ophthalmology 1986;93:1259.

Wise JB: Iris sphincterotomy, iridotomy, and synechiotomy by linear incision with the argon laser. Ophthalmology 1985;92:641.

Wise JB: Low-energy linear-incision neodymium:YAG laser

iridotomy versus linear-incision argon laser iridotomy. Ophthalmology 1987;94:1531.

Wise JB: Ten year results of laser trabeculoplasty. Does the laser avoid glaucoma surgery or merely defer it? Eye 1987;1:45.

Wise JB, Munnerlyn CR, Erickson PJ: A high-efficiency laser iridotomy-sphincterotomy lens. Am J Ophthalmol 1986;101:546.

Wise JB, Witter SL: Argon laser therapy for open-angle glaucoma. Arch Ophthalmol 1979;97:319.

Appendix I: Visual Standards

INDUSTRIAL VISUAL EVALUATION[*]

The following mathematical calculation of loss of visual efficiency is used for legal and industrial cases, particularly in determination of compensation for injury.[†]

Calculation of total visual efficiency is based on three factors of equal importance: percentage loss of visual acuity, percentage loss of visual field, and percentage loss of coordinated ocular movements. Percentage loss of visual acuity in one eye does not represent the individual's total disability; even a total loss of one eye would not represent a 50% disability if the remaining eye were normal. Many people lead normal lives with one eye.

For evaluation of industrial visual efficiency, therefore, three visual functions are measured and mathematically coordinated: (1) visual acuity, (2) visual field, and (3) ocular motility (diplopia field, binocular field).

Visual Acuity

Distance and near vision are weighted evenly.

For purposes of calculating total visual acuity loss, near visual acuity is equally as important as distance acuity.

Example: If the distance acuity is 20/80 and the subject can read Jaeger 6–

$$\frac{40 + 50}{2} = \frac{45\% \text{ visual acuity loss, or } 55\%}{\text{visual acuity efficiency}}$$

Visual Field

A white test object is used in 8 meridians as diagrammed on p 420. This can be done with a 3-mm ob-

---

[*]Modified and reproduced, with permission, from Arch Ind Health 1955;12:439. For further explanation of the reasons behind the statistics and a legal discussion, see Spaeth EB: Trans Am Acad Ophthalmol Otolaryngol 1957;61:592.
[†]The method described here may differ from government standards for defining reduced vision in assessing eligibility for compensation, which vary from state to state. The State Department of Industrial Relations (or its equivalent) can be contacted for data.

AMA Method of estimation of percentage visual loss (using best correcting spectacle lens)

Distance	
Distance Visual Acuity	% Loss
20/20	0
20/25	5
20/40	15
20/50	25
20/80	40
20/100	50
20/160	70
20/200	80
20/400	90

Near	
Jaeger Test Type	% Loss
1	0
2	0
3	10
6	50
7	60
11	85
14	95

ject at 0.33 m, using a perimeter. A full field represents 100% function. (Illumination should be at least 120 lux.)

Ocular Motility

The extent of diplopia in the various directions of gaze is best determined using a tangent screen at 1 meter. A small test light is used, and diplopia is plotted along the three meridians above the horizontal, 10, 20, and 30 degrees from fixation. Diplopia fields are also plotted on the horizontal meridians and the three meridians below, 10, 20, 30, and 40 degrees from the straight-ahead position. Diplopia within the central 20 degrees represents 100% loss of motility efficiency of one eye, since this condition usually requires patching one eye. If diplopia is not present in the central 20 degrees, loss of ocular motility is calculated from a field diagram showing percentage loss. This value is then subtracted from 100 and expressed as "80% motility efficiency," etc.

The inferior fields are weighted heavily, since this is

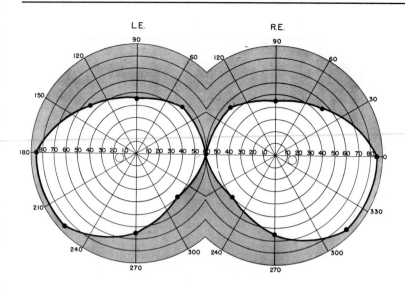

Minimum Legal Visual Field

Minimal Normal Field:

Temporally	85°
Down and temporally	85°
Down	65°
Down and nasally	50°
Nasally	60°
Up and nasally	55°
Up	45°
Up and temporally	55°
Full field	= 500°

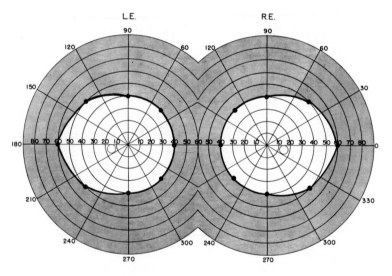

Twenty-eight Percent Loss

Moderate Loss of Field:

Temporally	60°
Down and temporally	50°
Down	40°
Down and nasally	40°
Nasally	40°
Up and nasally	40°
Up	40°
Up and temporally	50°
	360°

$$\frac{360 \times 100}{500} = \text{72\% field remaining, or 28\% field loss}$$

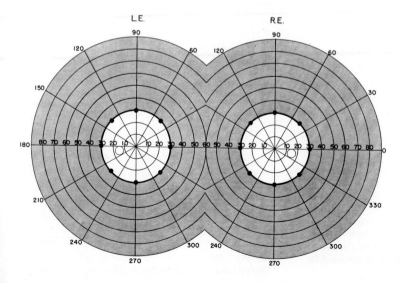

Fifty-two Percent Loss

Severe Loss of Field:

Temporally	30°
Down and temporally	30°
Down	30°
Down and nasally	30°
Nasally	30°
Up and nasally	30°
Up	30°
Up and temporally	30°
	240°

$$\frac{240 \times 100}{500} = \text{48\% field remaining, or 52\% field loss}$$

the position of the eyes in reading. Diplopia away from fixations in other quadrants is considered much less important.

Visual Efficiency (VE) of One Eye

The percentages of efficiency for the three measurements are multiplied to give the total visual efficiency.

Example: Visual acuity = 73%
Visual field = 57%
Motility = 90%

Visual Efficiency (VE) of Two Eyes

The two eyes are calculated separately; the better eye is weighted three times and the poorer eye once. Thus, one blind eye and one normal eye give 75% visual efficiency.

$$\frac{3 \times (\%VE\ better\ eye)\ +\ \%\ VE\ in\ worse\ eye}{4}$$

$$=\ binocular\ VE\ (\%)$$

Example: RE = 90%; LE = 30%.

$$\frac{3 \times 90 + 30}{4} = 75\%\ binocular\ VE$$

VISUAL STANDARDS FOR THE ARMED FORCES*

The visual acuity requirements outlined below apply for all branches of the services. For aircraft pilots, service academy candidates, and some other officer assignments, the requirements are much more strict.

Standards for Disqualification

Any strabismus of 40 prism diopters or more uncorrectable by lenses to less than 40 diopters is disqualifying, as is the presence of diplopia. Any active or progressive disease of the eyes is disqualifying even though the minimal visual standards can be met.

Minimal Standards

Distance visual acuity must correct to one of the following: (1) 20/40 in one eye and 20/70 in the other; (2) 20/30 in one eye and 20/100 in the other; (3) 20/20 in one eye and 20/400 in the other.

---

*Subject to change. Medical Officers for Recruitment at military hospitals or induction centers are supplied with the latest data.

Near visual acuity must correct to at least J-6 in the better eye.

VISUAL STANDARDS FOR DRIVERS' LICENSES IN THE USA

States have varying visual standards for persons applying for drivers' licenses. Failure to meet certain minimum standards may result in suspension of driving privileges or denial of license unless a certificate is obtained from an ophthalmologist or optometrist. In recent years there has been a trend toward higher standards and more frequent visual testing, especially in persons over age 70.

EDUCATIONAL VISUAL STANDARDS IN THE USA

Twelve percent of the students in elementary schools have significant eye difficulty, but no more than one in 1000 requires special educational facilities because of severe visual deficiencies. Although a medical examination is mandatory for schoolchildren in all states because of assessments required by Public Law 94–142, ophthalmologic examinations are seldom included. It has therefore been found necessary to devise procedures by which it will be possible, without a highly specialized staff, to give preliminary screening tests.

The Snellen test is the single most important test. Visual acuity tests may be given by nurses, parents, or trained volunteer teachers. Visual acuity testing of preschool children is far more important than visual acuity testing of school-age children. Testing should be performed as early as possible, preferably no later than 3½–4 years of age.

Even if a child has a significant visual handicap, it is best to try regular school. If the student cannot keep up with regular schoolwork, special "sight-saving" classes are necessary.

Education of Visually Handicapped Children

Education must be provided for partially seeing pupils at all school levels. (For educational purposes, a partially seeing child is one who has a corrected visual acuity of 20/70 or less in the better eye.) Experience indicates that it is best to establish the first class on an elementary school level, since the earlier help is given the better will be the prospect of success. In communities in which the school population is too small to warrant the establishment of more than one class, it may be advisable to give the advantages of the special class to children above the second grade, since much less close eye work is required in the first and second grades and a great deal of material in large, clear print is available for younger children. In general, well-motivated partially sighted children have good learning potential.

Education of Blind Children

Children with poor visual acuity who are unable to take advantage of ordinary visual educational methods are entered either in special schools for the blind, where emphasis is placed upon learning by touch (braille), or (preferably) in integrated schools where facilities are available for special training but where the child is not deprived of all contact with normal persons in the same age group.

Appendix II:
Practical Factors in Illumination

The physical aspects of illumination discussed below are of practical interest to the physician who may be called upon to evaluate the adequacy of light sources in factories, shops, schoolrooms, and homes. Of principal interest is light **intensity,** conventionally measured in lux. One lux is equal to 1 lumen per square meter. Lux can be measured directly with special light meters.

Proper illumination minimizes eyestrain and increases the speed and efficiency of reading. Poor lighting does not cause eye disease but increases eye fatigue. The most common error students make in adjusting their lighting arrangement is to place a desk lamp opposite them on the desk. From this position the light is reflected into the reader's eyes, causing glare. For reading, the best light source is an incandescent or fluorescent lamp coming from above that produces a diffuse light with a minimum of glare and shadows. For writing, the light source should be so adjusted that the shadow of the arm and hand on the page is eliminated.

The most common sources of light are daylight, incandescent light, and fluorescent light. Daylight is an excellent light source but quite variable, and it is difficult to control its intensity. Incandescent lamps simulate daylight and provide a steady, diffuse flow of light. Ordinary fluorescent tubes operate on an alternating current that causes flickering, but it is possible to link two fluorescent tubes in a couple so adjusted that when one is on the up-phase the other is on the down-phase, thus eliminating the flicker.

Illumination Factors Affecting Visibility

A. Intensity: The amount of illumination is directly related to reading efficiency. A reader employing 80 lux reads much more slowly and less efficiently than if a 500-lux source were utilized. The following minimum intensities are recommended (assuming that all undue reflections resulting in glare have been eliminated): reading black print on white paper, 500–650 lux; schoolrooms, 500–650 lux at the desk and 650–800 lux at the blackboard; passageways, halls, and closets, 80 lux; eye charts, 1350–1700 lux; operating room illumination at the point of surgery, 5000 lux.

There is a close relationship between a person's age and the magnification and illumination required. Because they have great powers of accommodation, children can read small print in semidarkness by holding the page close to their eyes. On the other hand, a 48-year-old, slightly farsighted presbyope cannot read under ordinary illumination without magnifying glasses because the power of accommodation has been lost. Using a stronger light bulb or taking the printed material into sunlight makes reading possible in such cases. The presbyope also can improve visual performance by holding printed matter farther away. ("I need longer arms.")

The basic requirement in illumination is to have enough light to see by. Once this is accomplished, the intensity of illumination and the magnification (eyeglasses) can be adjusted to increase the efficiency of visual performance.

The intensity of light on an object is inversely proportionate to the square of the distance from the light source. Therefore, if a reading lamp 0.6 m (2 feet) from the page is moved to a distance of 1.2 m (4 feet), there will be four times less light on the page.

B. Contrast: It is much easier to read black letters on a white page than black letters on a blue page. Eye fatigue is minimized when the surroundings are about 30–40% darker than the object being observed. Thus, in watching a television screen, it is best not to have a completely darkened room.

C. Diffuseness: Shadows and spotlight phenomena should be avoided. However, diffuseness is overdone by manufacturers of indirect lighting fixtures. Indirect "reading lamps" are usually inadequate because of the vastly decreased amount of illumination on the printed page. This can be demonstrated by observing the unwarranted amount of light cast on the ceiling by the average indirect reading lamp.

D. Age of Subject: Illumination requirements and age are closely related, as evidenced by the increased illumination required by the 45-year-old presbyope compared with a teenage daughter. Although it is not recommended, children in the age group from 7 to 16 can read adequately in semi-darkness, whereas the same person 30 years later may be able to read the telephone book only by "taking it to the window." Conversely, many people in the 50- to 65-year range who require full cor-rection for their presbyopia can still read fine print without glasses in sunlight.

In general, illumination should be sufficient to perform the task at hand efficiently and comfortably.

Appendix III:
Rehabilitation of the Visually Handicapped & Special Services Available to the Blind

State Services

The physician should be familiar with the many special services available to the blind. Services vary from state to state but may be illustrated by the diversified programs for the blind conducted by the State of California.[*]

A. Educational Services for the Blind:

1. California School for the Blind—A residential school for general education from kindergarten through the secondary grades; also provides field service, guidance, and assistance to preschool children and students in advanced courses.

2. California State Library—A repository for magazines and books in raised type (Moon and Braille), talking books and machines for use with the books, cassettes and tapes, games adapted for use by the blind, and writing appliances. These materials may be secured directly from the library or by mail (postage-free).

3. Office of Special Education—Coordinates the establishment and operation of special public school programs for visually handicapped children throughout the state. This program enables blind and partially seeing students to live at home and attend school with normal children.

4. Clearinghouse Depository for Handicapped Students—Instructional aids for visually handicapped students in public or nonprofit private schools that comply with the Civil Rights Act. Also serves as a referral service on educational materials for visually handicapped students.

B. Reader Services for Blind Students:
Provides reader services for blind students in high schools, junior colleges, vocational training schools, colleges, and universities.

C. Rehabilitation Services for the Blind:

1. Field rehabilitation services—Counselor-teachers provide services to the blind within their homes or in hospitals and other institutions so that individuals may learn the skills necessary to meet the demands of daily living. Counseling in adjustment to blindness is given to the visually disabled person and the family.

2. Orientation Center for the Blind (State of California Department of Rehabilitation)—Provides intensive orientation and prevocational training, including training in techniques of daily living and travel, physical conditioning, sensory training, instruction in braille, typing, and business methods, and training in hand and machine work, homemaking, and other vocationally useful skills. Limited residence facilities are available.

3. Vocational Rehabilitation Service—Provides, for the adult blind, vocational counseling to help work out suitable employment objectives, supervised vocational training, and job placement. The following services may also be provided if needed for employment and if the applicant is unable to pay for them: medical and surgical treatment, including hospitalization; prosthetic appliances and glasses; maintenance and transportation while undergoing treatment or training; and tools or equipment needed in training, job placement, or self-employment.

4. Business enterprise program—Assists blind persons to establish and operate vending stands, snack bars, and cafeteria or other businesses they may be qualified to operate.

D. Social Welfare Programs for the Blind:

1. Supplemental Security Income (SSI)—Financial assistance paid by state and federal governments to blind persons who, because of loss or impairment of sight, are unable to provide themselves with the necessities of life.

2. Aid to Potentially Self-Supporting Blind—Financial assistance by the county and state to the adult blind who, because of loss or impairment of sight, are unable fully to provide themselves with the necessities of life but who are working on a plan for self-support.

3. Prevention of Blindness—A program designed to prevent blindness or restore vision by providing necessary medical or surgical treatment through MediCal (Medicaid in other states) and other federal, state, and local funds.

4. Counseling and support programs—County Social Service Departments provide help to vi-

---

[*]The services referred to are those provided by public-sponsored agencies for the blind and do not include the many religious organizations, private or voluntary health and welfare agencies, sheltered workshops, and community and recreational facilities.

sually handicapped persons through locating needed services and, when necessary, paying for in-home chore workers.

E. Provisions for Prevention of Blindness, Preventive Medicine Services Branch (California State Department of Health):

1. Prevention of blindness in newborn infants–Enforces legal requirement of (1) silver nitrate or antibiotic prophylaxis for the eyes as a preventive measure against ophthalmia neonatorum; (2) prenatal serologic test of parents for syphilis; and (3) control of excessive use of oxygen in the care of premature infants as a preventive measure against retinopathy of prematurity.

2. Control of communicable diseases apt to cause loss of vision–Requires reporting, isolation, treatment, and control of ophthalmia neonatorum, trachoma, and syphilis.

3. Aid to Physically Handicapped Children (California Children's Service)–Provides for the necessary medical care of children suffering from eye conditions leading to loss of vision if the parents or legal guardians are unable to meet these costs in whole or in part.

F. Guide Dogs for the Blind: The State Board of Guide Dogs for the Blind (California State Department of Consumer Affairs) was established for the purpose of ensuring that guide dogs are trained and that their owners also are trained to use the dogs as guides. Minimum requirements, licensing, and supervision of guide dog schools are functions of the Board.

National Services

The following organizations will provide information and send literature and catalogs upon request:

(1) American Foundation for the Blind, 15 West 16th Street, New York 10011. Provides information on almost all phases of problems of the blind; sells special watches, home appliances, etc, for the blind.

(2) American Printing House for the Blind, 1839 Frankfort Avenue, PO Box 6085, Louisville, Kentucky 40206–0085. Prints and sells braille publications.

(3) Guide Dogs for the Blind, Inc., PO Box 1200, San Rafael, California 94915. Training of guide dogs and training of blind persons to use dogs as guides.

(4) The Hadley School for the Blind, Inc., 700 Elm Street, Winnetka, Illinois 60093. Provides free home-study courses from elementary level into college, vocational and avocational training, braille and other useful skills. Accredited by National Home Study Council, National Accreditation Council, and North Central Association of Colleges and Schools. Affiliate member of National University Extension Association.

(5) Howe Press of Perkins School for the Blind, 175 North Beacon Street, Watertown, Massachusetts 02172. Manufactures and distributes internationally the Perkins Brailler (portable braille typewriter) and braille paper. Also children's stories in a special braille edition, games, mathematical aids, braille maps, music, and braille writing appliances.

(6) Library of Congress. Extensive collection of books and magazines in braille, on disk, and on cassette available free to visually impaired United States citizens. Materials and playback equipment are distributed through a system of network libraries in each state. (Consult local library for specific addresses.) Music materials only are circulated directly from the Library (Division for the Blind and Physically Handicapped, 1291 Taylor Street, NW, Washington, DC 20542).

(7) Rehabilitation Services Administration, Division for the Blind and Visually Handicapped, US Department of Health and Human Services, 330 C Street, SW, Room 3229, Washington, DC 20201. Conducts a nationwide program for the vocational rehabilitation of the blind; provides pamphlets and other information regarding rehabilitation services available to the blind.

(8) Readers Digest. Publishes *Readers Digest* in Braille and on records for the Talking Book; may be secured from the American Printing House for the Blind.

(9) Recording for the Blind, Inc., 545 Fifth Avenue, Suite 204, New York 10017. Records textbooks and educational materials free of charge for blind persons for educational, vocational, or professional use.

(10) The Seeing Eye, Inc., PO Box 375, Morristown, New Jersey 07960. First organization in USA to provide guide dogs for qualified blind persons (1929).

(11) Central Blind Rehabilitation Center (124), Veterans Administration Hospital, Hines, Illinois 60141. Provides rehabilitation program lasting up to 18 weeks for veterans. VA Blind Rehabilitation Centers also located at Veterans Administration Hospitals in West Haven, Connecticut, and Palo Alto, California. Round trip transportation of veteran generally paid by Veterans Administration.

(12) Xavier Society for the Blind, 154 East 23rd Street, New York 10010, provides free periodical and library service in braille, large print, and cassette or open reel tape recordings to any interested blind or partially sighted reader. Catalogs available on request.

REFERENCES

American Foundation for the Blind. 1987-88 Catalog of Publications.

Carroll TJ: *Blindness.* Little, Brown, 1961.

Cholden L: *Psychiatric Aspects of Informing the Patient of Blindness.* American Academy of Ophthalmology and Otolaryngology, Instruction Section, Course No. 221, 1953.

Cholden L: *Some Psychiatric Problems in the Rehabilitation of the Blind.* Bulletin of the Menninger Clinic, Vol. 18, No. 3, May 1954.

Faye EE (editor): *Clinical Low Vision,* 2nd ed. Little, Brown, 1984.

Gloor B, Brückner R: *Rehabilitation of the Visually Disabled and the Blind at Different Ages.* University Park Press, 1980.

Hoehne CW, Cull JG, Hardy RE: *Ophthalmological Considerations in the Rehabilitation of the Blind.* Thomas, 1980. *If Blindness Occurs.* The Seeing Eye, Inc.

Mallinson GG (editor): *Blindness 1977–78.* American Association of Workers for the Blind, Inc., 1978.

Sekuler R, Kline D, Dimukes K: *Aging and Human Visual Function.* Alan R. Liss, 1982.

Stetten D Jr: Coping with blindness. N Engl J Med 1981;305:458.

US Department of Health, Education and Welfare: *Support for Vision Research: Interim Report of the National Advisory Eye Council, 1976.* National Institutes of Health, DHEW Publication No. (NIH) 76–1098.

Glossary of Terms Relating to the Eye*

Accommodation: The adjustment of the eye for seeing at near distances, accomplished by changing the shape of the lens through action of the ciliary muscle, thus focusing a clear image on the retina.

Agnosia: Inability to recognize common objects despite an intact visual apparatus.

Albinism: A hereditary deficiency of melanin pigment in the retinal pigment epithelium, iris, and choroid.

Amaurosis fugax: Transient loss of vision.

Amblyopia: Reduced visual acuity (uncorrectable with lenses) in the absence of detectable anatomic defect in the eye or visual pathways.

Ametropia: See Refractive error.

Amsler grid: A chart with vertical and horizontal lines used for testing the central visual field.

Angiography: A diagnostic test in which the vascular system is examined.

Aniridia: Congenital absence of the iris.

Aniseikonia: A condition in which the image seen by one eye differs in size or shape from that seen by the other.

Anisocoria: Unequal pupillary size.

Anisometropia: Difference in refractive error of the eyes.

Anophthalmos: Absence of a true eyeball.

Anterior chamber: Space filled with aqueous bounded anteriorly by the cornea and posteriorly by the iris.

Aphakia: Absence of the crystalline lens.

Aqueous: Clear, watery fluid that fills the anterior and posterior chambers.

Asthenopia: Eye fatigue from muscular, environmental, or psychologic causes.

Astigmatism: Refractive error that prevents the light rays from coming to a point focus on the retina because of different degrees of refraction in the various meridians of the cornea or crystalline lens.

Axis: The meridian specifying the orientation of a cylindric lens.

Binocular vision: Ability of the eyes to focus on one object and then to fuse two images into one.

Biomicroscope: See Slitlamp.

Bitot's spots: Keratinization of the bulbar conjunctiva near the limbus, resulting in a raised spot—a feature of vitamin A deficiency.

Blepharitis: Inflammation of the eyelids.

Blepharoptosis: Drooping of the eyelid.

Blepharospasm: Involuntary spasm of the lids.

Blind spot: "Blank" area in the visual field, corresponding to the light rays that come to a focus on the optic nerve.

Blindness: In the USA, the usual definition of blindness is corrected visual acuity of 20/200 or less in the better eye, or a visual field of no more than 20 degrees in the better eye.

Botulinum toxin: Neurotoxin A of the bacterium *Clostridium botulinum* used in very small doses to produce temporary paralysis of the extraocular or facial muscles.

Buphthalmos: Large eyeball in infantile glaucoma.

Canal of Schlemm: A circular modified venous structure in the anterior chamber angle that drains aqueous to the aqueous veins.

Canaliculus: Small tear drainage tube in inner aspect of upper and lower lids leading from the punctum to the common canaliculus and then to the tear sac.

Canthotomy: Usually implies lateral canthotomy—cutting of the lateral canthal tendon for the purpose of widening the palpebral fissure.

Canthus: The angle at either end of the eyelid aperture; specified as outer and inner.

Cataract: An opacity of the crystalline lens.

Cataract extraction: Removal of a cataract, either by removal of the lens complete with its capsule (intracapsular cataract extraction), or by removal of the lens contents after opening the capsule (extracapsular cataract extraction).

Chalazion: Granulomatous inflammation of a meibomian gland.

Chemosis: Conjunctival edema.

Choroid: The vascular middle coat between the retina and sclera.

Ciliary body: Portion of the uveal tract between the iris and the choroid. It consists of ciliary processes and the ciliary muscle.

Coloboma: Congenital cleft due to the failure of some portion of the eye or ocular adnexa to complete growth.

Color blindness: Diminished ability to perceive differences in color.

Concave lens: Lens having the power to diverge rays of light; also known as diverging, reducing, negative, or minus lens, denoted by the sign (−), used to correct myopia.

Cones and rods: Two kinds of retinal receptor cells. Cones are concerned with visual acuity and color discrimination; rods, with peripheral vision under decreased illumination.

Conjunctiva: Mucous membrane that lines the posterior aspect of the eyelids and the anterior sclera.

---

*See also Definitions of Strabismus, Chapter 12, and Glossary of Genetic Terms, Chapter 18.

Convergence: The process of directing the visual axes of the eyes to a near point.

Convex lens: Lens having power to converge rays of light and to bring them to a focus; also known as converging, magnifying, or plus lens, denoted by the sign (+), used to correct hyperopia or presbyopia.

Cornea: Transparent portion of the outer coat of the eyeball forming the anterior wall of the anterior chamber.

Corneal contact lenses: Thin lenses that fit directly on the cornea.

Corneal graft (keratoplasty): Operation to restore vision by replacing a section of opaque cornea with transparent cornea, either involving the full thickness of the cornea (penetrating keratoplasty) or only a superficial layer (lamellar keratoplasty). The donor cornea may be from the same human (autograft), another human (homograft), or another species (heterograft).

Cover test: A method of determining the presence and degree of phoria or tropia by covering one eye with an opaque object, thus eliminating fusion.

Cross cylinder: A specialized spherocylindrical lens used to measure astigmatism.

Crystalline lens: A transparent biconvex structure suspended in the eyeball between the aqueous and the vitreous. Its function is to bring rays of light to a focus on the retina. Accommodation is produced by variations in the magnitude of this effect. (Now usually called simply the lens.)

Cyclodestructive procedures: Surgical techniques to reduce aqueous production by destroying portions of the ciliary body in the treatment of intractable glaucoma, using cryotherapy (cyclocryotherapy), lasers (cyclophotocoagulation), ultrasound, or diathermy.

Cycloplegic: A drug that temporarily puts the ciliary muscle at rest, paralyzing accommodation.

Cylindrical lens: A segment of a cylinder the refractive power of which varies in different meridians, used to correct astigmatism.

Dacryocystitis: Infection of the lacrimal sac.

Dacryocystorhinostomy: A procedure by which a communication is made between the nasolacrimal duct and the nasal cavity to relieve an obstruction in the nasolacrimal duct, or sac.

Dark adaptation: The ability to adjust to decreased illumination.

Diopter: Unit of measurement of refractive power of lenses.

Diplopia: Seeing one object as two.

Ectropion: Turning out of the eyelid.

Emmetropia: Absence of refractive error.

Endolaser: Application of laser from a probe inserted into the globe.

Endophthalmitis: Extensive intraocular infection.

Enophthalmos: Abnormal retrodisplacement of the eyeball.

Entropion: A turning inward of the eyelid.

Enucleation: Complete surgical removal of the eyeball.

Epicanthus: Congenital skin fold that overlies the inner canthus.

Epiphora: Tearing.

Esophoria: A tendency of the eyes to turn inward.

Esotropia: A manifest inward deviation of the eyes.

Evisceration: Removal of the contents of the eyeball.

"E" test: A system of testing visual acuity in illiterates, particularly preschool children.

Exenteration: Removal of the entire contents of the orbit, including the eyeball and lids.

Exophoria: A tendency of the eyes to turn outward.

Exophthalmos: Abnormal protrusion of the eyeball.

Exotropia: A manifest outward deviation of the eyes.

Far point: The point at which the eye is focused when accommodation is completely relaxed.

Farsightedness: See Hyperopia.

Field of vision: The entire area that can be seen without shifting the gaze.

Floaters: Moving images in the visual field due to vitreous opacities.

Focus: A point to which rays of light are brought together to form an image; focal distance is the distance between a lens and its focal point.

Fornix: The junction of the palpebral and bulbar conjunctiva.

Fovea: Depression in the macula adapted for most acute vision.

Fundus: The posterior portion of the eye visible through an ophthalmoscope.

Fusion: Coordinating the images received by the two eyes into one image.

Glaucoma: Disease characterized by abnormally increased intraocular pressure, optic atrophy, and loss of visual field.

Gonioscopy: A technique of examining the anterior chamber angle, utilizing a corneal contact lens, magnifying device, and light source.

Hemianopia: Blindness in one-half the field of vision of one or both eyes.

Heterophoria (phoria): A tendency of the eyes to deviate.

Heterotropia: See Strabismus.

Hippus: Exaggerated spontaneous rhythmic movements of the iris.

Hordeolum, external (sty): Infection of the glands of Moll or Zeis.

Hordeolum, internal: Meibomian gland infection.

Hyperopia, hypermetropia (farsightedness): A refractive error in which the focus of light rays from a distant object is behind the retina.

Hyperphoria: A tendency of the eyes to deviate upward.

Hypertropia: A manifest upward deviation of one eye in relation to the other.

Hyphema: Blood in the anterior chamber.

Hypopyon: Pus in the anterior chamber.

Hypotony: Abnormally soft eye from any cause.

Injection: Congestion of blood vessels.

Iris: Colored, annular membrane, suspended behind the cornea and immediately in front of the lens.

Ishihara color plates: A test for color vision based on the ability to trace patterns in a series of multicolored charts.

Isopter: An object for testing visual fields. Isopters can be of different colors and sizes and are used to differentiate relative visual field defects from absolute defects.

Jaeger test: A test for near vision using lines of various sizes of type.

Keratic precipitate (KP): Accumulation of inflammatory cells on the posterior cornea in uveitis.

Keratitis: Inflammation of the cornea.

Keratoconus: Cone-shaped deformity of the cornea.

Keratomalacia: Corneal softening, usually associated with avitaminosis A.

Keratometer: An instrument for measuring the curvature of the cornea, used in fitting contact lenses.

Keratopathy, bullous: Swelling of the cornea with painful blisters in the epithelium due to excessive corneal hydration.

Keratoplasty: See Corneal graft.

Keratoprosthesis: Plastic implant surgically placed in an opaque cornea to achieve an area of optical clarity.

Keratotomy: An incision in the cornea. Radial keratotomy is a procedure in which radial incisions are made in the cornea to correct myopia.

Koeppe nodule: Accumulation of inflammatory cells on the iris in uveitis.

Lacrimal sac: The dilated area at the junction of the nasolacrimal duct and the canaliculi.

Lens: A refractive medium having one or both surfaces curved. (See also Crystalline lens.)

Limbus: Junction of the cornea and sclera.

Macula lutea: The small avascular area of the retina surrounding the fovea, containing yellow xanthophyll pigment.

Maddox rod: A red lens composed of parallel series of strong cylinders through which a point of light is viewed as a red line—used to measure phorias.

Magnification: The ratio of the size of an image to the size of its object.

Megalocornea: Abnormally large cornea (> 13 mm in diameter).

Metamorphopsia: Wavy distortion of vision.

Microphthalmos: Abnormally small eye with abnormal function (see Nanophthalmos).

Miotic: A drug causing pupillary constriction.

Mydriatic: A drug causing pupillary dilation.

Myopia (nearsightedness): A refractive error in which the focus for light rays from a distant object is anterior to the retina.

Nanophthalmos: Abnormally small eye with normal function (see Microphthalmos).

Near point: The point at which the eye is focused when accommodation is fully active.

Nearsightedness: See Myopia.

Nystagmus: An involuntary oscillation of the eyeball that may be horizontal, vertical, torsional, or mixed.

Ophthalmia neonatorum: Conjunctivitis in the newborn.

Ophthalmoscope: An instrument with a special illumination system for viewing the inner eye, particularly the retina and associated structures.

Optic atrophy: Optic nerve degeneration.

Optic disk: Ophthalmoscopically visible portion of the optic nerve.

Optic nerve: The nerve that carries visual impulses from the retina to the brain.

Orbital cellulitis: Inflammation of the tissues surrounding the eye.

Orthoptics: The study and treatment of defects of binocular visual function or of the muscles controlling movement of the eyeballs.

Oscillopsia: The subjective illusion of movement of objects that occurs with some types of nystagmus.

Palpebral: Pertaining to the eyelid.

Pannus: Infiltration of the cornea with blood vessels.

Panophthalmitis: Inflammation of the entire eyeball.

Papilledema: Swelling of the optic disk due to raised intracranial pressure.

Papillitis: Optic nerve head ischemia or inflammation that is ophthalmoscopically visible.

Partially seeing child: For educational purposes, a partially seeing child is one who has a corrected visual acuity of 20/70 or less in the better eye.

Perimeter: An instrument for measuring the field of vision.

Peripheral vision: Ability to perceive the presence, motion, or color of objects outside of the direct line of vision.

Phacoemulsification and phacofragmentation: Techniques of extracapsular cataract extraction in which the nucleus of the lens is disrupted into small fragments by ultrasonic vibrations, thus allowing aspiration of all the lens matter through a small wound.

Phakomatoses: A group of hereditary diseases characterized by the presence of spots, cysts, and tumors in various parts of the body—eg, Recklinghausen's disease, Von Hippel-Lindau disease, tuberous sclerosis.

Phlyctenule: Localized lymphocytic infiltration of the conjunctiva.

Phoria: See Heterophoria.

Photocoagulation: Thermal damage to tissues due to absorption of high levels of light (including laser) energy.

Photodecomposition: Tissue damage by direct separation of chemical bonds by absorption of very short wavelength ultraviolet light (eg, from excimer lasers).

Photodisruption: Tissue damage produced by the breakdown of "plasma," which is a state of ionization created by spot focusing a high-energy laser source (eg, neodymium:YAG).

Photophobia: Abnormal sensitivity to light.

Photopsia: Appearance of sparks or flashes within the eye due to retinal irritation.

Phthisis bulbi: Atrophy of the eyeball with blindness and decreased intraocular pressure, due to end-stage intraocular disease.

Placido's disk: A disk with concentric rings used to determine the regularity of the cornea by observing the ring's reflection on the corneal surface.

Poliosis: Depigmentation of the eyelashes.

Posterior chamber: Space filled with aqueous anterior to the lens and posterior to the iris.

Presbyopia ("old sight"): Physiologically blurred near vision, commonly evident soon after age 40, due to reduction in the power of accommodation.

Prism: A wedge of transparent material that deviates light rays without changing their focus.

Prism diopter: The unit of prism power.

Pseudoisochromatic charts: Charts with colored dots of various hues and shades forming numbers, letters, or patterns, used for testing color discrimination.

Pseudophakia: Presence of an artificial intraocular lens implant following cataract extraction.

Pterygium: A triangular growth of tissue that extends from the conjunctiva over the cornea.

Ptosis: Drooping of the eyelid.

Puncta: External orifices of the upper and lower canaliculi.

Pupil: The round hole in the center of the iris that corresponds to the lens aperture in a camera.

Refraction: (1) Deviation in the course of rays of light in passing from one transparent medium into another of different density. (2) Determination of refractive errors of the eye and correction by lenses.

Refractive error (ametropia): An optical defect that prevents light rays from being brought to a single focus on the retina.

Refractive index: The ratio of the speed of light in a vacuum to the speed of light in a given material.

Refractive keratoplasty: Surgery of the cornea to correct refractive errors.

Refractive media: The transparent parts of the eye having refractive power.

Retina: Innermost coat of the eye, consisting of the sensory retina, which is composed of light-sensitive neural elements connecting to other neural cells, and the pigment epithelium.

Retinal detachment: A separation of the neurosensory retina from the pigment epithelium and choroid.

Retinitis pigmentosa: A hereditary degeneration and atrophy of the retina.

Retinoscope: An instrument specially designed for refracting an eye objectively.

Rods: See Cones and rods.

Sclera: The white part of the eye—a tough covering that, with the cornea, forms the external protective coat of the eye.

Scleral spur: The protrusion of sclera into the anterior chamber angle.

Scotoma: A blind or partially blind area in the visual field.

Slitlamp: A combination light and microscope for examination of the eye.

Snellen chart: Used for testing central visual acuity. It consists of lines of letters or numbers, in graded sizes drawn to Snellen measurements.

Sphincterotomy: A surgical incision of the iris sphincter muscle.

Staphyloma: A thinned part of the coat of the eye, causing protrusion.

Strabismus (heterotropia, tropia): A manifest deviation of the eyes.

Sty: See Hordeolum, external.

Symblepharon: Adhesions between the bulbar and palpebral conjunctiva.

Sympathetic ophthalmia: Inflammation in both eyes following trauma.

Synechia: Adhesion of the iris to the cornea (anterior synechia) or lens (posterior synechia).

Syneresis: A degenerative process within a gel, involving a drawing together of particles of the dispersed medium, separation of the medium, and shrinkage of the gel. Specifically applied to the vitreous.

Tarsorrhaphy: A surgical procedure by which the upper and lower lid margins are united.

Tonometer: An instrument for measuring intraocular pressure.

Trabeculectomy: The preferred first-line procedure for surgically creating an additional aqueous drainage channel in the treatment of glaucoma.

Trabeculoplasty: Laser photocoagulation of the trabecular meshwork in the treatment of open-angle glaucoma.

Trachoma: A serious form of infectious keratoconjunctivitis.

Trichiasis: Inversion and rubbing of the eyelashes against the globe.

Tropia: See Strabismus.

Uvea (uveal tract): The iris, ciliary body, and choroid.

Uveitis: Inflammation of one or all portions of the uveal tract.

Visual acuity: Measure of the acuteness of vision; the finest of detail that the eye can distinguish.

Visual axis: An imaginary line that connects a point in space (point of fixation) with fovea centralis.

Vitiligo: Localized patchy decrease or absence of pigment on the skin.

Vitreous: Transparent, colorless mass of soft, gelatinous material filling the eyeball behind the crystalline lens.

Xerosis: Drying of tissues lining the anterior surface of the eye.

Zonule: The numerous fine tissue strands that stretch from the ciliary processes to the crystalline lens equator (360 degrees) and hold the lens in place.

Zonulolysis: Lysis of the zonule, as with chymotrypsin, to facilitate removal of the lens in intracapsular cataract surgery.

SUBJECT INDEX

NOTE: Page numbers in bold face type indicate a major discussion. A *t* following a page number indicates tabular material and an *i* following a page number indicates an illustration. Drugs are listed under generic names. When a drug trade name is listed, the reader is referred to the generic drug name.

Abducens nerve, 25, 282
Abducens nucleus lesion, 282
Abducens palsy, 238–239, 282
AC/A ratio. *See* Accommodative convergence to accommodation (AC/A) ratio
Acanthamoeba, keratitis due to, **132–133**
Accommodation, 374–375
Accommodative convergence to accommodation (AC/A) ratio, high, esotropia due to, 237
Acetazolamide, **66**
Acne rosacea, 324
  conjunctivitis in, **114–115**
  skin lesions in, 115*f*
Acquired immunodeficiency syndrome (AIDS), **316–317**
  posterior uveitis in, 156
  retinal changes in, 317*f*
Actinomyces israelii, canaliculitis from, 90*f*
Acute multifocal posterior placoid pigment epitheliopathy (AMPPPE), 190–191
Acyclovir, **71–72**
Adenovirus
  keratitis due to, 136
  type 3, acute follicular conjunctivitis due to, 104*f*
  type 8, conjunctivitis due to, mononuclear cell reaction in, 105*f*
Adrenergic drugs, **63, 65**. *See also* Mydriatics
  adverse effects of
    ocular, 75*t*
    systemic, 74*t*
Afferent pupillary defect, 276, 277*f*
  swinging penlight test for, 33–34
After-cataract, **170–171**
Age
  illumination requirements and, 413–414
  posterior uveitis and, 152–153
AIDS. *See* Acquired immunodeficiency syndrome (AIDS)
Alacrima, 88
Albinism, 323, 342
  oculocutaneous, pedigree of, 351*f*

Alleles, 348
Alomide. *See* Lodoxamide tromethamine
Alpha-adrenergic agonists, **66**
Alternate cover test, 230
Amaurosis
  fugax, 288–289, **297–298**, 299*f*
    causes of, 299*t*
  Leber's congenital, 198
Amaurotic pupillary response, 278*f*
Amblyopia, 229, 346
  methyl alcohol, **267–268**
  prevention of, **385–386**
  tobacco-alcohol, **266–267**
  treatment of, 233–234
Ametropia, 375
Amikacin, for endophthalmitis, dosages of, 69*t*
Amikin. *See* Amikacin
Amiodarone, ocular complications of, 325, 326*f*
Amphotericin B, **71**
  for endophthalmitis, dosages of, 69*t*
AMPPPE (acute multifocal posterior placoid pigment epitheliopathy), 190–191
Amsler grid, 47, 48*f*
Ancef. *See* Cefazolin
Anesthetics
  local, injected, **62–63**
  topical, 40, **62**
    adverse effects of
      ocular, 75*t*
      systemic, 74*t*
Angiography, orbital, 247
Angioid streaks, 191–192
Angioma
  of conjunctiva, 121
  retinal, 204
    in von Hippel-Lindau disease, 205*f*, 291–292
Angiomatosis, retinocerebellar. *See* von Hippel-Lindau disease
Angle kappa, 226
Aniridia, 221, 342
Aniseikonia, 243, 378
Anisometropia, 229, **377–378**
  amblyopia from, prevention of, 385–386

Ankylosing spondylitis, 320, 332–333
  acute iridocyclitis in, 332*f*
  anterior uveitis in, 150–151
Anomalous trichromats, 204
Anophthalmos, 341
Anterior chamber, estimation of depth of, by oblique illumination, 212*f*
Anterior chamber angle, 11, 12*f*, 14*f*
  normal, anatomic and gonioscopic view of, 212*f*
Anterior membrane dystrophies, 139
Anterior segment. *See* Eye(s), anterior segment of
Anti-infective agents, **69–72**. *See also specific type or agent*
  for endophthalmitis, dosages of, 69*t*
  mixed with corticosteroids, **68**
Anti-inflammatory agents
  nonsteroidal. *See* Nonsteroidal anti-inflammatory agents (NSAIDs)
  steroidal. *See* Corticosteroids
Antibiotics
  combination, 70*t*
  topical, **69–70**
Anticholinergic agents. *See also* Cycloplegics
  adverse effects of
    ocular, 75*t*, 325–326
    systemic, 74*t*
Anticholinesterase drugs, **65**
  adverse effects of
    ocular, 75*t*
    systemic, 74*t*
Antidepressants, ocular complications of, 326
Antifungal agents, topical, **71**
Antimicrobials. *See* Anti-infective agents
Antibiotics
  adverse effects of
    ocular, 75*t*
    systemic, 74*t*
  systemic, topical preparations of, **70**
Antiviral agents, **71–72**
  adverse ocular effects of, 75*t*
Apraclonidine hydrochloride, **66**
  for glaucoma, 214
Aqueous, 11
  composition of, 208

Aqueous *(cont.)*
formation and flow of, 208–209
outflow of, 209
facilitation of, in treatment of
glaucoma, 216
physiology of, **208–211**
suppression of production of, in
treatment of glaucoma, 214
Arachnodactyly, 320, 322*f*
Arcus senilis, 138
Areolar tissue, 16
Argyll Robertson pupil, 274
Armed forces, visual standards for, 411
Arteriosclerosis, 300–301
Arteriovenous malformation
occipital hematoma from, 273*f*
proptosis from, 250–251
Arteritis
giant cell, 320, 335
idiopathic, of Takayasu, 320
Arthritis
juvenile rheumatoid, 319
uveitis in, 150
rheumatoid, 319, 332–333
nodular scleritis associated with,
162*f*, 333*f*
scleral thinning in, 333*f*
Ascaris lumbricoides, conjunctivitis
due to, 108–109
Asteroid hyalosis, 178–179
Asthenopia, 243
Astigmatism, **376–377**
irregular, 376
oblique, 376
of oblique incidence, 369
operation to correct, 145
regular, 376
types of, 377*f*
against the rule, 376, 377*f*
with the rule, 376, 377*f*
Ataxia-telangiectasia, 292
Atherosclerosis, 300
Atropine sulfate, **63–64**
for amblyopia, 234
Autoimmune disease
marginal keratitis in, 134
ocular disorders associated with,
318–320
Axenfeld, intrascleral nerve loops of,
161
Axenfeld's syndrome, 221
Azathioprine, 325*t*

Bacitracin, 69
Bárány rotating chair, 286
Basilar artery, occlusion of, 289
Behçet's disease, 320, 321*f*, 335–336
Benoxinate hydrochloride, **62**
Beriberi, 312
Best's disease, 195
Beta-adrenergic blocking drugs, **65–
66**
adverse effects of
ocular, 75*t*

systemic, 74*t*
for glaucoma, 214
Betagan. *See* Levobunolol hydrochlo-
ride
Betaxolol hydrochloride, **65**
Betoptic. *See* Betaxolol hydrochloride
Bielschowsky test, 242*f*
Bietti's band-shaped nodular dystrophy (keratopathy), 118, 138
Binocular movement, development of,
228
Binocular vision, 229
Birdshot retinochoroidopathy, 191
Blenorrhea, inclusion. *See* Conjunctivitis, inclusion
Blepharitis
anterior, **79–80**
contact, mild conjunctivitis secondary to, 112
posterior, **80**
Blepharochalasis, **82**
Blepharoconjunctivitis
molluscum contagiosum, **107**
varicella-zoster, **107**
Blepharophimosis, 83
Blepharoptosis, **83–85**
in chronic trachoma, 103*f*
classification of, 83–84
treatment of, 84–85
Blepharospasm, **82–83**
Blind
financial assistance programs for,
400
rehabilitation of, **398–400**
special services available to,
415–416
Blind children, education of, 412
Blindness, **396–400**
in babies with normal ocular and
neurologic examination, **343–346**
causes of, **397–398**
color. *See* Color blindness
costs of avoiding, 398
definition of, 396
night, congenital stationary, pedigree of, 350*f*
prevalence of, 396, 397*t*
prevention and treatment of,
397–398
Botulinum toxin
for heterophoria, 244
for strabismus, 234
Bourneville's disease, 292–293
Boutonneuse fever, conjunctivitis due
to, 108
Braille, 399–400
Brightness acuity testing, 47–48
Brown's syndrome, 242–243
Bulbar conjunctiva, 5
Bulk modulus K, 211
Buphthalmos, 221*f*
Bupivicaine hydrochloride, **63**
Burns, **360–361**
chemical, 360–361
thermal, 361

Busulfan, pigmentary retinopathy
from, 328

**Calcific emboli, amaurosis fugax
from, 297**
Caloric stimulation, in nystagmus, 286
Canalicular system, disorders of, **89–90**
Canaliculitis, 89–90
from *Actinomyces israelii*, 90*f*
conjunctivitis secondary to, 117
Candida, 316
albicans, corneal ulcer caused by,
129*f*
conjunctivitis due to, 108
Carbachol, topical, **64–65**
Carbocaine. *See* Mepivicaine hydrochloride
Carbonic anhydrase inhibitors, **66–67**
for glaucoma, 214
Carcinoid conjunctivitis, 117
Carcinoma
associated with xeroderma pigmentosum, 87
basal cell, of eyelid, 86, 87*f*
of conjunctiva, 121
sebaceous gland, of eyelid, 87
squamous cell, of eyelid, 86–87
Carotid artery, occlusion of, 288–289,
302
Carotid artery-cavernous sinus fistula,
251, 302–303·
Carteolol hydrochloride, **66**
Caruncle, 5
Cat-scratch disease, conjunctival, 119
Cataract, **165–172**
after-, **170–171**
age-related (senile), **167**, 168*f*
in diabetics, 308
postoperative care for, 172
associated with systemic disease,
170
blindness from, 397
childhood, **167–169**
acquired, 168
clinical findings in, 167–168
congenital, 167–168
zonular type, 168*f*
prognosis for, 169
treatment of, 169
diabetic, 308
punctate dot, 170*f*
secondary to intraocular disease,
170
surgery for, **171–172**
intraocular lens in, 171–172
posterior capsulotomy after, 406
postoperative care in, 172
toxic, 170
traumatic, **169–170**
types of, 166*f*
Cefamandole, for endophthalmitis,
dosages of, 69*t*
Cefazolin, for endophthalmitis,
dosages of, 69*t*

Ceftazimide, for endophthalmitis, dosages of, 69*t*
Cellulitis, orbital, 249–250
Cerebellum, 283
Cerebral artery
  middle, occlusion of, 289
  posterior, occlusion of, 289
Cerebromacular degeneration, **293**
Cerebrovascular disorders, **288–291**
Chalazion, **79**
Chandler's syndrome, 223
Check ligaments, 7, 17*f*
Chemosis, in bacterial conjunctivitis, 98
Chiasmatic glioma, 271–272
Chibroxin. *See* Norfloxacin
Chickenpox, 315. *See also* Varicella-zoster
Child abuse, trauma from, 346
Chlamydia
  conjunctivitis from, **101–104**
    in newborn, 344. *See also* Ophthalmia neonatorum
  keratitis from, 135–136
Chlorambucil, 325*t*
Chloramphenicol
  ocular complications of, 326
  topical, **70**
Chloroquine, ocular complications of, 326–327
Chlorothiazide, xanthopsia from, 327
Cholesterol emboli, amaurosis fugax from, 297, 299*f*
Cholinergic drugs, **64–65**
  adverse effects of
    ocular, 75*t*
    systemic, 74*t*
  for glaucoma, 216
Chorioretinal atrophy, peripheral, 198
Chorioretinitis, vitiliginous, 191
Chorioretinopathy, central serous, **188–189**
Choroid, 9
  colobomas of, 341, 342
  congenital abnormalities of, 342
  cross section of, 12*f*
  embryology of, 27
  hemangioma of, 158–159
  lesions to, in posterior uveitis, 153
  malignant melanoma of, 159*f*
  metastases to, 160
  nevus of, 158, 159*f*
  rupture of, 359*f*
    in traumatic maculopathy, 193*f*
  sympathetic ophthalmia involving, giant cells and lymphocytes in, 157*f*
Choroidal infarction, 297
Choroidopathy, geographic helicoid peripapillary, 191
Chromatic aberration, 367, 369
Chromosomal abnormalities, **351–352**
Chromosomes, 348
  abnormal number of, syndromes associated with, **352**

sex, 348
  abnormalities involving, 352
Cicatricial pemphigoid, **113**, 334
Ciliary body, 8–9
  embryology of, 27
  medulloepithelioma of, 159
Ciliary muscle, 8–9
Ciliary staphyloma, 161*f*
Ciloxan. *See* Ciprofloxacin
Ciprofloxacin, topical, **70**
Circle of least confusion, 370
Cleocin. *See* Clindamycin
Climatic droplet keratopathy, 118, 138
Clindamycin, for endophthalmitis, dosages of, 69*t*
Coatings, for low-vision aids, 392–393
Cogan's dystrophy, 139
Colchicine, 325*t*
Coloboma, 341
  of eyelid, **81**
  of iris, 342
Color blindness, **204**
  red-green, pedigree of, 351*f*
Color vision
  defects in, **204**
  testing of, 48
Coma, 369
Commotio retinae, 193
Computed tomographic (CT) scans, 59
  of orbit, 245, 246*f*, 247*f*
Cone monochromatism, 204
Cone-rod dystrophies, 194, 195*f*
Confrontation testing, 33
Congenital infections, ocular damage due to, prevention of, **384**
Conjugate planes, 366
Conjugate points, 366
Conjunctiva, **5–6**
  blood supply, lymphatics, and nerve supply of, 6
  bulbar, 5
  degenerative diseases of, **117–118**
  disorders of, **95–121**
  exudation of, 98
  follicles in. *See also* Conjunctivitis, follicular
    in bacterial conjunctivitis, 98
    in trachoma, 101*f*
  histology of, 5–6
  hyperemia of, 97
  miscellaneous disorders of, **118–119**
  palpebral, 5, 17
  papillae of
    in bacterial conjunctivitis, 98
    "cobblestone," in vernal conjunctivitis, 110*f*, 331*f*
    in trachoma, 101*f*
  pseudomembranes and membranes in, 98
    in epidemic keratoconjunctivitis, 105*f*
  tumors of, **120–121**
    benign, **120–121**
    malignant, 121

Conjunctival cat-scratch disease, 119
Conjunctival dysplasia, 121
Conjunctival epithelial cells, cytoplasmic inclusion body in, in trachoma, 102*f*
Conjunctival epithelium, 5
Conjunctival intraepithelial neoplasia, 121
Conjunctival lymphedema, congenital, **118**
Conjunctival stroma, 6
  adenoid layer of, 6
  fibrous layer of, 6
Conjunctivitis, **95–118**
  acute hemorrhagic, **106–107**
  allergic, **109–112**
    due to delayed hypersensitivity reactions, 111–112
    due to immediate humoral hypersensitivity reactions, 109–111
    treatment of, drugs used in, 67–68, 72
  associated with systemic disease, **116**
  bacterial, **99–100**
    acute, 99–100
      mucopurulent (catarrhal), 99–100
      purulent, 99
    chronic, 100
    clinical findings in, 99–100
    complications and sequelae in, 100
    course and prognosis of, 100
    laboratory findings in, 100
    in newborn, 344. *See also* Ophthalmia neonatorum
    polymorphonuclear reaction in, 100*f*
    subacute, 100
    treatment of, 100
  butcher's, 108–109
  candidal, 108
  carcinoid, 117
  caterpillar hair, **114**
  causes of, 96–97*t*
  chemical/irritative, **113–114**
    in newborn, 344. *See also* Ophthalmia neonatorum
  chlamydial, **101–104**
    in newborn, 344. *See also* Ophthalmia neonatorum
  cytology of, 95
  due to autoimmune disease, **112–113**
  due to infectious agents, **95–109**
  follicular
    acute viral, **104–107**
      due to adenovirus type 3, 104*f*
      caused by inclusion conjunctivitis, 104*f*
    chronic, **114**
    molluscum contagiosum of lid margin with, 107*f*
  fungal, **108**

Conjunctivitis *(cont.)*
  giant papillary, **111**
  gonorrheal, 99*f*
  gouty, 117
  hay fever, **109–110, 330–331**
  herpes simplex virus, **106**
  iatrogenic, from topically applied
    drugs, **113–114**
  inclusion, **103–104**
    clinical findings in, 103–104
    differential diagnosis of, 104
    treatment of, 104
  ligneous, 98–99, **116**
  mild, secondary to contact blephari-
    tis, 112
  neonatal. *See* Ophthalmia neonato-
    rum
  Newcastle disease, **106**
  occupational, **114**
  parasitic, **108–109**
  rickettsial, **108**
  secondary to canaliculitis, 117
  secondary to dacryocystitis, 117
  secondary to neoplasms, 119
  signs of, 97–99
  symptoms of, 95–97
  in thyroid disease, 116–117
  of unknown cause, **114–116**
  vernal, **110–111, 331–332**
  viral, **104–108**
    acute, 104–107
    chronic, 107–108
    in newborn, 344. *See also* Oph-
      thalmia neonatorum
Connective tissue diseases, heritable,
    ocular disorders associated with,
    320–322
Conoid of Sturm, 370, 371*f*
Contact dermatitis, 336
Contact lenses. *See* Lens(es), contact
Contraceptives, oral, ocular complica-
    tions of, 327
Contrast, visibility and, 413
Contrast sensitivity
  test chart for, 50*f*
  testing of, 48–49
Convergence, testing for, 232–233
Convergence paralysis, 280
Convergence-retraction nystagmus,
    287
Cornea, 7, **123–145**
  blood staining of, 142
  changes to, in Graves' disease, 310
  congenital abnormalities of, 341
  degenerative conditions of,
    136–140
  diseases of
    laboratory studies in, 124
    physiology of symptoms of, 123
    recurrent erosion associated with,
      140
    symptoms and signs of, 123–
      124
  examination of, techniques for, 51
  foreign bodies on, 357–358

growth and development of, 28
iron lines in, 142
lesions of, morphologic diagnosis
    of, 124
miscellaneous disorders of,
    140–141
physiology of, 123
resistance to infection of, 123
scarring of
  in recurrent herpes simplex ker-
    atitis, 130*f*
  in trachoma, 103*f*
subepithelial opacities of, in herpes
    simplex keratitis, 130
transverse section of, 11*f*
trauma to, recurrent erosion associ-
    ated with, 140
Corneal abrasions, 357–358
Corneal annulus, 138
Corneal degeneration, **137–138**
  marginal, 137–138
  Salzmann's nodular, 138
  spheroid, 138
Corneal dehydrating agents, **72**
Corneal dystrophy, hereditary, **139–140**
  epithelial, 139
  posterior limiting membrane, 139
  recurrent erosion associated with,
    140
  stromal, 139
Corneal epithelium
  baring of, in dry eye syndrome, 93*f*
  debridement of, in herpes simplex
    keratitis, 131
Corneal erosion, recurrent, **140–141**
Corneal filaments, in dry eye syn-
    drome, 93*f*
Corneal grafts. *See* Corneal transplan-
    tation
Corneal implants, alloplastic, 145
Corneal pigmentation, **141–142**
Corneal surgery, refractive, **144–145,**
    378
  lasers in, 145, 406–407
Corneal topography system, comput-
    erized, 52*f*
Corneal transplantation, **143–144**
  graft reactions in, **336–337**
Corneal ulcers, **124–135.** *See also*
    Keratitis
  central, **124–133**
  dendritic, in herpes simplex kerati-
    tis, 130, 131*f*
  due to vitamin A deficiency,
    134–135, 312*f*
  geographic, in herpes simplex ker-
    atitis, 130
  marginal, 133
  peripheral, **133–135**
    in herpes simplex keratitis, 131
    in trachoma, 103*f*
Corticosteroids, 325
  adverse ocular effects of, 75*t*, 327,
    386
  glaucoma induced by, 223

topical, **67–68**
  mixed with anti-infective agents,
    68
Cosmetic soft contact lenses, 142–143
Cotton wool spots, 298*f*, 299*f*
  in lupus erythematosus, 334*f*
Cover test, 34
  in strabismus, 230, 231*f*
Cranial arteritis, 320
Cranial nerves III, IV, and VI, syn-
    dromes affecting, **283**
Craniofacial dysostosis, 343
Craniopharyngioma, 271
Critical angle, 365–366
Cromolyn sodium, **68**
Cross cylinder, 379
Crouzon's disease, 343
Cryptophthalmos, 341
CT scans. *See* Computed tomographic
    (CT) scans
Cup-to-disk ratio, 42*f*
  in end-stage glaucoma, 43*f*
Curvature of field, 369
Cyclodestructive procedures, for glau-
    coma, 217
Cyclogyl. *See* Cyclopentolate hy-
    drochloride
Cyclomydril. *See* Cyclopentolate hy-
    drochloride, with phenylephrine hy-
    drochloride
Cyclopentolate hydrochloride, **64**
  with phenylephrine hydrochloride,
    64
Cyclophosphamide, 325*t*
Cyclophotocoagulation, 405
Cycloplegics, **63–64**
  adverse effects of
    ocular, 75*t*
    systemic, 74*t*
  for glaucoma, 216
Cyclosporine, 325
Cyclotropia, 241
Cylinder axis notation, 371*f*
Cystic eye, congenital, 341
Cysticercosis, **158**
Cystinosis, **118,** 323
Cytomegalic inclusion disease,
    315
Cytotoxic agents, 325

Dacryoadenitis, 88
Dacryocystitis, **88–89**
  conjunctivitis secondary to, 117
  infantile, 89
Dacryocystorhinostomy, 89
Daranide. *See* Dichlorphenamide
Dark adaptation, testing of, 57
Decongestants, **72**
Demecarium bromide, **65**
Dermatitis
  contact, 336
  herpetiformis, **115**
Dermatochalasis, **82**
Dermatomyositis, 318

Dermoids, 343
　of conjunctiva, 120
　of orbit, 250
Deuteranopia, 204
Deviation
　primary, 226, 227*f*
　secondary, 226, 227*f*
Devic's disease, 260
Diabetes mellitus, **306–309**
Diabetic retinopathy. *See* Retinopathy, diabetic
Diamox. *See* Acetazolamide
Dichlorphenamide, **66**
Diktyoma, 159
Dilating drops. *See* Cycloplegics; Mydriatics
Diopter, 367–368
Dipivefrin, for glaucoma, 214, 216
Diplopia, 229
　binocular, 30
　monocular, 30
　from orbital injury, 361
Disposable soft contact lenses, 143
Dissociated vertical deviation, 242
Distichiasis, 81
Divergence, testing for, 233
Doll's head maneuver, 277–278
Dorzolamide hydrochloride, **66–67**
Double vision. *See* Diplopia
Downbeat nystagmus, 287
Downgaze nystagmus, 287
Down's syndrome, 352
Drivers' licenses, visual standards for, 411
Drug toxicity, optic neuropathy from, 267
Drugs. *See specific type or agent*; Medications
Drusen, 187
Dry eye syndrome. *See* Keratoconjunctivitis sicca
Duane's retraction syndrome, **241–242**, 282–283
Ductions, 226, 227*f*
　testing for, 232
Duranest. *See* Etidocaine hydrochloride
Dye solutions, diagnostic, **72**. *See also specific agent*
Dyslexia, 346

Eales' disease, **313**
Eccentric fixation, 229–230
Echothiophate iodide, **65**
Ectoderm
　neural, 25
　surface, 25
Ectopia lentis, **173**
Ectropion, **81**
Education
　of blind children, 412
　visual standards for, 411–412
　of visually handicapped children, 411–412

Edwards' syndrome, 352
Electro-oculography (EOG), 56
Electronic devices, for blind, 400
Electroretinography (ERG), 55–56
Embryotoxon, anterior, 138
Emmetropia, 375
Endocarditis, subacute infective, 305
Endocrine diseases, ocular disorders associated with, **309–312**
Endophthalmitis, 183–184
　treatment of, antimicrobials for, dosages of, 69*t*
Entoptic phenomena, 49
Entropion, **80–81**
EOG. *See* Electro-oculography (EOG)
Epiblepharon, 80
Epicanthus, 17, **81**
　tarsalis, 81*f*
Epidermoid cysts, orbital, 250
Epidermolysis bullosa, **116**
Epikeratophakia, 145
Epinephrine, **65**
　for glaucoma, 214, 216
Episclera, 7
Episcleritis, **161**
Epithelial cells
　basal, 5–6
　superficial, 5
Epithelioma, intraepithelial, 121*f*
Epitheliopathy, acute multifocal posterior placoid pigment (AMPPPE), 190–191
Equal-pressure balloons, 210*f*
ERG. *See* Electroretinography (ERG)
Erythema multiforme, **115**, 116*f*, 323
Erythromycin, **69**
Eserine. *See* Physostigmine salicylate & sulfate
Esotropia, **236–239**
　nonparetic, 237–238
　　accommodative, 237
　　nonaccommodative, 237
　paretic, 238–239
　partially accommodative, 237–238
Ethmoid bone, 2
Etidocaine hydrochloride, **63**
Exfoliation syndrome, 222
Exophthalmometry, **57–58**
Exophthalmos
　in Graves' disease, 310
　pulsating, following orbital injury, 362
Exotropia, **239–240**
　constant, 240
　intermittent, 239–240
Extracapsular extraction, 171, 172*f*
Extraocular abnormalities. *See also specific type*
　congenital, **343**
　diagnosis of, **57–60**
Extraocular movements. *See* Eye movements

Extraocular muscles, **15–16**
　attachment of, shifting point of, in strabismus, 235
　blood supply of, 16
　choice of, for surgery, in strabismus, 236
　embryology of, 27
　fibrosis of, congenital, blepharoptosis from, 83
　field of action of, 228
　functions of, 227–228
　nerve supply of, 15–16
　palsies of
　　in diabetes, 309
　　symptoms and signs of, 283
　resection and recession of, in strabismus, 235
　synergistic and antagonistic, 228
　yoke pairs of, 228
Extraocular structures, vessels and nerves of, 19*f*
Eye movements, **276–279**
　abnormalities of, **279–283**
　anatomy of, 278–279
　binocular, development of, 228
　classification and examination of, 277–278
　disjunctive
　　supranuclear syndromes involving, **280**
　　testing for, 232–233
　fast, 278
　　brainstem centers for, 278–279
　　cortical centers for, 279
　physiology of, 278
　slow, 278
　　brainstem centers for, 279
　　cortical centers for, 279
　testing of, 34
Eyeball, 4
　congenital abnormalities of, 341
　contusions of, **358–359**
　growth and development of, 28
　penetration of, 183, **358–359**
　rupture of, 183, **358–359**
Eyebrows, 16
Eyelashes, 17
Eyelids, **16–20**
　abrasions and lacerations of, 356–357
　anatomic deformities of, **80–85**, 341
　appearance of, abnormalities in, 30
　blood supply and lymphatics of, 20
　cosmetic micropigmentation of, 85
　embryology of, 25
　eversion of, 35–37
　infections and inflammations of, **78–80**
　margins of, 17
　retractors of, 18–19
　sensory nerve supply of, 20
　surgical anatomy of, **78**
　tumors of, **85–87**
　　benign, **85–86**
　　laser vaporization of, 406
　　malignant, **86–87**

Eye(s)
  abnormalities of. *See specific type*;
    Extraocular abnormalities; Ocu-
    lar abnormalities
  alignment of, testing of, 34
  ametropic, 31
  anatomy of, **1–25**
  anterior segment of
    developmental anomalies of, 221,
      342
    direct ophthalmoscopic examina-
      tion of, 43
    embryology of, 27
    examination of, in children, 341
    flow of aqueous in, 210*f*
  appearance of, abnormalities in, 30
  burns to, **360–361**
    chemical, 360–361
    thermal, 361
  congenital cystic, 341
  crossed. *See* Esotropia
  dryness of, 30
  embryology of, **25–28**
  emmetropic, 31
  examination of. *See also* Ophthal-
    mologic examination
    by nonophthalmologist, 45
  external landmarks of, 10*f*, 14–15,
    18*f*
  foreign bodies in, 359–360
  growth and development of, 28
  injuries to, **356–362**. *See also*
    Trauma
    occupational, 381
    prevention of, 362, **381–382**
  internal structures of, 8*f*
  irritation of, 30–31
  optics and, **373–375**
  pain in, 30
  posterior segment of, examination
    of, in children, 341
  posterior view of, 9*f*
  schematic, of Gullstrand, 374
  surface of, foreign bodies on,
    357–358
  vascular supply to, 4*f*, 5*f*, 296
    embryology of, 28
  venous drainage of, 6*f*

Facial tics, 82
Faden procedure, 235–236
Farsightedness. *See* Hyperopia
Fascia, 15, 16*f*
Fascia bulbi. *See* Tenon's capsule
Ferry's line, 142
Fine-needle aspiration, in orbital diag-
  nosis, 248
Fixation, eccentric, 229–230
Flash electroretinogram. *See* Elec-
  troretinography (ERG)
Flashing (flickering) lights, 30
  vitreous and, 176
Fleischer's ring, 142
Floating spots, 30

Floropryl. *See* Isoflurophate
Fluorescein angiography, **53–55**
Fluorescein sodium, **72**
Fluorescein staining, 37
  in dry eye syndrome, 93
  in evaluation of lacrimal system, 57
Focal length, 367
Focal point
  primary, 367
  secondary, 367
    position of, refractive errors as
      determined by, 376*f*
Focal resolution, impaired, management of, 394
Folliculosis, **114**
Foreign bodies
  corneal, 357–358
  intraocular, 359–360
Fortaz. *See* Ceftazimide
Frontal bone, 1–2
Frontal lobe, lesions of, abnormal eye
  movements from, 279
Fuchs' dystrophy, 139–140
Fuchs' heterochromic iridocyclitis,
  151
Fundus
  albipunctatus, 194–195
  flavimaculatus, 195
  normal, 42*f*
  photography of, 53
    with fluorescein. *See* Fluorescein
      angiography
  slitlamp examination of, 41–42
  view of, in direct and indirect oph-
    thalmoscopy, 45*f*
Fungal disease, ocular disorders associated with, **316**
Fungizone. *See* Amphotericin B
Fusion, 226
  sensory, 229
Fusion potential, testing for, 233

Galactosemia, 323
Gametes, 348
Gantrisin. *See* Sulfisoxazole
Garamycin. *See* Gentamicin
Gas-permeable contact lenses, 142
Gaze, primary position of, 228
  yoke muscles in, 228*t*
Genes, 348
Genetic carrier state, 352–353
Genetic counseling, 352
Genetic disease, prevention of,
  384–385
Genetic terms, glossary of, **353–354**
Genoptic. *See* Gentamicin
Genotype, 348
Gentacidin. *See* Gentamicin
Gentamicin
  for endophthalmitis, dosages of, 69*t*
  topical, **70**
Geographic helicoid peripapillary
  choroidopathy, 191
German measles, 316

Giant cell arteritis, 320, 335
Glare, 30
Glaucoma, **208–223**
  ciliary block, 223
  classified according to etiology,
    209*t*
  clinical assessment of, **211–214**
  congenital, **220–221**, 345
    primary, 221
  end-stage, cup-to-disk ratio in, 43*f*
  following ocular surgery, 223
  malignant, 223
  neovascular, 223
  pathology of, 211
  phacolytic, 222
  pigmentary, 221–222
  in posterior uveitis, 153
  primary, **217–220**
    angle-closure
      acute, 218–219
      chronic, 219–220
        laser treatment of, 404–405
      subacute, 219
    normal-pressure, 218
    open-angle, 217–218
      laser treatment of, 405
      prevention of, 385
  secondary, **221–223**
    to changes in lens, 222
    to changes in uveal tract,
      222–223
    to raised episcleral venous pres-
      sure, 223
    to trauma, 223
  steroid-induced, 223
  treatment of, **214–217**
    drugs used in, **64–67**
    laser, 216–217, **404–405**
    medical, 214–216
    surgical, 216–217
  in Vietnamese-Americans, 220
Glaucoma drainage surgery, 216–217
  laser suture lysis in, 405
Glaucomatous cupping, 213*f*, 214*f*
Glioma
  chiasmatic, 271–272
  optic nerve, 252, 271–272
Globe. *See* Eyeball
Glycerin, **67**
  for glaucoma, 216
Glyrol. *See* Glycerin
Goniolenses, 37*f*, 51, 53
Gonioscopy, 51, 53*f*
  in assessment of glaucoma,
    212–213
Goniotomy, 217
Gout, conjunctivitis in, 117
Gradenigo's syndrome, 283
Granular dystrophy, of corneal stroma,
  139
Granulomas, of conjunctiva, 99, 120
Granulomatosis, Wegener's, 319
Granulomatous diseases, ocular disor-
  ders associated with, **312–315**
Graphic ray tracing, 367

Graves' disease, **248–249**, **309–311**
  clinical findings in, 248, 310
  pathogenesis of ocular signs in, 310
  treatment of, 248–249, 310–311
Guide dogs, 399
Gullstrand, schematic eye of, 374
Gyrate atrophy, 198

Haemophilus aegyptius, **acute catarrhal conjunctivitis caused by, 99***f*
Haloes, 30
Hamartoma, astrocytic (glial), 204, 205*f*
Hand magnifiers, 391, 392*f*
Hansen's disease. *See* Leprosy
Hardy-Rand-Rittler pseudoisochromatic plates, 49*f*
Hay fever conjunctivitis, **109–110**, **330–331**
Head tilt test, 242*f*
Hemangioma
  capillary, of orbit, 251
  cavernous
    of eyelid, 86*f*
    of orbit, 251
    of choroid, 158–159
    of eyelid, 86
Hematologic disorders, ocular disorders associated with, **305–306**
Hepatolenticular degeneration, 323
Herbert's pits, 101
Hering's law, 228
Herpes simplex virus (HSV), **315**
  conjunctivitis caused by, **106**
  keratitis caused by, **129–132**
Herpes zoster, 315. *See also* Varicella-zoster
Herplex. *See* Idoxuridine
Hertel exophthalmometer, 58*f*
Heterochromia, 342
Heterophoria, 226, **243–244**
Heterotropia, 226
Hirschberg method, 232
Histiocytosis, orbital, 253
Histoplasmosis, **155**, 190
History
  family, 29
  ocular, **29–31**
    in low vision, 388
    in strabismus, 230
    past medical, 29
Homatropine hydrobromide, **64**
Hordeolum, **78–79**
Horner's syndrome, 84, **275–276**
HSV. *See* Herpes simplex virus (HSV)
Hudson-Ståhli line, 142
Humorsol. *See* Demecarium bromide
Hyaline degeneration, of sclera, 163
Hyperopia, 31*f*, 375–376
  accommodative esotropia due to, 237
  latent, 376
Hyperosmotic agents, for glaucoma, 216

Hypersensitivity reactions, conjunctivitis due to. *See* Conjunctivitis, allergic
Hypertelorism, 269, 270*f*
Hypertension, benign intracranial, 304–305
Hypertensive retinopathy, **301–302**, 303*f*, 304*f*
Hypertropia, **240–241**
Hyperviscosity syndromes, 305, 306*f*
Hyphema, **360**
Hypoparathyroidism, 311–312
Hypopyon, in posterior uveitis, 153
Hypothyroidism, 311

ICE syndrome. *See* **Iridocorneoendothelial (ICE) syndrome**
Idoxuridine, **71**
Illiterate E chart, 32*f*
Illumination, practical factors in, **413–414**
Immunologic diseases, **330–337**. *See also specific type*
Immunosuppressive agents, **324–325**
Impression cytology, in dry eye syndrome, 92–93
Industry, visual standards for, 409–411
Infranuclear pathways, lesions of, **280–283**
Infraorbital nerve, 24
Inheritance
  autosomal dominant, 349
  autosomal recessive, 349–350
  maternal, **350–351**
  mechanisms of, **348–349**
  Mendelian, **349–350**
  X-linked recessive, 350
Intercept, 379
Internuclear ophthalmoplegia, **280**
Intracapsular extraction, 171
Intraocular pressure
  devices for measuring, 211
  dynamics of, **209–211**
Intraocular tumors, **204–206**
  benign, 204
  malignant, 205–206
Intrascleral nerve loops of Axenfeld, 161
Iopidine. *See* Apraclonidine hydrochloride
Iridectomy, 216
Iridocorneoendothelial (ICE) syndrome, 223
Iridocyclitis. *See also* Uveitis
  in ankylosing spondylitis, 332*f*
  Fuchs' heterochromic, 151
  in Reiter's disease, 332*f*
Iridodonesis, 173
Iridotomy, 216
Iris, 7
  changes in, in diabetes, 309
  colobomas of, 341, 342
  congenital abnormalities of, 342
  growth and development of, 28

nevus of, 158, 159*f*
  plateau, 220
Iris atrophy, essential, 223
Iris nevus syndrome, 223
Iritis. *See* Uveitis, anterior
Ismotic. *See* Isosorbide
Isoflurophate, **65**
Isopters, 46–47
Isosorbide, **67**

Jaw-winking phenomenon, **84, 282**
Jenamycin. *See* Gentamicin
Joint disease
  affecting eye, 332–333
  uveitis associated with, 150–151
Jones I test, 57
Jones II test, 57

Kawasaki disease, **116**
Kayser-Fleischer ring, 142
Kefzol. *See* Cefazolin
Keith-Wagener retinopathy. *See* Hypertensive retinopathy
Keratitis. *See also* Corneal ulcers
  adenovirus, 136
  amebic, **132–133**
    treatment of, 127*t*
  bacterial, **126–129**
    treatment of, 127*t*
      drugs for, concentrations and dosages of, 128*t*
  chlamydial, 135–136
  endothelial, 124
  epithelial, 124, **135–136**
    drug-induced, 136
    principal types of, 125–126*t*
  exposure, 135
  fungal, **129**
    treatment of, 127*t*
      drugs for, concentrations and dosages of, 128*t*
  herpes simplex, **129–132**
    clinical findings in, 130–131
    treatment of, 131–132
  interstitial, **141**
  leprosy, 313*f*
  marginal, in autoimmune disease, 134
  neurotrophic, 135
  stromal, 124
  subepithelial, 124
  Thygeson's superficial punctate, **140**
  varicella-zoster, **132**
  viral, **129–132**, 136
Keratoconjunctivitis
  atopic, **111**, **331–332**
    chronic, corneal graft in, 336*f*
  epidemic, **105–107**
    iatrogenic, prevention of, 384
  measles, **107–108**
  phlyctenular, 134, 336
  sicca, **91–94**

Keratoconjunctivitis *(cont.)*
  sicca *(cont.)*
    associated with Sjögren's syndrome, **112**, 113*f*, 136
    baring of corneal epithelium in, 93*f*
    clinical findings in, 91–93
    complications of, 93
    corneal filaments in, 93*f*
    etiology and diagnosis of, 91, 92*t*
    treatment of, 93–94
  superior limbic, **116**
  vernal, **110–111**, **331–332**
Keratoconus, **136–137**
Keratomalacia, associated with xerophthalmia, 135*f*, 312*f*
Keratomileusis, 144
Keratopathy
  amiodarone, 326*f*
  band (calcific), 137–138
  climatic droplet, 118, 138
Keratophakia, 144–145
Keratoplasty, **143–144**
Keratotomy, radial, 144
Krimsky test, 232
Krukenberg's spindle, 141–142

Labrador keratopathy, **118, 138**
Lacrimal apparatus, **20–21, 87–90**
  blood supply and lymphatics of, 21
  embryology of, 25–27
  evaluation of, 57
  nerve supply of, 21
Lacrimal bone, 2
Lacrimal caruncle, 17
Lacrimal drainage system, 20*f*, 88
  disorders of, **88–90**
  evaluation of, 57
Lacrimal glands, 20–21, 87–88
  disorders of, **87–88**
  tumors of, 252–253
Lacrimal hypersecretion, 88
Lacrimal nerve, 24
Lacrimal punctum, 17
Lacrimal sac, 21
Lacrimation, paradoxic, 88
Lactoferrin, in tears, in dry eye syndrome, 93
Lamina cribrosa, 7
Larva migrans, visceral and ocular, comparison between, 155*f*
Laser interferometry, for assessment of potential vision, 49
Laser photomydriasis, 405–406
Laser sclerostomy, 406
Laser sphincterotomy, 405–406
Laser trabeculoplasty, 216
Lasers, **401–407**
  diagnostic imaging using, 407
  mechanisms of effects of, 401–402
  in refractive corneal surgery, 145, 406–407
  therapeutic applications of, **402–407**

in treatment of glaucoma, 216–217, **404–405**
Lattice degeneration, of retina, 198
Lattice dystrophy, of corneal stroma, 139
Laurence-Moon-Biedl syndrome, 323–324
Learning disabilities, 346
Leber's congenital amaurosis, 198
Leber's optic neuropathy, 268–269
Lens(es)
  biconvex, spherical aberration of, 370*f*
  characteristics of, rapid detection of, 373–374
  contact, **142–143**, 378
    as aid in vitreous examination, 175
    care of, 143
    hard, 142
    soft, 142–143
    wear of, ocular infection and, 383
  convex, as low-vision aids, 391
  cylindrical, 369–370
  of eye, 9, 13*f*
    changes in
      in diabetes, 308–309
      glaucoma secondary to, 222
    clear, surgical removal of, 145, 378–379
    dislocated, **173**
      glaucoma from, 222
    disorders of, **165–173**
      congenital, 342
      physiology of symptoms in, 165
    embryology of, 27
    growth and development of, 28
    intumescence of, glaucoma from, 222
  Goldmann three-mirror, 53
  intraocular, 171–172, 378
  planocylindrical, 369, 370*f*
  plus and minus, ray tracing through, 369*f*
  special, in slitlamp examination, 37–38
  spherical
    aberrations of, 369
    prismatic effect of, 373
  spherocylindrical, 370
    cross diagram and equivalent combinations for, 372*f*
  thick, in Gaussian optics, 368
  thin, equations of, 367
Leprosy, 313–314
  blindness from, 398
Leukemia, 305
  chronic myeloid, retinal changes in, 306*f*
Leukocoria, 345
Levator palpebrae superioris muscle, 18, 19–20
  aponeurosis of, blepharoptosis and, 84
  maldevelopment of, ptosis from, 83

Levobunolol hydrochloride, **66**
Levocabastine hydrochloride, **68**
Lidocaine hydrochloride, **62**
Light
  diffuseness of, visibility and, 413
  dispersion of, 365
    by various substances, 365*t*
  intensity of, visibility and, 413
  speed, frequency, and wavelength of, 364
  transmittance of, 365
Light reflex, 273–274
  normal, 276*f*
  path of, 275*f*
Lipodermoids, orbital, 250
Livostin. *See* Levocabastine hydrochloride
Loa loa, conjunctivitis due to, 108
Lodoxamide tromethamine, **68**
Low-vision aids, **390–393**
Lubricating agents, **72**
Lupus erythematosus, systemic, 318
  cotton wool spots in, 334*f*
Lyme disease, 324
Lymphadenopathy, preauricular, 99
Lymphangiectasis, **118**
Lymphangioma, orbital, 252
Lymphatic disorders, ocular disorders associated with, **305–306**
Lymphedema, congenital conjunctival, **118**
Lymphoid hyperplasia, of conjunctiva, 120
Lymphoma
  of conjunctiva, 120
  of orbit, 253
Lymphosarcoma, of conjunctiva, 121

Macula
  diseases of, **187–195**
  inflammatory disorders involving, **190–191**
Macular degeneration
  age-related, **187–188**
    exudative, 187–188
    nonexudative, 187
    prevention of, 385
  laser treatment of, 404
  myopic, 192–193
Macular dystrophy, **194–195**
  anatomic classification of, 194*t*
  of corneal stroma, 139
Macular edema, **189–190**
  cystoid, 189*f*
Macular hole, 192–193
Macular membranes, epiretinal, 193
Macular neuroretinopathy, acute, 191
Maculopathy, traumatic, 193–194
Maddox rod test, 230–231
  double, 241
Magnetic resonance imaging (MRI), 59–60
  of orbit, 245
Magnification, 368

Magnifiers, low-vision, 391, 392*f*
Malar bone, 2
Mandol. *See* Cefamandole
Mannitol, **67**
Map-dot-fingerprint dystrophy, 139
Marcaine. *See* Bupivicaine hydrochloride
Marcus Gunn pupil. *See* Afferent pupillary defect
Marcus Gunn syndrome, 84, 282
Marfan's syndrome, 320, 322*f*
Marie-Strümpell ankylosing spondylitis. *See* Ankylosing spondylitis
Marseilles fever, conjunctivitis due to, 108
Maxilla, 1–2
Measles, 316
  keratoconjunctivitis due to, **107–108**
Medial palpebral ligament, 21
Medications. *See also specific type or agent*
  eye, **62–72**
    adverse effects of
      ocular, 75*t*
      systemic, 74*t*
        ways to diminish, 74–75
    diagnostic, 40
    topical administration of, 76*f*
  systemic, adverse ocular effects of, 73*t*, **325–328**, 386–387
  visual loss due to, prevention of, **386–387**
Medulloepitheliomas, ciliary body, 159
Meesman's dystrophy, 139
Megalocornea, 341
Meiosis, 348
Melanoma
  malignant, of conjunctiva, 121
  malignant
    of choroid, 159*f*
    of eyelid, 87
    of uveal tract, 159–160
Meningioma, suprasellar, 271, 272*f*
Mepivicaine hydrochloride, **63**
Mesoderm, 25
Metabolic disorders
  hereditary, ocular disorders associated with, **323**
  ocular disorders associated with, **306–309**
Methanol poisoning, optic neuropathy from, 267–268
Methazolamide, **66**
Methicillin, for endophthalmitis, dosages of, 69*t*
Metipranolol hydrochloride, **66**
Miconazole, **71**
  for endophthalmitis, dosages of, 69*t*
Microphthalmos, 341
Midbrain, lesions of, abnormal eye movements from, 279–280
Migraine, 290–291
Miliary tuberculosis, 312

Miotics
  for glaucoma, 216
  for strabismus, 234
Mitosis, 348
MK-927, **66–67**
Mobility training, for blind, 399
Moll, glands of, 17
Molluscum contagiosum, of eyelid, 85
  conjunctivitis due to, **107**
Monistat. *See* Miconazole
Monochromatism, 204
Mononuclear cell reaction, in acute viral conjunctivitis, 105*f*
Mononucleosis, infectious, 316
Mooren's ulcer, 133–134
Moraxella liquefaciens, corneal ulcers caused by, 128
MRI. *See* Magnetic resonance imaging (MRI)
Mucocele, orbital, 250
Mucocutaneous lymph node syndrome, **116**
Mucormycosis, 250, 316
Müller's muscle. *See* Superior tarsal muscle
Multiple evanescent white dot syndrome, 191
Multiple sclerosis, **260–261**
  clinical findings in, 260–261
  course, treatment, and prognosis of, 261
Mumps, 316
Mutations, 353
Myasthenia gravis, **283–284**
  blepharoptosis from, 83
  immunosuppression for, retinitis from, 326*f*
Mycobacterium fortuitum-chelonei, corneal ulcers caused by, 129
Mycostatin. *See* Nystatin
Mydriacyl. *See* Tropicamide
Mydriatics, 40, **63**
  adverse systemic effects of, 74*t*
  for glaucoma, 216
Myelinated nerve fibers, papilledema mimicked by, 266*f*
Myokymia, superior oblique, 282
Myopia, 31*f*, 375
  macular degeneration in, 192
Myotonic dystrophy, blepharoptosis from, 83
Myxedema, 311

Nanophthalmos, 341
Nasolacrimal duct obstruction, congenital, 343
Natacyn. *See* Natamycin
Natamycin, **71**
National Registry of Drug-Induced Ocular Side Effects, 75
Near reflex, 274
  spasm of, 280
Nearsightedness. *See* Myopia
Nebcin. *See* Tobramycin

Neo-synephrine. *See* Phenylephrine hydrochloride
Neomycin, **69**
Neoplastic disease, ocular disorders associated with, 305–306, 307*f*
Neptazane. *See* Methazolamide
Nerve loops of Axenfeld, intrascleral, 161
Neural crest, 25
Neural integrator, tonic cells of, 278
Neuro-ophthalmology, **255–293**
Neurofibroma, orbital, 252
Neurofibromatosis, 252, **291**
Neuromyelitis optica, 260
Neuroretinopathy, acute macular, 191
Neutralization, point of, 379
Nevus
  of choroid, 158, 159*f*
  of conjunctiva, 120
  of eyelid, 85
  flammeus, of eyelid, 86
  of iris, 158, 159*f*
Newcastle disease conjunctivitis, **106**
Nicotinic acid deficiency, 312
Nocardia, corneal ulcers caused by, 129
Nodal point, 367
Nonsteroidal anti-inflammatory agents (NSAIDs), **68**
Norfloxacin, topical, **70**
Novocaine. *See* Procaine hydrochloride
NSAIDS. *See* Nonsteroidal anti-inflammatory agents (NSAIDs)
Nuclear pathways, lesions of, **280–283**
Nystagmus, **285–288**
  acquired pendular, 288
  classification of, 286
  congenital, 286–287
  convergence-retraction, 287
  downbeat, 287
  end point, 286
  gaze-evoked, 288
  horizontal, 287–288
  latent, 287
  mimics of, 288
  optokinetic, 286
  pathologic, 286–287
  periodic alternating, 288
  physiologic, 286
  physiology of symptoms of, 285–286
  seesaw, 287
  upbeat, 287
  vestibular, 288
  voluntary, 287–288
Nystatin, **71**

Oblique muscle(s), **15**
  inferior, 15
  superior, 15
Occipital lobe, lesions of, abnormal eye movements from, 279

Occlusion therapy, 233–234
Ocuflox. *See* Ofloxacin
Ocular abnormalities. *See also specific type*
   congenital, **341–343**
   diagnosis of, **50–57**
Ocular adnexa, **16–21**. *See also specific structure*
   external examination of, 34
Ocular disease. *See also specific type*
   early detection of treatable, **385**
Ocular ferning test, in dry eye syndrome, 92
Ocular herpes. *See* Conjunctivitis, herpes simplex virus
Ocular hypertension, 218
Ocular infection. *See also specific type*
   iatrogenic, prevention of, **384**
   prevention of, **382–383**
Ocular ischemia
   acute, **297–298**
   chronic, **302–303**, 304*f*
Ocular motility
   in industrial evaluation, 409–411
   testing of, 34
Ocular muscles. *See Extraocular muscles*
Ocular rosacea, **114–115**, 324
Ocular secretions, 31
Oculoglandular disease, **119**
Oculomotor nerve, 23, 280–281
Oculomotor palsy, 84, 281
   cyclic, 281–282
Oculomotor synkinesis, 281
Ocupress. *See* Carteolol hydrochloride
Ofloxacin, topical, **70**
Onchocerciasis, **158**
   blindness from, 398
Ophthaine. *See* Proparacaine hydrochloride
Ophthalmia
   neonatorum, **118–119**, **344**
      prevention of, 383
   nodosum, **114**
   sympathetic, **156–157**, **335**
Ophthalmodynamometry, 60
Ophthalmologic examination, **29–60**
   basic, **31–45**
   in low vision, 388–389
   neonatal, **339–340**
   pediatric, **339–341**
      schedule for, 339
   specialized, **45–60**
Ophthalmomyiasis, 109
Ophthalmoplegia
   chronic progressive external, 83, 284
   complete (sudden), 283
   in Graves' disease, 310
   internuclear, **280**
Ophthalmoscopy
   comparison of direct and indirect, 44–45
   direct, **40–43**
   indirect, **43–45**
   of newborn, 340

Optic chiasm, 23, 24*f*
   disorders of, **271–272**
Optic cup, 25
Optic disk
   assessment of, in glaucoma, 213
   glaucomatous cupping of, 213*f*, 214*f*
   tilted, 269, 270*f*
Optic disk infarction, 297, 298*f*
Optic nerve, **21–23**
   anomalies of, 269
   atrophy of, **265–266**
      clinical findings in, 266
      congenital/infantile hereditary, 269
      etiologic classification of, 265–266
      with neurodegenerative diseases, 269
   blood supply of, 22*f*, 23
   disorders of, **257–270**. *See also* Optic neuropathy
      congenital, 342–343
      etiologic classification of, 259*t*
   embryology of, 28
   hypoplasia of, 269, 270*f*, 342–343
   sheaths of, 21–23
   trauma to, 268
Optic nerve glioma, 252, 271–272
Optic neuritis, **257–260**
   clinical findings in, 257–259
   differential diagnosis of, 259–260
   in multiple sclerosis, 260–261, 262*f*
Optic neuropathy
   in diabetes, 309
   in Graves' disease, 310
   ischemic, **261–262**
      acute, 263*f*
      chronic, 264*f*
   Leber's, 268–269
   toxic-nutritional, **266–268**
Optic vesicle, 25
Opticrom. *See* Cromolyn sodium
Optics, **364–380**
   algebraic method in, 367–368
   calculations used in, **366–374**
OptiPranolol. *See* Metipranolol hydrochloride
Oral contraceptives, ocular complications of, 327
Orbicularis oculi muscle, 16
Orbit, **1–4**
   apex of, 2–3
   blood supply of, 3–4, 5*f*, 6*f*
   bones of, 1*f*, 2*f*
   contusions of, 362
   cystic lesions involving, **250**
   diagnostic studies of, **245–248**
   diseases and disorders of, **248–253**
      congenital, 343
      physiology of symptoms in, 245
   evaluation of, **57–59**
   infections of, 249–250
   inflammatory disorders of, **248–249**
   injuries to, **361–362**
      penetrating, 362

   pulsating exophthalmos following, 362
   pseudotumor of, 249
   tumors of, **251–253**
      metastatic, 253
      primary, 251–253
      secondary, 253
      vascular abnormalities involving, **250–251**
   walls of, 1–2
Orbital apex syndrome, 283
Orbital cellulitis, 249–250
Orbital fissure, superior, 2–3
Orbital fracture, 361–362
   blowout, 361*f*
Orbital septum, 17–18
Orthophoria, 226
Orthoptics, 234
Oscillopsia, 30
Osmitrol. *See* Mannitol
Osmoglyn. *See* Glycerin
Osmotic agents, **67**
Osteogenesis imperfecta, 321
Oxygen, role of, in retinopathy of prematurity, 327

Pain
   ocular, 30
   periocular, 30
   retrobulbar, 30
Palatine bone, 2
Palpebrae. *See* Eyelids
Palpebral conjunctiva, 5, 17
Palpebral fissure, 17
Pannus, trachomatous, 101*f*
Panum's area, 229
Papilledema, 259*f*, **262–265**
   mimicked by myelinated nerve fibers, 266*f*
Papillitis, 259*f*
Papillomas
   of conjunctiva, 120
   of eyelid, 85
Parasympatholytic agents. *See* Cycloplegics
Parasympathomimetic agents. *See* Cholinergic drugs
Paratrachoma. *See* Conjunctivitis, inclusion
Parinaud's oculogandular syndrome, **119**
Patau's syndrome, 352
Pattern ERG (PERG). *See* Electroretinography (ERG)
Pearl diver's keratopathy, 118, 138
Pellagra, 312
Pemphigoid, cicatricial, **113**, 334
Pemphigus vulgaris, 334–335
Perimeters
   computerized automated, 47, 48*f*
   Goldmann, 47
Perimetry, **45–47**
   kinetic, 46–47
   static, 46

Periocular tissues, appearance of, abnormalities in, 30
Peter's anomaly, 221
Phacoemulsification, 171
Phacofragmentation, 171
Phacolytic glaucoma, 222
Phakomatoses, **291–293**
Pharyngoconjunctival fever, **104–105**
Phenobarbital, ocular complications of, 327
Phenothiazines, ocular complications of, 327
Phenotype, 348
Phenylephrine hydrochloride, **63**
  with cyclopentolate hydrochloride, **64**
Phenytoin, ocular complications of, 327
  fetal, 328
Phlyctenular keratoconjunctivitis, 134, 336
Phlyctenules, 99, 336f
Phlyctenulosis, **111–112**
Phoria. See Heterophoria
Phoropter, 32f
Phospholine iodide. See Echothiophate iodide
Photo-evaporation, 402
Photocoagulation, 401–402
Photodecomposition, 402
Photodisruption, 402
Photomydriasis, laser, 405–406
Photopsia, 179
Photorefraction, 386
Physostigmine salicylate and sulfate, **65**
Pigment dispersion syndrome, 222
Pigment epithelium, hemorrhages under, 297
Pigmentary glaucoma, 221–222
Pilocarpine hydrochloride & nitrate, **64**
Pinguecula, **117**
Pinhole test, 32
Pinkeye. See Conjunctivitis, bacterial
Pituitary adenoma, 271f
Pituitary tumors, 271
Plateau iris, 220
Platelet-fibrin emboli, amaurosis fugax from, 297
Plica semilunaris, 17
Pneumatotonometer, 40
Point of neutralization, 379
Poliomyelitis, 315
Polyarteritis nodosa, 318–319, 335
Polycoria, 342
Polymyxin B, **70**
Pons, lesions of, abnormal eye movements from, 280
Pontocaine. See Tetracaine hydrochloride
Port wine stain. See Nevus flammeus
Position of minimum deviation, 370, 372f
Posterior fixation procedure, 235–236

Posterior polymorphous dystrophy, 140
Postphlyctenulosis, 112f
Potential acuity meters, 49–50
Prenatal diagnosis, 352
Prentice position, 370, 372f
Preretinal hemorrhage, 296
Presbyopia, 375
Preservatives, adverse ocular effects of, 75t
Pressure, hydrostatic, 209–210
Pressure dynamics, **209–211**
Presumed ocular histoplasmosis syndrome, 190
Principal plane, 367
Prism base notation, 371f
Prism diopters, 226, 372, 373f
Prism reflex method, 232
Prism test, in strabismus, 230
Prisms, **370–373**
  calibration of, 372f
  Fresnel, 374f
  in treatment of heterophoria, 243–244
  in treatment of strabismus, 234
Procaine hydrochloride, **63**
Proparacaine hydrochloride, **62**
Proptosis, from arteriovenous malformation, 250–251
Protanopia, 204
Pseudo-exfoliation syndrome, 222
Pseudoesotropia, 238–239
Pseudomonas, corneal ulcers caused by, 126
Pseudoptosis, in conjunctivitis, 98
Pseudotumor cerebri, 304–305
Psoriasis, conjunctivitis in, **115**
Pterygium, **117–118**
Pthirus pubis, conjunctivitis due to, 109
Ptosis. See Blepharoptosis
Pubic louse. See Pthirus pubis
Pulseless disease, 320
Pupillary pathways, neuroanatomy of, 273–274
Pupil(s)
  Argyll Robertson, 274
  disorders of, **273–276**
    congenital, 342
  examination of, 33–34
  light reflex of. See Light reflex
  Marcus Gunn. See Afferent pupillary defect
  near reflex of. See Near reflex
  tonic, 274
Purtscher's retinopathy, 194

Q fever, conjunctivitis due to, 108
Quinacrine, ocular complications of, 327–328
Quinine, ocular complications of, 327–328

Radiation
  ocular complications of, 328
  ultraviolet, ocular effects of, 382
Radiology, ophthalmic, 59
Raeder's paratrigeminal syndrome, 275–276
Random dot stereograms, 233
Ray tracing
  graphic, 367
  through plus and minus lenses, 369f
  trigonometric, 366–367
Rectus muscles, 15
Red reflex examination, 43
Reduction-division meiosis, 348
Reflection
  laws of, 365
  total, 365–366
Refraction, 31, 32f
  cycloplegic, 379–380
  index of, 364
    thermal coefficient of, 364–365
    for various substances, 365t
  laws of, 365
  methods of, **379–380**
  objective, 379
  in pediatric examination, 340–341
  subjective, 379
  sudden changes in, in diabetes, 309
Refractive corneal surgery, **144–145**, 378
  lasers in, 145, 406–407
Refractive errors, 31, **375–379**
  correction of, **378–379**
  natural history of, 377
  in strabismus, 230
Reiter's disease, **116**, 320, 332–333
  acute iridocyclitis in, 332f
Retina, 11–13
  angiograms of, 54f, 55f
  changes to, in Graves' disease, 310
  colobomas of, 341
  congenital abnormalities of, 342
  embryology of, 27–28
  examination of, 186–187
  hole in, posttraumatic, 358f
  layers of, 14f
  lesions to, in posterior uveitis, 153
  peripheral, diseases of, **196–199**
  physiology of, 186
  Toxoplasma cysts in, 154f
Retinal arterial macroaneurysm, **203–204**
Retinal artery occlusion
  branch, **202**
  central, **202**
Retinal correspondence, anomalous, 229
Retinal degenerations, **197–198**
Retinal detachment, **180–182**, 181f, **196–197**
  rhegmatogenous, 196
  serous and hemorrhagic, 196–197
  traction, 182, 196
    surgery for, 185f
  from vitreous collapse, 178f

Retinal detachment *(cont.)*
with vitreous contracture, surgery for, 185*f*
vitreous membrane with, 177*f*, 178*f*
Retinal hemorrhage, 296–297
Retinal infarction, 297, 298*f*, 299*f*
acute, 302*f*
Retinal ischemia, transient. *See* Amaurosis fugax
Retinal necrosis syndrome, acute, 315
Retinal tears, 179–180, 181*f*
laser treatment of, 403
Retinal vascular diseases, **199–204**
Retinal vein occlusion
branch, **203**, **300**, 301*f*
laser treatment of, 403
central, **202–203**, **298–300**
laser treatment of, 403
Retinal vessels, sclerotic, appearance of, 301
Retinitis
in immunosuppressed patient, 326*f*
pigmentosa, 197–198
punctata albescens, 195
Retinoblastoma, **205–206**, 345
after radiotherapy, 206*f*
endophytic, 205*f*
genetics of, 353
Retinocerebellar angiomatosis. *See* Von Hippel-Lindau disease
Retinochoroidopathy, birdshot, 191
Retinopathy
diabetic, **199–202**, 306–308
background, 199
laser treatment of, 402–403
nonproliferative, **199–201**
preproliferative, 200
prevention of ocular damage from, 386
proliferative, **201–202**, 308*f*
hypertensive, **301–302**, 303*f*, 304*f*
of prematurity, **197**, **344–345**
role of oxygen in, 327
stages of, 197*t*
Purtscher's, 194
solar, 194, 382
Retinoschisis
degenerative, 198–199
reticular, 199
X-linked juvenile, 194
Retinoscopic reflex, 379
movement of, 380*f*
Retrochiasmatic visual pathways, 23
Rhabdomyosarcoma, orbital, 252
Riboflavin deficiency, 312
Rieger's syndrome, 221
Rocky Mountain spotted fever, conjunctivitis due to, 108
Rod monochromatism, 204
Rosacea. *See* Acne rosacea
Rose bengal, **72**
Rose bengal staining
in dry eye syndrome, 92*f*, 93
in evaluation of lacrimal system, 57

Roth's spots, 297
Rubella, 316
Rubeola. *See* Measles
Rubeosis iridis, 309

Saccadic generator, burst cells of, 278
Salivary glands, accessory, mononuclear infiltration of, in Sjögren's syndrome, 113*f*
Salzmann's nodular degeneration, 138
Sanders-Retzlaff-Kraff (SRK) equation, 378
Sarcoidosis, **157**, 312, 313*f*, **331**
Sarcoma, of eyelid, 87
Schirmer test, 57, 91
Schistosoma haematobium, conjunctivitis due to, 109
Sclera, 7
blue, 160
in osteogenesis imperfecta, 321
diseases and disorders of, **160–163**
embryology of, 27
hyaline degeneration of, 163
Scleral depression, 44, 46*f*
Scleral ectasia, 160
Scleritis, **161–163**
anterior, 162–163
causes of, 162*t*
laboratory workup for, 162*t*
necrotizing, 162–163
nodular, 161*f*
associated with rheumatoid arthritis, 162*f*
posterior, 162
Scleroderma, 318
Sclerostomy, laser, 406
Scopolamine hydrobromide, **64**
Scotoma
central, management of, 394
centrocecal
in methyl alcohol amblyopia, 268*f*
in nutritional amblyopia, 267*f*
peripheral, management of, 394–395
in strabismus, 229
Scurvy, 312
Secretions, ocular, 31
Sedative tranquilizers, ocular complications of, 328
Seesaw nystagmus, 287
Semicircular canals, stimulation of, in nystagmus, 286
Semilunar fold, 5
Sensorcaine. *See* Bupivicaine hydrochloride
Sex chromosomes, 348
abnormalities involving, 352
Sezolamide hydrochloride, **66–67**
Shaken baby syndrome, 346
Shear modulus G, 211
Sherrington's law, 228
Sickle cell disease, 305

Simultaneous confrontation testing, 33
Sinus mucocele, orbital, 250
Sjögren's syndrome, 319
keratoconjunctivitis sicca associated with, **112**, 113*f*
Slitlamp examination, **34–38**
adjunctive techniques of, 35–38
basic techniques of, 34–35
of vitreous, 175
Snellen chart, 31–32
Solar retinopathy, 194, 382
Spasmus nutans, 287
Spectacle aids, low-vision, 391
Spectacles, 378
for strabismus, 234
Sphenoid bone, 2
Spherical aberration, 367, 369
of biconvex lens, 370*f*
Spheroidal degeneration, 118, 138
Sphincterotomy, laser, 405–406
SRK (Sanders-Retzlaff-Kraff) equation, 378
Stand magnifiers, 391, 392*f*
Staphcillin. *See* Methicillin
Staphylococcus, corneal ulcers caused by, 129
Staphyloma, 160–161
ciliary, 161*f*
Stargardt's disease, 195
Stereopsis, 229
testing for, 233
Stevens-Johnson syndrome, **115**, 116*f*, 323
Still's disease. *See* Arthritis, juvenile rheumatoid
Stocker's line, 142
Stoxil. *See* Idoxuridine
Strabismus, **226–244**, 345–346
amblyopia from, prevention of, 385
angle of, determination of, 230–232
classification of, 236
convergent, **236–239**. *See also* Esotropia
divergent, **239–240**. *See also* Exotropia
examination for, **230–233**
motor aspects of, 227–228
physiology of, **227–230**
sensory aspects of, 229–230
special forms of, **241–243**
treatment of, **233–236**
in children, timing of, 233
medical, 233–234
surgical, 235–236
A and V patterns in, 240
Strain, 210–211
Streptococcus
α-hemolytic, corneal ulcers caused by, 129
group A, corneal ulcers caused by, 128–129
pneumoniae, corneal ulcers caused by, 126
Sturge-Weber syndrome, 292
Sturm, conoid of, 370, 371*f*

Subarachnoid hemorrhage, 290
Subconjunctival hemorrhage, **118**
Subdural hemorrhage, 289–290
Subhyaloid hemorrhage, 290*f*
Subretinal hemorrhage, 297
Sulamyd. *See* Sulfacetamide sodium
Sulfacetamide sodium, **71**
Sulfisoxazole, **71**
Sulfonamides, **70–71**
Superior oblique myokymia, 282
Superior oblique tendon sheath syndrome, 242–243
Superior orbital fissure syndrome, 283
Superior tarsal muscle, 18
Suppression, 229
 testing for, 233
Supranuclear pathways, lesions of, **279–280**
Suprasellar meningiomas, 271
Sutures, adjustable, in strabismus surgery, 236
Swinging penlight test, 33–34
Sympathomimetic agents. *See* Adrenergic drugs; Mydriatics
Synechiae
 anterior, 148*f*
  peripheral, 223
 posterior, 148*f*
Syneresis, of vitreous, 179
Syphilis
 acquired, 314
 congenital, 314
  interstitial keratitis due to, **141**
Systemic diseases, ocular disorders associated with, **296–328**
 prevention of, **386**
Systemic lupus erythematosus, 318, 333
 cotton wool spots in, 334*f*

Taenia solium, conjunctivitis due to, **109**
Takayasu, idiopathic arteritis of, 320
Tamoxifen, ocular complications of, 328
Tangent screen, 47
Tardive dyskinesia, 82
Tarsal plates, 16–17
Tay-Sachs disease, 293*f*
Tear film
 break-up time of, in dry eye syndrome, 91–92
 layers of, 90
Tear lysozyme assay, in dry eye syndrome, 93
Tear osmolality, in dry eye syndrome, 93
Tear production, evaluation of, 57
Tear replacement agents, **72**
Tearing, 30–31
 in conjunctivitis, 97–98
Tears, **90–94**
 bloody, 88

composition of, 90–91
 "crocodile," 88
Telescopes, low-vision, 391–392, 393*f*
Temporal arteritis, 320
Tenon's capsule, 6–7, 16*f*
Tension (tensile stress), 210
Terrien's disease, 137
Terson's syndrome, 194
Tetracaine hydrochloride, **62**
Tetracyclines, topical, **70**
Thelazia californiensis, conjunctivitis due to, 108
Therapeutic soft contact lenses, 143
Thin lens equations, 367
Thyroid disease, conjunctivitis in, 116–117
Thyroid function tests, 309*t*
Thyroid gland disorders, **309–311**
Tilted disk, 269, 270*f*
Timolol maleate, **65**
 systemic side effects of, 72–74
Timoptic. *See* Timolol maleate
Tints, for low-vision aids, 392–393
Tobacco-alcohol amblyopia, 266–267
Tobramycin
 for endophthalmitis, dosages of, 69*t*
 topical, **70**
Tobrex. *See* Tobramycin
Tonic pupil, 274
Tono-Pen, 40
Tonometers
 Goldmann, 39
 Perkins, 40
 Schiotz, 38–39
Tonometry, **38–40**
 applanation, 39–40
 in assessment of glaucoma, 211–212
 noncontact, 40
 Schiotz, 38–39
Torsion, 227
Toxocariasis, **155–156**
Toxoplasmosis, **154–155**, **314–315**
 acquired, 314–315
 congenital, 314
Trabeculodysgenesis, 221
Trabeculoplasty, laser, 216
Trachoma, **101–103**
 blindness from, 397–398
 clinical findings in, 101–102
 complications and sequelae of, 102
 course and prognosis of, 103
 differential diagnosis of, 102
 laboratory findings in, 102
 treatment of, 102–103
Tranquilizers, ocular complications of, 327–328
Trauma, **356–362**. *See also structure affected*
 cataract from, **169–170**
 from child abuse, 346
 glaucoma secondary to, 223
 immediate management of, 356
 initial examination of, 356
Trephine, Castroviejo disposable, 144*f*

Trichiasis, 80
Trichinella spiralis, conjunctivitis due to, 109
Trichromats, anomalous, 204
Trifluridine, **71**
Trigeminal nerve, 24
Trigger mechanisms, control of, in herpes simplex keratitis, 132
Trigonometric ray tracing, 366–367
Trisomy 13, 352
Trisomy 18, 352
Trisomy 21, 352
Tritanopia, 204
Trochlear nerve, 23–24, 282
Trochlear paralysis, 282
Tropia. *See* Heterotropia
Tropicamide, **64**
Tuberculosis, 312
Tuberculous uveitis, **157**, 312
Tuberous sclerosis, 292–293
Tumors. *See specific type and structure affected*
Typhus, conjunctivitis due to, 108

Ultrasonography
 A scan, 59
 B scan, 59
  in orbital evaluation, 58–59, 245
  of vitreous, 175–176
Ultraviolet radiation, ocular effects of, 382
Uncover test, 230
Upbeat nystagmus, 287
Upgaze nystagmus, 287
Urea, **67**
Ureaphil. *See* Urea
Uveal tract, **7–9**
 disorders of, **147–160**
  glaucoma secondary to, 222–223
  physiology of symptoms of, 147
 tuberculosis of, **157**, 312
 tumors involving, **158–160**
  glaucoma from, 223
Uveitis, **147–158**
 anterior, **150–152**
  causes of, 151*t*
 associated with joint disease, 150–151
 in childhood, 344
 clinical findings in, 148–149
 course and prognosis of, 149–150
 differential diagnosis of, 149
 diffuse, **156–158**
  causes of, 156*t*
 glaucoma from, 222–223
 granulomatous
  and nongranulomatous, differentiation of, 148*t*
 treatment of, 149, 150*t*
 heterochromic, 151
 intermediate, **152**
 lens-induced, 151, 334

Uveitis *(cont.)*
 nongranulomatous, treatment of,
  149
 posterior, **152–156**
  causes of, 152*t*
  diagnosis and clinical features of,
   152–154
 sympathetic, **156–157**
 treatment of, 149
 tuberculous, **157**, 312

Vancocin. *See* **Vancomycin**
Vancomycin, for endophthalmitis,
 dosages of, 69*t*
Varicella-zoster, **315**
 blepharoconjunctivitis due to, **107**
 keratitis due to, **132**
Vascular disease
 ocular disorders associated with,
  296–305
 retinal, **199–204**
  pathologic appearances in,
   296–300
Vasoconstrictors, **72**
Venography, orbital, 247
Vergences, 227
Vernal keratoconjunctivitis, **110–111**,
 331–332
Versions, 227
 testing for, 232
Vertebrobasilar arterial system, vascular insufficiency of, 289
Vertex distance, change of, 368–369
Vestibular nystagmus, 287
Vestibulo-ocular responses, 277–278
Vidarabine, **71**
Vietnamese-Americans, glaucoma in,
 220
Vira-A. *See* Vidarabine
Viral diseases, ocular disorders associated with, **315–316**
Viroptic. *See* Trifluridine
Vision
 abnormalities of
  diagnosis of, examination techniques for, **45–50**
  ocular history and, 29–30
 blurred/hazy, management of, 394
 central, testing of, 31–32
 color. *See* Color vision
 double. *See* Diplopia
 loss of
  functional, 50
  ocular history and, 29–30
  percentage of, AMA method of
   evaluation of, 409
 low, **388–395**

activities adversely affected by,
  389*t*
 management of, **393–395**
  training programs for, 395
 optical aids for, **390–393**
 testing of, 32–33
 near, testing of, 389
 peripheral, testing of, 32–33
 potential, assessment of, 49–50
 testing of, **31–33**
  in children, **340**
Visual aberrations, ocular history and,
 30
Visual acuity, 375
 corrected, 32
 development of, 340*t*
 in industrial evaluation, 409
 in strabismus, 230
 uncorrected, 32
Visual confusion, 229
Visual distortion, 30
Visual efficiency, industrial, 409–411
Visual evoked response, 56–57
Visual field
 analysis of, in localizing lesions in
  visual pathways, 257, 258*f*
 assessment of
  in glaucoma, 213–214
  in industrial evaluation, 409, 410
 changes in, in glaucoma, 215*f*
Visual impairment. *See also* Blindness; Vision, low
 categories of, 396*t*
Visual pathway(s), 255–257
 retrochiasmatic, lesions of,
  272–273, 274*f*
 topography of, 256
Visual standards, **409–412**
 for armed forces, 411
 for drivers' licenses, 411
 educational, 411–412
 industrial, 409–411
Visually handicapped children, education of, 411–412
Vitamin A deficiency, 312
 corneal ulcers due to, 134–135,
  312*f*
Vitamin B deficiency, 312
Vitamin C deficiency, 312
Vitamins, eye disease and, **312**
Vitelliform dystrophy, 195
Vitreoretinopathy, proliferative,
 182–183
Vitreous, 13–14
 disorders of, **176–184**
  congenital, 342
 embryology of, 28
 examination of, **175–176**

foreign body in, 359*f*
 persistent hyperplastic primary, 342
 reduction of volume of, in treatment
  of glaucoma, 216
Vitreous abscess. *See* Endophthalmitis
Vitreous bands/opacities, laser cutting
 of, 406
Vitreous collapse, 178*f*, **179**, 180*f*
 posterior, 179*f*
Vitreous contracture, retinal detach-
 ment with, surgery for, 185*f*
Vitreous detachment, 175*f*
Vitreous floaters, **176–178**
Vitreous hemorrhage, 176*f*, **180**
 acute, 181*f*
 chronic, 181*f*
 removal of, 185*f*
Vitreous inflammation, **183–184**
Vitreous loss, 183
Vitreous membrane, 177*f*, 178*f*
Vitreous surgery, **184–185**
Vitritis, in posterior uveitis, 153
Vogt-Koyanagi-Harada syndrome,
 323, 324*f*, **335**
Von Hippel-Lindau disease, 205*f*,
 291–292

**Warfarin, fetal ocular abnormalities
 from, 328**
Wegener's granulomatosis, 319
White dot syndrome, multiple evanes-
 cent, 191
Wilson's disease, 323
Working distance, 379
Worth four-dot test, 233
Wyburn-Mason syndrome, 292

X-linked juvenile retinoschisis, 194
X-rays, 59
 of orbit, 248
Xanthelasma, 85, 86*f*
Xanthopsia, from chlorothiazide, 327
Xeroderma pigmentosum, carcinoma
 associated with, 87
Xerophthalmia, 135, 312*f*
 blindness from, 398
Xylocaine. *See* Lidocaine hydrochlo-
 ride

Young's modulus E, 211

Zeis, glands of, 17
Zovirax. *See* Acyclovir
Zygomatic bone, 2

Basic Science Textbooks

Biochemistry
Examination & Board Review
Balcavage & King
1995, ISBN 0-8385-0661-5, A0661-7

Color Atlas of Basic Histology
Berman
1993, ISBN 0-8385-0445-0, A0445-5

1996 First Aid for the USMLE Step 1
Bhushan, et al.
1996, ISBN 0-8385-2597-0, A2597-1

Jawetz, Melnick, & Adelberg's
Medical Microbiology, 20/e
Brooks, Butel, & Ornston
1995, ISBN 0-8385-6243-4, A6243-8

Manual for Human Dissection
Photographs with Clinical
Applications
Callas
1994, ISBN 0-8385-6133-0, A6133-1

Concise Pathology, 2/e
Chandrasoma & Taylor
1995, ISBN 0-8385-1229-1, A1229-2

Introduction to Clinical Psychiatry
Elkin
1996, ISBN 0-8385-4333-2, A4333-9

Medical Biostatistics & Epidemiology
Examination & Board Review
Essex-Sorlie
1995, ISBN 0-8385-6219-1, A6219-8

Fundamentals of Medical Cell Biology
and Histology
Fuller
1996, ISBN 0-8385-1384-0, A1384-5

Review of Medical Physiology, 17/e
Ganong
1995, ISBN 0-8385-8431-4, A8431-7

First Aid for the USMLE Step 2
A Student-to-Student Guide
Go, Curet-Salim, & Fullerton
1996, ISBN 0-8385-2591-1, A2591-4

Medical Epidemiology, 2/e
Greenberg, Daniels, Flanders, Eley, &
Boring
1996, ISBN 0-8385-6206-X, A6206-5

Basic Histology, 8/e
Junqueira, Carneiro, & Kelley
1995, ISBN 0-8385-0567-8, A0567-6

Basic & Clinical Pharmacology, 6/e
Katzung
1995, ISBN 0-8385-0619-4, A0619-5

Pharmacology
Examination & Board Review, 4/e
Katzung & Trevor
1995, ISBN 0-8385-8067-X, A8067-9

First Aid for the Match
Le, Bhushan, & Amin
1996, ISBN 0-8385-2596-2, A2596-3

Medical Microbiology & Immunology
Examination & Board Review, 4/e
Levinson & Jawetz
1996, ISBN 0-8385-6225-6, A6225-5

Clinical Anatomy
Lindner
1989, ISBN 0-8385-1259-3, A1259-9

Pathophysiology of Disease
McPhee, Lingappa, Ganong, & Lange
1995, ISBN 0-8385-7815-2, A7815-2

Harper's Biochemistry, 23/e
Murray, Granner, Mayes, & Rodwell
1993, ISBN 0-8385-3562-3, A3562-4

Pathology
Examination & Board Review
Newland
1995, ISBN 0-8385-7719-9, A7719-6

Basic Histology
Examination & Board Review, 3/e
Paulsen
1996, ISBN 0-8385-2282-3, A2282-0

Basic & Clinical Immunology, 8/e
Stites, Terr, & Parslow
1994, ISBN 0-8385-0561-9, A0561-9

Correlative Neuroanatomy, 22/e
Waxman & deGroot
1995, ISBN 0-8385-1091-4, A1091-6

Clinical Science Textbooks

Clinical Neurology, 3/e
Aminoff, Greenberg, & Simon
1996, ISBN 0-8385-1383-2, A1383-7

Understanding Health Policy:
A Clinical Approach
Bodenheimer & Grumbach
1995, ISBN 0-8385-3678-6, A3678-8

(more on reverse)

Clinical Cardiology, 6/e
Cheitlin, Sokolow, & McIlroy
1993, ISBN 0-8385-1093-0, A1093-2

Fluid & Electrolytes
Physiology & Pathophysiology
Cogan
1991, ISBN 0-8385-2546-6, A2546-8

Basic & Clinical Biostatistics, 2/e
Dawson-Saunders & Trapp
1994, ISBN 0-8385-0542-2, A0542-9

Basic Gynecology and Obstetrics
Gant & Cunningham
1993, ISBN 0-8385-9633-9, A9633-7

Review of General Psychiatry, 4/e
Goldman
1995, ISBN 0-8385-8421-7, A8421-8

**Principles of Clinical
Electrocardiography, 13/e**
Goldschlager & Goldman
1990, ISBN 0-8385-7951-5, A7951-5

Basic & Clinical Endocrinology, 4/e
Greenspan & Baxter
1994, ISBN 0-8385-0560-0, A0560-1

Occupational Medicine
LaDou
1990, ISBN 0-8385-7207-3, A7207-2

Primary Care of Women
Lemcke, Pattison, Marshall, & Cowley
1995, ISBN 0-8385-9813-7, A9813-5

Clinical Anesthesiology, 2/e
Morgan & Mikhail
1996, ISBN 0-8385-1381-6, A1381-1

Dermatology
Orkin, Maibach, & Dahl
1991, ISBN 0-8385-1288-7, A1288-8

**Rudolph's Fundamentals of
Pediatrics**
Rudolph & Kamei
1994, ISBN 0-8385-8233-8, A8233-7

**Genetics in Clinical Medicine and
Primary Care**
Seashore
1995, ISBN 0-8385-3128-8, A3128-4

Smith's General Urology, 14/e
Tanagho & McAninch
1995, ISBN 0-8385-8612-0, A8612-2

Clinical Oncology
Weiss
1993, ISBN 0-8385-1325-5, A1325-8

General Ophthalmology, 14/e
Vaughan, Asbury, & Riordan-Eva
1995, ISBN 0-8385-3127-X, A3127-6

CURRENT Clinical References

**CURRENT Critical Care Diagnosis &
Treatment,**
Bongard & Sue
1994, ISBN 0-8385-1443-X, A1443-9

**CURRENT Diagnosis & Treatment in
Cardiology**
Crawford
1995, ISBN 0-8385-1444-8, A1444-7

**CURRENT Diagnosis & Treatment in
Vascular Surgery**
Dean, Yao, & Brewster
1995, ISBN 0-8385-1351-4, A1351-4

**CURRENT Obstetric & Gynecologic
Diagnosis & Treatment, 8/e**
DeCherney & Pernoll
1994, ISBN 0-8385-1447-2, A1447-0

**CURRENT Diagnosis & Treatment in
Gastroenterology**
Grendell, McQuaid, & Friedman
1996, ISBN 0-8385-1448-0, A1448-8

**CURRENT Pediatric Diagnosis &
Treatment, 12/e**
Hay, Groothuis, Hayward, & Levin
1995, ISBN 0-8385-1446-4, A1446-2

**CURRENT Emergency Diagnosis &
Treatment, 4/e**
Saunders & Ho
1993, ISBN 0-8385-1347-6, A1347-2

**CURRENT Diagnosis & Treatment in
Orthopedics**
Skinner
1995, ISBN 0-8385-1009-4, A1009-8

**CURRENT Medical Diagnosis &
Treatment 1996**
Tierney, McPhee, & Papadakis
1996, ISBN 0-8385-1465-0, A1465-2

**CURRENT Surgical Diagnosis &
Treatment, 10/e**
Way
1994, ISBN 0-8385-1439-1, A1439-7

LANGE Clinical Manuals

Dermatology
Diagnosis and Therapy
Bondi, Jegasothy, & Lazarus
1991, ISBN 0-8385-1274-7, A1274-8

Practical Oncology
Cameron
1994, ISBN 0-8385-1326-3, A1326-6

Office & Bedside Procedures
Chesnutt, Dewar, Locksley, & Tureen
1993, ISBN 0-8385-1095-7, A1095-7

Psychiatry
Diagnosis & Therapy 2/e
Flaherty, Davis, & Janicak
1993, ISBN 0-8385-1267-4, A1267-2

Neonatology
*Management, Procedures, On-Call
Problems, Diseases and Drugs, 3/e*
Gomella
1994, ISBN 0-8385-1331-X, A1331-6

Practical Gynecology
Jacobs & Gast
1994, ISBN 0-8385-1336-0, A1336-5

Drug Therapy, 2/e
Katzung
1991, ISBN 0-8385-1312-3, A1312-6

Ambulatory Medicine
The Primary Care of Families
Mengel & Schwiebert
1993, ISBN 0-8385-1294-1, A1294-6

Poisoning & Drug Overdose, 2/e
Olson
1994, ISBN 0-8385-1108-2, A1108-8

Internal Medicine
Diagnosis and Therapy, 3/e
Stein
1993, ISBN 0-8385-1112-0, A1112-0

Surgery
Diagnosis & Therapy
Stillman
1989, ISBN 0-8385-1283-6, A1283-9

Medical Perioperative Management
Wolfsthal
1989, ISBN 0-8385-1298-4, A1298-7

LANGE Handbooks

**Handbook of Gynecology &
Obstetrics**
Brown & Crombleholme
1993, ISBN 0-8385-3608-5, A3608-5

HIV/AIDS Primary Care Handbook
Carmichael, Carmichael, & Fischl
1995, ISBN 0-8385-3557-7, A3557-4

Pocket Guide to Diagnostic Tests
Detmer, McPhee, Nicoll, & Chou
1992, ISBN 0-8385-8020-3, A8020-8

Handbook of Poisoning
*Prevention, Diagnosis & Treatment,
12/e*
Dreisbach & Robertson
1987, ISBN 0-8385-3643-3, A3643-2

**Handbook of Clinical Endocrinology,
2/e**
Fitzgerald
1992, ISBN 0-8385-3615-8, A3615-0

Clinician's Pocket Reference, 7/e
Gomella
1993, ISBN 0-8385-1222-4, A1222-7

Surgery on Call, 2/e
Gomella & Lefor
1996, ISBN 0-8385-8746-1, A8746-8

Internal Medicine On Call
Haist & Robbins
1991, ISBN 0-8385-4052-X, A4052-5

Obstetrics & Gynecology On Call
Horowitz & Gomella
1993, ISBN 0-8385-7174-3, A7174-4

**Pocket Guide to Commonly
Prescribed Drugs**
Levine
1993, ISBN 0-8385-8023-8, A8023-2

Handbook of Pediatrics, 17/e
Merenstein, Kaplan, & Rosenberg
1994, ISBN 0-8385-3657-3, A3657-2

 Appleton & Lange • P.O. Box 120041 • Stamford, CT • 06912-0041 • 1-800-423-1359